The Central Nervous System

The Central Nervous System

STRUCTURE AND FUNCTION

Per Brodal

New York   Oxford
OXFORD UNIVERSITY PRESS
1992

Oxford University Press

Oxford   New York   Toronto
Delhi   Bombay   Calcutta   Madras   Karachi
Kuala Lumpur   Singapore   Hong Kong   Tokyo
Nairobi   Dar es Salaam   Cape Town
Melbourne   Auckland

and associated companies in
Berlin   Ibadan

Originally published in Norwegian under the title
SENTRALNERVESYSTEMET with subtitle BYGNING OG FUNKSJON
Copyright © 1991 by TANO.

Copyright © 1992 by Oxford University Press, Inc.

Published by Oxford University Press, Inc.,
200 Madison Avenue, New York, New York 10016

Library of Congress Cataloging-in-Publication Data
Brodal, Per.
[Sentralnerversystemet. English]
The central nervous system : structure and function / Per Brodal.
p. cm.   Translation of: Sentralnervesystemet, c1990.
Includes bibliographical references and index.
ISBN 0-19-505518-7 (alk. paper)
1. Neuroanatomy. 2. Central nervous system—Anatomy.   I. Title.
[DNLM: 1. Central Nervous System—physiology.   WL 300 B8645c]
QM451.B78613   1992
612.8—dc20   DNLM/DLC
for Library of Congress   91-45315

3 5 7 9 8 6 4 2

Printed in the United States of America
on acid-free paper

PREFACE

This book is a translation of the Norwegian textbook *Sentralnervesystemet*. Its forerunner was written by my father, Alf Brodal and published in four editions from 1949 to 1982, aiming to encompass the progress in neurobiology during that period. Our original plan was to produce a fifth edition mainly by adding new material where necessary, but the pace of progress in neurobiological research has increased so much in the last ten years that I found that the book needed more than simple updating. A textbook that has been in use for such a long time in a rapidly developing field sooner or later reaches a point where updating is no longer sufficient if one wants to maintain a coherent presentation. Thus, the present version, planned from the start to appear in English as well as in Norwegian, has been completely rewritten. Almost all the illustrations are new and were produced especially for this book.

The book is intended primarily for use by students of medicine, physiotherapy, and psychology, that is, in undergraduate neuroscience courses for students needing a knowledge of the nervous system as a basis for later clinical learning and practice. Some of the material presented goes beyond what is usually included in the curriculum of any

of these groups. Thus, I hope that the book will also prove useful for graduate students and clinicians needing updating in neurobiology. More advanced material is printed in small type and placed so that it should not disturb reading of the main text.

Though changed in many ways, the book has the same aim as when my father first wrote it: to help readers achieve an understanding of the relationship between structure and function of the nervous system. Knowledge of structure is a prerequisite for understanding the normal working of the brain and the symptoms of neurological disease. Structure without function, however, is of limited interest. Therefore, although the main emphasis is on the structure of the central nervous system, throughout the book structure is correlated with function as revealed by physiological, clinical, psychological, and other methods.

During the preparation of the book, I have received help and advice from several colleagues, for which I am truly grateful. Eric Rinvik has read most of the chapters and given valuable comments and support. Jan Jansen, Jon Storm-Mathisen, Paul Heggelund, Ole Petter Ottersen, and Kirsten Osen have each read selected parts and provided constructive criticism and advice.

I also gratefully acknowledge the expert help of Kari Ruud, Anne Schreiner, and Lillan Eliassen, who have made all the line-drawings, and of Gunnar Lothe and Carina Ingebrigtsen, who produced the photographic work.

Finally, the careful scrutiny of the English and innumerable improvements of style by Miss Ellen Johannessen are greatly appreciated.

September 1991   P.B.

CONTENTS

INTRODUCTION, xiii

I MAIN FEATURES OF STRUCTURE AND FUNCTION

1. *Cellular Elements of Nervous Tissue and Their Functions*, 5

Structure of the Neuron, 5
Glial Cells, 18
Basis of Excitability and Impulse Propagation, 20
Synaptic Transmission, 29
Neurotransmitters, 34
Coupling of Neurons: Pathways for Impulses, 40
Some Aspects of Neural Development, 45
Restitution after Damage to the Central Nervous System, 50

2. *The Different Parts of the Nervous System*, 54

Prenatal Development, 55
The Spinal Cord, 56
The Brain Stem, 65
The Cerebrum, 75
The Cerebellum, 80
The Coverings of the Brain, 82

The Cerebral Ventricles and the Cerebrospinal Fluid, 85
The Blood Supply of the Central Nervous System, 91

3. *How Are the Structure and Function of the
   Nervous System Studied?, 97*

Some General Features of Neurobiological Research, 98
Methods, 99

II SENSORY SYSTEMS

4. *The Somatosensory System, 113*

Exteroceptors: Cutaneous Sensation, 113
Proprioceptors: Deep Sensation, 119
The Sensory Fibers and the Dorsal Roots, 128
Central Parts of the Somatosensory System, 135

5. *The Visual System, 155*

Structure of the Eye, 155
The Retina, 158
Organization of the Visual Pathways, 166
The Visual Cortex, 172

6. *The Auditory System, 179*

The Cochlea, 179
The Auditory Pathways, 185
The Auditory Cortex, 190

7. *The Olfactory System, 192*

Receptors for Smell, 192
Central Pathways for Olfactory Impulses, 193
The Terminal Areas of the Olfactory Tract, 193
Olfactory Impulses and Reflexes, 194

III MOTOR SYSTEMS

8. *The Peripheral Motor Neurons, 199*

Motoneurons and Muscles, 199
Reflexes, 209
Muscle Tone, 218

9. *Central Motor Pathways, 222*

The Pyramidal Tract (The Corticospinal Tract), 222
Other Descending Pathways to the Spinal Cord, 230
Control of Automatic Movements, 234
Motor Cortical Areas and the Control of Voluntary Movements, 237
Symptoms Caused by Interruption of Central Motor Pathways, 242

10. *The Basal Ganglia, 246*

Structure and Connections of the Basal Ganglia, 246
Functions of the Basal Ganglia, 257
Diseases of the Basal Ganglia, 257

11. *The Cerebellum, 262*

Subdivisions, Structure, and Connections of the Cerebellum, 263
Cerebellar Functions and Symptoms in Disease, 278

IV THE BRAIN STEM AND THE CRANIAL NERVES

12. *Reticular Formation, 285*

Structure and Connections of the Reticular Formation, 285
Functions of the Reticular Formation, 294

13. *Cranial Nerves, 302*

General Organization of the Cranial Nerves, 302
The Hypoglossal Nerve, 307
The Accessory Nerve, 309

The Vagus Nerve, 309

The Glossopharyngeal Nerve, 312

The Vestibulocochlear Nerve: The Sense of Equilibrium, 313

The Facial and Intermediate Nerves, 323

The Sense of Taste, 326

The Trigeminal Nerve, 328

The Abducent, Trochlear, and Oculomotor Nerves, 331

Control of Eye Movements, 336

V THE AUTONOMIC NERVOUS SYSTEM

14. Peripheral Autonomic Nervous System, 345

General Organization of the Autonomic System, 345

Peripheral Parts of the Sympathetic System, 349

Peripheral Parts of the Parasympathetic System, 354

Functional Aspects of the Autonomic Nervous System, 357

Neurotransmitters in the Autonomic Nervous System, 361

Sensory Innervation of Visceral Organs, 363

15. Central Autonomic System: Hypothalamus, 368

Autonomic Centers in the Brain Stem, 368

Structure and Connections of the Hypothalamus, 368

Functional Aspects, 373

The Hypothalamus and the Endocrine System, 375

The Hypothalamus and Mental Functions, 378

VI THE CEREBRAL CORTEX AND LIMBIC STRUCTURES

16. Limbic Structures, 383

The "Limbic System," 383

The Cerebral Cortex and "Limbic Functions":
The Cingulate Gyrus, 384

The Amygdaloid Nucleus, 386

The Septal Nuclei, 388

The Hippocampal Formation, 389

17. Cerebral Cortex, 398

Structure of the Cerebral Cortex, 398
Connections of the Cerebral Cortex, 406
Functions of the Cerebral Cortex, 413

LITERATURE, 425

INDEX, 439

INTRODUCTION

The essential building block of the nervous system is the nerve cell, specialized for rapid conveyance of signals over long distances and in a very precise manner. Together, billions of nerve cells in the brain form complicated and highly organized networks for *communication* and *information processing*.

The nervous system receives a wealth of information from one's surroundings and body. From all this information, it extracts the essentials, stores what may be needed later, and emits a command to muscles or glands if an answer is appropriate. Sometimes the answer comes within milliseconds, as a reflex or automatic response. At other times it may take considerably longer, requiring cooperation among many parts of the brain and involving conscious processes. In any case, the main task of the nervous system is to ensure that the organism adapts optimally to the environment.

The nervous system is equipped with sense organs, *receptors,* that react to various forms of sensory information or *stimuli.* Regardless of the mode of stimulation (the form of energy), the receptors "translate" the energy of the stimulus to the language spoken by the nervous system, that is, nerve impulses. These are tiny electric discharges rapidly conducted along the nerve processes.

Thus, signals are conveyed from the receptors to the regions of the nervous system where information processing takes place.

The nervous system can elicit an external response only by acting on *effectors,* which are either *muscles* or *glands. The response* is in the form of either movement or secretion. Obviously, muscle contraction can have various expressions, from communication through speech, facial expression, and bodily posture, to walking and running, respiratory movements, and changes of blood pressure. But one should bear in mind that the nervous system can only act on muscles and glands to express its "will." Conversely, if we are to judge the activity going on in the brain of another being, we have only the expressions produced by muscle contraction and secretion to go by.

On an anatomic basis we can divide the nervous system into *the central nervous system (CNS),* consisting of the brain and the spinal cord, and the *peripheral nervous sytem* (PNS), which connects the central nervous system with the receptors and the effectors. Although without sharp transitions, the PNS and the CNS may both be subdivided into parts that are concerned primarily with the regulation of visceral organs and the internal milieu, and parts that are concerned mainly with the more or less conscious adaptation to the external world. The first is called the *autonomic* or *visceral nervous system;* the second is usually called *somatic nervous system.* The latter, also called the *cerebrospinal* nervous system, receives information from sense organs capturing events in our surroundings (vision, hearing, receptors in the skin) and controls the activity of voluntary muscles (made up of cross-striated skeletal muscle cells). In contrast, the autonomic nervous system controls the activity of involuntary muscles (smooth muscle and heart muscle cells) and gland cells. The autonomic system may be further subdivided into the *sympathetic system,* mainly concerned with mobilizing the resources of the body when demands are increased (as in emergencies), and the *parasympathetic system,* which is devoted more to the daily maintenance of the body.

The higher an animal is on the scale of evolution, the more complicated is its central nervous system. The tasks carried out by the CNS are correspondingly complex and varied, reaching a maximal development in humans, whose brain provides enormous flexibility and adaptability compared with the brains of lower animals. This evolutionary development depends in part on development of the sense organs, in particular those providing information about events taking place at some distance (vision, hearing, and to some extent, smell). By means of these senses, the range of experience is vastly increased, and the animal can adapt in advance to external events. Thus, the animal may predict on the basis of previous experience what is going to happen and alter its behavior accordingly (escape from enemies, search for food or partner, and so on). For more primitive animals the amount and variety of sensory information that has to be integrated to give an appropriate response is limited. The development of new and specialized senses means, of course, that more information reaches the brain. This would be of little use, however, if the brain had not increased its capacity to process information. Thus, what we see in evolution is that as the size of the brain increases dramatically, many more nerve cells are needed for the greater number of impulse pathways and interconnections. The brain is increasingly *differentiated,* in the sense that it can handle a wider variety of information and also vary its responses over a much wider range than is the case in lower animals. The more an animal organizes its activities on the basis of previous experience, and the more it is freed from the dominance of immediate sensations, the more complicated are the processes required of the central nervous system.

The higher processes of integration and association—that is, what we call mental processes—are first and foremost a function of the cerebral cortex. Consequently, this part of the brain shows the most marked relative increase in number of nerve cells as we go from lower to higher vertebrates. In lower mammals (such as the rat) the modest cerebral cortex is mostly engaged in receiving sensory messages or in sending out commands to the muscles. In higher species, especially anthropoid apes and humans, large parts of the cortex are engaged in comparing and integrating the vast amount of immediate information with that stored from previous experiences. Nevertheless, the basic principles underlying the structure and function of this most elaborate part of the brain are the same as for the more primitive parts, and cannot be understood without knowledge of them.

The Central Nervous System

I

Main Features of Structure and Function

General information about the structure and function of the nervous system forms a necessary basis for treatment of the specific systems in subsequent parts of this book. Chapter 1 describes nervous tissue and its properties, and also incorporates a brief survey of the development of the nervous system with particular reference to how its incredibly complicated and precise patterns of connections may arise. Chapter 2 gives an overview of the macroscopic, and to some extent microscopic, structure of the nervous system. Chapter 3 treats some general approaches to neurobiological research, and some of the methods that have been used to obtain the information presented in this book.

1

Cellular Elements of Nervous Tissue and Their Functions

The nervous system is built up of nerve cells, *neurons,* and special kinds of supporting cells, *glial cells.* The nerve cells are responsible for the functions that are unique to the nervous system, whereas the glial cells primarily serve the needs of the neurons. Neurons are characterized by their ability to respond to stimuli with an electrical discharge, a *nerve impulse,* and, further, by their fast conduction of the nerve impulse over long distances. In this way, signals can be transmitted in milliseconds from one place to another, either within the central nervous system or between it and other organs of the body. The functions of the glial cells are still incompletely known. It is established, however, that they are responsible for isolating neuronal processes and controlling the environment of neurons and that they take part in repair processes. Glial cells also play important roles during the embryological development of the nervous system.

STRUCTURE OF THE NEURON
Neurons Have Long Processes

Like other cells, a neuron has a cell body with a nucleus surrounded by cytoplasm with various organelles. The cell body is also called the *perikaryon* or *soma.* Long processes extend from the cell body. The number and length of the processes can vary, but they are of two main kinds. There are usually several *dendrites,* whereas there is only one *axon* (Fig. 1.1). The dendrites usually branch and form dendritic "trees" with a large surface to receive signals from other nerve cells. Each neuron has only one axon, which is specially built to conduct the nerve impulse from the cell body to other cells. The axon may have many ramifications, enabling its parent cell to influence many other cells.

To study the elements of nervous tissue, one has to use thin sections that can be examined under the microscope. Different staining methods make it possible to distinguish the whole neuron or parts of it from the surroundings (Figs. 1.2 and 1.3). It then becomes evident that the morphology of neurons may vary, with regard to both the size of the perikaryon and the number, length, and branching of dendrites. The size of the dendritic tree is related to the number of contacts the cell can receive from other nerve cells. Dendrites often have small spikes, *spinae* or *spines,* that further increase the receiving surface of the neuron (Figs. 1.1 and 1.7). The axons also vary, from those

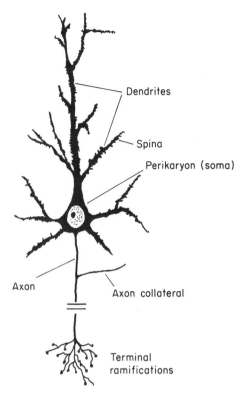

Fig. 1.1. *A neuron.* Half-schematic drawing of a neuron (pyramidal cell) from the cerebral cortex. Note the two types of processes emerging from the perikaryon. Small spikes on the dendrites are called spines (spina, plural spinae).

that ramify and end close to the perikaryon to those that extend for more than 1 meter. These structural differences are closely connected to functional differences.

Communication between Nerve Cells Takes Place at Synapses

The terminal branches of an axon have club-shaped enlargements called *boutons* (Figs. 1.1 and 1.4). The term *terminal bouton* is often used when the bouton sits at the end of an axon branch. In other instances, the bouton is just a thickening along the course of the axon, with several such *en passage* boutons along one terminal branch. In any case, the bouton is found close to the surface membrane of another cell, usually on the dendrites or the perikaryon. Such a place of

close contact between a bouton and another cell is called a *synapse.* In the peripheral nervous system, synapses are formed between boutons and muscle cells. *The synapse is where information is transmitted from one neuron to another.* This transmission does not occur by direct propagation of the nerve impulse from one cell (neuron) to the other, but by liberation of signal molecules that subsequently influence the other cell. Such a signal molecule is called a *neurotransmitter* or, for short, a *transmitter* (the term *transmitter substance* is also used). The neurotransmitter is (at least partly) located in small vesicles in the bouton called *synaptic vesicles* (Figs. 1.4 and 1.5). How the synapse and the transmitters work is treated later in this chapter. At the moment we will restrict ourselves to the structure of the synapse.

The membrane of the bouton is separated from the membrane of the other nerve cell by a narrow cleft about 20 nm wide (that is, 2/100,000 mm). This *synaptic cleft* cannot be observed in the light microscope. Only when electron microscopy of nervous tissue became feasible in the 1950s could it be demonstrated that neurons are indeed anatomically separate entities. In the electron microscope, one can observe that the membranes facing the synaptic cleft are thickened. This is due to accumulation of specific proteins that are of crucial importance for transmission of the synaptic signal. Many of these protein molecules are receptors for neurotransmitters; others form channels for passage of charged particles, as discussed later. The membrane of the bouton facing the cleft is called the *presynaptic membrane,* and the membrane of the cell that is contacted is called the *postsynaptic membrane.* We also use the terms *pre- and postsynaptic neurons.*

Synapses formed on the cell soma are called *axosomatic,* while synapses on dendrites are called *axodendritic* (Figs. 1.6 and 1.7). Boutons may also form a synapse with an axon (usually close to a terminal bouton), and such synapses are called *axoaxonic.* In general, the placement of the synapse tells us something about how strong its particular

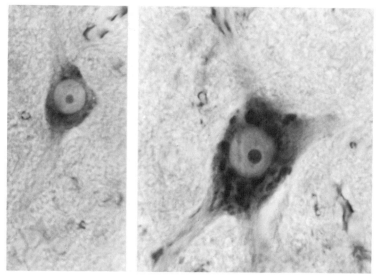

Fig. 1.2. *Neuronal perikarya* (cell bodies). Photomicrograph of section of the spinal cord stained to show cell bodies (Nissl staining). The stain (thionine) binds primarily to nucleic acids (DNA in the nucleus and RNA in the cytoplasm and nucleolus). The deeply stained clumps in the cytoplasm represent aggregates of rough endoplasmic reticulum (rER), formerly called Nissl granules. Two motor neurons, one large and one small, are shown. Only the proximal parts of the dendrites are stained. Magnification, ×800.

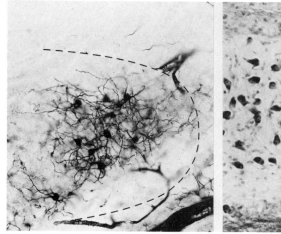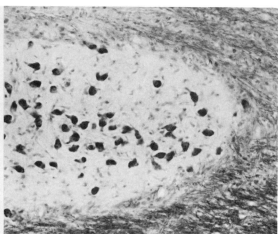

Fig. 1.3. *Neurons.* Photomicrographs of sections stained with two different methods. To the **right**, only the cell bodies (perikarya) of a group of neurons are stained and visible in the section. The dark region surrounding the group of neurons is made up of myelinated fibers that are also stained. The section to the **left** is from the same cell group, but treated in accordance with the Golgi method so that the dendrites as well as the cell bodies are visualized. Magnification, ×150.

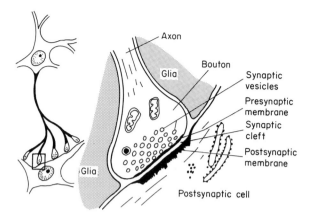

Fig. 1.4. *A synapse.* Schematic drawing based on electron micrographs.

influence may be. A synapse on the cell soma is usually more powerful than a synapse far out on a dendrite. Every neuron as a rule has many thousands of synapses on its surface, and it is the sum of their influences that determines how active the postsynaptic neuron will be at any moment.

Neurons Are Rich in Organelles for Oxidative Metabolism and Protein Synthesis

When seen in a microscopic section, the *nucleus* of a neuron is characterized by its large size and light staining (that is, the chromatin is extended, indicating that much of the genome is in use). There is also a prominent nucleolus (Figs. 1.2 and 1.8). These features make it easy to distinguish a neuron from other cells (such as glial cells), even in sections in which only the nuclei are clearly stained. In the neuronal cytoplasm there are many *mitochondria,* an indication of the high metabolic activity of nerve cells. They depend entirely on aerobic adenosine triphosphate (ATP) production and cannot (unlike most other cell types) utilize anaerobic ATP synthesis. Glucose is the substrate

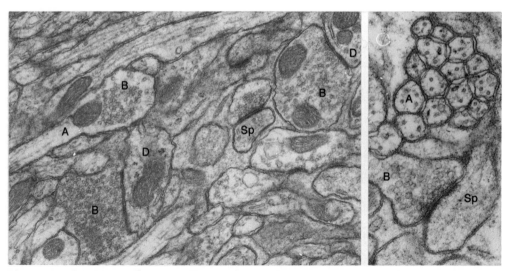

Fig. 1.5. *Synapses.* Electron micrographs showing boutons (B) in synaptic contacts with dendrites (D), and dendritic spines (Sp). A bundle of unmyelinated axons (A) is seen in the electron micrograph to the **right.** Magnifications, ×20,000 and ×40,000.

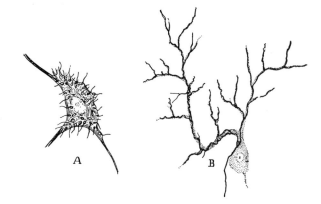

Fig. 1.6. *Two types of synaptic contacts.* **A.** Numerous club-shaped boutons on a cell body (axosomatic synapses). **B.** An axon follows the dendritic tree closely, and forms numerous boutons with synapses *en passage.*

for ATP production in the mitochondria of nerve cells, which cannot (unlike muscle cells, for example) use fat.

Neuronal somata also contain conspicuous amounts of *free ribosomes* and *rough endoplasmic reticulum (rER)* for synthesis of proteins. Large clumps of rER are seen light microscopically in the cytoplasm of neurons over a certain size (Fig. 1.2). These were called (tigroid granules or *Nissl bodies* long before their true nature was known. There are also as a rule several Golgi complexes, which modify proteins before they are exported or inserted in membranes. The large neuronal production of proteins probably reflects their enormous surface membrane containing many protein molecules that must be constantly renewed. These proteins have a number of important functions that will be considered later.

Neurons Have a Cytoskeleton That Also Serves Transport Functions

The somata and processes of neurons contain thin threads, *neurofibrils,* that can be observed in specially stained microscopic sections (Fig. 1.9). While originally thought to be related to impulse conduction, the neurofibrils are now known to be of importance for the *shape of neurons,* forming a *cytoskeleton,* and for *transport of substances in the neuronal processes.*

Electron microscopic and biochemical analysis have shown that the cytoskeleton consists of various kinds of fibrillary proteins, making threads of three main kinds: (1) actin filaments (microfilaments) and associated protein molecules, (2) microtubules (narrow tubes) and associated proteins, and (3) so-called intermediary filaments (neurofilaments).

Actin (microfilaments) is present in the axon, among other places. There it plays an important role during development. When the axon elongates, actin serves to produce movements of the so-called *growth cone* at the tip of the axon (in general, actin is present in cells capable of movement, such as muscle cells). In addition, actin is probably of importance in maintaining the shape of the axon when fully grown.

Microtubules and microtubule-associated proteins (MAPs) are present in all kinds of neuronal processes and are most likely important for their shape. Of special interest is the relation of microtubules to the transport of substances in the axonal cytoplasm (axoplasm). There is a continuous movement of organelles, proteins, and other particles in the axons, both in the direction from the cell body to the terminals of the axon and in the opposite direction. The first is called *anterograde axonal transport,* and movement toward the cell body is called *retrograde axonal transport.* By anterograde transport, substances that are synthesized only in the cell body can be moved to the axon terminals; these include mitochondria and various proteins of importance for synaptic transmission. By retrograde transport, signal molecules taken up by the axon termi-

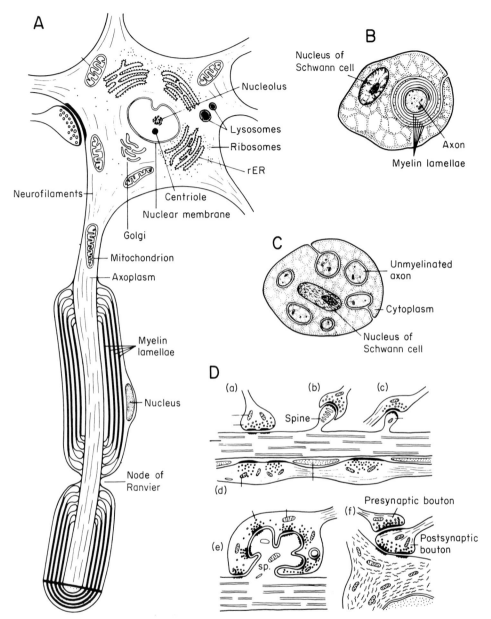

Fig. 1.7. *Ultrastructure of the neuron.* Schematic drawings based on electron microscopic observations. **A.** Perikaryon with proximal parts of the dendrites and the axon (myelinated). Various kinds of organelles are shown. The node of Ranvier is where two segments of myelin meets. **B.** Cross section of axon in the process of becoming myelinated. The myelin sheath consists of lamellae formed by the membrane of a glial cell or a Schwann cell. **C.** Unmyelinated axons (in the peripheral nervous system), surrounded by Schwann cell cytoplasm. **D.** Various kinds of synaptic contacts. A bouton may form a synapse directly on (**a**) the shaft of the dendrite, or (**b, c,** and **e**) on a spine, (**d**) the axon may also have several boutons *en passage,* (**f**) an axoaxonic synapse (a synapse between two boutons).

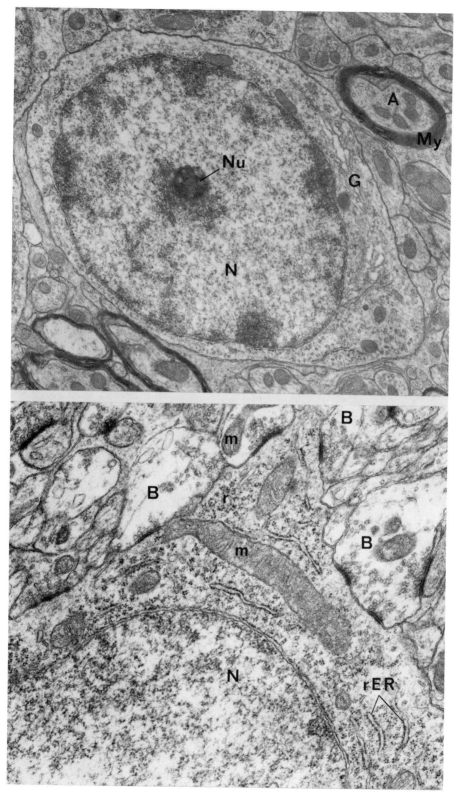

Fig. 1.8. *Ultrastructure of the neuron.* Electron micrograph showing the cell body of a small neuron (**above**) and parts of a larger neuron (**below**). Note the presence of rough endoplasmic reticulum (rER), free ribosomes (r), mitochondria, (m), and Golgi complex (G). Boutons (B) forming axosomatic synapses are also present. N = nucleus, Nu = nucleolus, A = axon, My = myelin. Magnifications, ×9,000 and ×15,000, respectively.

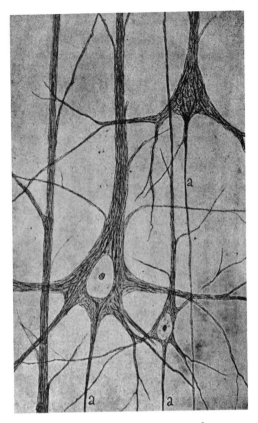

Fig. 1.9. *Neurofibrils.* Drawing of neurons from the cerebral cortex, as appearing in sections stained with heavy metals to visualize neurofibrils. From Cajal (1911).

nals can reach the cell body and thereby alter its activity (for example, increased or decreased synthesis of transmitters and receptor molecules). Retrograde transport also serves to bring axonal particles that need to be broken down (for example, "worn-out" mitochondria) to the cell body, where there are lysosomes.

By injection of radioactively labeled substances that are taken up by neurons, it has been demonstrated that axonally transported material moves in at least two different phases. One is rapid, with particles moving more than 5 mm per hour; the other is considerably slower. Injections into nervous tissue of substances that are transported axonally and later can be detected in tissue sections are widely used to trace neuronal connections—that is, to reveal the "wiring pattern" of the brain (see Chapter 3).

Many Axons Are Isolated to Increase the Speed of Impulse Propagation

The velocity with which the nerve impulse travels depends on the diameter of the axon, among other factors. In addition, how well the axon is insulated is of crucial importance. Many axons have an extra insulation (in addition to the axonal membrane) called a *myelin sheath.* Such axons are therefore called *myelinated,* to distinguish them from those without a myelin sheath, which are called *unmyelinated.*

Many of the tasks performed by the nervous system require very rapid conduction of signals. If unmyelinated axons were to do this, they would have to be extremely thick. Nerves bringing signals to the muscles of the hand, for example, would be impossibly thick, and the brain would also have to be much larger. Insulation is thus a very efficient way of saving space and expensive building materials. Efficient insulation of axons is in fact a prerequisite for the dramatic development of the nervous system that has taken place in vertebrates as compared with invertebrates.

Oligodendroglia and Schwann Cells Make Myelin

The *myelin sheaths* mentioned above consist mainly of lipids, with smaller amounts of proteins. Together, the material ensheathing the axons is called *myelin.* The myelin sheath forms a cylinder around axons (Figs. 1.7, 1.10, and 1.11), reducing the loss of current from the axon to surrounding tissue fluid during impulse conduction. This contributes to the much higher conduction velocity in myelinated than in unmyelinated axons (see p. 29). The thickest myelinated axons conduct at about 120 m/sec.

Myelin is whitish owing to its high lipid content. With special methods for staining lipids, the myelin sheaths can be observed in the light and electron microscopes (Figs. 1.10, 1.11, and 1.14). In longitudinal sections one can then see that the myelin sheath is interrupted at intervals (Fig. 1.7), forming

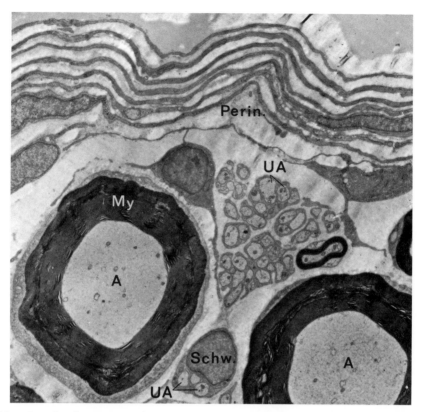

Fig. 1.10. *Peripheral nerve.* Myelinated and unmyelinated axons and the perineurium. Electron micrograph of cross section of the sciatic nerve. Note the large difference in diameter among various myelinated axons (My = myelin, A = axon). The thickness of the myelin sheath increases apace with the increase in axonal diameter. In between the myelinated axons there are numerous unmyelinated ones (UA) and occasional fibroblasts (f). Schwann cells (Schw.) are also associated with unmyelinated axons. The perineurium (Perin.) is formed by several lamellae of flattened cells. Magnification, ×4,000.

so-called *nodes of Ranvier.* With the electron microscope, it can be seen that the axolemma (the axonal membrane) is "naked" at the node; that is, it is exposed to the interstitial fluid. Thus, only at the node of Ranvier can current in the form of ions pass from the axon to the interstitial fluid (and in the opposite direction). This arrangement makes it possible for the nerve impulse to "jump" from node to node, thus increasing the speed of propagation (see p. 29).

Electron microscopically, the myelin sheath has been shown to consist of numerous layers of cell membrane. The layers or *lamellae* are formed when a special kind of glial cell wraps itself around the axon (Fig. 1.7B). During this process, the cytoplasm of the glial cell is squeezed away so that the layers of cell membrane lie closely apposed. The nodes of Ranvier exist because the glial cells forming myelin lie in a row along the axon, each cell making myelin only for a restricted length, or *segment,* of the axon. In the central nervous system, or CNS, myelin is made by *oligodendrocytes* (oligodendroglia), whereas *Schwann cells* are responsible in the peripheral nervous system. The structure of the myelin sheath is nevertheless the same in both places. Oligodendrocytes and Schwann cells are not identical, however. One difference is that a single oligodendrocyte usually sends out processes to produce myelin segments for several axons, whereas each Schwann cell forms a myelin segment only for one axon. The length between two nodes of Ranvier in the peripheral nervous system

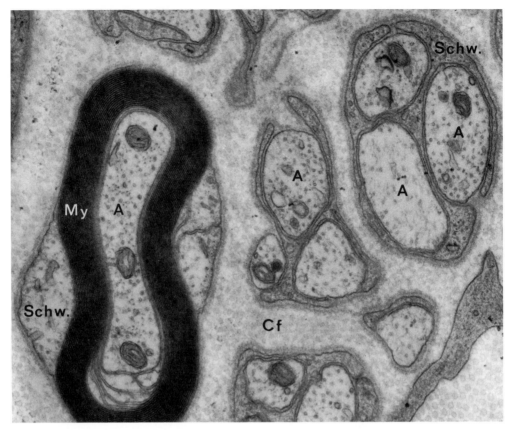

Fig. 1.11. *Myelinated and unmyelinated axons.* Detail from Figure 1.10. Note the myelin lamellae (My), formed by Schwann cells (Schw.). The unmyelinated axons (A) are completely sur-rounded by Schwann cells. Between the axons are numerous collagen fibrils (Cf). Magnification, ×30,000.

may be up to 0.5 mm or more. The *myelination of the axons* starts prenatally, but many neural pathways in man are not fully myelinated until two years after birth. The process of myelination is closely related to functional maturation.

The *unmyelinated* axons conduct much more slowly (at less than 1 m/sec) than the myelinated ones. This is because they are thinner and they lack the extra insulation provided by the myelin sheath. In the central nervous system, unmyelinated axons are often found closely packed in bundles without any glial cells separating them (Fig. 1.5). In the peripheral nervous system, however, unmyelinated axons are always ensheathed in Schwann cells that do not make layers of myelin (Fig. 1.11). Several axons become embedded in the cytoplasm of the Schwann cells by invagination of the Schwann cell membrane. This arrangement probably serves to protect the axon from potentially harmful substances in the interstitial fluid. Such protection is not necessary in the central nervous system, since the composition of the interstitial fluid is governed in other ways.

Demyelinating Diseases Block Impulse Conduction

In *demyelinating diseases* of the nervous system, the myelin sheaths degenerate. The commonest among these diseases is *multiple sclerosis*, typically affecting young adults. Its cause is still unknown, but the symptoms are caused by isolated, apparently randomly distributed regions of inflammation and demyelination. In such regions (*plaques*), impulse conduction in the axons is severely slowed or halted, leading to motor and sensory disturbances. For some reason, the optic nerve is often the first to be affected, resulting in reduced vision. Typically, the symptoms are intermittent, in pace with fluctuation of the inflammatory process. Thus periods of marked symptoms (such as paresis of extremities) are followed by periods of partial recovery. The improvement of symptoms is due to partial remyelination of the affected regions. As the disease progresses, however, not only the myelin sheaths but also the axons may degenerate, leading to permanent and progressive disability.

Peripheral Nerves Are Built for Protection of the Axons

Fresh nervous tissue is rather soft and almost jellylike, having virtually no mechanical strength in itself. Protection of the central nervous system against external mechanical forces is provided by its location in the skull and vertebral canal, and furthermore, by its "wrapping" in membranes of connective tissue. For peripheral parts of the nervous system, the situation is different. Often located superficially, the bundles of axons and groups of nerve cells are exposed to various mechanical stresses. They are also subject to considerable stretching by movements of the body. Axons can be stretched only slightly before their impulse conduction suffers, and they may even break. To prevent this, peripheral nerves contain large amounts of dense connective tissue with numerous collagen fibers arranged largely longitudinally (Figs. 1.10 and 1.11). The collagen fibers, specialized to resist stretching, protect the axons effectively. The presence of connective tissue in peripheral nerves explains why the nerves become so much thicker on leaving the skull or the vertebral canal.

The connective tissue components of peripheral nerves are arranged in distinctive layers. An external thick layer of mostly longitudinally running collagen fibers is called the *epineurium*. Internal to this layer, the axons are arranged into smaller bundles, *fascicles,* wrapped in the *perineurium* (Fig. 1.10). The rather sparse amount of collagen fibers and fibroblasts within the fascicles constitutes the *endoneurium.* The perineural sheath is special in that it contains several

layers of flattened cells. The cells, which in some respects resemble epithelial cells, are connected by various kinds of junctions, indicating that the perineurium constitutes a barrier preventing certain substances from reaching the interior of the fascicles with the axons. Experimental data indicate that this is indeed the case. It does not seem surprising that peripheral nervous tissue also needs some extra mechanisms to ensure that the environment is kept optimal for conducting impulses.

Projection Neurons and Interneurons

Some neurons influence cells that are far away, and their axon is correspondingly long (more than a meter for the longest). They are called *projection neurons* or Golgi type 1 (Fig. 1.12). Neurons conveying signals from the spinal cord to the muscles are examples of projection neurons; others are neurons in the cerebral cortex with axons contacting cells in the brain stem and the spinal cord. The axons of projection neurons as a rule send out branches, *collaterals,* in their course (Figs. 1.12, 1.27, and 17.5). Thus, one projection neuron may send signals to neurons in various other parts of the nervous system.

The other main type of neuron is the *interneuron* (Golgi type 2), characterized by a short axon that branches extensively in the vicinity of the cell body. The name implies that an interneuron is intercalated between two other neurons. Even though, strictly speaking, all neurons with axons that do not leave the central nervous system are thus interneurons, the term is usually restricted to neurons with short axons that do not leave one particular neuronal group. The interneurons thus mediate communication between neurons within one group. Since interneurons may be "switched" on and off, the possible number of interrelations among the neurons within one group increases dramatically. The number of interneurons is particularly high in the cerebral cortex, and it is the number of interneurons that is so much higher in the human brain than in any other animal. The number of typical projec-

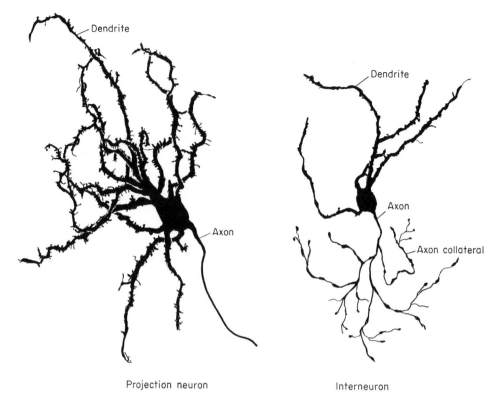

Projection neuron　　　　　　　　Interneuron

Fig. 1.12.　*Projection neuron and interneuron.* Examples from the brain stem of a monkey, based on sections treated according to the Golgi method.

tion neurons interconnecting the various parts of the nervous system, and interconnecting the latter with the rest of the body, as a rule varies more with the size of the body than with the stage of development.

The distinction between projection neurons and interneurons is not always very clear, however. Many neurons previously regarded as giving off only local branches have been shown by modern methods also to give off long axonal branches to more distant cell groups. Thus, they function both as projection neurons and interneurons. On the other hand, many of the "classical" projection neurons give off collaterals ending within the cell group in which the perikaryon is located (Fig. 17.5).

Most Neurons Are Multipolar

The kinds of neurons described above usually have several processes, and are therefore called *multipolar*. Special kinds of neurons, however, may be different. Thus, neurons conducting sensory signals from the receptors to the central nervous system have only one process that divides close to the cell body. One branch conducts impulses from the receptor toward the perikaryon; the other conducts impulses toward and into the central nervous system. Such neurons are called *pseudounipolar*[1] (Fig. 1.13). Some neurons have two processes, one conducting toward the perikaryon, the other away from it. Such neurons, present in the retina and some other locations, are called *bipolar*.

Neurons Are Collected in Nuclei and Ganglia

When examining sections from the *central nervous system* under the microscope, one sees that the perikarya of the neurons are

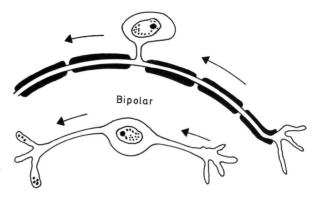

Fig. 1.13. *Pseudounipolar and bipolar neurons.*

not diffusely spread out but are collected in groups. Such a group is called a *nucleus* (Figs. 1.2 and 1.14). Neurons collected in this manner share many connections with other groups and constitute in certain respects a functional unit. In the *peripheral nervous system,* a corresponding collection of perikarya is called a *ganglion.*

Axons from the neurons of one nucleus usually have common targets and therefore run together, forming bundles. Such a bun-

dle of axons connecting one nucleus with another is called a *tract* (tractus) (Fig. 1.14). In the peripheral nervous system, a collection of axons is called a *nerve* (nervus).

Schematically, the large tracts of the nervous system are the main routes for nerve impulses—to some extent comparable to highways connecting big cities. In addition, there are numerous smaller pathways often running parallel to the "highways," and many smaller bundles of axons leave the big

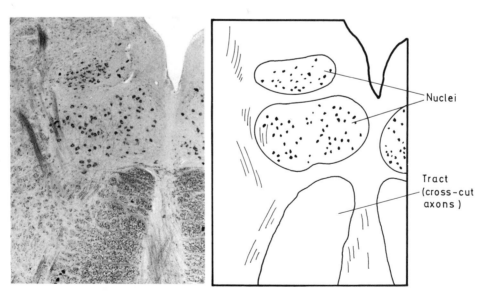

Fig. 1.14. *Nuclei and tracts.* Photomicrographs showing two nuclei in the brain stem (the hypoglossal nucleus and the dorsal motor nucleus of the vagus) and a tract (the medial lemniscus). In addition, some minor bundles of my-

elinated fibers can be seen. The sections are stained with thionine to visualize neuronal cell bodies (Nissl staining) and with another method that stains myelin. Magnification, ×75.

tracts to terminate in nuclei along the course. The number of smaller "footpaths" interconnecting nuclei is enormous, making possible (at least theoretically) the spread of impulses from one nucleus to almost any part of the nervous system. Normally, the spread of impulses is far from random, but rather is highly ordered and patterned. As a rule, the bigger tracts play more significant roles than the smaller ones in the main tasks of the nervous system. Consequently, diseases affecting such tracts usually produce marked symptoms that can be understood only if one has a fair knowledge of the main features of the wiring patterns of the brain.

Nuclei and Tracts Make Up Gray and White Matter

The surfaces made by cutting nervous tissue contain some areas that are whitish and others that have a gray color. The whitish areas consist mainly of myelinated axons, the myelin being responsible for the color. Such regions are called *white matter*. The gray regions, called *gray matter*, contain mainly perikarya and dendrites (and, of course, axons passing to and from the neurons). The neurons themselves have a grayish color. Owing to this difference in color, one can macroscopically identify the major nuclei (gray) and tracts (white) in brains that have been cut (see, for example, Fig. 2.28). This is dealt with in Chapter 2.

GLIAL CELLS

We have already encountered glial cells briefly. All are equipped with processes, but these are not responsible for the conduction of impulses. The significance of glial cells lies in their crucial role in the functioning of nerve cells. In fact, the number of glial cells is much higher than that of neurons. The name derives from the original, erroneous belief that the glial cells mainly served as "glue," keeping the neurons together.

Most of the tasks today ascribed to glia had been suggested by the turn of the century on the basis of microscopic observations

of their structure and relation to other elements of nervous tissue. Nevertheless, only by modern methods has it been possible to study directly the properties and functional roles of glia, and much still remains unknown. The study of glial cells has recently been greatly facilitated by immunocytochemical methods that identify certain cytoplasmic or surface molecules.

It is customary to group glial cells in three categories, *astrocytes (astroglia), oligodendrocytes (oligodendroglia),* and *microglial cells (microglia).* These are structurally and functionally different[2] (Fig. 1.15).

Astrocytes Contact Both Capillaries and Neurons

Astrocytes have numerous short or long processes and may be divided on this basis into two kinds: protoplasmic and fibrillary astrocytes, respectively. The processes extend in all directions (Fig. 1.16). Some contact the surface of capillaries with expanded "feet," and most of the capillary surface is covered by astrocytic processes (Fig. 1.15). The astrocytes are probably of importance for the capillary permeability to certain substances (see p. 92). Other processes contact neuronal surfaces; in this manner, parts not contacted by boutons are mainly covered by glia.

The intimate contact between astrocytes and neurons indicates that they may exchange substances, and several examples of this are known. One important function is apparently to remove or degrade neurotransmitters released from boutons into the interstitial space. This prevents accumulation of transmitters extracellularly, which would be deleterious to the neurons. Another task appears to be the regulation of extracellular K^+ ion concentration. This is important because neuronal excitability is strongly influenced by the extracellular potassium concentration, and prolonged neuronal activity may lead to the accumulation of K^+ extracellularly. Since the extracellular space in the brain is very limited, the potassium concentration could easily reach high values were it not for effective means of removal by glia.

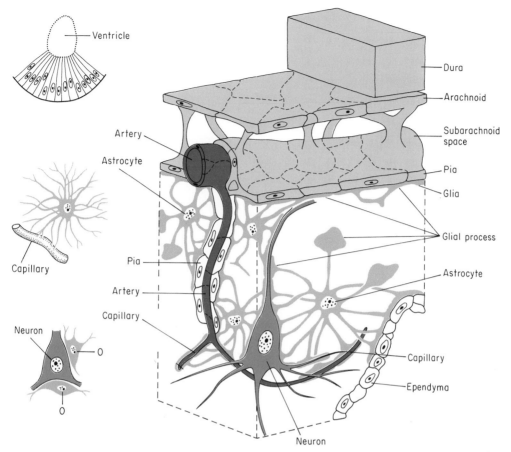

Fig. 1.15. *Glial cells.* Upper left: Ependymal cells lining the wall of the ventricular system. Middle left: Astrocyte. Lower left: Oligodendrocytes (o) close to the perikaryon of a neuron. Right: Scheme showing the three-dimensional arrangement of astrocytes and the vessels of the brain. Note that astrocytes are closely related to vessels, ependymal cells, and the innermost of the cerebral meninges (Pia).

There is also much evidence that glial cells are important during development of the nervous system—for example, by providing surfaces and scaffoldings for the axons to follow during outgrowth.

Astrocytes also form a continuous, thin sheet where nervous tissue borders connective tissue. Such a *limiting membrane* (membrana limitans) is found around the big vessels and on the inside of the coverings of the brain and spinal cord (meninges).

Oligodendrocytes Make Myelin Sheaths

Oligodendrocytes have relatively few and short processes (*oligo* = few, little). The cell body is often closely apposed to a neuronal perikaryon and for this reason oligodendrocytes are also called *satellite cells*. As mentioned above, oligodendrocytes are responsible for *myelination* of axons in the central nervous system, but their position in relation to nerve cell somata suggests that they also have other tasks.

Microglial Cells Are Phagocytes

The third kind of glial cell is called *microglia* because of its small size (Fig. 1.15). Microglial cells were first described light microscopically in sections treated with heavy metal impregnation methods. Estimates indicate

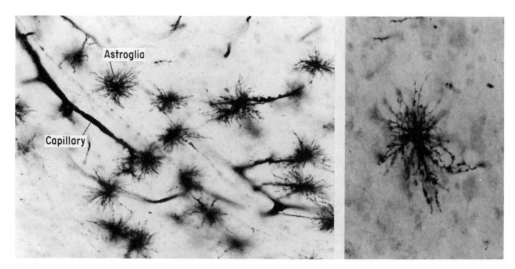

Fig. 1.16. *Astrocytes.* Photomicrograph of section from the cerebral cortex treated according to the Golgi method. Magnifications, ×200 and ×400.

that microglia may constitute 5%–20% of all glial cells, being fairly evenly distributed in all parts of the central nervous system. The identification of microglia is not as straightforward as that of the other glial types, however. There are no clear-cut ultrastructural features that characterize microglia, and some investigators have suggested that microglial cells represent only a variety of oligodendrocytes.

Originally, microglial cells were considered to be of mesodermal origin; that is, they had presumably invaded the nervous system during embryonic development. Although it has been debated for a long time, recent immunocytochemical studies support this view. Several surface markers (antigens) are common to blood monocytes and microglia, and cells that express such antigens first occur in the central nervous system (of rodents) in late embryonic development. After invading nervous tissue, the cells undergo morphological changes that make them closely resemble microglial cells as identified in the adult. The invasion of the CNS by monocytes may correspond in time to a period of cell death (during development a surplus of neurons is produced, with subsequent elimination of a large number during a restricted period of time).

Injury of the mature nervous system increases the number of microglialike cells, and they show marked phagocytic activity. It is not finally settled, however, whether the increased number of phagocytic cells is due to a new invasion of monocytes from the bloodstream, or to activation of phagocytes already present.[3]

Glial Cells Are Activated by Injury of Nervous Tissue

As mentioned above, there is good evidence that microglia can "eat" the debris after neurons and other elements of nervous tissue are destroyed by trauma, ischemia (lack of blood supply), or inflammation. Astrocytes also appear to have phagocytic properties, although less so than microglial cells. Astrocytes, however, are particularly active in forming a kind of scar tissue at the site of injury.

BASIS OF EXCITABILITY AND IMPULSE PROPAGATION

We have briefly mentioned some characteristic properties of neurons, such as their *excitability* and their ability to *conduct im-*

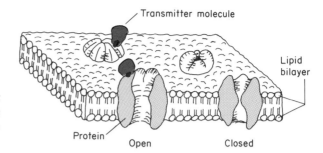

Fig. 1.17. *Ion channels.* Schematic representation of a small part of the lipid bilayer of the cell membrane with interspersed ion channels.

pulses. The term excitability means that the cell can react with a brief electrical discharge, an *action potential,* when sufficiently stimulated. The action potential (the nerve impulse) is conducted along the axon, and is a main factor in the communication among nerve cells and between nerve cells and the body. The action potential is due to movement of charged particles, *ions,* through the cell membrane. A prerequisite for such a current across the membrane is an electric potential between the inside and outside of the cell. This is called the *membrane potential* and is due to unequal distribution of positively and negatively charged particles on the two sides of the membrane.[4]

In the following discussion, we will treat main features of the basis for neuronal excitability and impulse conduction, and for communication between nerve cells at the synapses. For a more complete presentation of this subject, the reader should consult a textbook of physiology or a comprehensive textbook of neurobiology (e.g., Kuffler, Nicholls and Martin; Kandel and Schwartz; or Shepherd).

Excitability Depends on Ion Channels in the Neuronal Membrane

The normal stimulus for a neuron consists of the synaptic effect evoked by other neurons acting on it. The signal is conveyed from one neuron to the next by the presynaptic release of a neurotransmitter. This neurotransmitter binds briefly to *receptor molecules* in the postsynaptic membrane. Usually, the receptor is closely associated with *ion channels* in the membrane, which are opened when the transmitter binds to

the receptor (Figs. 1.17 and 1.18). Thus, a brief current is produced by ions passing through the membrane. There are many types of ion channels, each being selectively permeable to one or a few kinds of ions (most important being Na^+, K^+, Ca^{2+}, and Cl^-). By selectively controlling the opening of ion channels, the transmitters regulate the membrane potential and the excitability of the neuron.

The structure of several ion channels has now been determined. As a rule, they consist

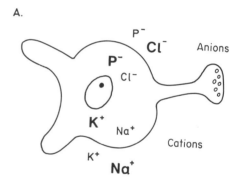

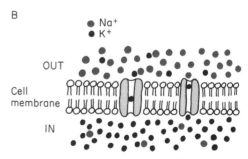

Fig. 1.18. *Ions of importance for the membrane potential.* **A.** Unequal distribution of some ions. **B.** Unequal distribution of K^+ ions is of particular significance for the resting membrane potential, whereas the unequal distribution of Na^+ is crucial for the action potential.

of several polypeptide subunits arranged around a central pore (Fig. 1.17). The subunits span the membrane and extend out on the external and internal faces of the membrane. Thus, molecules inside the cell also may influence the opening of the ion channel.

Ion Channels May Be Ligand-Gated or Voltage-Gated

When the opening of a channel is controlled by neurotransmitters (or other chemical substances), they are called *transmitter-gated* or *ligand-gated*. Binding of the transmitter to a specific site at the external face of a channel polypeptide may change the form of the polypeptides, thus changing the diameter of the channel. Usually, the channel is open only briefly after binding of a transmitter molecule.

Many channels are not controlled primarily by chemical substances but by the magnitude of the membrane potential, and are therefore called *voltage-gated*. Such channels are, for example, responsible for the action potential and thus for the propagation of impulses in the axons. Voltage-gated channels are responsible for the activation of nerves and muscles by external electrical stimulation. Thus, electrical stimulation of a peripheral nerve may produce muscle twitches by activating motor nerve fibers as well as sensations due to activation of sensory nerve fibers.

Cell Membrane Permeability Is Determined by Ion Channels

Ions can pass the cell membrane almost exclusively through specific ion channels, since their electrical charges prevent them from passing the lipid bilayer. It follows that the ease with which an ion may pass through the membrane—that is, the *membrane permeability*[5] to that particular kind of ion—depends upon how densely the channels are distributed in the membrane, and on their degree of opening.

The current of ions through the mem-

brane is, however, not only dependent on density and opening of channels. One additional important factor is the *concentration gradient* across the membrane for the ion: The steeper the gradient, the greater the flow of ions will be from high to low concentration (provided that the membrane is not totally impermeable to the ion). Furthermore, since ions are electrically charged particles, the *voltage gradient* across the membrane (that is, the membrane potential) will also be of importance. Thus, if the inside of the cell is negative in relation to the outside, positively charged ions (cations) on the outside will be exposed to a force attracting them into the cell, while inside cations will be subjected to forces that tend to drive them out. The strength of these attractive and expulsive forces depends on the magnitude of the membrane potential. Thus, the *concentration gradient and the membrane potential together determine the flow of ions through the membrane.*

The Membrane Potential

In a typical nerve cell, the potential across the cell membrane is stable at around 60 mV (millivolt) in the resting state—that is, as long as the cell is not exposed to any stimuli. We therefore use the term *resting potential* in this situation (in different kinds of nerve cells, the resting potential may vary from about 45 to about 75 mV). The resting potential is due to a small surplus of negatively charged ions, *anions*, inside the cell as compared with the outside, and it has arbitrarily been decided to define the *resting potential as negative*—for example, −60 mV.

The resting potential is primarily due to two factors. One is that the *cell membrane is selectively permeable*—that is, some kinds of ion may pass through the membrane with much greater ease than other kinds. The other factor is that the *concentration of certain ions differs greatly inside and outside the cell.* This unequal distribution of ions is established and maintained by energy-requiring "pumps" in the cell membrane that actively transport ions through the membrane

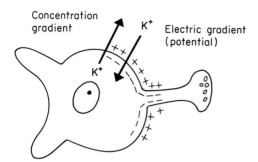

Fig. 1.19. *Forces acting on the K⁺ ions.*

against a concentration gradient. Several ions are unequally distributed (Fig. 1.18A), but to explain the membrane potential we may restrict ourselves for the moment to just K^+ (Fig. 1.18B). This is so because at rest only K^+ can pass the membrane with some ease, while the membrane is very slightly permeable to, for example, Na^+ (which is also very unequally distributed). For the time being, then, we will ignore the sodium ions. The concentration gradient will tend to drive K^+ out of the cell. This means that positive charges are lost from the inside of the cell, making the inside negative compared to the outside, and creating a membrane potential. The membrane potential reaches only a certain value, however, because it will oppose the movement of K^+ ions out of the cell. Two opposite forces are thus at work: the concentration gradient tending to drive K^+ out of the cell and the electrical gradient (membrane potential) tending to drive K^+ into the cell (Fig. 1.19). When the membrane potential is about 75 mV, these two forces are equally strong; that is, the flow of K^+ into the cell equals exactly the flow out. This is therefore called *the equilibrium potential for K^+*, and its magnitude is determined by the concentration gradient for potassium ions.

The resting potential in most neurons is, however, lower than the equilibrium potential for K^+. This is because, although not taken into consideration above, the cell membrane is slightly permeable to Na^+ (although only about 1/50th of the permeability to K^+). Thus, some positive charges (Na^+) pass into the cell driven by both the concen-

tration gradient and the membrane potential, making the inside of the cell less negative than the equilibrium potential for K^+. The membrane potential is thus changed somewhat in the direction of the equilibrium potential for Na^+, that is, $+55$ mV.

Even though the two opposite currents of K^+ and Na^+ in the resting state are small, they would over time lead to elimination of the concentration gradients of these ions across the membrane (Fig. 1.18B) were it not for the *sodium–potassium pump*. This pump actively expels Na^+ ions from the inside, in exchange for K^+ at the same rate as the ions leak through the membrane. Thus, as long as the cell is in the resting state, there is equilibrium between flow of ions in and out of the cell.

Not Only Na⁺ and K⁺ Are Unequally Distributed

For simplicity we have so far dealt with only two of the cations, K^+ and Na^+, because they are the most important ones for the membrane potential and also for the nerve impulse. However, several other kinds of ions are also unequally distributed. Of the anions, chloride ions (Cl^-) and negatively charged protein molecules (abbreviated to P^-) make up the bulk (Fig. 1.18). These are also unequally distributed, so that chloride is the major extracellular anion, whereas proteins are the major intracellular ones. The proteins are so big that they cannot pass the membrane—the membrane is impermeable to protein molecules. The membrane is, however, somewhat permeable to Cl^-. The concentration gradient tends to drive chloride into the cell, whereas the membrane potential tends to drive it out, making the net flow of Cl^- small. In fact, the equilibrium potential for Cl^-, -65 mV, is close to the resting potential of most nerve cells. Therefore, no active mechanism for pumping of chloride is needed.

The Sodium–Potassium Pump and the Unequal Distribution of Ions

The unequal distribution of ions is, as we have seen, of fundamental importance for the membrane potential. How is this unequal distribution produced in the first place, and how is it maintained? This was briefly alluded to above. Again, the selective permeability of the cell membrane is crucial. We may start with a hypothetical situation with only potassium chloride, KCl, inside the cell. This is in the form of K^+ and Cl^- ions. No other ions are present either inside or outside the cell. As mentioned above, the membrane is somewhat permeable to both ions, and they will therefore diffuse slowly out of the cell until the concentrations are equal on both sides of the membrane. Imagine that we now add a large number of negatively charged protein molecules, P^-, to which the cell membrane is impermeable, and an equal number of cations, which in this case are K^+ (cations must follow the anions in order to ensure electrical neutrality). The equilibrium between positive and negative charges inside the cell is thus not disturbed by adding KP. However, the concentration of K^+ becomes higher inside the cell than outside. Thus, some K^+ ions move out of the cell, driven by the concentration gradient, and Cl^- follows, driven by the electric potential (inside negative) that arises when K^+ ions move out. After a while, a new state of equilibrium is reached, at which the electrical gradient produced by the outward flow of K^+ ions equals the concentration gradient for K^+. When this equilibrium is reached, the concentration of K^+ is still higher inside than outside, while the concentration of Cl^- has become highest outside. This situation may appear to be stable. However, because of the protein molecules, which cannot pass the membrane, the total concentration of ions is higher inside than outside the cell. In this situation, water would flow into the cell by osmosis (the water concentration being lower inside than outside the cell). The cell would swell and ultimately disintegrate. This obviously does not happen with the cells in our body. The reason is that, unlike the hypothetical situation described above, the extracellular fluid contains NaCl (as Na^+ and Cl^-), making the total ion concentration equal outside and inside the cell. However, to prevent Na^+ from entering the cell (driven by both concentration and electrical gradients) and thus unsettling the osmotic balance, the cell membrane must have a very low permeability to Na^+. Although this permeability is low, however, it is not zero. Some Na^+ therefore would flow into the cell, and some K^+ would flow out (because the membrane potential would be lowered by cations coming into the cell) were it not for the sodium–potassium pump. In fact, all cells, not only nerve cells, are dependent on the activity of the sodium–potassium pump to maintain osmotic equilibrium between the intracellular and extracellular fluid compartments. Unique to nerve cells (and, for example, muscle cells) is that the pumping activity has to be in-

creased in relation to action potentials, since these are produced by an inward current of Na^+ ions and an outward current of K^+ ions. The activity of the pump is increased in pace with increases of the intracellular Na^+ concentration.

A significant part of our energy in the form of ATP is spent on driving the sodium–potassium pump. In the resting state of nerve cells it may constitute around one-third, whereas after high-frequency trains of action potentials it may increase to two-thirds of the total energy requirement.

Alteration of the Membrane Potential: Depolarization and Hyperpolarization

As mentioned above, in the resting state the membrane permeability for Na^+ is low. If for some reason Na^+ channels are opened so that the permeability is increased, Na^+ ions will flow into the cell and thereby reduce the magnitude of the membrane potential (that is, change it toward the equilibrium potential of Na^+ at $+55\,mV$). Such a reduction of the membrane potential is called *depolarization*. The membrane potential is made less negative by depolarization. Correspondingly, one may foresee that when the membrane permeability for K^+ is increased, the membrane potential will become more negative than the resting potential. This is called *hyperpolarization*. The same would be achieved by opening channels for chloride ions, enabling negative charges (Cl^-) to flow into the cell.

In conclusion, the membrane potential is determined by the relative permeability of the various ions that can pass the membrane. At rest, the membrane is primarily permeable to K^+, and the resting potential is therefore close to the equilibrium potential of K^+. As we will see in the following discussion, the action potential is caused by a sudden increase in the Na^+ permeability.

The Action Potential

The basis of the action potential is found in the presence of voltage-gated Na^+ channels, which are opened by depolarization of the membrane. Depolarization may be induced in several ways; for example, under artificial

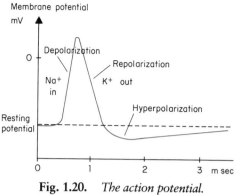

Fig. 1.20. *The action potential.*

conditions by direct electrical stimulation. Normally, however, it is caused by the action of neurotransmitters acting on transmitter-gated channels. Thus, depolarization is often started by opening of transmitter-gated Na^+ channels. Opening of the voltage-gated channels requires that the membrane be depolarized to a certain *threshold value*— that is, the threshold for producing an action potential (Fig. 1.20). When voltage-gated channels are opened, the permeability to Na^+ is increased compared to what was achieved by opening of transmitter-gated channels, and Na^+ flows into the cell driven by both the concentration gradient and the membrane potential. The membrane is more depolarized, this in turn opens more voltage-gated channels, and so on. Thus, the permeability to Na^+ increases in an explosive manner as soon as the membrane is depolarized to the threshold value. Even with all sodium channels fully open, however, the inward current of Na^+ ions stops when the membrane is depolarized to $+55$ mV; at that value the inward concentration force is equal to the outward electrical force (the membrane potential). As mentioned above, $+55$ mV is the equilibrium potential of Na^+. Figure 1.20 shows how, during an action potential, the membrane potential quickly changes to positive values and then returns almost as rapidly to about the resting value. This happens because the membrane again becomes impermeable to Na^+; the Na^+ *channels are closed or inactivated.* Thus at the peak of the action potential and for a short time afterward, no Na^+ can pass

through the membrane. In this situation with a positive membrane potential, K^+ is driven out both by the concentration gradient and the membrane potential (electrical force). Since no Na^+ can enter the cell, there is a net outward flow of positive charges, again making the interior of the cell negative. We say that the membrane is *repolarized.* The speed of repolarization is increased by the presence of voltage-gated K^+ channels, which open when the membrane is sufficiently depolarized. The opening of the voltage-gated K^+ channels is somewhat delayed compared with the Na^+ channels, but whereas the Na^+ channels inactivate after about 1 msec, the K^+ channels stay open for several milliseconds.

In summary, the action potential is caused by a brief inward current of Na^+ ions, followed by an outward current of K^+ ions. The whole sequence of depolarization–repolarization is generally finished in 1–2 msec.

One might perhaps think that an action potential would cause significant changes in the concentrations of Na^+ and K^+ on the two sides of the membrane. This, however, is not the case. The number of ions actually passing the membrane during an action potential is extremely small compared with the total number inside the cell and in its immediate surroundings. Even in an axon with a diameter of about 1 μm, with a very small intracellular volume compared to the membrane surface area, only 1 of 3000 K^+ ions moves out during the action potential. In addition, active pumping (the sodium–potassium pump) ensures that Na^+ is moved out and K^+ moved in between each action potential and in periods of rest. Even when the sodium–potassium pump is blocked experimentally, a nerve cell can produce several thousand action potentials before concentration gradients are reduced so much that the cell loses its excitability.

Nerve Cells Are Often Continuously Active: Frequency Coding

So far we have treated the action potential as a unitary phenomenon. In reality, many neurons produce trains of action potentials in rapid succession and then pause for a while before a new train of impulses is produced. The frequency of action potentials in some neurons may be more than 100 per second (Hertz), whereas in others it may be much lower. Each neuronal type has its characteristic frequency pattern, caused by differences in membrane properties and synaptic inputs. Neurons with high maximal impulse frequency especially tend to discharge in bursts, with trains of impulses interrupted by periods of rest.

The *code* for the information carried by an axon is the *frequency and pattern of action potentials,* since the strength of action potential always is the same.

Calcium and the Action Potential

Although not mentioned above, a cation other than Na^+, namely Ca^{2+}, may also contribute to the rising phase of the action potential. For Ca^{2+} too the extracellular concentration is much higher than the intracellular one, and there are voltage-gated calcium channels in the membrane.

Cellular influx of calcium can be visualized after intracellular injection of a substance that fluoresces when Ca^{2+} binds to it. During the action potential, calcium enters the cell, partly through Na^+ channels, partly through voltage-gated calcium channels, which have a more prolonged opening-closing phase than the sodium channels. There are also transmitter-gated calcium channels. In most neurons the contribution of Ca^{2+} to the action potential is nevertheless small compared with that of Na^+ (in certain other cells such as heart muscle, however, calcium is the ion largely responsible for the action potential). Because the calcium channels open and close more slowly than the Na^+ channels, an action potential produced by calcium currents lasts longer than one produced by flow of Na^+.

Another aspect of the functional role of calcium is that the *extracellular calcium concentration influences the membrane excitability.* This is most likely mediated through effects on the Na^+ and K^+ channels. Reducing the calcium concentration in the blood and interstitial fluid (hypocalcemia) lowers the threshold for evoking action potentials in neurons and muscle cells, whereas increasing the concentration (hypercalcemia) has the opposite effect. A typical symptom of hypocalcemia is muscle spasms due to hyperexcitability of nerves and muscles.

Calcium Is an Important Signal Molecule for Nerve Cells

Cellular influx of calcium has other and probably more important effects on most neurons than contributing directly to the action potential. Calcium is an important signal molecule in itself, functioning intracellularly as a second messenger and influencing other second messengers like cyclic adenosine monophosphate (cAMP). One well-known effect is that calcium influx into boutons is necessary for *release of neurotransmitters* (corresponding to conditions in secretory cells). We return to this below.

Another important effect calcium may have as a signal molecule is to produce (via intermediaries) changes of gene expression and protein synthesis. This may be crucial, for example, in relation to long-term changes in neuronal properties underlying learning and memory. Calcium influx can apparently be restricted to only certain parts of the neuronal membrane; for example, on part of a dendrite subjected to particularly strong synaptic influences. This may produce changes in the properties of the synapses only on this part of the neuron, whereas synapses at other sites remain unchanged.

The Refractory Period

After an action potential, it takes some time before the neuron can again produce an action potential in response to a stimulus. The cell is said to be in a *refractory* state. This ensures that the cell always gets at least a minimal period of rest between each action potential and thus puts an upper limit on the frequency with which the cell can fire. The length of the refractory period, and thus the maximal frequency of firing, varies considerably among different kinds of nerve cells.

Two conditions are responsible for the refractory period. One is the above-mentioned *inactivation of the voltage-gated Na^+ channels,* and the other is the fact that the *membrane is hyperpolarized immediately after the action potential* (Fig. 1.20). The inactivation of Na^+ channels means that they cannot be opened, regardless of the strength of the stimulus and the ensuing depolarization. The hyperpolarization is due to the fact that the K^+ channels remain open longer than required just to bring the membrane potential back to resting value. These two different mechanisms can explain why the refractory period consists of two phases. During the first phase, the *absolute refractory period,* the cell cannot be made to discharge however strong the stimulus may be; during the *relative refractory period,* stronger depolarization than normal is needed to produce an action potential.

Impulse Conduction in Axons

We will now consider how the action potential moves along the axon. The ability of the axon to conduct electrical current depends on several conditions, some of which are given by the physical properties of axons, which make them very different from, for example, copper wire, whereas other conditions vary among axons of different kinds. An axon is a poor conductor compared with the usual electrical conductors made of metal. This is because the axoplasm through which the current has to pass consists of a weak solution of electrolytes (that is, low concentrations of charged particles in water) that is not a particularly good conductor. In addition, the diameter of axons is small (from less than 1 to 20 μm) with a correspondingly enormous *internal resistance* to the current in the axon. Furthermore, the axonal membrane is not a perfect insulator, so that charged particles are lost from the interior of the axon as the current passes along the axon. The amount of current being lost is determined by the *membrane resistance* (that is, the resistance offered by the membrane to charged particles trying to pass). Finally, the axonal membrane (like all cell membranes) has an *electrical capacity;* that is, it can store a certain amount of charged particles, in the way a battery does. This further contributes to the rapid attenuation of a current that is conducted along an axon— the membrane has to be charged before the current can move on.

From the foregoing it can be concluded that *how well the current is conducted in an axon depends on its internal resistance (its diameter), the membrane resistance (how well insulated it is), and the capacity of the axonal membrane.* If the propagation of the

action potential along the axon took place only by passive, electrotonic movement of charged particles, the internal resistance and loss of charges to the exterior would cause the action potential to move only a short distance before it "died out." The solution to this problem is that the *action potential is regenerated while moving along the axon.* Thus, it is propagated with undiminished strength all the way from the perikaryon to the terminal boutons. *The strength of the action potential—that is, the magnitude of the changes of the membrane potential taking place—is the same regardless of the strength of the stimulus that produced it* (as long as the stimulus depolarizes the membrane to threshold). Increasing the strength of the stimulus increases the frequency of action potentials, whereas the magnitude of each action potential remains constant.

When the cell membrane close to the site where the axon leaves the cell body is depolarized to threshold, an axon potential is produced and is conducted passively a short distance along the axon. From then on, what happens differs somewhat in myelinated and unmyelinated axons. We will consider *unmyelinated axons* first (Fig. 1.21). The action potential is produced by positive charges entering the interior of the axon, which thus becomes positive relative to more distal parts of the axon. Positive charges then start moving in the distal direction (along the electrical gradient that has been set up). A corresponding current of positive charges moves in the opposite direction outside the axon, so that an electrical circuit is established. Movement of positive charges in the distal direction inside the axon means that the membrane is depolarized as the charges move along. This depolarization leads to the opening of enough voltage-gated Na^+ and K^+ channels to produce a "new" action potential. In this manner, the action potential moves along the axon at a speed that depends on the speed with which the charged particles (that is, ions) move inside the axon and on the time needed for full opening of the ion channels. The membrane capacity represents a further factor slowing the propagation, because the membrane has

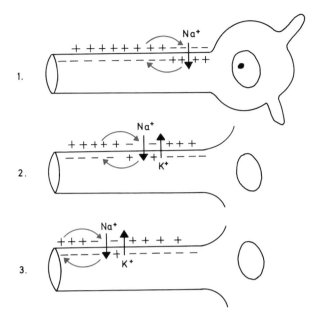

Fig. 1.21.   *Impulse conduction in unmyelinated axons.*

to be charged before there can be a net flow of charges through the membrane.

In essence, the action potential is propagated as a wave of depolarization, followed closely by a corresponding wave of repolarization. Where the membrane has just been through this cycle, it is in the refractory state for some milliseconds. This prevents the action potential from spreading "backward" toward the perikaryon, and ensures that under normal conditions the impulse conduction is unidirectional. If, however, the axon is artificially stimulated (for example, electrically) at some distance from the perikaryon, the action potential spreads both toward the perikaryon and toward the end ramifications.

In *myelinated axons,* the action potential is also regenerated along the axon (Fig. 1.22). But, in contrast to that in unmyelinated axons, *the action potential is regenerated only at each node of Ranvier*—that is, where the axon membrane lacks covering by the myelin sheath and is in direct contact with the extracellular fluid. As in unmyelinated axons, the action potential arises in the first part of the axon where it emerges from the perikaryon. The current then spreads

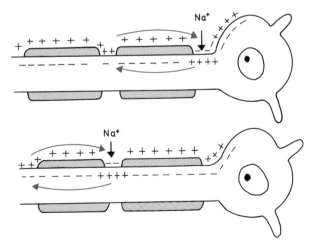

Fig. 1.22.   *Impulse conduction in myelinated axons.*

passively (electrotonically) to the first node of Ranvier. Here, the depolarization of the membrane leads to opening of voltage-gated channels and a "new" action potential. The density of voltage-gated sodium channels is particularly high in the axonal membrane at the node of Ranvier. The current can flow electrotonically as far as to the first node of Ranvier (and probably sometimes longer) because the axon is so well insulated by myelin, preventing loss of charges from the interior of the axon (myelin increases dramatically the resistance across the membrane and also reduces the membrane capacity). In addition, the axonal diameter is larger in myelinated than in unmyelinated axons, thus reducing the internal resistance.

In conclusion, in myelinated axons the action potential does not move smoothly and slowly along, as in unmyelinated axons, but instead "jumps" from one node of Ranvier to the next. While the impulse propagation is very rapid between nodes, at each node there is a delay due to the time required for opening of channels and establishment of sufficient flow of current.

Conduction Velocities in Myelinated and Unmyelinated Axons

The main reason why myelinated axons conduct so much more rapidly than unmyelinated ones is that the action potential needs to be regenerated only at certain sites. A figure for conduction velocity (in meters per second) in myelinated axons is obtained by multiplying the axonal diameter (in micrometers) by 6. An axon of 20 μm (the maximal diameter) thus conducts at approximately 120 m/sec, whereas the thinnest myelinated axons of about 3 μm conduct at 18 m/sec. In comparison, a typical unmyelinated axon of about 1 μm conducts at less than 1 m/sec.

SYNAPTIC TRANSMISSION

So far, we have discussed the basis of nerve impulses and how they are conducted over long distances. Now we will look into the synaptic transfer of the signal represented by an action potential. We will also examine what leads up to the discharge of an action potential.

Transfer of Signals between Nerve Cells Is Usually Chemically Mediated

We can sum up the signal transfer as follows (Fig. 1.23): First, an action potential reaches the nerve terminal (bouton) and depolarizes it. This *depolarization opens Ca^{2+} channels,* enabling Ca^{2+} to enter the bouton. Increase in intracellular Ca^{2+} concentration is a signal for *release of transmitter* from vesicles by exocytosis. The released transmitter binds briefly to *receptors* in the postsynaptic membrane. This leads directly or indirectly to alteration of the opening of ion channels and thus to transient changes in membrane permeability to certain ions and alteration of the membrane potential. The potential change arising as a result of such synaptic influence is called a *synaptic potential.* If the synaptic influence depolarizes the postsynaptic cell, the probability that the cell will fire action potentials is increased. This synaptic effect is called an *excitatory* synaptic potential. If the synaptic potential hyperpolarizes the cell, it is called an *inhibitory*

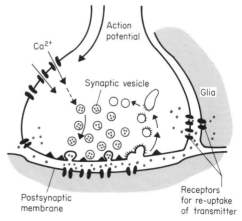

Fig. 1.23. *Impulse transmission at the synapse.* Schematic representation of some important features.

synaptic potential because the probability of the cell's firing is diminished.

Summation of Stimuli Is Necessary to Evoke an Action Potential

Not every impulse leading to transmitter release at a synapse evokes an action potential in the postsynaptic cell. As mentioned, the membrane has to be depolarized to a *threshold value* (Fig. 1.24) for an action potential to be evoked. A *subthreshold depolarization* (excitatory synaptic potential) nevertheless may be of functional significance. Thus, if the synaptic potential is followed by another depolarization before the membrane potential has returned to resting value, the second depolarization is added to the first one so that threshold is reached. This phenomenon is called *summation* (Fig. 1.24A). The summation may be in time, as in the example above, and is then called *temporal summation*, or it may be in space, then called *spatial*

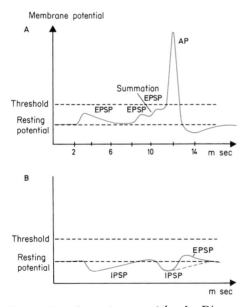

Fig. 1.24. *Synaptic potentials.* **A.** Diagram showing the time course and polarity of an EPSP. In this example, one EPSP alone does not depolarize the membrane to threshold for eliciting an action potential, but if one or more EPSP follows shortly after the first one, the threshold is reached (summation). **B.** Diagram showing the time course and polarity of an IPSP.

summation. In temporal summation, impulses may follow each other in rapid succession in one terminal, whereas in spatial summation, boutons at different places on the cell surface release transmitter and depolarize the cell almost simultaneously.

That summation can be an important mechanism for controlling the activity of nerve cells is due to the comparatively slow time course of synaptic potentials (in contrast to the time course of an action potential). The excitatory synaptic potential is caused by simultaneous opening of several types of cation channels (for Na^+ and Ca^{2+} going in, and K^+ going out). Because the cations outside the cell are driven in both by concentration gradients and by the membrane potential, whereas K^+ is driven out only by the concentration gradient, the inward current dominates initially and the membrane is depolarized. This, however, leads to an increased outward current of K^+. Depolarization in itself does not increase opening of transmitter gated-channels (unlike the case for voltage-gated channels responsible for the action potential). Therefore, the synaptic potential gradually increases and decreases (graded potential). From the site of the synapse, the current spreads passively (electrotonically) along the membrane of the postsynaptic cell, without being regenerated. Thus, because charges (ions) leak through the membrane, the current will gradually become weaker and weaker as it moves from the synapse.

Usually, action potentials do not arise in dendrites or the perikaryon, where most of the synapses are placed, but in the first part of the axon, where it leaves the cell body, the so-called *initial segment*.

The current produced at synaptic sites must spread electrotonically to the initial segment. If the depolarization of the membrane of the initial segment reaches threshold, an action potential arises in the usual manner by opening voltage-gated Na^+ channels. The threshold for evoking an action potential is usually much lower at the initial segment than elsewhere on the cell surface, explaining why action potentials as a rule do not arise in dendrites or the peri-karyon. The threshold differences are due to differences in the density of voltage-gated Na^+ channels.

Excitatory Synapses

As mentioned above, at a synapse where the transmitter depolarizes the postsynaptic membrane, an excitatory synaptic potential is evoked. Usually the term *excitatory post-synaptic potential (EPSP)* is used. If a new EPSP follows before the previous one is finished, summation of depolarizations occurs because more ion channels are open at the same time (Fig. 1.24A). Neurotransmitters producing EPSPs are called *excitatory transmitters,* and we also use the term *excitatory synapses*. One EPSP alone does not as a rule cause sufficient depolarization to give rise to an action potential, but for a short while the cell has increased responsiveness to further excitatory input. Thus repeated stimuli, or an increase in the number of synapses being active, may fire a cell that would not respond with an action potential to a single stimulus.

Inhibitory Synapses

At many synapses, the transmitter substances released reduce the probability of the postsynaptic cell responding with action potentials. One way in which such transmitters work is by *hyperpolarizing* the postsynaptic membrane transiently. Thus, more depolarization is needed to bring the membrane potential to threshold. The potential evoked at such synapses is called an *inhibitory postsynaptic potential (IPSP)*. This synaptic potential has a comparatively slow time course and lasts for many milliseconds (Fig. 1.24B). An EPSP occurring during an IPSP will have less probability of evoking an action potential. The postsynaptic cell is therefore inhibited, and we use the term *inhibitory transmitters* and *inhibitory synapses*.

The mechanism underlying hyperpolarization is usually opening of transmitter-gated K^+ or Cl^- channels. This leads to a flow of K^+ ions out of the cell, with the inside becoming more negative than earlier compared with the outside, or to Cl^- flowing into the cell, with the same effect on the membrane potential. A prerequisite for hyperpolarization to result from opening of K^+ or Cl^- channels is that the membrane potential at the outset is less negative than the equilibrium potentials for K^+ or Cl^-. The equilibrium potential of Cl^- is in fact close to the resting potential in many nerve cells. Nevertheless, even when there is no net flow of Cl^- into the cell, opening of chloride channels can reduce the effect of simultaneous excitatory transmitters. This is because Cl^- starts to flow into the cell as soon as the membrane is even slightly depolarized (because this makes the inside less negative) and thus opposes change of the membrane potential. In this manner, the inhibitory transmitter acts to short-circuit nearby excitatory synapses.

Facilitation: Repeated Action Potentials Can Lead to Increased Transmitter Release

When action potentials reach the nerve terminal at only brief intervals (high firing frequency), the amplitude of the ensuing postsynaptic potentials often increases (the amplitude of the presynaptic action potential remains the same under such conditions). One possible explanation of this phenomenon is that some of the Ca^{2+} that enters during one action potential remains when the next action potential reaches the bouton and again opens calcium channels. Thus the effect of Ca^{2+} on transmitter release is enhanced. Facilitation may last for seconds, so that as long as the interval between action potentials is shorter than this, the postsynaptic effect of each action potential may increase by repetitive stimulation.

Facilitation appears to be of importance for the nervous system's ability to store information and to change responses during learning (plasticity). However, other and more long-term cellular mechanisms than facilitation are also responsible for changes in synaptic effects during learning and information storage (see Chapter 16).

Axoaxonic Synapses Enable Presynaptic Control of Transmitter Release

A special kind of synaptic influence is mediated by the so-called *axoaxonic synapses* (Figs. 1.7D and 1.25). The *presynaptic* bouton makes synaptic contact with a *postsynaptic bouton,* which in turn contacts a perikaryon or a dendrite. Release of transmitter from the presynaptic bouton serves to regulate the amount of transmitter released by the postsynaptic bouton.

In one type of axoaxonic contact, action potentials in the presynaptic bouton lead to reduced transmitter release from the postsynaptic bouton; thus the effect is *inhibitory with regard to the neuron contacted by the postsynaptic bouton.* A prerequisite for this inhibitory effect to occur, however, is that the presynaptic bouton be depolarized (by an action potential) at the same time as or immediately before an action potential reaches the postsynaptic bouton. This phenomenon is termed *presynaptic inhibition* to distinguish it from the postsynaptic inhibition described above. Two mechanisms may be responsible for presynaptic inhibition. One is the opening of chloride channels in the membrane of the postsynaptic bouton, thereby short-circuiting it in the manner described above in connection with postsynaptic inhibition. In such a case, the action potential invading the postsynaptic bouton would elicit less depolarization than normally. Less depolarization means opening of fewer calcium channels, and since the amount of transmitter released is proportional to the influx

of Ca^{2+}, less transmitter will be released. Another mechanism for presynaptic inhibition may be direct influence on calcium channels by the transmitter released from the presynaptic bouton. Presynaptic inhibition has been found most frequently among fiber systems that transmit sensory information; for example, sensory fibers entering the spinal cord are subject to powerful presynaptic inhibition.

Presynaptic facilitation may be elicited at axoaxonic synapses by transmitters that lead to increased Ca^{2+} influx in the postsynaptic bouton. Increased calcium influx may be caused by closure of K^+ channels by the transmitter. This leads to prolongation of the action potential (the repolarization phase being slower), which enables more Ca^{2+} to enter the postsynaptic bouton.

In general, presynaptic influences make it possible to control selectively the signal transmission from one neuron to another, without affecting the general excitability of the postsynaptic neuron and thus its responsiveness to other synaptic inputs.

Why Do We Need Inhibitory Synapses?

Inhibitory synapses are present everywhere in the central nervous system and are of vital importance for its proper functioning. Inhibition is, for example, necessary to suppress irrelevant sensory information, thus enabling us to concentrate on certain events and leave others out. Inhibitory synapses also serve to increase the precision of sensory information by, for example, enhancing contrast between regions with different light intensity in visual images.

Inhibition is also necessary for another reason—namely, to dampen or interrupt excitation, which might otherwise lead to cell damage. As mentioned earlier, ions have to be pumped through the cell membrane in order to maintain osmotic equilibrium. If many neurons fire continuously with high frequency, even maximal pumping may be insufficient in this respect. Increased extracellular potassium concentration depolarizes neurons, thus further increasing the neuronal excitation; this in turn leads to more potassium extracellularly and so on.

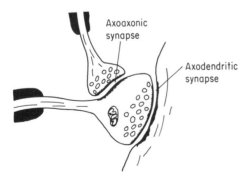

Fig. 1.25. *Presynaptic inhibition* is mediated by axoaxonic synapses.

Epileptic seizures are due to uncontrolled firing of groups of neurons, and drugs reducing the tendency for seizures generally increase the effect of inhibitory transmitters.

A Neuron Integrates Information from Many Others

We have seen that as a rule many impulses must reach a neuron almost simultaneously to make it fire—that is, to send an action potential through its axon. In other words, summation of excitatory synaptic effects is necessary. The stronger the sum of excitatory effects, the shorter the time necessary to depolarize the cell to the threshold for eliciting another action potential. Thus, the *frequency of action potentials, or firing frequency, is an expression of the total synaptic input to a neuron.* Total synaptic input here means the *sum of both excitatory and inhibitory synaptic influences.* Often a neuron is strongly influenced (many synaptic contacts) by one neuronal group but is in addition weakly influenced by many others. Thus, this particular neuron may be principally involved in signal transmission from one source (a nucleus, a set of receptors, etc.) but the efficiency of transmission may be facilitated or inhibited by many other cell groups. One example among many is the suppression of signal transmission from receptors related to pain perception.

The efficiency or strength of a certain synaptic input is not only related to the total number of synaptic contacts. The placement of a synapse on the neuronal surface is also of importance. Synapses close to the initial segment of the axon have a greater chance of eliciting (or preventing) an action potential than synapses far out on the dendrites (this is related to the loss of current during electrotonic spread of the synaptic potential over long distances). Thus, a centrally placed synapse may perhaps fire the neuron alone, whereas many peripherally placed synapses will have to cooperate to fire the cell. In this sense, synapses may be more or less *strategically* placed.

Synaptic Effects May Also Be Prolonged

So far we have considered only fast synaptic effects on the membrane potential, typically lasting only a few milliseconds. Recently, however, it has become clear that transmitters may have other kinds of effects as well.

One important finding is that *synaptic influences on channel opening may be slow and long-lasting,* so that, for example, the membrane may be kept depolarized for many seconds or even minutes (slow EPSP). A brief train of impulses in axons releasing such a transmitter from its terminals may keep the membrane depolarized for seconds after the train of impulses is ended. More intense stimulation may in some neurons produce depolarization lasting minutes. Such effects may be mediated by *transmitters that close K^+ channels* (there are several types of potassium channels: Some are voltage-gated, such as those opened during the action potential; some are regulated by intracellular Ca^{2+}, others are transmitter-gated). Closing of potassium channels reduces the membrane permeability to potassium and thereby the outward flow of K^+, and thus the membrane potential is lowered.

There are also *slow, long-lasting hyperpolarizing synaptic effects* (slow IPSP), which also may be mediated by the transmitter regulating the opening of potassium channels. To obtain a hyperpolarizing effect, the potassium channels have to be opened to increase the membrane permeability to K^+.

Certain kinds of transmitter-gated potassium channels shorten the hyperpolarization phase after an action potential—that is, the refractory period is shortened—and the cell may elicit action potentials with an increased frequency. Thus, if a neuron is under this kind of synaptic influence, another synaptic input operating on "ordinary" fast ion channels may drive the cell to a higher frequency than it otherwise could have done.

Slow synaptic effects are usually not due to direct binding of the transmitter molecule to the channel proteins. Rather, the transmitter binds to membrane receptors that trigger a train of intracellular events, involving second messenger molecules like Ca^{2+} or cAMP, and ultimately changing the opening of ion channels. To distinguish such long-lasting synaptic effects from the fast ones, we often use the term *modulatory synaptic effects* about the slow EPSPs and IPSPs, and we may also use the terms *modulatory transmitters* or *modulatory neuroactive substances*. When using the term modulatory, it is usually implied that the transmitter does not elicit action potentials on its own but regulates the neuronal sensitivity to other fast synaptic influences.

One transmitter may have fast excitatory effects at certain synapses and modulatory effects at others. This depends on the kind of receptor present in the postsynaptic membrane—for example, whether it is part of an ion channel or operates via intracellular second messengers.

Neurotransmitters May Alter the Metabolism of the Neuron

Transmitters, apart from regulating the excitability of neurons, can also influence the metabolic activity of the postsynaptic cell (via intracellular second messengers). This may be related to growth and development of neurons, since this has been shown in many instances to depend on synaptic activity. It probably also relates to plastic changes in neurons involved in learning and memory.

Such long-term (or even permanent) effects may, for example, be produced by changes in synthesis of receptor proteins and enzymes involved in transmitter synthesis. There may also be changes in the amount and activity of intracellular signal molecules. If, for example, the neuron after a certain synaptic influence liberates more transmitter at its terminals than previously, its effect on other neurons is strengthened. If, on the other hand, the density of receptor molecules in the neuronal membrane increases as a consequence of synaptic influence, the neuron may react more

strongly than earlier to a certain synaptic input.

Unusual Synapses: Electrotonic and Dendrodendritic Transmission

Although rare, at some synapses in the central nervous system, the pre-and postsynaptic elements are electrically rather than chemically coupled. Electron microscopically, such *electrotonic synapses* differ from chemical synapses in that the synaptic cleft is only 2 nm compared to about 20 nm. The cell contact formed is called a *nexus* or *gap junction,* and consists of channels that span the synaptic cleft. Thus, ions (electrical current) can pass directly and quickly from one cell to another with no synaptic delay. In invertebrates and lower vertebrates, electrotonic synapses are formed between neurons mediating short latency responses to stimuli (for example, escape reactions). Electrotonic synapses may also provide electrical coupling between many neurons in a group, so that their activity may be synchronized. Chemical synapses may occur close to electrical ones, and serve to uncouple the electrical synapse so that these apparently can be switched on and off.

Electrical coupling by gap junctions is much more common among glial cells than among neurons, and they occur regularly among cardiac, smooth-muscle, and epithelial cells.

There are also other unusual types of synapses. Contacts between dendrites with all the morphological characteristics of synapses have been observed in several places in the central nervous system. Such *dendrodendritic synapses* are often part of more complex synaptic arrangements. Through dendrodendritic synapses, adjacent neurons can influence each other without being connected with axons. The function of such synapses, however, is not fully understood.

NEUROTRANSMITTERS

Above we have described neurotransmitters (transmitters) in general in connection with synapses. We will now deal more specifically with the best-known neurotransmitters.

It Is Difficult to Prove That a Substance Functions as a Neurotransmitter

The term *neurotransmitter* or *transmitter* is used for chemical substances that are released at synapses and transmit a signal from one neuron to another. To prove that a substance present in a neuron actually functions as a neurotransmitter, however, is far from easy. Several complicated anatomic, neurophysiological, and pharmacological techniques are required to demonstrate that the neuron synthesizes the transmitter candidate, that it is stored in the nerve terminals, that it is released by depolarization, that the release is calcium-dependent, and that the released substance is directly responsible for the postsynaptic changes. There also should be specific mechanisms for removal of the substance from the synaptic cleft and its immediate vicinity. For these kinds of studies, we are critically dependent on the availability of specific agonists and antagonists—that is, substances that mimic or prevent the action, respectively, of only the transmitter candidate.

Only a few transmitter candidates have met all of these criteria when tested experimentally. For several others, the probability that they function as transmitters is high, and they are often described as transmitters without reservation. Strictly speaking, however, they should be termed *transmitter candidates* or *putative transmitters*.

As mentioned above, the effects of substances released at synapses are multifarious and not limited to excitation or inhibition mediated by regulation of ion channel permeability. The term *modulator* is therefore often used for substances that do not mediate the usual synaptic effects in the form of fast EPSPs and IPSPs. Modulators typically elicit slow, long-lasting changes of the membrane potential or metabolic changes in the postsynaptic cell, as discussed above.

The Two Main Groups of Chemical Transmitters

The neurotransmitters known today fall into two main chemical groups. One consists of *small molecules,* which with few exceptions (acetylcholine and ATP) are *amino acids* or *amines* (amino acids in which the carboxyl group is removed). The other group consists of larger molecules, namely *peptides* (short proteins consisting of about 5 to 30 amino acids). In general, the functions of these *neuroactive peptides or neuropeptides* are far less clarified than those of the small-molecular transmitters.

Whereas fast synaptic effects mediated by opening or closing of ion channels are produced by small-molecular transmitters, the neuroactive peptides appear to produce preferentially slow or long-lasting effects mediated by intracellular signal molecules. The numerous transmitters and transmitter candidates have an even larger variety of *receptor types* to act on. For the best-known transmitters, several receptor types (subtypes) have been described, mediating different effects on the postsynaptic cell. *One transmitter therefore does not have only one effect but several, dependent on the types of receptors present in the postsynaptic membrane.* Also, some receptors are localized to the *presynaptic membrane* and regulate the release of transmitters. The various receptors acted on by one particular transmitter are often differentially distributed in the nervous system. Therefore, it is usually not possible to assign one specific functional role to a particular transmitter.

Conditions are further complicated by the fact that *more than one transmitter may be present in one nerve terminal.* Most often, there is such *coexistence* of one small-molecular ("classical") neurotransmitter and one or several neuropeptides. It may therefore be difficult to decide which of the transmitters is responsible for the physiological or behavioral effects produced by stimulation of a certain group of nerve cells.

Acetylcholine

Acetylcholine is a small molecule synthesized by binding of choline to acetyl coenzyme A by the enzyme *choline acetyltranferase* (ChAT). The presence of this enzyme is characteristic for neurons containing acetylcholine, so-called *cholinergic neurons.* Acetylcholine is present in motor neurons in the spinal cord and brain stem–innervating skeletal muscle cells and in certain other neuronal groups in the central and the peripheral nervous system.

The actions of acetylcholine are especially well known for the cholinergic synapses between motor neurons and skeletal muscle cells. There, acetylcholine binds to *acetylcholine receptors,* which are part of a channel for cations (in its open state this channel enables Na^+, K^+, Ca^{2+} to pass). Opening of such channels elicits an action potential that spreads out in all directions to reach all parts of the muscle cell membrane. This is the signal that in turn leads to muscle contraction. Such acetylcholine receptors are also termed *nicotinic receptors* because the action of acetylcholine on striated muscle cells can be mimicked by nicotine. These receptors are blocked by *curare* and chemically similar synthetic compounds. By use of certain toxins (for example, the snake venom α-bungarotoxin) binding specifically and blocking the effect of acetylcholine, the structure and properties of the acetylcholine receptor have been determined in great detail.

Another kind of receptor for acetylcholine, the *muscarinic receptor,* is not stimulated by nicotine but by muscarine. This kind of receptor is blocked by *atropine.* Whereas skeletal muscle cells only contain nicotinic receptors, smooth-muscle cells are equipped with only muscarinic receptors. In the central nervous system, both kinds of receptors are present, even though muscarinic receptors appear to dominate quantitatively.

The effects produced by activation of muscarinic receptors are slower than those obtained by activating nicotinic ones. This is probably because effects of muscarinic receptor activation are mediated by several steps of intracellular signals. One effect is *closure of a particular kind of potassium channel.* This produces a slow, long-lasting depolarization of the postsynaptic membrane without itself eliciting action potentials. The cell is, however, facilitated, and the probability that other excitatory inputs will elicit action potentials is increased. In one particular cholinergic axonal pathway, brief electrical stimulation produces depolarization of the postsynaptic neurons for more than 300 msec, and repeated stimulation may lead to depolarization for seconds to minutes. Closure of another kind of potassium channel leads to shortening of the refractory period so that the neuron can increase its firing frequency.

Such slow effects of actylcholine are assumed to be of importance for higher mental functions closely related to the cerebral cortex (see Chapter 16: "The Basal Nucleus (Meynert) and Alzheimer's Disease".

Monoamines (Biogenic Amines)

The so-called *biogenic amines* or *monoamines* constitute a subgroup of the small-molecular transmitters. Among the monoamines, *norepinephrine (noradrenaline), epinephrine (adrenaline),* and *dopamine* are all synthesized from the amino acid tyrosine and are collectively called *catecholamines.* They are present in distinct cell groups both in the central and in the peripheral nervous system. Neurons containing norepinephrine are said to be *noradrenergic,* while those containing dopamine are *dopaminergic* (the same terminology is used for the receptors corresponding to these transmitters).

The other monoamines, *serotonin (5-hydroxytryptamine)* and *histamine,* are formed from the amino acids tryptophane and histidine, respectively.

The synaptic effects of the monoamines are complex. Slow changes of the membrane potential via intracellular signal molecules have been studied most. For example, in the cerebral cortex norepinephrine produces long-lasting depolarization by closure of a particular kind of potassium channel. As in the effects of acetylcholine on another kind of potassium channel, intracellular second messengers are involved.

One monoamine transmitter may have different effects on the postsynaptic cell, dependent on the kind of receptor present. Thus, there are several varieties of receptors for each of the catecholamines and for serotonin. For dopamine, there are D_1 and D_2 receptors with different properties and different distribution in the nervous system. There are two main receptor types, α and β, for norepinephrine and epinephrine. Their effects are often opposite, and they are also differentially distributed. For serotonin, several different receptor types have been characterized, with different and partly opposite effects. It is therefore not possible to say that a particular monoamine transmitter is either excitatory or inhibitory; it may be both, depending on the type of receptor present postsynaptically. Thus, serotonin, as one example, appears to have inhibitory actions at certain sites in the brain, whereas it is excitatory at other sites.

Excitatory Amino Acid Transmitters

This group contains the most ubiquitous excitatory transmitters. *Glutamate* is excitatory and acts directly on channels for Na^+ and K^+. Conditions are nevertheless more complicated than this, because there are at least three different receptor types for glutamate. This has been studied by use of various selective agonists and antagonists. Two of the receptors mediate fast depolarization and are called *kainate (K)* and *quiscualate (Q) receptors,* respectively, after the name of their specific agonists. The third type of glutamate receptor has different properties from the two others. It is closely linked to a voltage-gated Ca^{2+} channel. Depolarization produced by opening of this channel lasts considerably longer than depolarization elicited by stimulation of K and Q receptors. An agonist for this peculiar glutamate receptor is N-methyl-D-aspartate (NMDA), and it is therefore called the *NMDA receptor.* As a rule, NMDA receptors are located together with either K or Q receptors in the neuronal membrane. Thus, strong depolarization by stimulation of K or Q receptors may activate the voltage-gated NMDA receptor, leading to prolongation of the depolarization and Ca^{2+} flowing into the cell. This acts as a signal for intracellular changes, probably related to long-term alterations of synaptic signal transmission. This phenomenon is of particular interest in connection with the search for the cellular basis of learning and memory (see Chapter 16).

Aspartate also probably functions as an excitatory neurotransmitter with fast action. The evidence for its role as neurotransmitter is, however, less convincing than for glutamate.

Inhibitory Amino Acid Transmitters

Gamma-aminobutyric acid (GABA) is the most ubiquitous inhibitory transmitter, being present in virtually all parts of the central nervous system. GABA is synthesized from glutamic acid in one step by the enzyme glutamic acid decarboxylase (GAD). Most often, GABA appears to act by opening chloride channels, thus producing a brief hyperpolarizing current (IPSP). GABA may, however, also elicit hyperpolarization by opening of potassium channels. In this case the hyperpolarization lasts much longer and is mediated by intracellular signal molecules. By the use of agonists and antagonists, two kinds of GABA receptors have been characterized: $GABA_A$ and $GABA_B$, which are differently distributed. $GABA_A$ receptors are responsible for presynaptic effects of GABA—that is, in connection with presynaptic inhibition (p. 32). $GABA_A$ receptors mediate increases in chloride permeability, whereas the $GABA_B$ receptors appear to be responsible for the effects of GABA on the membrane permeability to potassium.

The GABA receptor consists of several subunits and is structurally similar to other ligand-gated receptors, which are integrated parts of ion channels. Also, the $GABA_A$ receptor has several binding sites, in addition to the one for GABA. Barbiturates and benzodiazepines, for example, bind to the $GABA_A$ receptor and enhance the effect of GABA. Whereas benzodiazepines increase the frequency of opening of Cl^- channels, the barbiturates prolong the time the channel stays open. The clinical use of these GABA agonists reflects that they act by enhancing inhibition at various places in the central nervous system: Benzodiazepines are used to reduce anxiety and provide muscle relaxation, and some derivatives are used as hypnotics. Barbiturates were formerly widely used as hypnotics, but are now used mainly to treat epilepsy and to induce general anesthesia. Another drug, baclofen, used to treat increased muscle tone (spasticity; see Chapter 8), apparently binds only to the $GABA_B$ receptor.

Another inhibitory amino acid transmitter is *glycine,* but its distribution is very restricted compared with that of GABA. Apart from being found in certain cell groups in the brain stem, glycine is most likely a transmitter for certain spinal interneurons inhibiting motor neurons (Fig. 3.5). Like GABA, glycine acts by opening chloride channels. Strychnine blocks the glycine receptors, and this probably explains why strychnine poisoning produces muscle spasms. Likewise, violent muscle spasms are provoked by the tetanus toxin, which inhibits synaptic release of glycine.

Neuroactive Peptides

More than 30 neuroactive peptides have so far been identified in the central nervous system, but many of them were first found in the peripheral nervous system and in the gut. Although there is firm evidence of a transmitter function for only a few neuropeptides, many of them have marked effects on physiological processes and behavior if administered locally in the central nervous system. Several of the neuropeptides elicit slow inhibitory or excitatory synaptic potentials when they are administered in minute amounts close to neurons, which would suggest a transmitter role. It is not clear, however, whether some of the neuropeptides function more like local hormones than like specific neurotransmitters.

It is a characteristic feature that *neuropeptides as a rule are colocalized in nerve terminals with small-molecular (classical) transmitters.* Two or more peptides may also coexist. Thus, one neuron may be expected to release several neuroactive substances simultaneously, some with fast synaptic actions, others with long-lasting effects. The released substances may also elicit intracellular responses related to growth and development. There is some evidence to suggest that the frequency of action potentials determines whether peptides are released.

One example of coexistence of a "classical" transmitter and a neuropeptide follows: Terminals of nerve fibers innervating salivary glands contain both acetylcholine and the neuropeptide vasoactive intestinal polypeptide (VIP). Both substances are released when the nerves are stimulated, but they act on different target cells: Acetylcholine elicits secretion from glandular cells, whereas VIP produces vasodilatation by relaxing smooth-muscle cells, thereby increasing blood flow to the organ at the same time as its secretion is increased.

Synthesis of Neurotransmitters

The *small-molecular neurotransmitters* are synthesized in the nerve terminals, the synthesis being catalyzed by enzymes transported axonally from the perikaryon. As a rule, the rate of transmitter synthesis is determined by the enzymatic activity. Thus, up- or down-regulation of the enzymatic activity represents one way of changing the properties of nerve cells—for example, with regard to learning. Activation of enzymes often requires that they be phosphorylated, and this may be a result of external stimuli that, via membrane receptors, induce increased intracellular concentration of second messengers (such as Ca^{2+} or cAMP).

Since the organelles necessary for protein synthesis are present only in the perikaryon, the *neuropeptides* have to be synthesized in the perikaryon and subsequently transported to the terminals. Accordingly, substances that block axonal transport, such as colchicine, lead to accumulation of neuropeptides in the perikaryon. Usually, the neuropeptides are produced as larger polypeptides (prepropeptides) that most likely are split into smaller units on their way to the terminals.

Transmitters Are Contained in Vesicles and Released in Quanta

We have previously described synaptic vesicles, aggregated near the presynaptic membrane of boutons (Fig. 1.23). Although the question is not finally settled, we assume that all transmitters, once they are ready for release, are localized in synaptic vesicles. The release then takes place by *exocytosis.* The vesicle moves toward the presynaptic membrane and the vesicle membrane fuses with the presynaptic membrane. This also opens the vesicle and the content of transmitter molecules enters the synaptic cleft. For some synapses, in particular those between motor nerve terminals and striated muscle cells (neuromuscular junction), there is convincing evidence that the transmitter (acetylcholine) is released in packets, or *quanta,* corresponding to the transmitter content of one vesicle. Calculations from experiments with such synapses indicate that one vesicle contains on the average 10,000 acetylcholine molecules. Release of one quantum elicits a so-called *miniature EPSP.* If stimulation is increased, so that more transmitter is released, the depolarization increases in steps correspondong to one miniature EPSP. The motor axon innervating a muscle cell ramifies into many terminal boutons. An action potential in the motor axon therefore invades all the boutons and leads to release of many quanta. Therefore, the subsequent EPSP becomes large enough to reach threshold for an action potential in the muscle cell. *Each bouton probably releases only one or a few quanta for each presynaptic action potential.* Conditions are probably similar in the central nervous system: Each action potential invading a bouton releases the transmitter content of none to a few vesicles. It should be noted that an action potential does not necessarily elicit transmitter release; it merely *increases the probablity of release.*

Transmitter Release Is Ca²⁺-dependent

Depolarization of the presynaptic membrane (by the action potential) is the normal event preceding transmitter release. The transmitter release is, however, dependent on Ca^{2+} entering the bouton (Fig. 1.23). Voltage-gated calcium channels are opened by depolarization. How increased intracellular calcium concentration is coupled to the movement of vesicles and the subsequent release of transmitter is not fully understood.

Axoaxonic synapses may regulate the opening of Ca^{2+} channels in the presynaptic membrane. This makes it possible for other neurons to influence the amount of transmitter released (see p. 32).

How the Action of Neurotransmitters Is Stopped

Synaptic signal transfer is characterized by a precisely timed start and stop, and this is fundamental to many of the functions of the nervous system. We have looked into the mechanisms responsible for precise timing of transmitter release. It is also necessary, however, that the transmitter, once released, be quickly removed from the synaptic cleft. Several different mechanisms are of importance for this task.

For many transmitters the most important factor seems to be simple diffusion out of the synaptic cleft. Experimentally, this has been shown to happen very quickly. In addition, *specific uptake mechanisms* actively transport the transmitter back into the bouton and into glial cells (Fig. 1.23). Examples of transmitters with specific uptake mechanisms are glutamate, GABA, and the monoamines. In such cases, the presynaptic membrane and glial membrane contain spe-

cific receptors and carriers ("pumps") to bind and transport the transmitter molecules. After entering the bouton, the transmitter may be used again, or enzymatically degraded. The latter is the case, for example, for norepinephrine, which is broken down by the enzyme monoamine oxidase.

The effect of acetylcholine can also be terminated in another manner—namely, by a specific enzyme present in the synaptic cleft that breaks down the transmitter. This enzyme is called *acetylcholine esterase (AchE)*. *Neuropeptides* in general also appear to be subject to this kind of removal by specific *peptidases*.

Transmitter Systems

Some neuronal groups are special because they consist of a relatively small number of cells that send axons to large parts of the central nervous system. This happens because the axons ramify extensively. Furthermore, it is characteristic that in most of these groups the neurons contain one of the monoamines. Four monoamines—*norepinephrine, serotonin, dopamine, and histamine*—and, in addition, *acetylcholine* appear to be the main transmitters in cell groups with such widely branching axons.

These groups, each containing one of the mentioned transmitters, form more or less distinct entities. For example, neurons containing dopamine form nuclei that are clearly separate from nuclei containing neurons with norepinephrine. Some of these cell groups are treated more specifically in Chapters 12, 16, and 17. Here we will limit ourselves to brief descriptions.

Norepinephrine is first and formost localized to neurons forming distributed cell groups in the so-called reticular formation of the brain stem. Many of the neurons form a distinct group in the pons, the *nucleus locus coeruleus* (Fig. 12.6).

Dopamine is mostly confined to a large nucleus in the mesencephalon, the *substantia nigra*, and some smaller cell groups in its vicinity (Figs. 10.8 and 10.9).

Serotonin is mostly found in neurons forming a series of nuclei close to the midline in the brain stem, the *raphe nuclei* (nuclei raphe) (Fig. 12.5).

Acetylcholine is particularly prominent in somewhat diffusely organized cell groups in the brain stem and in basal parts of the forebrain, the latter forming the *basal nucleus (of Meynert)* (nucleus basalis Meynert) (Fig. 16.8).

Histamine is mainly found in a small cell group in the hypothalamus, the *tuberomammillary nucleus* (nucleus tuberomammillaris).

Such transmitter-specific cell groups with their widespread axonal ramifications would seem likely to play special functional roles, different from most other neuronal groups with more limited and specific axonal connections. They are, for example, hardly fit to provide precise information about time and space. It seems more likely that they make possible a homogeneous influence on many different parts of the nervous system by exerting general excitatory or inhibitory effects. This probably serves to modulate the excitability of the target neurons, and thus their responsiveness to other inputs carrying specific information. Such assumptions are consistent with the fact that, for example, norepinephrine and acetylcholine both appear to have mostly slow (modulatory) synaptic effects in the central nervous system. Rather diffuse, modulatory synaptic effects are probably of importance in relation to the level of consciousness, different stages of sleep, attention, motivation, and mood. Monoamine-containing neuronal groups also appear to influence general changes in the excitability of motor neurons and neurons that carry sensory information.

Nevertheless, it is an oversimplification to regard each transmitter-specific group as a functional entity and to use terms such as "the serotonin system," "the dopamine system," and so on. First, within each group there are subgroups differing in where they send their axons. Second, the axonal ramifications from each group are not as diffuse as they appeared to be from earlier studies. Thus, in the cerebral cortex, fibers containing serotonin, dopamine, or norepinephrine are largely differentially distributed. Third, not all neurons in the apparently transmitter-specific cell groups contain the same transmitter, and furthermore, in addition to a monoamine transmitter, most neurons also contain one or more neuropeptides. The effects obtained by stimulation of one of these cell groups therefore cannot be ascribed to one transmitter only. Finally, it should also be recalled that the effects of one transmitter depend on the receptor type present postsynaptically and that there is more than one receptor type for each transmitter.

Drugs Acting on the Nervous System

Most drugs acting on the nervous system do so by influencing *synaptic transmission*. They may affect synthesis, release, or degradation of transmitters, or the transmitter receptors. There are drugs that have one or more of these actions with regard to one or several transmitters.

Most transmitters are present in many parts of the nervous system, differing both physiologically and anatomically. It therefore should not be surprising that even drugs apparently influencing the actions of only one transmitter nevertheless have multifarious effects.

We have already mentioned drugs with generalized sedative effects (barbiturates, benzodiazepines, and others) that appear to act primarily on GABA receptors. Some of these drugs are particularly effective in reducing anxiety (anxiolytic drugs) but in addition have hypnotic effects. Others have primarily hypnotic effects. Such differences probably reflect relatively specific binding of the drugs to different cell groups that differ with regard to their subtype of GABA receptors.

Drugs that are effective in treating serious mental illness (psychoses) appear to be characterized generally by prominent effects on dopamine receptors, acting by reducing the postsynaptic sensitivity to the transmitter. Dopamine, however, is present in nuclei and tracts involved in a variety of functions—for example, in motor control and in cognitive processes and emotions. Motor disturbances therefore are commonly seen as a side effect in patients treated with antipsychotic drugs (neuroleptics). Correspondingly, mental disturbances may occur as a side effect in patients with Parkinson's disease treated with dopamine precursors to alleviate their motor symptoms.

Drugs that have proved effective in treating serious depressive disorders appear to act largely by inhibiting the reuptake or degradation of monoamine transmitters (particularly norepinephrine and serotonin). Such drugs often alleviate depression but in addition can cause several unwanted side effects (for example, by also acting on cholinergic neurotransmission).

COUPLING OF NEURONS: PATHWAYS FOR IMPULSES

In addition to the properties of synapses, which determine the transfer of signals among neurons, the function of the nervous system depends on how the various neuronal groups (nuclei) are interconnected (often called the *wiring pattern* of the brain). This determines the pathways that signals may take and the possibilities for cooperation among neuronal groups. Thus, although each neuron is to some extent a functional unit, it is only by proper cooperation that neurons can fulfill their tasks. We will describe here some typical examples of how neurons are interconnected, since such general knowledge is important for understanding the specific examples of connections to be dealt with in later chapters.

Divergence and Convergence Are Fundamental Principles in the Organization of the Nervous System

The simplest example of an impulse pathway is that of the axon of one neuron contacting another neuron that does not receive any other connections (Fig. 1.26A). Such simple arrangements do not exist in the central nervous system, however. Here the connections are frequently arranged so that sig-

nals from one neuron are distributed to many other (because the axon sends off collaterals; Fig. 1.26B). In the scheme in Figure 1.26B, it can be seen that all of the neurons that are synaptically contacted by the first one themselves contact several others (in reality, many more than shown here). The end result is that the signal coming from one neuron is transmitted to many others (again, in reality, signals from one group of neurons are transmitted to many other groups). This is an example of the *divergence of connections* that is very common in the nervous system. Thus, information of a particular kind is distributed to many, often functionally diverse, neuronal groups.

Another principle, *convergence of connections*, is shown schematically in Figure 1.26C. In this case, one neuron (*m*) is synaptically contacted by many other nerve cells (*s*, *p*, and *v*). The sum of excitatory and inhibitory synaptic effects at any given moment determines the activity of the neuron *m*. This neuron is said to represent the *final*

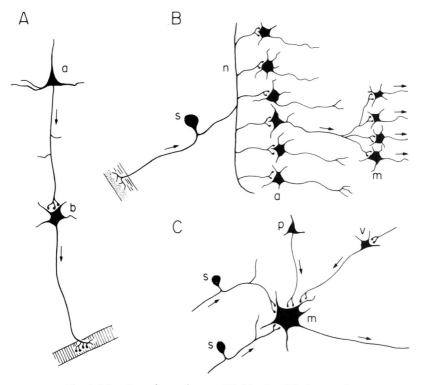

Fig. 1.26. *Impulse pathways.* Highly simplified examples.

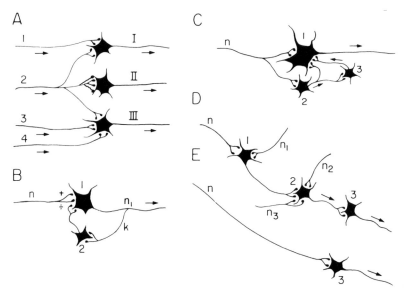

Fig. 1.27. *Impulse pathways.* Highly simplified examples.

common path for the neurons contacting it, since it *integrates* the information from various sources into a unified response. Examples of such a final common path are the motor neurons in the cord, which send their axons to skeletal muscle cells. The frequency at which action potentials are sent to the muscle cell is determined by the sum of all synaptic inputs to the motor neuron.

The signals may not necessarily pass all the way along pathways consisting of several neurons coupled serially (as in Figs. 1.26B and 1.27D). As discussed earlier in this chapter, *summation* of synaptic effects is as a rule necessary for an action potential to be elicited in the postsynaptic neuron. One example is shown in Figure 1.27A. We imagine that an excitatory signal comes from axon 2. This axon has many boutons that contact the neuron *II,* and together they make the neuron fire an action potential. Axon 2 makes only a few synaptic contacts with neurons *I* and *III* and is on its own unable to make them fire action potentials. If, however, neurons *I* and *III* at the same time receive synaptic inputs from axons *1, 3,* and *4,* summation may be sufficient to fire the neurons. In this way we may explain why only a few of the many neurons in a nucleus fire action potentials when receiving im-

pulses from an afferent axonal tract. Neurons not eliciting action potentials may nevertheless be depolarized almost to threshold for action potentials and may fire if they receive an additional excitatory input. In such instances, a weak additional excitatory input may elicit a disproportionally large increase in the number of neurons firing.

Many Neurons Are Continuously Active

In the examples mentioned above, the neurons stop firing as soon as excitatory synaptic inputs from other neurons end. In other instances, however, activity in the form of action potentials goes on long after activity has ended in afferent pathways to a nucleus. In fact, most parts of the central nervous system are virtually never totally "silent"—there is always some impulse traffic. In the cerebral cortex, for example, even during sleep there is considerable neuronal activity. *Such neuronal behavior may be partly explained by the membrane properties of many neurons but also by the presence of numerous interneurons.* An example is shown in Figure 1.27C. The axon *n* excites neuron *1,* which in response fires an action potential. At the same time, the interneuron

2 is also excited and fires an action potential, which in turn excites both neurons 1 and 3. Because of the synaptic delay of a few milliseconds and the time required for impulse conduction in the axons of the interneuron, cell 1 receives excitation in three succeeding waves and may itself fire several action potentials in response. With this kind of arrangement (which in reality would be much more elaborate and complicated than in this example), one impulse (or a brief train of impulses) may set up prolonged impulse activity in a group of neurons.

We mentioned above that the *membrane properties* of neurons may contribute to the activity of neurons in the absence of excitatory synaptic inputs. Such neurons are said to discharge spontaneously and to have autorhythmicity or *pacemaker* properties. The frequency and pattern of their firing is nevertheless regulated up or down by afferent synaptic inputs.

Inhibitory Neurons Serve as "Brakes"

In the examples given above, the interneurons were excitatory. Many interneurons, however, are inhibitory. An example is shown in Figure 1.27B. In this case, firing of neuron 1 leads to subsequent inhibition of itself, by way of the inhibitory interneuron 2. This is called *recurrent inhibition*. In this manner the frequency of action potentials in neuron 1 is prevented from becoming too high. Recurrent inhibition may also ensure that the neuron fires only a few action potentials with high frequency, with a subsequent pause. The typical pattern of activity for this particular neuron is repeated, brief bursts of action potentials. Interneuron 2 is, however, subject to other synaptic influences (although not shown in Fig. 1.27B) that may excite or inhibit it. In this way the recurrent inhibition may be increased or decreased by other neuronal groups; the "brake" may be switched on and off. Recurrent inhibition is found in many places in the nervous system, such as the spinal cord, where it regulates the motor neurons governing the contraction of skeletal muscle.

Signaling by Disinhibition

Inhibition may not only reduce neuronal activity but under certain circumstances may also lead to increased activity. This happens when inhibitory neurons inhibit other inhibitory neurons, which in their turn inhibit excitatory neurons. The result of increased activity of the first inhibitory neuron is reduced inhibitory input to the excitatory neuron, and thus an increased excitatory output from the latter. This phenomenon is called *disinhibition*. If, for example, an inhibitory interneuron has some axonal terminals on an inhibitory neuron and other terminals on an excitatory neuron, it may at the same time excite some neurons and inhibit others. This may be used to switch impulse traffic in the direction required by the situation. Such a mechanism may be of importance, for example, when the central nervous system has to select different combinations of muscles to perform various movements.

Interneurons Provide Flexibility of Responses

Figure 1.27D exemplifies another way in which neurons may be interconnected. An action potential in axon *n* activates neuron 1, which in its turn activates neuron 2, and so on. One might perhaps imagine that the same information could have been transferred more economically by the simple connection shown in Figure 1.27E. The intercalated neurons in Figure 1.27D give a delay in impulse propagation, which in itself is a disadvantage. The main point, however, is that the interrupted pathway provides greater flexibility of response from neuron 3 in response to an input in axon *n*. Neuron 3 is not governed dictatorially by axon *n*, in contrast to the situation in Figure 1.27E, because interneurons 1 and 2 are under the influence of other neurons. Thus the impulse traffic from *n* to neuron 3 may be facilitated or inhibited. Usually, the axons contacting the interneurons (n_1 and n_2) come from nuclei in parts of the central nervous system

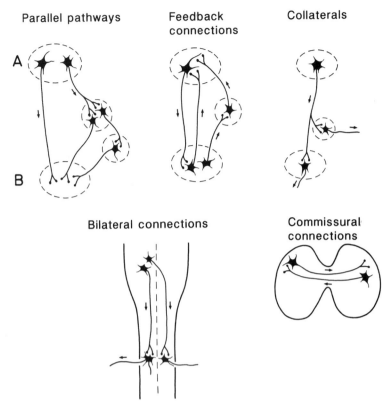

Fig. 1.28. *Examples of simple neuronal coupling diagrams.*

other than axon *n*. Thus, impulses from very different parts of the nervous system may influence the impulse transmission from *n* to neuron *3*. Identical sensory stimuli, for example, may thus elicit quite different responses, depending on the situation in many, often distant, parts of the nervous system. Such response flexibility is typical of the brains of higher animals, which are characterized by their large number of interneurons.

Nuclei in the Central Nervous System Are Interconnected

Many of the examples given above concern local wiring patterns—that is, within groups of neurons. Figure 1.28 gives examples of interconnections among nuclei that are at some distance. At the upper left is shown two *parallel pathways* between the two nuclei *A* and *B*. One pathway is direct, the other synaptically interrupted (there are

often several pathways of the latter kind). Parallel pathways are common in the central nervous system—for example, for transmission of sensory information. Although their functional significance is not always clear, parallel pathways may be of practical importance after partial brain injury. If, for example, the direct pathway between *A* and *B* is interrupted, the indirect one may at least partly take over the tasks formerly performed by the direct one.

Feedback connections between two nuclei represent another common arrangement. When one nucleus sends axons to another, the latter as a rule sends some axons back. In this manner the first nucleus is informed of the outcome of the impulses emitted to the second one. If the influence was too strong, the message back may serve to reduce activity, and vice versa if the influence was too weak. The significance of such feedback connections lies in their ability to *stabilize the functioning of the nervous system*. Thus, many of the symptoms appearing in neurological diseases are due to the failure of stabilizing feedback mechanisms.

Another important general feature is that most nuclei have connections with both sides of the brain: the so-called *bilateral connections* (Fig. 1.28). Some tracts supply both sides with approximately the same number of axons (that is, equal numbers of crossed and uncrossed axons), whereas other tracts are predominantly crossed (contralateral), with only a few axons supplying the same (ipsilateral) side. That there must be extensive cooperation between the two sides of the central nervous system is made even more evident by the vast number of *commissural connections*—that is, direct connections between corresponding parts in the two halves (Fig. 1.28). Such connections occur at all levels of the central nervous system. The most prominent one connects the two halves of the cerebral hemispheres (corpus callosum, Figs. 2.27 and 2.28) and contains probably around 180 million axons in man.

Cell Populations, Not Individual Cells, Determine What the Nervous System Can Do

For simplicity, we have considered so far mainly connections between individual nerve cells. This can be justified because the general principles are the same whether the connections are between two or several thousand neurons. It is nevertheless important to realize that the tasks performed by the nervous system do not depend on the function of single cells but on the collective activity of *populations of neurons*. It is not necessary that *all* neurons within such a population or group behave correctly; rather, it is a question of a sufficiently high probability for the neurons to send the right signal. If there are many neurons sharing the job, the chance is good that a sufficient number of them at any time will behave correctly. Many of the tasks of the nervous system can still be performed even if the responsible neuronal populations are numerically reduced.

Only when the demand on performance is very high may it become apparent that something is wrong. If, however, the number undergoes further reduction, a point may be reached at which obvious functional deficits occur rather abruptly, even though the disease process may have been progressing slowly for years.

SOME ASPECTS OF NEURAL DEVELOPMENT

The fully developed nervous system consists of incredibly complex networks of connections. There are many billions of neurons in the human brain, and each neuron is connected probably on the average with several thousand others. The number of possible combinations of synaptic contacts is therefore astronomic. Indeed, a section of nervous tissue stained to reveal all neuronal processes may appear as a chaotic jungle. Nevertheless, we have ample evidence that this is very far from the case: Strict order exists everywhere, and the mutual connections between neuronal groups are far from random. Improved methods have made it increasingly clear that precise order prevails even in parts of the nervous system formerly believed to possess only a crude localization. Individual nuclei, formerly regarded as structural and functional units, have also been shown to consist of subdivisions differing with regard to connections and other characteristics. Even for the individual neuron, afferent axons from different sources may terminate on different parts of the dendritic tree.

How do these complicated and highly organized networks arise during development of the individual? We know that, with regard to the main patterns of connections, most are laid down already prenatally. With few exceptions, no new neurons are formed after birth, but the outgrowth of processes and establishment of synaptic contacts go on for a long time. What are the factors guiding the migration of neurons in early embryonic life, and, in particular, what guides the outgrowing axons so that they find their correct target neurons, often at a considerable distance? How do the axons "know" with which neurons, among the many they encounter during growth, they are to establish synaptic contact? These questions are all related to how the *specificity* of neural connections is established. Each neuron and group of neurons is also specific with regard to morphology, content of neurotransmitters, and the expression of ion channels and receptors in their membrane.

Although we still lack final answers to these questions, considerable progress has been made during recent years in the field of developmental neurobiology. With increasing use of methods from molecular biology, we will be able to identify more and more of the cellular markers and signal substances governing neural development. Identification of genes for the regulation of cell multiplication, growth, and differentiation (oncogenes) has opened new possibilities also for the understanding of neural development.

The Structure of the Nervous System Is Genetically Determined But Also Plastic

How neurons are collected into nuclei and how the nuclei are interconnected are largely genetically determined; our genome contains the "recipe" for the structure of the nervous system in considerable detail. Thus, to a large extent, each individual neuron contains the information that determines its final size, the shape of its dendritic tree, its axonal ramifications, the types of neurotransmitters, and so on. This can be verified when neurons grow in cell culture. Nevertheless, the full range of features characteristic of a particular neuronal type is usually not expressed in culture. The normal development of a neuron is also dependent on *epigenetic factors*—that is, influence from other neurons in its vicinity. In addition, *proper use of the neurons and their interconnections* also plays an important role. The nervous system is *plastic*; that is, it may

modify its structure and performance in response to altered external requirements. The fact that we are able to learn and memorize tells us that, in some way or another, the nervous system is modifiable. In light of the crucial role of synaptic transmission for all information processing in the brain, it seems a priori very likely that modifications take place at the synpatic level. Much experimental evidence supports this assumption, and there is also evidence that modifications of performance are accompanied by structural changes. Such plasticity is of crucial importance for the recovery of function that usually occurs after damage to the nervous system.

In the following, we will look at certain salient features of the development of the nervous system as well as some of the evidence for neuronal plasticity.

The Earliest Stages: Induction and Cell Proliferation

In early embryonic life, the nervous system develops as a tube, formed by infolding of the ectoderm at the dorsal side of the embryo (Fig. 2.3). This early *induction* of the ectodermal cells to start on a new line of development depends on diffusible substances from the underlying tissue. Then a prolonged period of cell division among the primitive neuroblasts follows. This is the phase of *cell proliferation*. Cell divisions take place while the cells remain in a position close to the canal inside the neural tube. The number of divisions each cell undergoes is genetically determined.

Second Stage: Migration and Differentiation

To reach their final position in the nervous system, the primitive neurons start to *migrate* away from their position close to the inside of the neural tube. After reaching their final location, the neurons start to aggregate into groups, representing the future nuclei. For most neurons the *differentiation* starts with the outgrowth of processes after the migration is finished. By differentiation, we mean development of structural and functional features that makes neurons different from each other. Very early in differentiation the dendritic tree starts to develop. Fully grown, this is often highly characteristic. At the same time as the neuronal processes develop, the neuronal membranes undergo changes, and the neurotransmitter and other specific synaptic properties of the neurons begin to be expressed.

Growth of Axons and Establishment of Specific Connections

The next step in the development of the nervous system is the outgrowth of axons and *establishment of specific synaptic connections*. During this phase the axons must find their way and recognize the neurons with which they are going to establish synaptic contact. While growing, the axons encounter many neurons without establishing synaptic contacts. After arriving in the target region, only some of the many neurons receive synaptic contacts from the ingrowing axon. Several factors play a role in these processes. Trial and error seems to be of only limited importance, since there are many examples of the growth being goal-directed, with few or no aberrations. To some extent, axons grow along glial processes laid down in advance. This represents a kind of *mechanical guidance*. Moreover, axons have a tendency to grow along other axons, so that if a few "pioneer" axons have arrived safely, others may simply follow their course. But these factors cannot explain how axons, if necessary, may circumvent an experimentally placed obstacle and still reach the correct target. In some instances neurons that have been transposed to another location before outgrowth of axons nevertheless obtain synaptic contact with the correct target. In such cases, the axons must be able to grow in the right direction through strange territory. This could be most easily explained if there are gradients of specific chemical sub-

stances in the tissue, and the axons always grow in the direction of increasing concentrations of such substances. There is also evidence to suggest the existence of chemical markers along the trajectory of the axonal growth.

With regard to how the axons recognize the appropriate target neurons among many others, some kind of *chemoaffinity* between axonal terminals and target neurons is most likely present. The chemoaffinity may be caused by specific surface markers or receptors expressed only by certain subsets of neurons. Various candidate molecules have been identified by immunocytochemical techniques. Typically, such molecules are expressed only during certain phases of development—for example, during synapse formation—and then disappear. *Cell adhesion molecules* (CAMs) make cells "sticky," and if they are present on the surface of certain neurons and not on others at a certain time, they may contribute to the establishment of selective contacts.

Selective Cell Death and Trophic Factors

Many more neurons are formed in embryonic life than the number present in the mature nervous system. In fact, many neurons are eliminated at the time their axons are establishing synaptic contacts. This is called the *phase of selective cell death* and has been observed in many parts of the nervous system. It appears to be common that about half of the neurons in a nucleus are eliminated during this phase. For example, this is the case with the motor neurons in the spinal cord. The elimination is very rapid, apparently finished within days in some systems.

The elimination of neurons is probably related to the size of the target group of neurons; if this is experimentally expanded, more of the neurons in a nucleus supplying it with axons survive. On the other hand, by reducing the number of neurons in the target nucleus, the elimination is increased.

The most likely explanation is that the neurons need some kind of trophic substance to survive. This substance is provided by the neurons in the target nucleus. But the amount of trophic substance is probably limited and only sufficient to keep a proportion of the neurons sending axons to the target nucleus alive. Thus, neurons innervating a certain target neuronal group (or other target organ, such as muscle) have to *compete* for the trophic substance.

It has long been known that a *nerve growth factor* (NGF) is present in the peripheral nervous system. NGF stimulates outgrowth of axons from autonomic ganglion cells and sensory neurons. It is a protein and is present and produced in target organs of the neuronal types mentioned. By the use of specific antibodies against NGF, axonal outgrowth can be inhibited. It can also be demonstrated in cell cultures that axons grow toward and into regions containing NGF, whereas axons retract from regions devoid of NGF.

For some neuronal types in the brain, a protein called *brain-derived neurotrophic factor* (BDNF) may play a role corresponding to that of NGF in the peripheral nervous system. Presumably, more neurotrophic factors will be discovered in the future.

Synapse Elimination and Withdrawal of Axon Collaterals

Elimination of axon collaterals takes place in some systems at a later stage than the selective cell death. This phenomenon, which may be compared with pruning a tree so that only the most viable branches remain, has been most studied with regard to the innervation of skeletal muscles. In early development, each muscle cell receives synaptic contacts from several motor neurons—so-called *polyneural innervation*. Gradually, however, synapses are eliminated so that in the end there remain on each muscle cell only synapses belonging to a single motor neuron. The factors governing this elimination are not fully understood, but it occurs only if the motor neurons start to send impulses

to the muscles. For the central nervous system, too, there is evidence that normal activity is necessary for elimination of the apparent surplus of axon collaterals. The elimination is, perhaps, a way of increasing the precision of neural interconnections.

Synapse Formation Depends on Function

We have mentioned that neuronal *activity* is necessary for proper development of the axonal ramifications and for synapse formation. During this process, certain connections survive and possibly expand, whereas others are eliminated. There is, however, evidence that in the central nervous system impulse activity in itself is not enough for proper development. The pattern of impulses has to be natural, which probably means that it must contain *meaningful information* to be of consequence for synapse formation.

Examples of Relationship between Activity and Development of Normal Neuronal Connections

As an example, we may choose data from studies of the pathways from the retina to the visual cortex. Under normal conditions these connections are organized so that neuronal groups influenced primarily from one or the other eye are kept separate in the cortex. The ensuing bands of neurons with different properties in this respect are termed *ocular dominance columns*.

By blocking all impulse activity in the visual pathways by application of tetrodotoxin to the retina of kittens, the ocular dominance columns do not develop. They may, however, be established also in this situation if the nerves leading impulses from the eye to the visual cortex are stimulated electrically. Electrical stimulation is effective, however, only if the signals arrive with a small time difference from the two eyes, which is how signals arrive under normal conditions.

Another example concerns development of connections from the eye to visual centers in the goldfish. If the fish is exposed only to diffuse light (devoid of any informative value) during the phase in which axons from the retina establish synaptic contacts, the topopgraphical pattern of connections becomes abnormal. Thus, normal

Striate area   Parietal association cortex

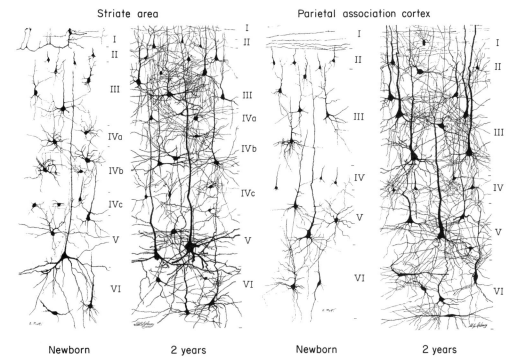

Newborn   2 years   Newborn   2 years

Fig. 1.29.   *Development of the human cerebral cortex postnatally.* Drawings based on Golgi sections from the visual cortex showing the increase in dendritic arborizations from birth and until the age of 2 years. The increase in dendritic arborization is most likely related to increase in number of synapses per neuron. From Conel (1939).

patterned activity is necessary also to produce an orderly map of the visual field in the brain of the goldfish.

It should be emphasized that when we say normal activity is necessary for the formation of proper neuronal connections, this does not as a rule concern development of the major tracts of the nervous system but rather the final adjustment of synapse distribution, and of the number and effectiveness of the synapses. Proper activity appears to be particularly important for the connections established by interneurons. These "details" are of course of crucial importance for the functioning of the neuronal groups and the nervous system as a whole.

Even though many synapses are eliminated at an early stage, there is a dramatic increase in the number of synapses postnatally. This increase is particularly prominent in the human cerebral cortex. Figure 1.29 shows the increase in dendritic arborizations

in the visual cortex from birth to 2 years of age. We take for granted here that the increase in dendritic arborizations—that is, increased dendritic surface—is closely linked to an increased number of synapses. There is in fact good evidence that this is true. Thus, Figure 1.30 shows the increase in number of synapses in the visual cortex of cats from the time of birth until the adult number is achieved. The most marked increase takes place at the time the kitten opens its eyes about 8 days postnatally.

Further experiments have strengthened the assumption that the increase in synapse number is, in part, dependent on proper use of the visual system. As an example: One group of rats was kept in the dark for 1 month after birth. Then half the group was transferred to an environment with normal light, while the other half remained in the dark. One month later the animals were killed and their brains examined under the microscope. Results showed that there were

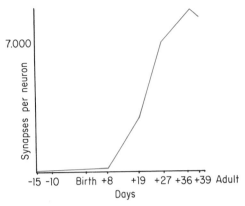

Fig. 1.30. *Increase in number of synapses postnatally.* Synapses per neuron increase dramatically shortly after birth in the cat. Note that the steep rise in synapse number starts at the time the kittens open their eyes. Based on Cragg (1972).

about 30% more synapses in the visual cortex of the rats exposed to light than in those reared only in the dark. Other experiments, some of them in primates, indicate that later increased stimulation cannot fully compensate for the lack of proper early use of the visual system—that is, use of the system during the phase when the development normally is particularly rapid.

We have here examples of the *normal cooperation between genetic factors and environmental factors in the development of the nervous system.* A postnatal phase with genetically determined increased synapse formation probably must coincide with use of the system to ensure optimal development. Normally, these events coincide, as shown in the visual cortex of the cat, where there is a strong increase in synapse formation at the same time as the kitten opens its eyes (it should be noted that a large part of the increase seen in Fig. 1.30 occurs even in the absence of light, thus proving it genetically determined). We use the term *critical period of development* for this phenomenon. From observations of the development of normal infants, we know that new skills are learned at a certain age (with individual variations). If the skill is not achieved at that age, later learning cannot be expected to give equally good results. Probably in man as well, genet-ically determined synapse formation must coincide with use-dependent stimulation of the systems to obtain optimal functional results. In a wider context, all *learning,* whether in the child or in the adult, probably depends on changes in the number, distribution, and functioning of synapses.

Examples of Use-Dependent Synapse Formation

Other examples of how normal use influences the development of the nervous system include the following: Rats growing up in a "natural" environment with lots of space and "toys" have larger dendritic trees in the cerebral cortex than rats kept in small, standard laboratory cages. This may be taken to indicate that increased use of the brain is reflected both in its structure and in its performance. Comparison of rats performing various kinds of motor activities showed differences in the number of synapses per neuron in the cerebellar cortex (the cerebellum is of importance for the coordination of movements). Interestingly, an increased number of synapses was not correlated with high motor activity per se but with activities that implied learning of new motor skills. Stereotyped repetition of already-learned motor acts had no effect on the number of synapses.

Differences in brain size and weight between domesticated and wild members of the same animal species also indicate that environmental factors are of importance for the development of the brain. Thus, wild animals have larger brains than their tame relatives. The difference must arise early because animals born in the wild and later captured have the same brain weight as the wild ones. Nevertheless, there are no genetic differences, because the reduction in brain size occurs even in the first generation of individuals kept in captivity. It seems reasonable to suggest that such differences are related to differences in the amount of learning: Animals living in freedom in their proper habitat are subjected to much more varied challenges than those living in a cage.

RESTITUTION AFTER DAMAGE TO THE CENTRAL NERVOUS SYSTEM

It is well known that marked functional recovery can occur after damage to the central nervous system, even though we know that neurons that are lost cannot be replaced. Lately, we have become increasingly aware of the possibilities for functional recovery and the importance of stimulating the process. An increased therapeutic optimism has gained support from experimental studies in animals.

Early Phase of Rapid Recovery

After acute damage to neural tissue, secondary changes occur in the tissue surrounding the damaged area, such as disturbed local circulation and edema. This occurs, for example, after crushing of neural tissue and bleeding caused by head injuries, and after vascular occlusion caused by thrombosis or an embolus. Thus, neurons outside the damaged region may also become temporarily or permanently nonfunctional. If, for example, the edema subsides quickly and the circulation improves in the zone around the permanently damaged region, many neurons regain their normal activity. This is probably why there often is a marked improvement in the patient's condition during the first weeks after the accident. For example, an arm that was totally paralyzed the day after a stroke may in a few weeks be only slightly weaker and more clumsy than before the stroke.

Ischemic Cell Damage

The cell damage following an *ischemic episode*— that is, a period with reduced or abolished blood supply—probably is only indirectly caused by the lack of oxygen and glucose. The cell damage appears to be related to the fact that lack of oxygen causes a marked release of excitatory amino acid transmitters (particularly glutamate). This opens calcium channels, with subsequent massive influx of Ca^{2+} ions that in turn initiate uncontrollable intercellular reactions leading to cell death. One active line of research today is therefore to find ways of reducing neuronal excitability shortly after an ischemic episode—for example, with drugs blocking glutamate receptors. Animal experiments indicate that if this is achieved, the brain may tolerate much longer periods of circulatory arrest than the few minutes that

today are the upper limit before irreversible damage arises.

Protracted Phase with Slow Recovery

Further improvement in a patient's condition after brain damage may go on for months and even years, but at a reduced rate compared with the early rapid phase of recovery. This long-term process cannot be explained in the same manner as the rapid phase, and we still do not have a clear understanding of the mechanisms involved. It is very likely, however, that cell groups and pathways that before the damage took little part in a certain functional task gradually may take over and functionally replace the lost neurons. This cannot be expected to make up for the lost neurons and connections entirely, however, and indeed functional capacities are very seldom *completely* recovered after brain damage. If other parts of the nervous system take over, it seems likely that tasks may be solved in different ways than previously. This is also in agreement with common observations; for example, movements may be performed by using different sets of muscles and different strategies than before.

Another factor of potential relevance to recovery of function deserves to be mentioned. It has been shown experimentally that normal axons may send out new branches, so that neurons in the vicinity that have lost their afferents may be supplied with new ones. This phenomenon is called *collateral sprouting*. In experiments where the afferent axons to a neuronal group are cut (deafferentation), the axons degenerate and the boutons are removed by phagocytic activity of glial cells. In a relatively short time, however, these vacant synaptic sites may be filled with new boutons. This is probably caused by a trophic substance becoming available from the neurons that have lost their afferents. The trophic substance then stimulates nearby normal axons to send out sprouts. Collateral sprouting would mainly be of local importance in restoring neuronal activity. There is no evidence that it can restore connections between more distant cell groups.

There is no way collateral sprouting can restore the original pattern of innervation since the neurons responsible for that are gone. There would inevitably be a loss of specificity of connections compared with the normal situation. It is of interest that the restitution of function seen after brain damage is usually characterized by a loss of precision; for example, the force of movements may be well restored, whereas the ability to perform delicate movements never returns.

Collateral sprouting may not always be functionally beneficial. For example, after a stroke that damages the motor pathways descending from the cerebral cortex, the vacant synaptic sites on motor neurons in the cord may be filled by axon collaterals from sensory neurons. This would not help to improve the voluntary control of the muscles but might rather contribute to the hyperreactivity of the muscles to sensory stimuli that is characteristic in such cases (spasticity; see p. 220).

Restitution of Function Is a Learning Process

Regardless of whether the long-term restitution is caused by other neuronal groups taking over or by collateral sprouting (or as is probable, both), there is good reason to believe that basically the improvement is the result of a *learning process,* subjected to the same rules that underlie learning in an intact nervous system. All learning probably involves changes in the properties of existing synapses, formation of new ones, and removal of inappropriate ones. Such a process is bound to take time, especially in a brain that has been deprived of many neurons. Also, the importance of *motivation,* crucial in all learning, should not be overlooked when treating patients with brain damage. It is important, for example, that they feel that the training program is relevant to their daily life activities. Repetitions of apparently meaningless fragments of more complex motor or cognitive tasks may not be optimal in this respect. Recall the example given above of increases in the number of synapses in the cerebellum in animals continuously learning new tasks, while rote repetition had no such effect.

Restitution May Be More Complete in the Immature Than in the Mature Nervous System

The capacity for plastic changes is generally greater in the immature than in the mature nervous system. This is probably only partly due to the properties of the individual neurons, which may be more apt to send out new collaterals and remove others in the immature nervous system. Another factor may be of greater importance. Various parts of the young brain, particularly of the cerebral cortex, are not yet fully engaged in the tasks they are destined for. Therefore they may more easily be recruited for other purposes if necessary. For example, the right hemisphere may partly take over the processing of language if the left hemisphere (which normally does this) is damaged at an early age; that is, before the right hemisphere is fully engaged in other tasks. But if the damage to the left hemisphere comes after the right one has become fully occupied, there may be little the right hemisphere can do to help.

Even in the immature brain of an infant, connections that are already established are apparently not replaced if damaged. Thus, if the left motor cortex (sending fibers to the right spinal cord) is removed in monkeys shortly after birth, the remaining right motor cortex is not able to supply the denervated right half of the spinal cord with axons. Behaviorally, these monkeys never learn (with their right hand) the kinds of movements that depend on direct connections from the cerebral cortex to the cord. This is because these connections are already established at birth in monkeys. Reports of apparent reestablishment of long fiber tracts after early injury are probably based on experiments in which the injury was inflicted *before* the axons from the relevant cell groups had reached their targets. In such instances, the outgrowing axons may also innervate other cell groups than they normally do. This may be due to a lack of normal competition among outgrowing fiber tracts.

NOTES

1. In this case the process conducting toward the cell body should be termed a *dendrite,* in accordance with the usual definition. Both with regard to structure and function, however, this process must be regarded as an *axon.*

2. In addition to these three kinds, there are some other specialized forms of glial cells. The surface of the cavities inside the central nervous system (ventricles; see Chapter 2) is lined with a layer of cylindrical cells called *ependyma.* There are also special kinds of glial cells in the retina (Müller cells), the cerebellum (Bergman cells), and in posterior pituitary (pituicytes).

3. There are important immunological similarities between microglia in normal nervous tissue and the macrophage-like cells occurring after injury. Both types express, for example, receptors for the Fc part of the immunoglobulin molecule and other surface receptors, suggesting that both are of importance for antigen presentation and subsequent phagocytosis. It is also interesting that the morphology of certain cells of the immune system, such as Langerhans cells in the skin, resembles that of microglia. It is finally shown (in mice) that microglial cells express the CD4 antigen, which in humans binds HIV-1 (the virus responsible for AIDS).

4. Neither membrane potentials nor action potentials are properties unique to nerve cells. All cells have a membrane potential, although usually of less magnitude than that of neurons. Muscle cells and endocrine gland cells also produce action potentials in relation to contraction and secretion, respectively.

5. To express the membrane permeability of a particular kind of ion more precisely, we use the term *conductance.* The conductance is the inverse of the membrane resistance. In an electrical circuit the current is $I = V/R$, where V is the voltage and R is the resistance (Ohm's law). This may be rewritten by using conductance (g) instead of R, as $I = gV$. Thus, one may obtain quantitative measures of membrane permeability under various conditions. For our purpose, however, it is sufficient to use the less precise term *permeability.*

2

The Different Parts
of the Nervous System

The central nervous system is well protected against external forces, as it lies inside the skull and the vertebral canal. In addition to this bony protection, the central nervous system is wrapped in three membranes of connective tissue, with fluid-filled spaces between the membranes. It is in fact loosely suspended in a fluid-filled container. Since the specific weight of nervous tissue is only slightly higher than that of water, the brain and spinal cord almost float. This further serves to reduce the impact of external forces on the brain and spinal cord.

The central nervous system can be subdivided anatomically into different parts (Figs. 2.1 and 2.2). The *spinal cord* lies in the vertebral canal, whereas the *brain* is located in the cranial cavity. The brain is further subdivided into the *brain stem,* which constitutes the upward continuation of the spinal cord; the *cerebellum* ("little brain"); and the *cerebrum* or *cerebral hemispheres.* The cerebellum and cerebrum largely cover the brain stem and constitute the major part of the brain in higher mammals, and particularly in humans.

In this chapter we will give an overview of the main features of the anatomy of the central nervous system, with brief mention of the functional significance of the various parts. Structure and function of many of these parts will be treated in more depth in the later chapters dealing with functional systems. It will then be assumed, however, that the reader is familiar with the names and the locations of the major cell groups of the central nervous system. After some comments on the prenatal development of the central nervous system, we start with a description of the spinal cord, since conditions are simplest there.

Some Anatomic Terms Used in This Book

The term *medial,* toward the midline, and *lateral,* away from the midline, are used to describe the relative position of structures in relation to a midsagittal plane of the body. The terms *cranial* or *rostral,* toward the head or nose, and *caudal,* toward the tail, are used to describe the relative position of structures along a longitudinal axis of the body. Thus, for example, nucleus *A* in the brain stem may lie medial to and rostral to nucleus *B,* which in turn lies lateral to and caudal to *A.*

The terms *ventral* and *dorsal* are used to describe the relative position of structures in relation to the front (venter = belly) and the back (dorsum) of the body, respectively. *Anterior* (front) and *posterior* (rear) are most often used interchangeably with ventral and dorsal (except for the human forebrain, where anterior means to-

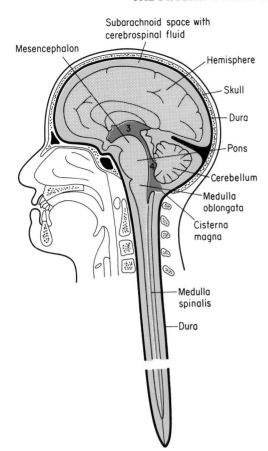

Subarachnoid space with
cerebrospinal fluid

Mesencephalon

Hemisphere

Skull

Dura

Pons

Cerebellum

Medulla
oblongata

Cisterna
magna

Medulla
spinalis

Dura

Fig. 2.1. *The central nervous system seen in a midsagittal section.*

ward the nose and ventral means toward the base of the skull).

PRENATAL DEVELOPMENT

The Central Nervous System Develops as a Long Tube

In the earliest stages of development, the embryo is like a somewhat elongated disk. The disk is covered on the upper or dorsal side and along the edges by primitive epithelium, the *ectoderm*. The first sign of development of the nervous system is the formation of a longitudinal infolding of the ectoderm (Fig. 2.3). This *neural groove* is subsequently closed, starting in the middle part, and thus forms the *neural tube*. The wall of the tube is formed by primitive neuroepithelial cells, which develop into neurons and glial cells. A

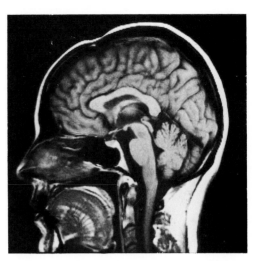

Fig. 2.2. *Magnetic resonance image* (MRI) at a level corresponding to the drawing in Figure 2.1. Most of the structures seen in Figure 2.1 can be identified in this picture. Courtesy of Dr. S. J. Bakke.

canal remains in the center. The inside of the wall of the neural tube, facing the canal, becomes covered by a special kind of glial cell, the *ependymal cells* (Fig. 1.15). The canal is

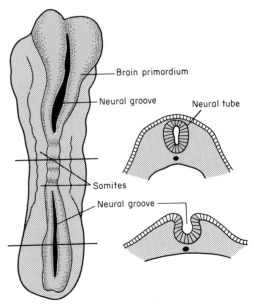

Brain primordium

Neural groove

Neural tube

Somites

Neural groove

Fig. 2.3. *Early stages in the development of the central nervous system.* Drawing of a 22-day-old human embryo, approximately 1 mm long. The central nervous system is indicated in red. Based on Hamilton, Boyd, and Mossman (1972).

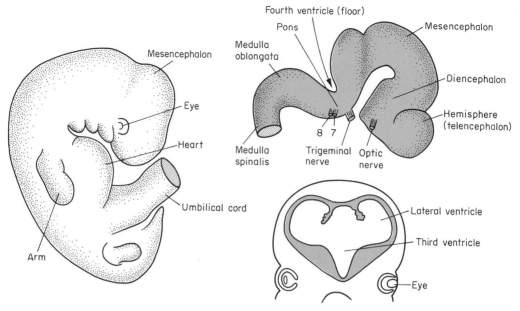

Fig. 2.4. *Development of the central nervous system.* To the **left,** a drawing of a 36-day-old human embryo, approximately 11 mm long. To the **right,** the neural tube at the same stage. Based on Hamilton, Boyd, and Mossman (1972).

filled with fluid, the *cerebrospinal fluid,* which is produced by vascular tufts, the *choroid plexus,* invaginated into the canal from its wall.

During further embryonic development, the cranial part of the neural tube develops much more than the rest and gives rise to the brain, whereas the caudal part, later developing into the spinal cord, remains straight. Various subdivisions of the cranial part grow at different rates, so that the neural tube forms several expansions (vesicles) and foldings (Fig. 2.4). The diameter of the central cavity (canal) also becomes highly variable in the various parts of the cranial end, forming four interconnected dilatations called *cerebral ventricles* (Figs. 2.1, 2.3, and 2.38). The ventricles, together with the narrow canals joining them and the canal extending throughout the spinal cord, form the *ventricular system.* The spinal cord remains straight, but the thickness of the wall increases so that, finally, there is only a narrow *central canal* that connects cranially with the ventricular system in the brain stem (Fig. 2.1). The ventricular system of the

brain and the cerebrospinal fluid are treated in more detail later in this chapter.

THE SPINAL CORD

In humans the spinal cord is a 40 to 45 cm-long cylinder of nervous tissue, of approximately the same thickness as a little finger. It extends from the lower end of the brain stem (at the level of the upper end of the first cervical vertebra) down the vertebral canal (Figs. 2.1 and 2.5) to the upper margin of the second lumbar vertebra (L_2). Here the cord has a wedge-shaped end called the *medullary conus* (or simply conus). In children the spinal cord extends more caudally, however, and reaches to the third lumbar vertebra in the newborn. This difference between the position of the lower end of the spinal cord in adults and infants is caused by the vertebral column growing more rapidly than the spinal cord. In early embryonic life, the neural tube and the primordium of the vertebral column are equally long.

The spinal cord is somewhat flattened in

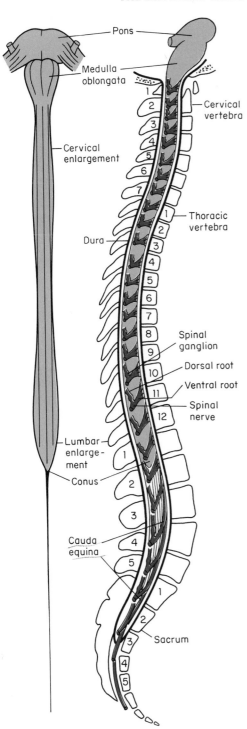

the anteroposterior direction and is not equally thick along its length. In general, the thickness decreases caudally, but there are two marked intumescences (Fig. 2.5), the *cervical and lumbar enlargements* (intumescentia cervicalis et lumbalis). The intumescences supply the extremities with sensory and motor nerves, hence the increased thickness.

In the midline along the anterior aspect of the cord, there is a longitudinal furrow or *fissure* (ventral median fissure, Fig. 2.6). Some of the vessels of the cord enter through this fissure and penetrate deeply into the substance of the cord. At the posterior aspect of the cord there is a corresponding, but more shallow, furrow in the midline (the posterior median sulcus). In addition, on each side there are shallow, longitudinal sulci anteriorly and posteriorly (the anterior and posterior lateral sulci). These laterally placed sulci mark where the spinal nerves connect with the cord.

The color of the spinal cord is whitish because the outer part consist of axons, many of which are myelinated. The consistency of the cord, as of the rest of the central nervous system, is soft and jellylike.

Spinal Nerves Connect the Spinal Cord with the Body

Axons mediating communication between the central nervous system and other parts of the body make up the *peripheral nerves*. The axons (nerve fibers) leave and enter the cord in small bundles called *rootlets* (Fig. 2.7). Several adjacent rootlets unite to a thicker strand, called a *root* or nerve root. In this manner, rows of roots are formed along the dorsal and ventral aspects of the cord—the *ventral (anterior) roots* and the *dorsal (posterior) roots*, respectively. Each dorsal

Fig. 2.5. *The spinal cord.* To the **left,** the cord from the ventral side. Note the cervical and lumbar enlargements. To the **right,** the cord and the vertebral column from the side, but the right halves of the vertebrae have been removed to ex-

pose the vertebral canal with its contents. Below the first–second lumbar vertebrae, the vertebral canal contains only nerve roots (the cauda equina). Note that the roots unite to form the spinal nerves.

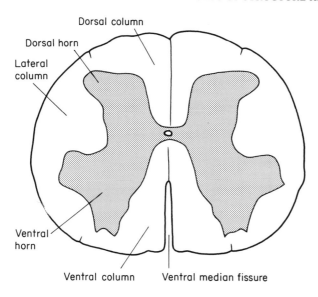

Fig. 2.6. *Cross section of the spinal cord at a lumbar level.* Note the central H-shaped region of gray matter and the subdivision of the surrounding white matter into funiculi.

root has a swelling, the *spinal ganglion,* which contains the cell bodies of the sensory axons entering the cord through the dorsal root (Figs. 2.5 and 2.7). A dorsal and a ventral root unite to form a *spinal nerve* (nervus spinalis). The spinal ganglion lies in the intervertebral foramen just where the dorsal and ventral roots unite (Fig. 2.8).

There is an important functional difference between the ventral and dorsal roots: *The ventral roots consist of efferent (motor) fibers, and the dorsal roots of afferent (sensory) fibers.*

In total, 31 spinal nerves are present on each side, forming symmetrical pairs (Fig. 2.5). They all leave the vertebral canal

through the intervertebral foramina on each side. As mentioned, the ventral and dorsal roots unite at the level of the intervertebral foramen to form the spinal nerves. The spinal nerves are numbered (as a general rule) in accordance with the number of verbebrae above the nerve. We therefore have 12 pairs of thoracic nerves, 5 pairs of lumbar nerves, and 5 pairs of sacral nerves. In humans, there is only one pair of coccygeal nerves. There are 7 cervical vertebrae but 8 pairs of cervical nerves, because the first cervical nerve leaves the vertebral canal above the first cervical vertebra (Fig. 2.5). Therefore, the numbering of the cervical nerves does not follow the general rule given above.

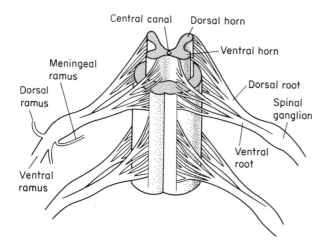

Fig. 2.7. *Two segments of the spinal cord* (seen from the ventral aspect). In the upper part, the white matter has been removed. The dorsal and ventral roots emerge from the posterior and anterior lateral sulci, respectively, and unite to form spinal nerves. Note the location of the spinal ganglion at the site where the roots unite.

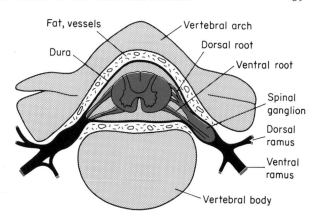

Fig. 2.8. *Cross section of the vertebral column* showing the positions of the spinal cord and the spinal nerves. Note the location of the spinal ganglion in the intervertebral foramen. The spinal cord is surrounded by the cerebrospinal fluid contained within the dura. Outside the dura, there is fat and a venous plexus, also serving as soft padding for the cord and the spinal nerves.

The spinal cord extends caudally only to the level of between the first and the second lumbar vertebrae. Whereas the upper spinal nerves pass approximately horizontally from the cord to the intervertebral foramen, the lower ones have to run obliquely downward in the vertebral canal to reach the corresponding intervertebral foramen, the distance between the site of exit from the cord and the site of exit from the canal increasing steadily (Fig. 2.5). *Below the conus, the vertebral canal contains only spinal nerve roots running longitudinally.* This collection of dorsal and ventral roots is called the *cauda equina* (the horsetail).

The Spinal Cord Is Divided into Segments

The part of the spinal cord giving origin to a pair of spinal nerves is called a *spinal segment*. There are, therefore, as many segments as there are spinal nerves. They are numbered accordingly, the first cervical segment originating to the first cervical nerves, and so on. There are no surface markings of the cord to indicate borders between the segments, but the rootlets nevertheless outline them rather precisely (Fig. 2.7).

The cervical enlargement (intumescence) corresponds to the fourth cervical (C_4) through the second thoracic (T_2) segments, the lumbar enlargement to the first lumbar (L_1) through the second sacral (S_2) segments.

The difference in rostrocaudal level between the spinal segments and the exit from the vertebral canal of the spinal nerves is of practical importance. Thus, identical symptoms may be provoked by a process close to the cord at one level and by one close to the intervertebral foramen at a considerably lower level (as should be clear from the above; however, this does not concern the nerves in the cervical region).

The Spinal Cord Consists of Gray and White Matter

When cut transversely, the fresh spinal cord can be seen to consist of an outer zone of white matter and a central, H-shaped region of gray matter (Fig. 2.6). The arms of the H, extending dorsally and ventrally, are called the *dorsal horn* (cornu posterius) and *ventral horn* (cornu anterius), respectively. The gray matter extends as a column through the length of the spinal cord (Fig. 2.6). The *central canal* is seen as a narrow opening in the center of the cord. The central canal ends blindly in the caudal end of the cord, whereas it continues rostrally into the ventricular system of the brain.

The *white matter* of the cord contains axons running longitudinally. Some of these axons convey signals from the cord to higher levels of the central nervous system, others from higher levels to the cord. Finally, a large proportion of the fibers serve the signal traffic, and hence cooperation, between the segments of the cord. Since the first two groups of axons become successively more numerous in the rostral direction, the proportion of white to gray matter increases from caudal to rostral.

The white matter is divided into *funiculi*, or *columns*, by drawing lines in the transverse plane from the sulci on the surface of the cord to the center (Fig. 2.6). Thus, in each half of the cord, the white matter is divided into a *ventral* or *anterior funiculus*, a *lateral funiculus*, and a *dorsal or posterior funiculus*. For the latter, the term *dorsal column* is used most frequently.

The Spinal Gray Matter Contains Three Main Types of Neurons

Among neurons in the gray matter of the spinal cord, there are both morphological and functional differences. *Three main types may be identified according to where they send their axons:* (1) neurons sending their axons *out of the central nervous system;* (2) neurons sending their axons *to higher levels of the central nervous system* (such as the brain stem); and (3) neurons sending their axons *to other parts of the spinal cord.* We will now consider in some detail each of these three groups.

Efferent Fibers from the Cord Control Muscles and Glands

The cell bodies of the first kind of neuron listed above are located in the ventral horn and at the transition between the dorsal and ventral horns. The *motor neurons* or *motoneurons* have large, multipolar perikarya and are in the ventral horn proper (Figs. 1.2, 2.9, 2.10, 2.12, and 8.2). The dendrites extend for a considerable distance in the gray matter. The axons leave the cord through the ventral root, follow the spinal nerves, and end in *skeletal muscles* (muscles that are controlled voluntarily). The motoneurons are further discussed in Chapter 8.

There is also another group of neurons that sends its axons out of the cord through the ventral root. These supply *smooth muscles* and *glands* with motor signals, and be-

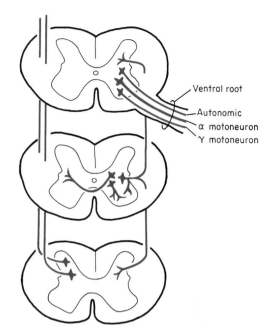

Fig. 2.9. *Three main types of neurons in the spinal cord.* Schematic drawing shows neuronal types classified in accordance with where their axons terminate: (1) Motoneurons; α and γ are two different types of motoneuron supplying skeletal muscles. (2) Sensory neurons; their axons ascend in the white matter (see also Fig. 2.11). (3) Interneurons; their axons are confined to the spinal cord.

long to the *autonomic nervous system.* The autonomic system controls the vascular smooth muscles and visceral organs throughout the body. The cell bodies lie in the *lateral horn* (Fig. 2.10). Most of them form a long, slender column, the *intermediolateral cell column.* This column is present only in the thoracic and upper two lumbar segments of the cord and belongs to the *sympathetic part of the autonomic nervous system.* A corresponding, smaller group of neurons is present in the sacral cord (S_3–S_4) and belongs to the *parasympathetic part of the autonomic nervous system.*

The motor neurons and those in the intermediolateral cell column (and those in the sacral cord) are under synaptic influence from higher levels of the central nervous system.

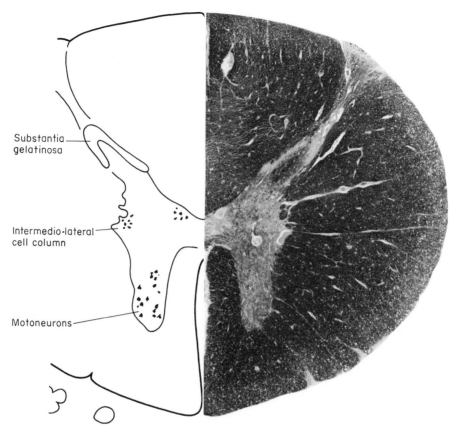

Substantia gelatinosa

Intermedio-lateral cell column

Motoneurons

Fig. 2.10. *Cross section of the spinal cord at the thoracic level.* Photomicrograph of a section stained so that myelinated axons appear dark. The large motoneurons in the ventral horn have also been stained (Nissl staining) and are just visible (owing to shrinkage, the motoneurons are surrounded by a clear zone).

Sensory Neurons in the Cord Are Influenced from the Dorsal Roots and Convey Signals to the Brain

The second main type of spinal neuron mentioned above sends axons to higher levels of the central nervous system. Their perikarya are mainly located in the dorsal horn and in the transition zone between the dorsal and ventral horn (Figs. 2.9 and 2.11). Their job is to inform the brain of the activities of the spinal cord, and especially about what is going on in the body. To fulfill the latter task, the neurons must receive signals from *sense organs—receptors—*in various parts of the body (in the skin, muscles, viscera, and so on). *Sensory,* or *afferent,* nerve fibers con-

ducting impulses from the receptors enter the spinal cord through the dorsal roots and ramify, forming terminal boutons in the gray matter of the cord (Figs. 2.11 and 4.10). The sensory neurons have their perikarya in the spinal ganglia and are therefore called *spinal ganglion cells.* These are morphologically special, since they have only one process, which divides shortly after leaving the cell body: One peripheral process connects with the sense organs, and the other extends centrally and enters the spinal cord (Figs. 1.13 and 4.10). In accordance with the usual definition of axons and dendrites, the peripheral process (conducting toward the cell body) should be called a dendrite, whereas the central process is an axon. Both pro-

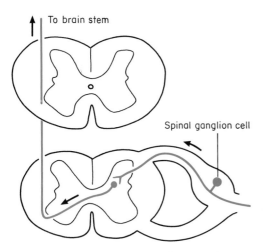

Fig. 2.11. *Sensory neuron in the gray substance of the spinal cord.* The neuron, which sends its axon to the brain stem, is synaptically contacted by sensory afferents entering the cord through the dorsal root (pseudounipolar ganglion cell). The presentation is very simplified—in reality, every sensory neuron is contacted by numerous dorsal root afferents.

cesses are, however, morphologically and functionally axons (for example, by conducting action potentials and by being myelinated).

The dorsal root fibers form synaptic contacts—in part directly, in part indirectly via interneurons—with neurons in the spinal cord, sending their axons to various parts of the brain. Such axons, destined for a common target in the brain, are grouped together in the spinal white matter, forming *tracts* (tractus). Such tracts are named after the location of the cell bodies and after the target organ. A tract leading from the spinal cord to the cerebellum, for example, is named the spinocerebellar tract (tractus spinocerebellaris).

Interneurons Enable Cooperation between Different Cell Groups in the Cord

The axons of the third type of spinal neuron do not leave the spinal cord. Usually, the axons ramify extensively and establish synaptic contacts with many other neurons in the cord, within the segment in which the cell body is located and in segments above and below (Fig. 2.9). Such neurons are called *spinal interneurons*, to emphasize that they are intercalated between other neurons (see Chapter 1, p. 15).[1] Many spinal interneurons are found in an intermediate zone between the dorsal and ventral horns and receive major synaptic inputs from sensory fibers in the dorsal roots. Many of these interneurons establish synaptic contacts with motoneurons in the ventral horn, thus mediating motor responses to sensory stimuli. Most interneurons, however, receive additional strong inputs from other spinal interneurons and from the brain.

As mentioned, spinal interneurons also send collaterals to terminate in segments of the cord other than the one in which their cell body and local ramifications are found. Such collaterals enter the white matter, run there for some distance, and reenter the cord at another segmental level, to ramify and establish synaptic contacts in the gray matter. Axons of this kind in the white matter are called *propriospinal fibers* (that is, fibers "belonging" to the spinal cord itself), to distinguish them from long ascending and descending fibers connecting the cord with the brain. *Propriospinal neurons* is, therefore, another term used for spinal interneurons.[2]

Propriospinal neurons provide opportunities for cooperation among the various spinal segments. In many instances it is necessary for the activity of many segments, each controlling different groups of muscles, to be closely coordinated. Some propriospinal connections are very long, interconnecting segments in the cervical and lumbar parts of the cord that control muscles in the forelimb and hindlimb, respectively. Cooperation between the forelimbs and hindlimbs is necessary, for example, during walking.

The Spinal Gray Matter Can Be Divided into Zones Called Rexed's Laminae

Systematic observations with the microscope of transverse sections of the spinal cord stained to visualize cell bodies show

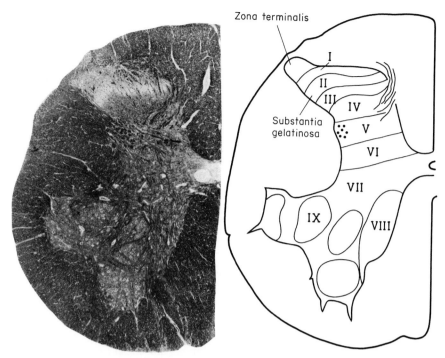

Fig. 2.12.   *Cross section of the spinal cord at the lumbar level* (lumbar intumescence). Photomicrograph of section stained to show myelin and neuronal perikarya. The drawing shows the borders between Rexed's laminae. Note the groups of motoneurons in the ventral horn (α and γ motoneurons) constituting lamina IX. The zona terminalis (tract of Lissauer) consists primarily of thin dorsal root fibers.

that neurons with different sizes and shapes are also differently distributed (Fig. 2.12). Essentially, neurons with common morphological features are collected into transversely oriented bands or zones. What appear as bands in the transverse plane are, three-dimensionally, longitudinal plates. This laminar pattern is most clear-cut in the dorsal horn, whereas in the ventral horn neurons are collected into regions forming longitudinal columns rather than plates (Fig. 8.1). Nevertheless, the columns in the ventral horn as well as the plates in the dorsal horn are termed *laminae*. This pattern was first described in 1952 by the Swedish neuroanatomist Rexed, and has since proved to be of great help for investigations of the spinal cord. Altogether, Rexed described 10 laminae; laminae 1–6 constitute the dorsal horn, whereas lamina 9 is made up of columns of motoneurons in the ventral horn.

Experimental studies of the connections of the spinal cord and of the functional properties of single spinal neurons have shown that the various laminae differ in these respects. Thus, the laminae may be regarded, at least to some extent, as the nuclei of the spinal cord. We will return to Rexed's laminae when dealing with the functional organization of the spinal cord in Chapters 4, 8, and 9.

It should be emphasized that, even though the laminae of the cord in certain respects are functionally distinct entities, the anatomic identification of a lamina is based solely on the location of the neuronal perikarya. The dendrites of these neurons, however, often extend into neighboring laminae (Fig. 2.13). Therefore, not only axons terminating within a lamina but also those ending in neighboring ones may be expected to influence the spinal neurons within one particular lamina.

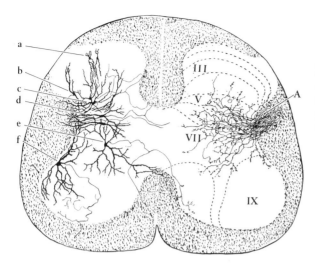

Fig. 2.13. *Dendritic arborizations of spinal neurons extend beyond the lamina of their perikarya.* Composite drawing based on observations in many Golgi-impregnated transverse sections from the spinal cord of the cat. The dendrites extend far, not only in the transverse plane as shown here but also longitudinally. To the right are the terminal ramifications of axons descending to the cord from higher levels of the central nervous system. From Scheibel and Scheibel (1966).

The Spinal Nerves Form Plexuses

The dorsal (sensory) and ventral (motor) roots join to form spinal nerves, as described above. Each spinal nerve then divides into several branches just outside the intervertebral foramen (Figs. 2.7 and 2.8). The thickest one, the *ventral ramus* (ramus ventralis), passes ventrally. A thinner branch, the *dorsal ramus* (ramus dorsalis), bends in the dorsal direction. In contrast to the spinal roots, *the ventral and dorsal branches (rami) contain both sensory and motor fibers.* This is caused by mixing of fibers from dorsal and ventral roots as they continue into the spinal nerves.

The dorsal rami innervate muscles and skin on the back, whereas the ventral rami innervate skin and muscles on the ventral aspect of the trunk and neck and, in addition, the extremities. Thus, the ventral rami innervate much larger parts of the body than the dorsal rami, which explains why the ventral ones contain more nerve fibers and are considerably thicker than the dorsal ones.

Some of the ventral rami join each other to form *plexuses* (Fig. 8.10). This will be discussed further in Chapter 8.

Each spinal nerve also sends off a small branch, the *meningeal ramus,* which passes back through the intervertebral foramen to reenter the vertebral canal. These branches supply the meninges of the spinal cord with sensory and autonomic (sympathetic) fibers.

The Spinal Cord Consists of Cooperating Subunits That Are Controlled from the Brain

Each segment of the spinal cord is to some extent a functional unit, since, as we will see in Chapter 4, a pair of spinal nerves relates to a particular "segment" of the body. A spinal segment may be regarded as the "local government" of a part of the body: It receives sensory information from its own district, processes this information, and issues orders through motor nerves to muscles and glands to ensure adequate responses. However, just as local governing bodies in our society must take orders from higher governing bodies (for example, county versus national governments), the spinal segments have only limited independence. Many of the functional tasks of the spinal cord are under strict control and supervision from higher levels of the central nervous system. This control is mediated by fibers from the brain stem and cerebral cortex, which descend in the white matter of the cord and terminate in the gray matter of the spinal segments that are to be influenced. The brain also ensures that the activity of the various spinal segments is coordinated, so that it serves the body as a whole and not only a small part. To be able to carry out this co-ordination, the brain must continuously receive information about conditions in all the "local districts" of the body and in the spinal segments related to them. This information is mediated by long, ascending fibers in the white matter of the cord terminating in the brain stem. The local cooperation among spinal segments is taken care of by the numerous propriospinal fibers coming from spinal interneurons.

THE BRAIN STEM

The brain stem represents the upward (rostral, cranial) continuation of the spinal cord (Fig. 2.1). It consists of several portions with, in part, clear-cut surface borders between them (Fig. 2.14). Whereas the lowermost (caudal) part of the brain stem is structurally similar to the spinal cord, the upper parts are

more complicated. The subdivisions of the brain stem are as follows (from caudal to rostral): the *medulla oblongata* (often just called medulla), the *pons* (the bridge), the *mesencephalon* (the midbrain), and the *diencephalon*.

The Brain Stem Contains the Third and Fourth Ventricles

A continuous, fluid-filled cavity varying in diameter stretches through the brain stem (Fig. 2.3). It is the upward continuation of the thin central canal of the spinal cord, and it continues rostrally into the cavities of the cerebrum (Fig. 2.1). Together, these cavities constitute the *ventricular system of the brain and spinal cord*. The cavity in the brain stem has two dilated parts. One, the *fourth ventricle*, is at the level of the medulla and pons, whereas the *third ventricle* is situated in the diencephalon (Fig. 2.38). We will return to the ventricular system later (p. 85).

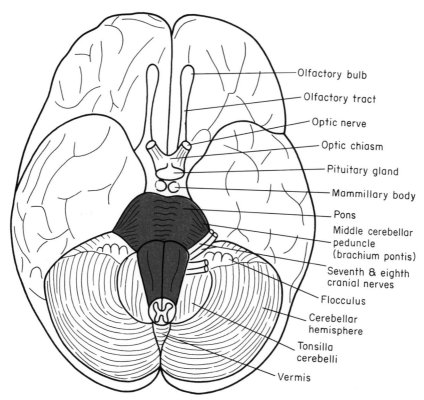

Olfactory bulb
Olfactory tract
Optic nerve
Optic chiasm
Pituitary gland
Mammillary body
Pons
Middle cerebellar peduncle (brachium pontis)
Seventh & eighth cranial nerves
Flocculus
Cerebellar hemisphere
Tonsilla cerebelli
Vermis

Fig. 2.14. *The basal aspect of the brain.* Only some of the cranial nerves are shown.

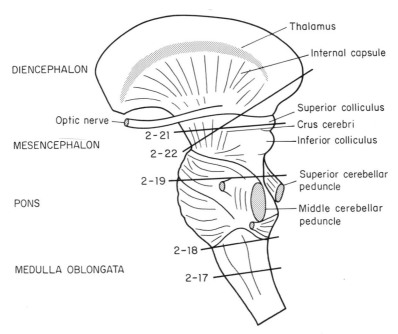

Fig. 2.15. *The brain stem* seen from the left side. The levels of sections shown in several of the following figures are indicated.

The Brain Stem Has Similarities to the Spinal Cord: The Cranial Nerves

Examination of the *internal structure of the brain stem* (Figs. 2.18–2.22 and 2.25) shows that it is more complicated than that of the spinal cord. Even though in both the brain stem and the cord gray matter is generally located centrally, surrounded by a zone of white matter, the gray matter of the brain stem is subdivided into several regions separated by strands of white matter. The white matter of the brain stem consists of myelinated fibers, as in other parts of the central nervous system. The regions with gray matter contain various nuclei—that is, groups of neurons with common tasks. Many of the nuclei belong to the *cranial nerves*. There are a total of *12 pairs* of cranial nerves, which, with the exception of the first, all emerge from the brain stem (Fig. 2.16). They correspond to the spinal nerves but show a more complex and less regular organization. Thus, there is no clear separation of sensory (dorsal) and motor (ventral) roots. The cranial nerves are numbered from rostral to caudal, in accordance with where they emerge on the surface of the brain stem. Fig-

ure 2.37 shows the places on the base of the skull where the cranial nerves leave through small holes or fissures.

Many of the cranial nerves contain fibers that conduct impulses out of the brain stem; that is, the fibers are efferent or motor. These

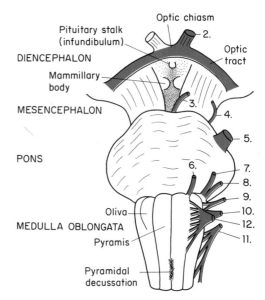

Fig. 2.16. *The cranial nerves.* The brain stem is seen from the ventral side.

fibers belong to neurons with their perikarya in nuclei that are called *motor cranial nerve nuclei*. They correspond to the groups (columns) of neurons in the ventral and lateral horns of the spinal cord. The cranial nerves, like the spinal nerves, also contain sensory, afferent fibers bringing impulses from sense organs. The brain stem cell groups in which these afferent fibers terminate are, accordingly, called *sensory cranial nerve nuclei*. They correspond to the laminae of the spinal dorsal horn. The sensory fibers entering the brain stem have their perikarya in ganglia just outside the brain stem, *cranial nerve ganglia,* corresponding to the spinal ganglia of the spinal nerves. Most cranial nerves are mixed; that is, they contain both motor and sensory fibers, but a few are either purely sensory or purely motor.

The only cranial nerve not emerging from the brain stem is the *first cranial nerve,* the *olfactory nerve* (nervus olfactorius). This consists of short axons coming from sensory cells in the roof of the nasal cavity, which, immediately after penetrating the base of the skull, terminate in the *olfactory bulb* (bulbus olfactorius) (Fig. 2.14). The other cranial nerves are briefly mentiond below in connection with a description of the main structural features of the brain stem. More thorough treatment of the cranial nerves and their central connections is found in Chapters 5, 6, 7, and 13.

The Reticular Formation Extends through Central Parts of the Brain Stem

Among the cranial nerve nuclei and other clearly delimited cell groups, there are more diffuse collections of neurons. In microscopic sections stained to visualize the neuronal processes, a networklike pattern is seen. The old anatomists therefore termed these parts—present in the core of most of the brain stem— the *reticular formation* (formatio reticularis, Figs. 2.17–2.19, 2.21,

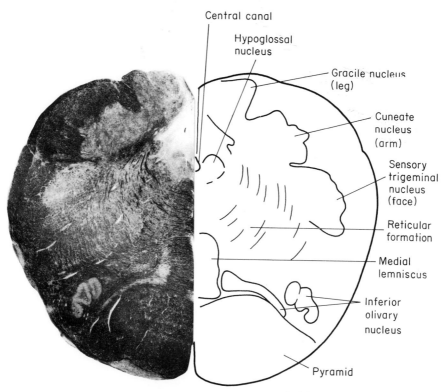

Central canal
Hypoglossal nucleus
Gracile nucleus (leg)
Cuneate nucleus (arm)
Sensory trigeminal nucleus (face)
Reticular formation
Medial lemniscus
Inferior olivary nucleus
Pyramid

Fig. 2.17. *Lower part of the medulla oblongata.* Cross section. See Figure 2.15 for exact level. The **left** half is a photomicrograph of a section with darkly stained myelinated fibers (Woelke method); that is, white matter appears dark and gray matter light.

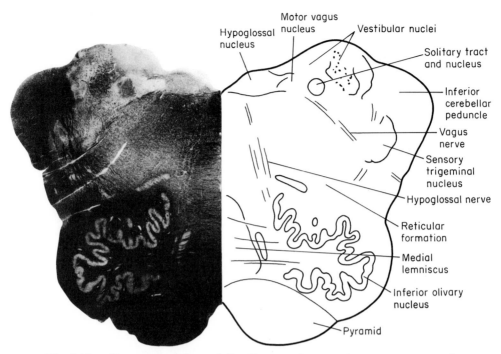

Fig. 2.18. *Upper part of the medulla oblongata.* Cross section. See Figure 2.15 for exact level. Myelin staining as in Figure 2.17.

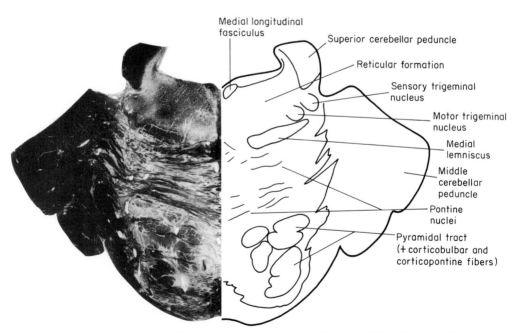

Fig. 2.19. *Upper part of the pons.* Cross section; myelin-stained. See Figure 2.15 for exact level.

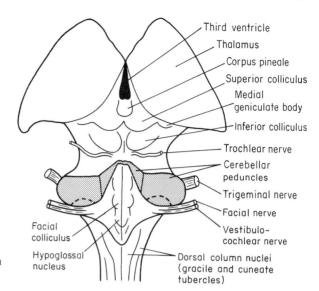

Fig. 2.20. *The brain stem* seen from the dorsal aspect.

and 12.1). In reality, however, the reticular formation is not one homogeneous structure but rather a comglomerate of cell groups with different connections and functional tasks. Some parts of the reticular formation are, for example, primarily concerned with control of circulation and respiration; other parts are particularly concerned with regulation of sleep and wakefulness. But the collective term, the reticular formation, is still in common use, and it may be practical to

retain it to denote parts of the brain stem with certain common anatomic features, without implying that they have common functional tasks. The reticular formation is treated more comprehensively in Chapter 12.

The Medulla Oblongata

Ventrally in the midline, the medulla has a longitudinal sulcus, which is a continuation

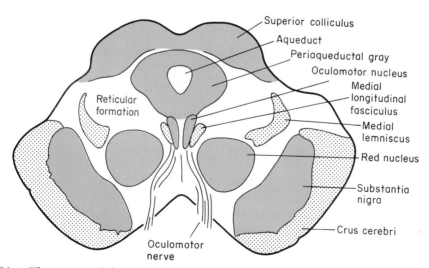

Fig. 2.21. *The mesencephalon.* Cross section. The major nuclei are indicated in red and the major tracts in gray. See Figure 2.15 for exact level.

of the ventral (anterior) median fissure of the cord. The sulcus ends abruptly at the lower end of the pons (Fig. 2.16). The so-called *pyramids* protrude on each side of the longitudinal sulcus. Each pyramid is formed by a thick bundle of axons belonging to the *pyramidal tract*. This important fiber tract conveys signals from the cerebral cortex to the spinal cord (the pyramidal tract is discussed in Chapter 9). Close to the lower end of the medulla, on the transition to the cord, bundles of fibers can be seen to cross the midline, forming the *pyramidal decussation*. Lateral to the pyramids is an oval protrusion (the olive) formed by a large nucleus (the inferior olivary nucleus). This nucleus sends its efferents to the cerebellum (see Chapter 11). Between the olive and the pyramid is a row of small bundles of nerve fibers, which are the rootlets of the *hypoglossal nerve* (the twelfth cranial nerve, nervus hypoglossus). This nerve supplies the striated muscles of the tongue with motor fibers. Lateral to the olive, the rootlets of the *glossopharyngeal* and *vagus nerves* (ninth and tenth cranial nerves, nervus glossopharyngeus and nervus vagus) leave the brain stem. These two nerves supply the pharnyx, the larynx, and most of the viscera with motor and sensory fibers. The *accessory nerve* (eleventh cranial nerve, nervus accessorius) runs cranially along the lateral aspect of the medulla. Most of its fibers come from the upper cervical spinal segments but enter the cranial cavity to leave the skull together with the glossopharyngeal and vagus nerves. The accessory nerve supplies two muscles in the neck with motor fibers.

Figure 2.17 shows a *cross section through the lower part of the medulla*, at a level below the caudal end of the fourth ventricle. The section is stained so that regions with white matter (myelinated fiber tracts) are dark, whereas gray matter (nuclei) appears light. The ventrally located bundle of cross-sectioned fibers is the *pyramidal tract*, forming the pyramid (Fig. 2.16), and containing about 1 million fibers. Dorsal to the pyramid lies a highly convoluted band of gray matter, the *inferior olivary nucleus* (often called the

inferior olive). The *dorsal column nuclei*, the *gracile and cuneate* (nucleus gracilis and nucleus cuneatus), are located dorsally in the medulla. The efferent fibers from these nuclei arch ventrally and take up a position close to the midline dorsal to the pyramids, where they form a triangular area of cross-sectioned fibers. This is an important sensory tract, the *medial lemniscus* (lemniscus medialis), leading from neurons in the dorsal column nuclei to nuclei in the diencephalon. The dorsal column nuclei receive afferent fibers that ascend in the dorsal columns (or dorsal funiculi) and convey impulses from receptors (sense organs) in the skin and muscles and around joints. Close to the midline, just ventral to the central canal, lies the *hypoglossal nucleus*, consisting of the perikarya of the motor fibers that form the hypoglossal nerve. The efferent fibers of the hypoglossal nucleus pass ventrally and leave the medulla at the lateral edge of the pyramid. Lateral to the motor cranial nerve nuclei are found several sensory cranial nerve nuclei, among them the big *sensory trigeminal nucleus* that receives sensory impulses from the face, carried in the *trigeminal nerve* (the fifth cranial nerve). Note how the nuclei transmitting sensory impulses from the leg, arm, and face are distributed from medial to lateral in the dorsal part of the medulla (Fig. 2.17).

A cross section through the *upper (cranial) part of the medulla oblongata* (Fig. 2.18) shows partly the same fiber tracts and nuclei as the section at a lower level (Fig. 2.17). In addition, we may notice the big *vestibular nuclei* situated dorsally and laterally under the floor of the fourth ventricle (these nuclei also extend cranially into the pons; see Fig. 13-16). They receive sensory impulses from the vestibular apparatus in the inner ear via the vestibular nerve (the eighth cranial nerve). One of the main efferent pathways from the vestibular nuclei forms a distinct tract, the *medial longitudinal fasciculus* (fasciculus longitudinalis medialis), close to the midline under the floor of the fourth ventricle (Fig. 2.19). This tract terminates in the motor nuclei of the cranial nerves supplying the eye muscles, thus conveying influences on eye movements from the receptors for equilibrium. Furthermore, Figure 2.18 shows the *motor and sensory nuclei of the vagus,* and some of the fibers of the vagus nerve, which pass laterally and ventrally, to leave the medulla lateral to the olive (compare with Fig. 2.16).

The Pons

The pons forms a bulbous protrusion at the ventral aspect of the brain stem, with clear-cut transversely running fiber bundles (Figs. 2.15 and 2.16). It is sharply delimited both caudally and cranially. The transverse fiber bundles are formed by fibers from large cell groups in the pons, the pontine nuclei (Fig. 2.19), and terminate in the cerebellum. The fiber bundles join at the lateral aspect of the pons to form the *middle cerebellar peduncle* (brachium pontis) (Figs. 2.15 and 2.19).

Several cranial nerves leave the brain stem at the ventral aspect of the pons. At the lower (caudal) edge, just lateral to the midline, a thin nerve emerges on each side. This is the *abducens nerve* (the sixth cranial nerve, nervus abducens) carrying motor fibers to one of the external eye muscles (rotates the eye laterally). Still at the lower edge of the pons, but more laterally, two other cranial nerves leave the brain stem. Most ventrally lies the *facial nerve* (seventh cranial nerve, nervus facialis), bringing motor impulses to the mimetic muscles of the face (it also contains some other kinds of fibers, to be considered in Chapter 13). Closely behind the facial nerve lies the *vestibulocochlear nerve* (the eighth cranial nerve, nervus vestibulocochlearis). It carries sensory impulses from the sense organs for equilibrium and hearing in the inner ear. The largest of all the cranial nerves is the *trigeminal nerve* (the fifth cranial nerve, nervus trigeminus). It leaves the brain stem laterally at middle levels of the pons. The largest portion of the nerve consists of sensory fibers from the face, whereas a smaller (medial) portion contains motor fibers destined for the masticatory muscles.

In a *cross section through the pons,* the large *pontine nuclei* can be easily seen (Fig. 2.19). As mentioned, the neurons of the pontine nuclei send their axons to the cerebellum (see Chapter 11). Bordering the pontine nuclei dorsally lies the *medial lemniscus,* which has turned around and moved laterally compared with its location in the medulla (see Fig. 2.17). In the lower part of the pons, the nucleus of the abducens nerve, the *abducens nucleus,* is located dorsally and medially, whereas the *facial nucleus* lies more ventrally and laterally (Fig. 13.18). Figure 13.18 also shows the course taken by the efferent fibers of the abducens and facial nuclei (forming the sixth and seventh cranial nerves, respectively).

A *cross section through the middle–upper part of the pons* (Fig. 2.19) shows the *sensory trigeminal nucleus* laterally (this nucleus extends as a slender column through the medulla, pons, and mesencephalon; see also Figs. 2.17–2.19, and 13.2). Medial to the sensory nucleus lies the *motor trigeminal nucleus* (masticatory muscles), but this nucleus is present only in the pons.

The Medulla and Pons Seen from the Dorsal Side

At the dorsal side of the medulla oblongata, at caudal levels, there are two longitudinal protrusions, the *gracile and cuneate tubercles* (Fig. 2.20). These are formed by the *dorsal column nuclei,* mentioned above (they are relay stations in pathways for sensory information from the body to the cerebral cortex). The most medial one of these nuclei, the *gracile nucleus,* receives impulses from the leg and lower part of the trunk, whereas the laterally situated *cuneate nucleus* receives impulses from the arm and upper part of the trunk. Further laterally, another oblong protrusion (tuberculum cinereum) is formed by the *sensory trigeminal nucleus* (relay station for sensory impulses from the face).

Rostral to the upper end of the dorsal column nuclei, there is a flattened, diamond-shaped area, the *rhomboid fossa* (fossa rhomboides), extending rostrally onto the posterior face of the pons (Fig. 2.20). This constitutes the floor of the fourth ventricle (Fig. 2.38). Laterally and rostrally the rhomboid fossa is delimited by the *cerebellar peduncles* (these have been cut in Fig. 2.20). Some of the cranial nerve nuclei and some fiber tracts form small protrusions medially at the floor of the fourth ventricle—notably the hypoglossal nucleus and the root fibers of the facial nerve (forming the facial colliculus) (Fig. 13.18 shows the peculiar route taken by the facial root fibers).

The Mesencephalon (Midbrain)

The part of the brain stem rostral to the pons, the mesencephalon, is relatively short (Figs. 2.1, 2.15, and 2.24). Ventrally, an almost half-cylindrical protrusion is present on each side of the midline—the *cerebral peduncle* or the *crus cerebri* (Fig. 2.16).[3] Crus cerebri consists of nerve fibers descending from the cerebral cortex to the brain stem and spinal cord—among these fibers are those of the pyramidal tract. The fibers continue into the pons, where they spread out into several smaller bundles among the pontine nuclei (Fig. 2.19).

In the furrow between the two crura, the *oculomotor nerve* emerges (third cranial nerve, nervus oculomotorius) (Fig. 2.16). As the name implies, the nerve carries motor impulses to muscles that move the eye. The oculomotor nerve innervates four of the six extraocular (striated) muscles and, in addition, two smooth internal muscles that regulate the diameter of the pupil and the curvature of the lens.

At the *dorsal side of the mesencephalon* there is a characteristic formation of four small, rounded protrusions, two on each side of the midline (Fig. 2.20). These are called the *colliculi* (corpora quadrigemina) and consist of, on each side, the *superior colliculus* and the *inferior colliculus*. They contain nuclei that are centers for visual (superior) and auditory (inferior) reflexes. The inferior colliculus is also a relay station in the pathways that bring auditory impulses to awareness.

Below the inferior colliculi there emerges on each side a thin fiber bundle, the *trochlear nerve* (fourth cranial nerve, nervus trochlearis). This is the only cranial nerve that emerges on the dorsal side of the brain stem. It supplies one of the extraocular muscles with motor fibers.

In *cross sections of the mesencephalon* (Figs. 2.21 and 2.22), the crus cerebri can be recognized ventrally, and the superior colliculus dorsally. In the midline just ventral to the colliculi there is a small hole, which is a cross section of the *aqueduct* (aquaeductus cerebri). This a narrow canal interconnecting the third and fourth ventricles (Figs. 2.1, 2.21, and 2.24). Surrounding the aqueduct is a region of gray matter called the *periaqueductal gray substance* (substantia grisea centralis), which is of importance for sensations of pain (this will be discussed further in Chapter 4). Ventral to the periaqueductal gray, close to the midline, we find the *oculomotor nucleus* (or nucleus of the oculomotor nerve). Further ventrally lies the large *red nucleus* (nucleus ruber)—so named because of its slightly reddish color. Just dorsal to the crus and ventral to the red nucleus is the *substantia nigra* (the black substance). The neurons of the substantia nigra contain a dark pigment, making the nucleus clearly visible macroscopically. The red nucleus and the substantia nigra are both of importance for the control of our movements.

Figure 2.22 shows how the mesencephalon merges with the diencephalon rostrally without any clear transition.

The Diencephalon Consists of the Thalamus and the Hypothalamus

The diencephalon is not clearly delimited because in early embryonic life it fuses with the primordium of the cerebral hemispheres. The *optic nerve* (the second cranial nerve, nervus opticus) with afferent fibers from the retina ends in the diencephalon.

The largest part of the diencephalon is oc-

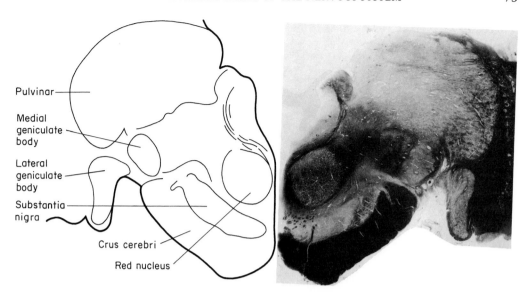

Pulvinar

Medial geniculate body

Lateral geniculate body

Substantia nigra

Crus cerebri

Red nucleus

Fig. 2.22. *The transition between the mesencephalon and the diencephalon.* Oblique frontal section; myelin staining. See Figure 2.15 for exact plane and level of the section.

cupied by the *thalamus*, situated on each side of the *third ventricle* (Figs. 2.23, 2.28, and 2.32). The thalamus consists of many smaller nuclei and is a *relay station for almost all information transmitted from the lower parts of the central nervous system to the cerebral cortex* (notably most kinds of sensory information). Each thalamus is ap-

proximately egg-shaped with a flattened side toward the third ventricle (Figs. 2.23 and 2.24). Lateral to the thalamus lies a thick sheet of white matter, the *internal capsule* (capsula interna). It consists mainly of fibers connecting the cerebral cortex with the brain stem and the spinal cord (Figs. 2.15 and 2.25). The crus cerebri is a caudal con-

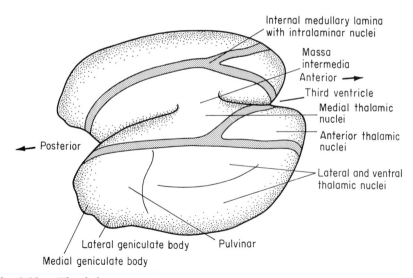

Internal medullary lamina with intralaminar nuclei

Massa intermedia

Anterior →

Third ventricle

Medial thalamic nuclei

Anterior thalamic nuclei

Lateral and ventral thalamic nuclei

← Posterior

Lateral geniculate body   Pulvinar

Medial geniculate body

Fig. 2.23. *The thalamus.* Drawing of the thalami of both sides, to indicate their three-dimensional form.

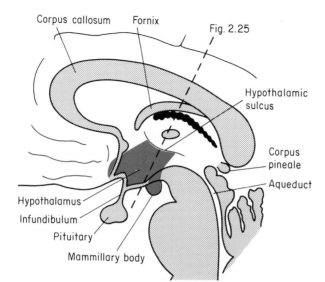

Fig. 2.24. *The hypothalamus.* Drawing of midsagittal section showing the upper parts of the brain stem. The hypothalamus is indicated in red.

tinuation of many of the fibers of the internal capsule.

In Figure 2.25 (showing a frontal section of the brain), it can be seen that the thalamus is subdivided by narrow bands of white matter forming a Y—the *internal medullary lamina* (lamina medullaris interna) (see also Fig. 2.23). As a result, three major thalamic nuclei can be identified, the *medial thalamic nucleus* (nucleus medialis thalami), the *lateral thalamic nucleus,* and the *anterior thalamic nucleus.* On closer (microscopic) inspection, each of these consists of several smaller nuclei, which connect to different parts of the cerebral cortex. In addition to the three main nuclei mentioned, the thala-

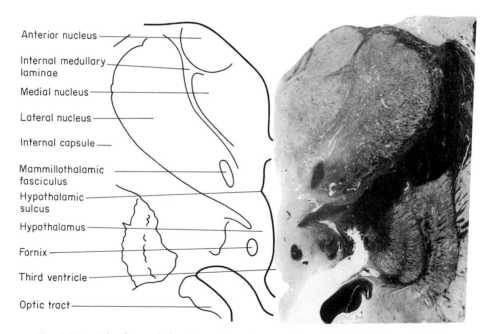

Fig. 2.25. *The diencephalon.* Frontal section; myelin staining. See Figure 2.24 for exact orientation and level of the section.

mus includes one large nucleus in its posterior part, the *pulvinar* (Figs. 2.22 and 2.23), and two nuclei partly covered by the pulvinar, the *lateral geniculate body* (corpus geniculatum laterale) and the *medial geniculate body* (corpus geniculatum mediale). The latter two nuclei are relay stations for visual and auditory impulses, respectively. Thus, fibers of the *optic nerve* end in the lateral geniculate body.

The optic nerves from the two eyes unite just underneath the diencephalon and form the *optic chiasma* (chiasma opticum), in which there is a partial crossing of the optic nerve fibers (Figs. 2.14 and 2.16). In their further course from the optic chiasma to the lateral geniculate body, the fibers form the *optic tract* (Figs. 2.16 and 2.25).

Anterior and inferior to the thalamus lies the *hypothalamus* (Fig. 2.24), which is particularly involved with *central control of the autonomic nervous system*—that is, with control of the visceral organs and the vessels. The hypothalamus forms the lateral wall of the anterior part of the third ventricle. The border between the thalamus and the hypothalamus is marked by the shallow *hypothalamic sulcus* (Figs. 2.24 and 2.25). The *mammillary body* (corpus mammillare), a special part of the hypothalamus, protrudes downward from its posterior part (Figs. 2.14 and 2.24). The *fornix* is a thick, arching bundle of fibers originating in the cerebral cortex (in the so-called hippocampal region) and terminating in the mammillary bodies. The major efferent pathway of the mammillary body goes to the thalamus, forming a distinct fiber bundle, the *mammillothalamic tract* (fasciculus mammillothalamicus) (Fig. 2.25). In front of the mammillary bodies, the floor of the third ventricle bulges downward like a funnel and forms the stalk of the pituitary gland, the *infundibulum*. The region between the mammillary bodies and the infundibulum is called the *tuber cinereum*. It contains cell groups influencing the activity of the pituitary gland.

The *pituitary* (Figs. 2.14 and 2.24) consists of a posterior lobe, developed from the central nervous system, and an anterior lobe, developed from the epithelium in the roof of the mouth. The anterior lobe, secreting several hormones that control important bodily functions, is itself under the control of the hypothalamus. This is further discussed in Chapter 15.

THE CEREBRUM

The cerebrum has an ovoid shape and fills most of the cranial cavity. Whereas its convexity—that is, its upper and lateral surfaces—are evenly curved, the basal surface is uneven. In the center of the basal surface, the brain stem emerges (Figs. 2.14 and 2.27). The cerebrum is almost completely divided in two by a vertical slit, the *longitudinal cerebral fissure* (fissura longitudinalis cerebri), so that it consists of two approximate halfspheres or *cerebral hemispheres*. Each of the cerebral hemispheres contains a central cavity, the *lateral ventricle* (Figs. 2.28 and 2.38). The lateral ventricles are continuous with the third ventricle through a small opening, the *interventricular foramen* (Fig. 2.39). The lateral ventricles are surrounded by masses of white matter with some embedded nuclei. The surface of the hemisphere is covered everywhere by a 3 to 5 mm–thick layer of gray substance, the *cerebral cortex* (cortex cerebri). The structure, connections, and functions of the cerebral cortex are covered most completely in Chapter 17, but some main features are briefly described here because knowledge of them is necessary for the chapters dealing with sensory and motor systems.

The neurons of the cerebral cortex receive impulses from lower parts of the central nervous system, most of which are relayed through the thalamus. In addition, there are numerous *association fibers*—that is, fibers interconnecting neurons in various parts of the cerebral cortex of one hemisphere. Finally, a vast number of *commissural fibers* interconnects neurons in the two hemispheres. Most of the commissural fibers are collected into a thick plate of white matter, the *corpus callosum,* which joins the two hemispheres across the midline (Fig. 2.27). The fibers in the corpus callosum enable impulses to travel from one hemisphere to the other and thus ensure that the right and left hemispheres can cooperate (discussed further in Chapter 17). A few commissural fibers pass in the *anterior commissure* (commissura anterior) (Fig. 2.27).

The Surface of the Hemisphere Is Highly Convoluted and Forms Gyri and Sulci

During embryonic development, the cerebral hemispheres fold as they grow in size (Fig. 2.40). This leads to a great increase in their surface area and thus in the amount of cortex relative to their volume (only about a third of the total cortical surface is exposed). The furrowed, walnutlike appearance of the cerebral hemispheres of man and some higher mammals is highly characteristic (Figs. 2.26 and 2.27). The folding of the hemisphere produces deep *fissures* and more shallow *sulci*. Between the sulci, the surface of the cortex forms rounded *gyri*. Apart from the fissure that divides the two hemispheres along the midline, the *longitudinal cerebral fissure*, the largest fissure in each hemisphere is the *lateral cerebral fissure* or the Sylvian fissure (Fig. 2.26). This fissure follows a course upward and backward, and extends deep into the hemisphere (Fig. 2.28). The small gyri in the bottom of the lateral fissure form the *insula* (the island). More sulci and gyri will be mentioned when dealing with the lobes of the cerebrum.

The pattern of the fissures and the larger sulci in the human brain is fairly constant. Nevertheless, variations are great enough to make it impossible to know exactly where a certain sulcus is located only from landmarks on the outside of the skull. The smaller sulci and gyri are subject to considerable individual variations.

The Hemisphere Can Be Divided into Four Lobes

With more or less sharply defined borders (formed by fissures and sulci), one can distinguish four lobes of the cerebral hemispheres. They are named in accordance with the bone of the skull under which they are located. The *frontal lobe* (lobus frontalis) (Fig. 2.26) lies in the anterior cranial fossa above

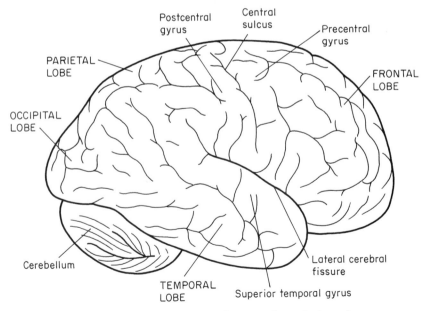

Fig. 2.26. *The right cerebral hemisphere seen from the lateral aspect.*

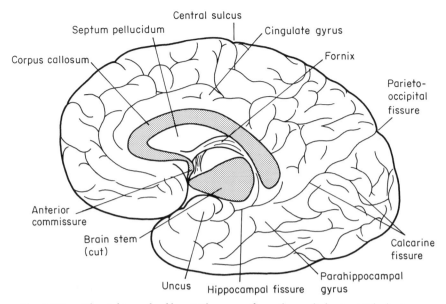

Fig. 2.27. *The right cerebral hemisphere seen from the medial aspect.* The brain stem has been removed.

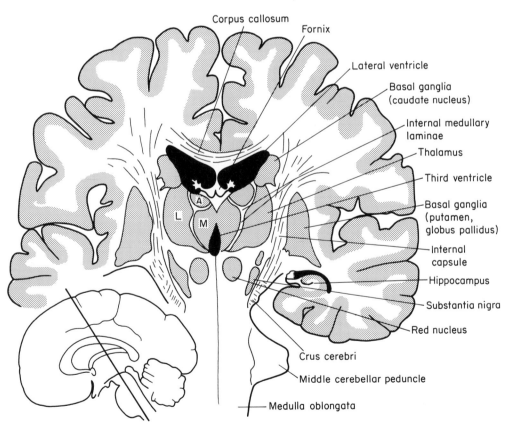

Fig. 2.28. *The cerebral hemispheres and the brain stem.* Oblique frontal section. Compare with Figure 2.29.

77

the orbit. The frontal lobe is separated from the *parietal lobe* (lobus parietalis) by the *central sulcus,* which extends from the medial edge of the hemisphere laterally to the lateral fissure. Below the lateral fissure lies the *temporal lobe* (lobus temporalis). Neither the parietal nor the temporal lobe has any clearly defined border posteriorly toward the *occipital lobe.* The occipital lobe lies above the cerebellum, which is located in the posterior cranial fossa (Fig. 2.1). On the medial aspect of the hemisphere, the border between the parietal and the occipital lobe is marked by the *parieto-occipital fissure* (fissura parieto-occipitalis) (Fig. 2.27).

Anatomically and functionally, the cerebral cortex can be divided into different regions, which do not, however, coincide with the different lobes. Here only a few points will be mentioned. The gyrus in front of the central sulcus, the *precentral gyrus* (gyrus precentralis) (Fig. 2.26), coincides fairly closely with the *motor cortex* (MI), which is of special significance for the execution of voluntary movements. If this gyrus is destroyed in one hemisphere, pareses ensue in the opposite side of the body. Many of the fibers in the pyramidal tract come from the precentral gyrus, and, as mentioned above, most of these fibers cross the midline on their way to the spinal cord. The *postcentral gyrus,* situated just posterior to the central sulcus, is the major receiving region for sensory impulses from the skin, musculoskeletal system, and the viscera. This region is called the *somatosensory cortex* (SI). The tracts that conduct impulses from the sense organs to the cortex are also crossed. Thus, destruction of the postcentral gyrus on one side leads to reduced sensibility (for example, of the skin) on the opposite side of the body. We have previously mentioned the medial lemniscus, which is part of the pathways from the sense organs to the postcentral gyrus. The fibers of the medial lemniscus terminate in the lateral thalamic nucleus (Fig. 2.25), and the neurons in this nucleus send their axons to the postcentral gyrus.

The *visual cortex*—that is, the main cortical region receiving information from the eyes—is located in the occipital lobe around a deep fissure, the *calcarine fissure* (fissura calcarina) (Fig. 2.27). The impulses start in the retina and are conducted in the optic nerve and the optic tract to the thalamus (the lateral geniculate body) (Figs. 2.22 and 2.23) and from there to the visual cortex. The visual cortex can be distinguished from the surrounding parts of the cortex in sections perpendicular to the surface: It contains a thin whitish stripe running parallel to the surface (caused by a large number of myelinated fibers). Because of the stripe, this part of the cortex was named the *striate area* by the early anatomists (see also Fig. 5.15).

The *auditory cortex*—that is, the cortical region receiving impulses from the cochlea in the inner ear—is located in the temporal lobe (in the superior temporal gyrus) (Figs. 2.26 and 6.10). The pathway for auditory impulses is synaptically interrupted in the thalamus (the medial geniculate body) (Figs. 2.22 and 2.23).

The *olfactory cortex* is a small region on the medial aspect of the hemisphere near the tip of the temporal lobe. It is part of the so-called *uncus* (Fig. 2.27) and extends somewhat onto the adjoining *parahippocampal gyrus.* The olfactory cortex receives fibers from the *olfactory bulb* (bulbus olfactorius) through the *olfactory tract* (tractus olfactorius) (Fig. 2.14). The parahippocampal gyrus and adjoining cortical regions are of particular interest with regard to *learning and memory* (this will be treated further in Chapter 16). The cortex of the parahippocampal gyrus extends into the *hippocampal fissure,* forming a longitudinal elevation, the *hippocampus* (Figs. 2.28 and 2.32). The hippocampus belongs to the phylogenetically oldest parts of the cerebral cortex and has a simpler structure than the newer parts.

The Cerebral Cortex Consists of Six Cell Layers

When the cerebral cortex is examined in a microscopic section cut perpendicular to the surface, it can be seen that the neuronal cell bodies (perikarya) are not randomly distributed (Figs. 17.1 and 17.2). They are arranged into *layers* or *laminae* parallel to the surface. Each layer is characterized by a certain shape, size, and packing density of the perikarya (compare with the Rexed's laminae of the spinal cord). The layers are numbered from the surface inward to the white matter. *Lamina 1* is cell-poor and consists largely of dendrites from neurons with perikarya in deeper layers and of axons with boutons making synapses on the dendrites. *Layers or laminae 2 and 4* are made up of predominantly small, rounded cells and are therefore also called the *external and internal granular layer,* respectively. These two layers have in common that they largely have a receiving function: Many of the afferent fibers to the cerebral cortex terminate and form synapses in layers 2 and 4. Fibers conveying sensory information from lower levels of the central nervous system end predominantly in layer 4, and consequently this layer is particularly well developed in the sensory cortical regions mentioned above. *Layers or laminae 3 and 5* contain cells that are larger than those in layers 2 and 4, and the cell bodies tend to be of pyramidal shape, hence the name pyramidal cells. Many of the pyramidal cells in layer 5 send their axons to the brain stem and spinal cord, where they influence motor neurons. Layer 5 is therefore especially well developed in the motor cortex in the precentral gyrus. The pyramidal neurons in lamina 3 send their axons primarily to other parts of the cerebral cortex, either in the same hemisphere (association fibers) or to cortex in the hemisphere of the other side (commissural fibers). The perikarya of *layer 6* are smaller and more spindle-shaped than those in lamina 5. Many of the neurons send their axons to the thalamus, enabling the cerebral cortex to influence the impulse traffic from the thalamus to the cortex (feedback connections).

There are also numerous *interneurons* in the cerebral cortex, providing opportunity for cooperation between the various layers (interneurons with "vertically" oriented axons) and between neurons in different parts of one layer (interneurons with "horizontally" oriented axons). The layers are obviously not independent units.

The Cerebral Cortex Can Be Divided into Many Areas on a Cytoarchitectonic Basis

We have mentioned above that some layers may be particularly well developed in certain regions of the cortex—for example, layer 4 in the sensory receiving areas and layer 5 in the motor cortex. There are many more differences when all layers all over the cortex are systematically compared. Such *cytoarchitectonic* differences (that is, differences in perikaryal size, shape, and packing density) form the basis of a parcellation of the cerebral cortex of each hemisphere into approximately 50 *cortical areas* (areae). Maps of the cerebral cortex showing the positions of the various areas were published by several investigators around the turn of the century and are still in use. The most widely used map was published by the German anatomist Brodmann (Fig. 17.3). Such cytoarchitectonically defined areas have later been shown, in many cases, to differ also with regard to connections and functional properties. The numbering of the cortical areas may appear illogical. For example, the motor cortex in the precentral gyrus corresponds to area 4 of Brodmann. This borders posteriorly on area 3 but on area 6 anteriorly. Area 3 borders on area 1, which borders on area 2, and so on (Fig. 17.3). It is not necessary, however, to learn the position of more than a few of the cortical areas, and these will be dealt with in connection with the various functional systems in Parts II–VI.

The Basal Ganglia

The interior of the hemispheres contains regions with a gray substance. Largest among these are the so-called *basal ganglia,*[4] which perform important tasks related to *control of movements.* Other nuclear groups (the amygdaloid nucleus, the septal nuclei,

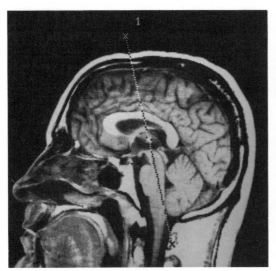
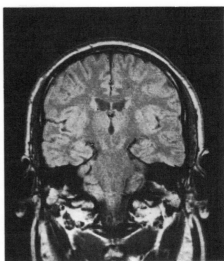

Fig. 2.29. *Magnetic resonance image* (MRI) with plane of sectioning corresponding to that in Figure 2.28. Almost all of the structures that can be identified in a section of a fixed brain can be recognized in the MRI. Courtesy of Dr. S. J. Bakke.

and the basal nucleus) are treated in Chapter 16, and the basal ganglia are discussed in Chapter 10. Here we will mention only a few main points with regard to the anatomy of the basal ganglia.

The basal ganglia receive massive afferent connections from the cerebral cortex and acts, by way of their efferent fibers, primarily back on motor regions of the cortex. Sections through the hemispheres show that the basal ganglia consist of two main parts (Figs. 2.28, 2.29, and 2.30). In a horizontal section (Fig. 2.28) one large part lies lateral to the internal capsule, and a smaller medial to the internal capsule and anterior to the thalamus. The largest part is called the *lentiform nucleus* (nucleus lentiformis) because of its shape. It consists of two closely apposed parts: The lateral or external part is called the *putamen,* and the medial or internal part is called the *globus pallidus.* The part of the basal ganglia situated medial to the internal capsule is called the *caudate nucleus* (nucleus caudatus). The name describes its form—a large part of the nucleus is indeed formed like a long, curved tail (Figs. 2.32 and 10.1). The caudate nucleus consists of an anterior bulky part, the *caput* (head), and a progres-

sively thinner *cauda* (tail). The cauda extends first backward and then down and forward into the temporal lobe, located in the wall of the lateral ventricle. Figure 2.40 shows how this peculiar form can be explained on the basis of the embryonic development of the cerebral hemispheres.

THE CEREBELLUM

The cerebellum (the "little brain") is first and foremost of importance for the execution of movements; like the basal ganglia, it belongs to the motor system. The cerebellum is located in the posterior cranial fossa, dorsal to the brain stem (Figs. 2.1 and 2.33). It is connected with the brain stem anteriorly by way of three stalks of white matter on each side: *the inferior, middle, and superior cerebellar peduncles* (Figs. 2.15 and 2.17). In general, the inferior cerebellar peduncle or *restiform body* (corpus restiforme) contains fibers carrying impulses from the spinal cord to the cerebellum, whereas the middle cerebellar peduncle or the *brachium pontis* conveys information from the cerebral cortex. The superior cerebellar peduncle or the *bra-*

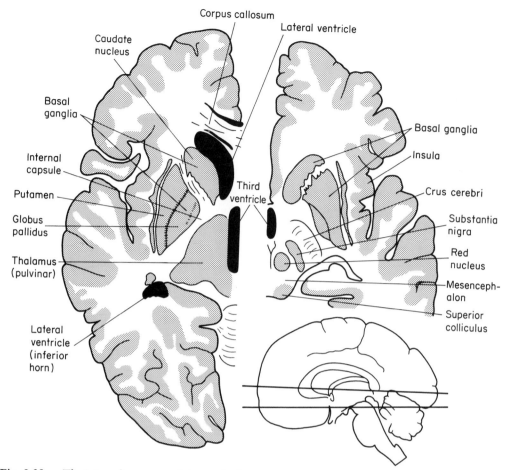

Caudate nucleus

Corpus callosum

Lateral ventricle

Basal ganglia

Basal ganglia

Insula

Internal capsule

Putamen

Third ventricle

Crus cerebri

Globus pallidus

Substantia nigra

Red nucleus

Thalamus (pulvinar)

Mesencephalon

Superior colliculus

Lateral ventricle (inferior horn)

Fig. 2.30. *The internal structure of the cerebral hemispheres.* Drawings of two horizontal sections at slightly different levels, the right section lowest. Compare with Figure 2.31.

chium conjunctivum contains most of the fibers conveying impulses out of the cerebellum—that is, the cerebellar efferent fibers.

Like the cerebrum, the cerebellum is covered by a layer of gray substance, the *cerebellar cortex* (cortex cerebelli), with underlying white matter. Enclosed in the white matter are regions of gray matter, the *central (deep) cerebellar nuclei* (Fig. 11.12). From the neurons in these nuclei come the majority of efferent fibers conveying information from the cerebellum to other parts of the central nervous system.

The cerebellar surface is extensively folded, forming numerous narrow sheets or *folia* that are predominantly oriented transversely (Fig. 2.33). The fissures and sulci between the folia are partly very deep; the deepest among them divide the cerebellum into *lobes* (this is further treated in Chapter 11). In addition, the cerebellum can be subdivided macroscopically on another basis. In the posterior part of the cerebellum a narrow middle region is situated deeper than the much larger lateral parts (Fig. 2.33B). This middle part of the cerebellum is called the *vermis* (worm) and is present also in the anterior part of the cerebellum, although not as clearly distinguished from the lateral parts as posteriorly. The lateral parts are called the *cerebellar hemispheres.* A small bulbous part on each is connected medially with a thin stalk to the vermis. This part is called the *flocculus* (Fig. 2.33B) and lies close

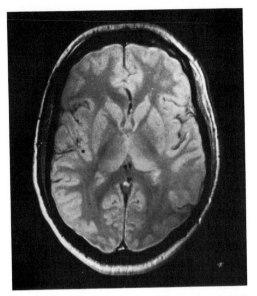

Fig. 2.31. *Magnetic resonance image* (MRI). Same direction and level of sectioning as in the left half of Figure 2.30. Courtesy of Dr. S. J. Bakke.

to the middle cerebellar peduncle, just posterior to the seventh and eighth cranial nerves.

A midsagittal section through the cerebellum (Fig. 2.33C) shows clearly the deep sulci and fissures. The white substance forms a treelike structure and is called the *arbor vitae* (the tree of life—perhaps not very fitting, since the cerebellum is not necessary for life). The fourth ventricle, extending into the cerebellum like the apex of a tent, is also evident in the midsagittal section.

THE COVERINGS OF THE BRAIN

The central nervous system is enclosed in three connective tissue membranes, the *meninges*. The innermost one is the vascular *pia mater* (usually just called *pia*). It follows the surface of the brain and spinal cord closely, and extends into all sulci and depressions of

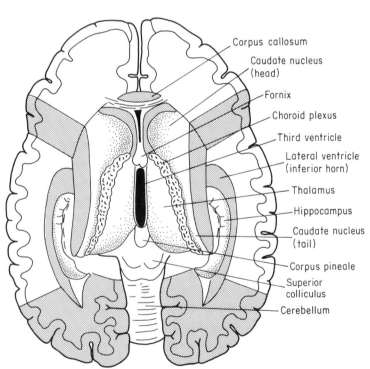

Corpus callosum
Caudate nucleus (head)
Fornix
Choroid plexus
Third ventricle
Lateral ventricle (inferior horn)
Thalamus
Hippocampus
Caudate nucleus (tail)
Corpus pineale
Superior colliculus
Cerebellum

Fig. 2.32. *The internal structure of the cerebral hemispheres.* Parts of the hemispheres are removed to open the lateral ventricles. In the anterior part, the caudate nucleus can be seen to form the bottom and lateral wall of the ventricle. In the temporal horn of the ventricle, the hippocampus forms the medial wall.

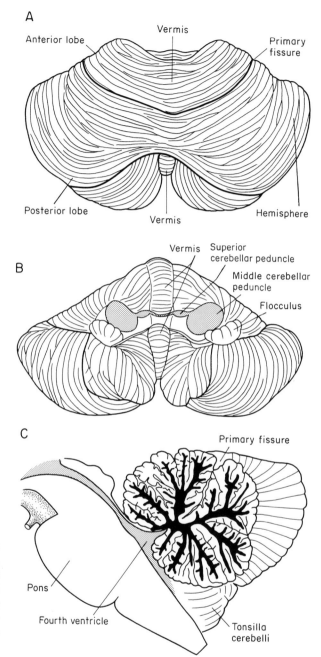

Fig. 2.33. *The cerebellum.* **A.** Seen from the rostral–posterior aspect. **B.** Seen from the ventral aspect (the side facing the brain stem). **C.** Midsagittal section showing the cerebellar cortex as a thin layer with white matter underneath (indicated in black in the drawing).

the surface (Figs. 2.34 and 2.35). Thin vessels pass from the pia into the substance of the brain and supply the external parts, such as the cerebral cortex, with blood (the deeper parts of the brain are supplied by vessels entering the brain at its basal surface). The next membrane, the *arachnoid*, does not follow the uneven surface of the brain but extends across depressions, fissures, and sulci. Between the pia and the arachnoid exists a narrow space, the *subarachnoid space*, which is filled with *cerebrospinal fluid* (Figs. 2.1, 2.34, and 2.35). Numerous thin threads of connective tissue connect the pia with the arachnoid, thus spanning the subarachnoid space. The depth of the subarachnoid space

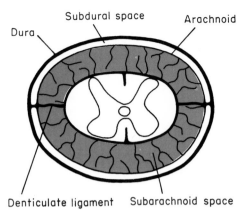

Fig. 2.34. *The meninges and subarachnoidal space of the spinal cord.*

varies from place to place because the arachnoid, as mentioned, does not follow the surface of the brain. Where it crosses larger depressions, the subarachnoid space is considerably widened, forming so-called *cisterns* filled with cerebrospinal fluid. Several cisterns are found around the brain stem, but the largest one, the *cisterna magna* or *cerebellomedullary cistern*, is located posterior to the medulla below the cerebellum (Figs. 2.1 and 2.2). The cerebrospinal fluid enters the cisterna magna from the fourth ventricle (Figs. 2.1 and 2.39).

The subarachnoid space is continuous around the whole central nervous system.

Substances released into the subarachnoid space at one place are therefore quickly spread out. A *subarachnoid hemorrhage*, for example, most often caused by rupture of a vessel at the base of the brain, quickly leads to all of the cerebrospinal fluid being mixed with blood. Thus, if a sample of cerebrospinal fluid is taken from the dural sac at lumbar levels, it will be bloody.

The outermost membrane, the *dura mater* (usually just called the *dura*), is thick and strong because it consists of dense connective tissue (Figs. 2.1, 2.34, and 2.35). The dura covers closely the inside of the skull and constitutes also the periosteum. The arachnoid follows the inside of the dura closely so that there is only a very narrow space between these two meninges, the *subdural space* (Figs. 2.34 and 2.35). The dura extends down into the vertebral canal to enclose the spinal cord. It extends further down than the cord, however, forming a sac around the roots of the lower spinal nerves (the cauda equina). This dural sac extends down to the level of the second sacral vertebra. Thus below the level of the first–second lumbar vertebra (the lower end of the cord) the dural sac contains only spinal nerve roots and cerebrospinal fluid (Figs. 2.1 and 2.5). This is a safe place to enter the subarachnoid space with a needle (lumbar punc-

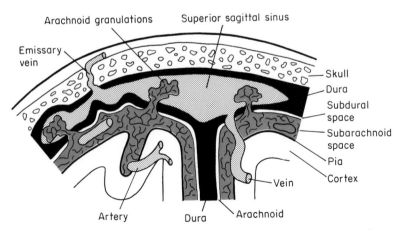

Fig. 2.35. *The meninges, the subarachnoidal space, and the superior sagittal sinus.* Schematic drawing of a frontal section through the head, with the skull and the brain. See also Figure 1.15.

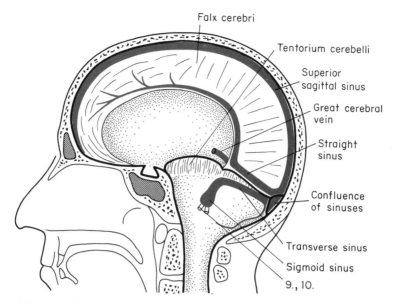

Falx cerebri

Tentorium cerebelli

Superior sagittal sinus

Great cerebral vein

Straight sinus

Confluence of sinuses

Transverse sinus

Sigmoid sinus

9., 10.

Fig. 2.36. *Folds of the dura and the venous sinuses.* The folds serve to minimize movements of the brain and also contain venous sinuses (red).

ture) to take samples of the cerebrospinal fluid, since there is no danger of harming the cord.

In a few places *the dura forms strong infoldings,* serving to restrict the movements of the brain within the skull. Large movements can stretch and damage vessels and nerves connecting the brain with the skull (one of the possible effects of head injuries). From the midline, the *falx cerebri* extends down between the two hemispheres (Fig. 2.36). Posteriorly, the falx divides into two parts that extend laterally over the superior face of the cerebellum and attach to the temporal pyramid (Fig. 2.37). These two folds meet in the midline and form the *cerebellar tentorium.* In the anterior part of the tentorium, there is an elongated opening for the brain stem. If the pressure in the skull above the tentorium increases (due to bleeding, a tumor, or brain edema), part of the temporal lobe may be pressed down (herniate) between the tentorium and the brain stem, harming the brain stem temporarily or permanently.

The spinal cord is anchored to the meninges partly by the spinal nerves and partly by

two thin bands, the *denticulate ligaments,* extending laterally from the cord to the arachnoid and dura (this is not a continuous ligament but one that forms 21 lateral extensions from the cord to the dura). The spinal cord nevertheless moves considerably up and down in the dural sac with movements of the vertebral column (the length of the vertebral canal varies by almost 10 cm from maximal flexion, when it is longest, to maximal extension).

THE CEREBRAL VENTRICLES AND THE CEREBROSPINAL FLUID

We have mentioned the ventricular system several times above in connection with treatment of the various parts of the brain. Here we will consider the ventricular system as a whole, along with the cerebrospinal fluid.

The Location and Form of the Ventricles

The thin central canal of the cord continues upward into the brain stem. There the canal

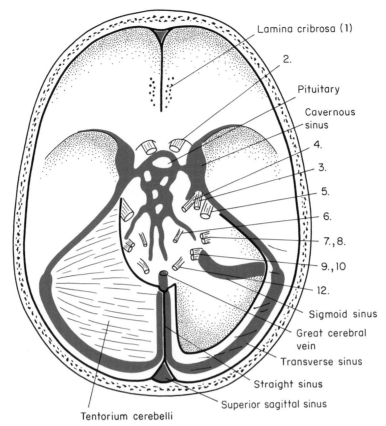

Fig. 2.37. *The tentorium cerebelli and the large venous sinuses at the base of the skull. At the right side, the tentorium is partly removed. The cra-* nial nerves and their sites of exit from the skull are also shown.

widens to form the fourth ventricle at the posterior aspect of the medulla and pons (Figs. 2.1, 2.38, and 2.39). The floor of the fourth ventricle is formed by the diamond-shaped *rhomboid fossa* (Fig. 2.17). The lateral walls of the ventricle are formed by the cerebellar peduncles. The ventricle has a tentlike form with the apex projecting into the cerebellum and two lateral evaginations (recessus lateralis).

The *third ventricle* is a thin slitlike room between the two thalami (Figs. 2.32, 2.38, and 2.39). During embryonic development, the primordia of the hemispheres become closely apposed to the diencephalon. The loose masses of connective tissue between the hemispheres form an approximately horizontal plate that constitues the roof of

the third ventricle. The choroid plexus is attached to the inside of the roof (Fig. 2.39).

The *two lateral ventricles* represent the first and second ventricles, but these terms are not used. From a central part in the parietal lobe, the lateral ventricles have processes called *horns* into the three other lobes: an *anterior* (frontal) horn, a *posterior* (occipital) horn, and an *inferior* (temporal) horn extending downward and anteriorly into the temporal lobe (Figs. 2.32 and 2.38). The anterior horn is the largest and is bordered medially by the septum pellucidum[5] (Fig. 2.39), whereas the head of the caudate nucleus bulges into it from the lateral side. The central part of the ventricle lies just above the thalamus (Fig. 2.32). The inferior horn starts at the transition between the central

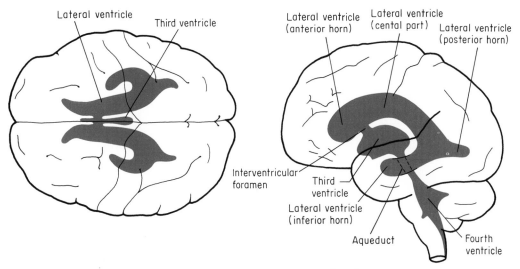

Fig. 2.38. *The ventricular system of the brain.*

part and the posterior horn and follows the temporal lobe almost to its tip. Medially in the inferior horn there is an elongated elevation, the *hippocampus* (Fig. 2.32), formed by invagination of the ventriclar wall from the medial side by the hippocampal fissure (Fig. 2.27).

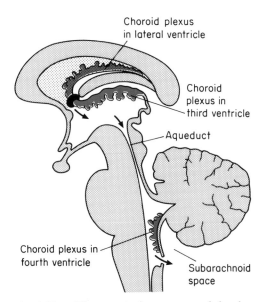

Fig. 2.39. *The ventricular system and the choroid plexus.* The flow of the cerebrospinal fluid is indicated with arrows in the drawing. All ventricles contain choroid plexus.

The form of the lateral ventricles can be understood on the basis of the embryonic development of the cerebrum (Fig. 2.40). Both the lateral ventricles and the nervous tissue in its walls (such as the caudate nucleus and the hippocampus) eventually obtain a curved shape.

The Cerebrospinal Fluid Is Produced by Vascular Plexuses in the Ventricles

All of the ventricles are filled with a clear, watery fluid, the *cerebrospinal fluid* (CSF). Most of the fluid is produced by vascular tufts, the *choroid plexus*. This is present in all four ventricles (Fig. 2.39), but the largest amount is found in the lateral ventricles. The plexuses are formed in early embryonic life by invaginations of the innermost meninx (the pia mater) at sites where the wall of the neural tube is very thin (Fig. 2.41). An elaborate structure of thin, branching protrusions or villi arises here (Fig. 2.42). The choroid plexuses are attached to the wall of the ventricles with a thin stalk (tela choroidea). The surface of the villi is covered by simple cuboid epithelium (which is continuous with the ependyma covering the inside of the ventricles). The epithelial cells have microvilli that increase their surface in con-

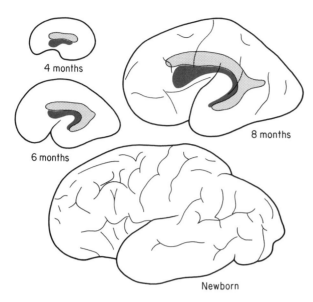

Fig. 2.40. *Development of the cerebral hemispheres and the lateral ventricles.* The characteristic arched shape of the ventricles can be explained by the manner in which the hemispheres fold during their growth in embryonic life. The caudate nucleus, located in the wall of the lateral ventricle, is indicated in red. All structures in the wall of the ventricles attain the curved shape. The figure also shows the development of gyri and sulci. Compare the pattern in the newborn and in the adult (Fig. 2.26). Based on Hamilton, Boyd, and Mossman (1972).

tact with the cerebrospinal fluid. The interior of the villi is composed of loose connective tissue with numerous capillaries of the fenestrated type, which are rather leaky. Therefore the hydrostatic pressure inside the capillaries produces a net flow of water with solutes (and a fair amount of proteins) into the interstitial space of the villi. This protein-rich fluid cannot leave the villi directly, however, since the epithelial cells covering the villi are attached to each other with tight junctions. The transport of water through the epithelium appears to be caused by active transport of sodium. Thus, the pumping of sodium produces an osmotic gradient so that water diffuses from the interior of the villi into the ventricles. Other ions, such as chloride and bicarbonate, follow the water passively.

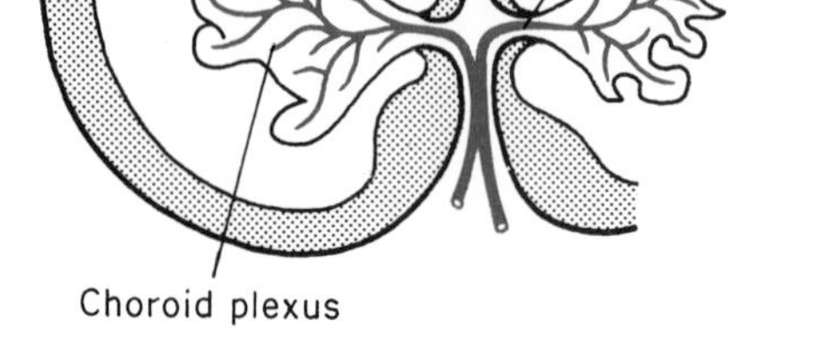

The epithelium of the choroid plexus represents a barrier between the blood and the cerebrospinal fluid, the *blood–cerebrospinal fluid barrier.* Thus, many substances that can leave the capillaries of the choroid plexus cannot enter the cerebrospinal fluid. This is obviously important, because neurons are extremely sensitive to changes in the composition of their environment. We will later describe a similar barrier between the blood in the brain capillaries and the brain interstitium.

Fig. 2.41. *Embryonic development of the choroid plexus.* Schematic drawing of a frontal section through the cerebral hemispheres at an early stage, showing how the choroid plexus is formed by invaginations of the pia into the ventricles.

Composition and Function of the Cerebrospinal Fluid

The concentration of sodium, potassium, and several other ions is about the same in the cerebrospinal fluid as in the blood (there are, however, some minor differences). The

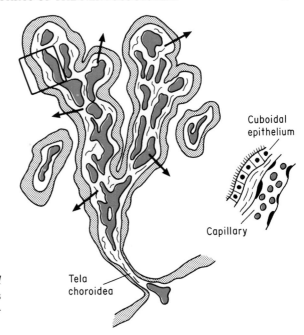

Cuboidal
epithelium

Capillary

Fig. 2.42. *The structure of the choroid plexus,* exemplified by one villus. Arrows indicate the flow of fluid from the capillaries to the ventricles.

Tela
choroidea

concentration of glucose is about two-thirds that in the blood. A major difference concerns proteins: There is normally very little protein in the cerebrospinal fluid (less than 0.5% of the plasma protein concentration).

Water and soluble substances are freely exchangeable between the cerebrospinal fluid and the interstitial fluid of the nervous tissue because the ependyma is freely permeable to water and even small protein molecules. It is, therefore, not surprising that many of the neurotransmitters, peptides, and other neuroactive substances can be found in the cerebrospinal fluid. Some substances, notably hormones synthesized in the anterior pituitary, are apparently actively secreted into the cerebrospinal fluid and thus reach it not only by passive diffusion. The functional role of the various neurotransmitters and peptides present in the cerebrospinal fluid is not yet known.

Determination of the presence and concentration of various neuroactive substances in the cerebrospinal fluid is nevertheless of great interest, because it represents an indirect way of examining the extracellular fluid of the brain, which is very difficult to examine directly. Owing to the free permeability of the ependymal layer, the concentration of a substance in the cerebrospinal fluid presumably corresponds closely to that in the extracellular fluid of the nervous tissue—that is, in the immediate vicinity of the neurons.

We mentioned at the beginning of this chapter that, because the brain almost floats in it, the cerebrospinal fluid has important *protective functions.* This buoyancy reduces the weight of the brain to about 50 g, which means less traction on vessels and nerves connected to the central nervous system. Furthermore, the effect on the brain of blows to the head is dampened because water has to be pressed aside before the brain hits its hard surroundings (the skull).

Another possible functional role of the cerebrospinal fluid can be deduced from the fact, mentioned above, that water and solutes can pass freely between it and the extracellular fluid (interstitium) of the nervous tissue. Thus, accumulation of substances in the nervous tissue (such as potassium ions during prolonged periods of intense neuronal activity) may be minimized by diffusion into the cerebrospinal fluid. In general, it appears likely that the cerebrospinal fluid *con-*

tributes to the maintenance of a constant composition of the neuronal environment. This is important, for example, for the excitability of the neurons. As discussed in Chapter 1, glial cells also have important roles in this respect.

Circulation and Drainage of the Cerebrospinal Fluid

About one-half liter of cerebrospinal fluid is produced each day, yet the total volume of fluid in the ventricles and the subarachnoid space is less than 150 ml. Thus, the total amount is renewed several times a day. This means that effective means of drainage must exist.

The fluid produced in the lateral ventricles flows into the third ventricle through the *interventricular foramen* (of Monro) (Fig. 2.39). From there the fluid flows through the narrow *cerebral aqueduct* to the fourth ventricle. More fluid is added by the choroid plexuses in the third and fourth ventricles. The fluid leaves the ventricular system and enters the subarachnoid space (more specifically the cisterna magna) through three openings in the roof of the fourth ventricle—one in the midline posteriorly (the foramen of Magendie) and two laterally (the lateral recesses or foramina of Luschka) (Figs. 2.1 and 2.39). The fluid then spreads out over the entire surface of the brain and spinal cord. From the base of the brain, there is an upward stream along the lateral aspects of the hemispheres toward the midline. Here, most of the cerebrospinal fluid empties into venous sinuses. This happens by way of small evaginations of the arachnoid (arachnoid villi) into the venous sinuses. Several villi together form macroscopically visible protrusions called *arachnoid granulations,* which are particularly prominent along the superior sagittal sinus (Fig. 2.35). The passage of fluid from the subarachnoid space to the venous sinuses is probably caused by a difference in hydrostatic pressure—the pressure being higher in the subarachnoid space (about 15 cm H_2O) than in the sinuses (7–8 cm H_2O). Some of

the cerebrospinal fluid is drained via other routes, such as lymphatic vessels in cranial and spinal nerves.

Diseases Affecting the Ventricles and the Cerebrospinal Fluid

Because the central nervous system and the cerebrospinal fluid are located in a closed container with rigid walls, the pressure inside the container increases if, for some reason, the amount of substance inside it increases. The intracranial pressure is the same for the nervous tissue and the cerebrospinal fluid, but it can be measured most conveniently in the latter. For each heartbeat, for example, the pressure inside the cerebral ventricles increases slightly because more blood is pumped into the brain. Correspondingly, the pressure increases on coughing and straining because the drainage of venous blood from the cranial cavity and the vertebral canal is reduced and the volume inside increases. *Regardless of cause, any intracranial expansive process leads to increased intracranial pressure.* When the pressure increases, the blood pressure has to be increased to maintain cerebral blood flow. Thus, abnormally elevated blood pressure, usually combined with slowing of the heart rate, is one of the signs of severely increased intracranial pressure. However, if the increase is above a certain level, the cerebral blood flow is reduced, and the functioning of the brain suffers (with signs of confusion and eventually loss of consciousness). This happens, for example, in patients with *brain edema.* This is a dangerous complication of acute brain damage caused by, for example, head injuries. The edema is caused by extravasation of fluid from the brain capillaries. Similarly, an intracranial hemorrhage, which may arise from vessels inside or outside the brain substance, can also cause a dangerous increase of the intracranial pressure. If the expansive process is located in the posterior fossa (below the tentorium cerebelli), the tonsilla cerebelli (Fig. 2.33C) may be dislocated downward into the foramen magnum and thus compress the medulla (tonsillar herniation). If the expansive process is located above the tentorium cerebelli (in the middle or anterior fossa), the uncus of the temporal lobe (Fig. 2.27) can be dislocated downward beneath the edge of the tentorium and compress the brain stem at the level of the mesencephalon (Fig. 2.28). Both forms of herniation may lead to serious brain damage or death.

If the amount of cerebrospinal fluid is increased in the ventricles, the pressure usually increases as well. A condition with an increased amount of cerebrospinal fluid is called *hydrocephalus*. Most often, this is caused by obstruction of the drainage of the cerebrospinal fluid—for example, by closure of the aqueduct (inflammation, tumor, bleeding) or the outlets from the fourth ventricles. If this happens in an adult, in whom the sutures of the skull have grown firmly together, the intracranial pressure increases markedly, with dramatic symptoms. If, however, the condition arises in early childhood before the sutures are closed, the size of the head grows abnormally, with the skull yielding to the increased intracranial pressure. This may continue for some time with surprisingly few signs of cerebral dysfunction, but the development of the brain will eventually suffer, with results such as mental retardation. Hydrocephalus in children may be treated by shunting the cerebrospinal fluid directly into a big vein outside the skull. A thin tube is inserted through a small hole in the skull into the lateral ventricle and is then directed under the skin, usually to where the internal jugular and the subclavian veins meet. In this manner, damage to the brain may be prevented.

Examination of the cerebrospinal fluid can provide valuable information about neurological diseases. A sample of the fluid is usually withdrawn with a thin needle from the subarachnoid space in the dural sac—that is, below the level of the second lumbar vertebra. This way there is no risk of damaging the spinal cord (Figs. 2.1 and 2.5). When the tip of the needle is in the subarachnoid space, the intracranial pressure can also be determined. Examination of the fluid, in part under the microscope, can give information about possible bleeding into the subarachnoid space and about infections and inflammations of the brain itself (encephalitis) or the meninges (meningitis). In the latter case there are numerous leukocytes in the cerebrospinal fluid. The concentration of proteins, normally very low, may increase in certain diseases (for example, in multiple sclerosis, in which the proteins are antibodies against components of the nervous tissue).

The shape and size of the ventricles can now be determined noninvasively in living subjects by use of computer tomography (CT) and magnetic resonance imaging (MRI) (Figs. 2.2, 2.29, and 2.31). Atrophy of the nervous tissue of the brain—for example, the atrophy of the cerebral cortex occurring in dementia—leads to dilatation of the ventricles, whereas expansive, space-occupying processes like hemorrhages and tumors may distort and compress the ventricles.

THE BLOOD SUPPLY OF THE CENTRAL NERVOUS SYSTEM

Of all cell types in our body, neurons are the most sensitive to interruption of their supply of oxygen (anoxia). Only a few minutes' stop in the blood flow may produce neuronal death. The oxygen consumption of the brain is high even at rest. Therefore, the blood supply of the central nervous system is ample, and the brain receives about 15% of the cardiac output at rest. Regulatory mechanisms ensure that the brain gets what it needs—if necessary, at the expense of all other organs. The arteries of the brain lie within the cranial cavity and are mostly devoid of anastomoses (connections) with arteries outside the skull. Therefore, other arteries cannot take over if the intracranial ones are narrowed or occluded.

The Blood–Brain Barrier Prevents Many Substances from Entering the Brain

In most organs of our body, small-molecular substances pass the capillary wall with relative ease, and their concentration is therefore similar in the blood plasma and in the interstitial fluid. The composition of the interstitial (extracellular) fluid of the brain differs, however, from that in most other organs. The *blood–brain barrier* (we have previously mentioned a similar barrier between the blood and the cerebrospinal fluid) is due to special, selective properties of the brain capillaries. Many small molecules cannot pass the capillary wall at all, whereas others pass with greater ease than in other organs. Thus, *there is not only a barrier intercalated between the blood and the brain but also specific transport mechanisms for certain substances that the brain needs.*

The barrier properties of the brain capillaries appear to be caused mainly by very extensive *tight junctions* between the endothelial cells. Substances therefore have to pass through the plasma membrane of the capillaries to enter the brain interstitium.[6] Water-soluble substances are thus effectively prevented from passing (except via specific uptake-mechanisms), whereas lipid-soluble substances can pass the plasma membrane with ease. This is of consequence for whether a drug may gain access to the brain; only lipid-soluble drugs can as a rule reach therapeutic concentrations in the brain. Certain drugs—such as barbiturates used for induction of anesthesia—are highly lipid-soluble and act rapidly. Other drugs, such as penicillin, have low lipid solubility and pass the blood–brain barrier only with difficulty.

Glucose is an example of a substance with high water solubility that nevertheless reaches high concentrations in the brain (this is necessary because the neurons depend almost solely on glucose as a source of energy). The reason is that the plasma membrane of the brain endothelial cells is equipped with carrier proteins that transport glucose actively. Similar active mechanisms exist for other water-soluble substances that the brain needs.

There is evidence that the special barrier properties of the brain capillaries depend upon influence from surrounding astrocytes. As mentioned earlier, all brain capillaries are surrounded by astrocyte processes (Fig. 1.15D), and these probably induce the special morphological and functional features of the brain capillaries.

In several different, unrelated *diseases of the brain, the blood–brain barrier becomes less effective.* At the ultrastructural level the capillaries are changed with loss of tight junctions as a prominent feature, and at the same time there are also changes of the astrocytes.

The blood–brain barrier appears first and foremost to have *protective functions.* Many foreign substances that would be harmful to the neurons are kept out. Also, neuroactive substances in the bloodstream, such as neurotransmitters and peptides (produced in the peripheral nervous tissue, endocrine organs,

and the gut) are prevented from reaching the brain. For example, fluctuations of the plasma level of norepinephrine or serotonin are not accompanied by similar fluctuations in the brain, which would have disturbed its normal functioning.

It is also likely that the endothelial cells of the brain actively pump several ions that are present in different concentrations in the blood plasma and in the extracellular fluid of the brain (Na^+, K^+, Ca^{2+}, and others). Even more than other cells, neurons depend on precise control of the concentrations of such ions for their normal functioning (for example, their excitability is increased by an increase of the extracellular potassium concentration).

The Brain Receives Arterial Blood from the Internal Carotid and the Vertebral Arteries

Broadly speaking, the internal carotid artery supplies most of the cerebral hemispheres, whereas the vertebral artery supplies the brain stem and the cerebellum.

The *internal carotid artery* (arteria carotis interna) enters the cranial cavity through a canal at the base of the skull (the carotid canal in the temporal bone) and then divides into three branches (Fig. 2.43). The *ophthalmic artery* passes to the orbit through the optic canal and thus does not supply the brain itself (although, strictly speaking, the retina is part of the central nervous system). The *anterior cerebral artery* runs forward over the optic nerve and along the medial aspect of the hemispheres. Its branches reach only a short distance onto the convexity of the hemispheres (Fig. 2.45). The *middle cerebral artery* is the largest branch. It curves laterally into the lateral cerebral fissure and follows this backward and upward (Figs. 2.44 and 2.45). On its way, numerous branches are given off that supply most of the cerebral cortex on the convexity of the hemispheres, notably the *motor* and *somatosensory cortical areas,* except for their most medial parts (with neuronal groups concerned with the motor and sensory func-

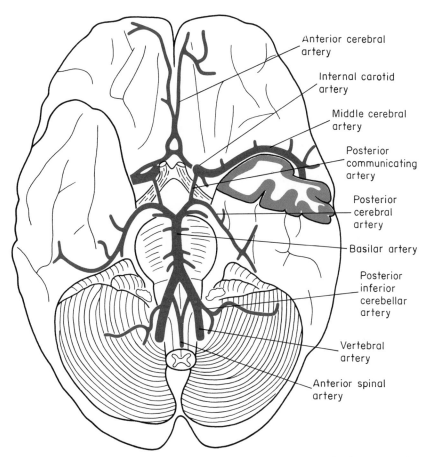

Anterior cerebral artery

Internal carotid artery

Middle cerebral artery

Posterior communicating artery

Posterior cerebral artery

Basilar artery

Posterior inferior cerebellar artery

Vertebral artery

Anterior spinal artery

Fig. 2.43. *The main arteries of the brain.* Note anastomoses between branches of the internal carotid artery and the vertebral artery and between the two anterior cerebral arteries. These anastomoses form an arterial circuit at the base of the brain.

tions of the legs; see Figs. 9.4 and 9.8), which are supplied by the anterior cerebral artery. The deep parts of the cerebrum, such as the *basal ganglia* and the *internal capsule,* are supplied by their own branches from the middle cerebral artery (Fig. 2.44).

The *vertebral artery* (Fig. 2.43) enters the posterior fossa after ascending through the transverse foramina of the cervical vertebrae. When passing from the atlas through the foramen magnum, the artery is highly convoluted, enabling it to follow the large movements in the upper cervical joints without being overstretched or compressed. Nevertheless, by extreme movements—particularly in elderly people with sclerotic arteries—the vertebral artery may be temporarily occluded. This may lead to loss of

consciousness due to lack of blood supply to the brain stem. Backward bending of the head combined with rotation is particularly apt to compress the vertebral artery. The vertebral arteries of the two sides unite at the lower level of the pons to form the *basilar artery* (Fig. 2.43). The vertebral arteries and the basilar artery send off numerous branches to supply the medulla oblongata, the pons, the mesencephalon, and the cerebellum. One of these, the *posterior inferior cerebellar artery* (PICA), supplies the lateral part of the medulla and parts of the cerebellar hemispheres.

At the upper end of the pons, the basilar artery divides into its two end branches, the *posterior cerebral arteries.* These curve posteriorly around the mesencephalon and con-

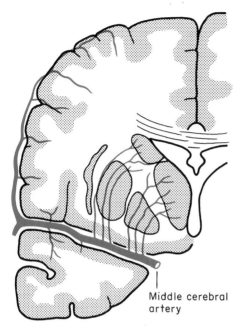

Middle cerebral
artery

Fig. 2.44. *The course of the middle cerebral artery.* In the depth of the lateral fissure, it gives off branches to the internal capsule and the basal ganglia.

tinue at the medial side of the hemisphere to the occipital lobe (Figs. 2.43 and 2.45). The posterior cerebral artery supplies large parts of the occipital lobe, notably the *visual cortex,* and the inferior aspect of the temporal lobe.

There Are Communications between the Vertebral and Carotid Arteries and between the Arteries of the Two Sides

At the base of the brain there is a connection on each side between the middle and the posterior cerebral arteries, the *posterior communicating artery* (arteria communicans posterior) (Fig. 2.43). This means that if one of the two main arterial trunks (the internal carotid or the vertebral artery) is narrowed or even occluded, the other may to some extent compensate for the loss (as long as the communicating artery is open). There is also a corresponding communicating artery between the two anterior cerebral arteries (Fig. 2.43). In this manner a circle of anastomosing arteries is formed at the base of the skull,

the *circle of Willis,* which may be of great clinical significance. It may explain, for example, how some people may have a totally occluded internal carotid artery on one side without any neurological signs.

The Spinal Cord Receives Arteries at Many Levels

In general, the arteries of the cord are arranged with one artery running in midline anteriorly, the *anterior spinal artery,* and one on each side running along the rows of posterior roots, the *posterior spinal arteries* (Fig. 2.46). All three arteries begin cranially as branches of the vertebral arteries but receive contributions from small arteries entering the vertebral canal along with the spinal nerves.

The *venous blood* is collected in a venous plexus at the surface of the cord. This plexus empties into another, larger plexus at the surface of the dura, the *epidural plexus* (Fig. 2.8). From there the blood is emptied into veins outside the vertebral canal.

The Venous Blood Is Collected in Sinuses and Leaves the Skull in the Internal Jugular Vein

The cerebral veins can be divided into deep and superficial types. The latter partly accompany the arteries on the surface of the brain. All of the veins empty into large *venous sinuses* that are formed by folds of the dura (Figs. 2.36 and 2.37). At the base of the skull there are several sinuses, among them the *cavernous sinus* lateral to the pituitary gland. The superficial veins at the dorsal parts of the hemispheres run upward and medially and empty into the large *superior sagittal sinus* in the upper margin of the falx cerebri. Where the falx cerebri meets the tentorium cerebelli, the superior sagittal sinus divides into two parts, the *transverse sinuses.* These follow a transverse course laterally along where the tentorium is attached to the occipital bone. The *sigmoid sinus*—forming the direct continuation of the transverse sinus—empties into the *internal jugu-*

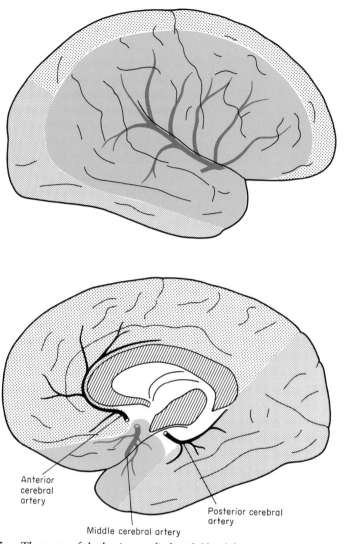

Anterior
cerebral
artery

Middle cerebral artery

Posterior cerebral
artery

Fig. 2.45. *The parts of the brain supplied with blood from the main arterial branches.*

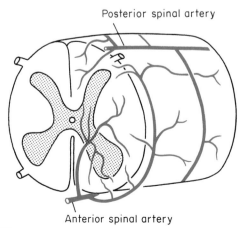

Posterior spinal artery

Anterior spinal artery

Fig. 2.46. *The arterial supply of the spinal cord.*

lar vein at the jugular foramen. The internal jugular vein leaves the skull and continues downward into the neck.

Most of the blood in the deep cerebral veins collects into the *great cerebral vein* of Galen (vena cerebri magna) (Fig. 2.37). This comes out from the inferior side of the posterior end of the corpus callosum and empties into the *straight sinus* (sinus rectus) in the midline of the tentorium. The sinus rectus drains into the superior sagittal sinus at the *confluence* region, from which the transverse sinus originates (Fig. 2.37).

Unlike the arteries, the cerebral veins have numerous anastomoses. At some locations there are also *emissary veins* that form connections between intracranial and extracranial veins (Fig. 2.35).

Veins draining into the sinuses from the subarachnoid space—for example, along the superior sagittal sinus—are called *bridging veins* (Fig. 2.35). They constitute some of the few attachments that exist between the convexity of the hemispheres and the skull. Head injuries that lead to sudden displacement of the brain inside the skull may cause bridging veins to tear, with venous bleeding as a result. This results in a *chronic subdural hematoma,* which expands very slowly (due to an osmotic effect of the decomposing blood of the hematoma). The name implies that the blood collects between the dura and the arachnoid, in the subdural space. The blood remains localized, in contrast to what happens when the bleeding occurs in the subarachnoid space. The symptoms arising from a subdural hematoma may be due to pressure on the underlying parts of the brain (for example, paresis if the hematoma overlies the motor cortex), or they may be due to increased intracranial pressure with more nonspecific symptoms, such as headache and confusion.

NOTES

1. Strictly speaking, most neurons in the central nervous system are interneurons according to this definition—including, for example, spinal neurons with axons ascending to the brain. In practice the term interneurons is nevertheless restricted to neurons with an axon ramifying in the vicinity of the cell body, thus synaptically coupling neurons within one nucleus.

2. It was formerly believed that propriospinal neurons—that is, spinal neurons with axons entering the white matter but not leaving the spinal cord—and interneurons represented two distinct cell groups. Recent studies have, however, shown that spinal interneurons have local (intrasegmental) branches as well as collaterals destined for other segments (intersegmental).

3. The *pedunculus cerebri*, strictly speaking, includes both the crus cerebri and parts of the mesencephalon dorsal to the crus except the colliculi (connectively termed the *tectum*). The region between the crus cerebri and the tectum is called the *tegmentum* and includes the periaqueductal gray, the red nucleus, and the substantia nigra. Previously, however, the crus cerebri and pedunculus cerebri were both applied to the ventralmost, fiber-rich part.

4. The name basal ganglia is unfortunate and has been retained from a time when all collections of neurons were called ganglia, regardless of whether they were located inside or outside the central nervous system. Today we use the term ganglion only of collections of neurons *outside* the central nervous system, as discussed in Chapter 1.

5. Between the septum pellucidum of the two sides there is a thin slit that has nothing to do with the ventricles. The slit was originally continuous with the room between the two hemispheres, but has been closed by the corpus callosum growing across the two hemispheres. Downward, the slit is closed by the fornices lying close together.

6. In the capillary walls of most other organs, there are slits—as a result of less extensive tight junctions between the endothelial cells—where water can flow.

3

How Are the Structure and Function of the Nervous System Studied?

Many approaches have been used to study the structure and function of the nervous system, from straightforward observations of its macroscopic appearance to determination of the function of single neuronal molecules. Recent years have witnessed a tremendous development of methods, so that problems can be approached today that formerly were a matter of speculation only. The number of neuroscientists has also increased almost exponentially, and they are engaged in problems ranging from molecular genetics to behavior. The mass of knowledge in the field of neurobiology has increased accordingly, and, more importantly, the understanding of how our brains work has improved considerably. Nevertheless, the steadily expanding amount of information has made it more difficult than before for each scientist to have a comprehensive knowledge of more than his or her own field. The rapid advancement of user-friendly computer systems for accessing the voluminous literature may help in this respect.

Traditionally, methods used for neurobiological research were grouped into those dealing with structure (neuroanatomy) and those aiming at disclosing the function of the structures (neurophysiology, neuropsy-

chology). The borders, however, are far from sharp, and it is typical of modern neuroscience that anatomic, physiological, biochemical, pharmacological, psychological, and other methods are combined. Furthermore, the introduction of modern computer-based imaging techniques has opened exciting possibilities for studying the relation between structure and function in the living human brain. The number of methods used in modern neuroscience is so large that only a few will be mentioned here. More and more of the methods originally developed in cell biology and immunology are being applied to the nervous system, and we now realize that neurons are not so different from other cells as was once assumed.

Here we will discuss a selection of methods that form the basis of most of what is presented in this book. The emphasis will be on methods that show the "wiring pattern" of the brain, and those that reveal the relationship between structure and function. Although knowledge of structure alone does not tell us how the brain operates or how its various parts function, such knowledge is nevertheless a prerequisite for sound interpretations of findings obtained with other methods.

SOME GENERAL FEATURES OF NEUROBIOLOGICAL RESEARCH

Animal Experiments Have Been Crucial for Progress

Only a minor part of our present knowledge of the nervous system is based on observations in man; most has been obtained in experimental animals. In humans we are usually limited to comparison of symptoms caused by naturally occurring diseases with the findings made at postmortem examination of the brain. Two cases are seldom identical, and the structural derangement of the brain is often too extensive to enable unequivocal conclusions. In animals, on the other hand, the experimental conditions can be controlled, and the experiments may be repeated, to reach reliable conclusions. The properties of the elements of neural tissue can be examined directly—for example, the activity of single neurons can be correlated with the behavior of the animal. Parts of the nervous system can also be studied in isolation—for example, by using tissue slices that can be kept viable in vitro for hours. This enables recordings and experimental manipulations to be done, with subsequent structural analysis of the tissue. Studies in invertebrates with a simple nervous system have made it possible to discover fundamental mechanisms underlying synaptic function and the functioning of simple neuronal networks.

When addressing questions about functions specific to the most highly developed nervous systems, however, experiments must be performed in higher mammals, such as cats and monkeys, with a well-developed cerebral cortex. Even from such experiments, inferences about the human nervous system must be drawn with great caution. Thus, even though the nervous systems in all higher mammals show striking similarities with regard to their basic principles of organization, important differences exist in the relative development of the various parts. Such anatomic differences indicate that there are functional differences as well. Therefore, results based on the study of humans, as done in clinical neurology, psychiatry, and psychology, must have the final word when it comes to functions of the human brain. But because the clinician seldom can experiment, he must often build his conclusions on observations made in experimental animals. He must decide whether findings obtained in patients or normal volunteers can be explained on such a basis. If this is not possible, the clinical findings may raise new problems that require studies in experimental animals to be solved. Basically, however, the methods used for study of the human brain are the same as those used in the study of experimental animals.

Experiments on animals are often criticized from an ethical point of view. The question of whether such experiments are acceptable, however, cannot be entirely separated from the broader question of whether mankind has the right to determine the lives of animals by using them for food, by taking over their territories, and so forth. With regard to using animals for scientific purposes, one has to realize that a better understanding of man as a thinking, feeling, and acting being requires, among other things, further animal experiments. Even though cell cultures and computer models may replace some, in the foreseeable future we will still need animal experiments. Computer-based models of the neuronal interactions taking place in the cerebral cortex, for example, usually turn out to require further animal experiments to test their tenability. Improved knowledge and understanding of the human brain is, however, also mandatory if we want to improve the prospects for treatment of the many diseases affecting the nervous system. Until today, these diseases— most often leading to severe suffering and disability—have only occasionally been amenable to effective treatment. Modern neurobiological research nevertheless gives hope, and many promising results have appeared in the last few years. Again, this would not have been possible without animal experiments.

Yet there are obviously limits to what can be defended ethically, even when the purpose is to alleviate human suffering. Strict rules have been made by the governmental authorities and the scientific community itself to ensure that only properly trained persons perform animal experiments and that the experiments are conducted so that discomfort and pain are reduced to a minimum. Most international neuroscience journals require that the experiments they publish have been conducted in accordance with such rules.

There Are Sources of Error in All Methods

Even though we will not treat systematically the sources of error inherent in the various methods to be discussed in this book, it should be realized that all methods have their limitations. One source of error when doing animal experiments is to draw premature conclusions about conditions in humans. In general, all experiments aim at *isolating* structures and processes so that they can be observed more clearly. However necessary this may be, it also means that many phenomena are only studied out of their natural context. Conclusions with regard to how the parts function in conjunction with all of the others must therefore be speculative.

Purely anatomic methods also have their sources of error and have led to many erroneous conclusions in the past about connections between neuronal groups. Such errors may in turn may lead to misinterpretations of physiological and psychological data. The study of man also entails sources of error—for example, of a psychological nature. Thus, the answers and information given by a patient or a volunteer are not always reliable; the patient may, for example, want to please the doctor and answers accordingly.

Scientific "Truths" Must Be Revised from Time to Time

That our methods have sources of error and that our interpretations of data are not always tenable are witnessed by the fact that

our concepts of the nervous system must be revised regularly. Reinterpretations of old data and changing concepts are often made necessary by the introduction of new methods. As in all areas of science, conclusions based on the available data should not be regarded as final truths but as more or less probable and preliminary interpretations. Natural science is basically concerned with posing questions to nature. How understandable and unequivocal the answers are depends on the precision of our questions and how relevant they are to the problem we are studying—stupid questions receive stupid answers. It is furthermore fundamental to science—although not always easy for the individual scientist to live up to—that conclusions and interpretations be made without any bias and solely on the strength of the facts and the arguments. It should be irrelevant whether the scientist is a young student or a Nobel laureate.

METHODS
Comparative Studies

Comparison of functional specialization and the development of particular parts of the nervous system in different species has given us much insight, and is still a useful and robust method in neuroscience. When a part of the brain is particularly well developed in a species with certain behavioral characteristics and only slightly developed in other species lacking these characteristics, conclusions about the correlation between structure and function can be drawn with some confidence. Such comparative studies have now been extended from purely anatomic ones down to the molecular level.

Dissection and Microscopic Examination Laid the Foundation for Knowledge of the Structure of the Nervous System

Our first knowledge of the structure of the nervous system and its subdivision into different parts was gained by simple macroscopic observation and dissection. The names of the major subdivisions as we use them today stem from such investigations with simple and primitive methods, made before there was any knowlege of the construction of the nervous tissue. A better understanding of the building elements of the nervous system and their interconnections was first made possible with the invention of the light microscope in the middle of the nineteenth century. Thus, tissue that was fixed, cut in thin sections, and stained to differentiate among structural elements could be examined. By the turn of the century, the main features of the microscopic structure and many of the interconnections of the major cell groups were known. This was partly achieved with staining methods that predominantly stain cell bodies, *Nissl staining,* which was used for *cytoarchitectonic* characterization of the gray substance, such as dividing the cerebral cortex in different areas and the brain stem in numerous separate nuclei (Figs. 1.14 and 17.1–17.3). Partly, methods visualizing primarily the *myelin sheaths* (Fig. 2.17) enabled the early anatomists to follow the course of the major fiber tracts. Methods that visualized neurons by impregnating them with the salts of heavy metals (of silver and gold) made it possible to study also the dendrites and axonal ramifications. The *Golgi method* (intro-

duced by the Italian anatomist Camillo Golgi) was particularly powerful in this respect and is widely used even today. With the Golgi method, only a small percentage of all neurons within a region are impregnated, which provides a clearer view of the neuronal processes (Figs. 1.3 and 17.5). In young animals, before the fiber tracts are myelinated, axons can be followed for considerable distances after Golgi impregnation. It was then possible to formulate basic rules with regard to how neurons are interconnected and communicate. The great Spanish neuroanatomist Ramón y Cajal expressed particularly clearly, on the basis of his own careful observations, that neuronal impulse traffic is one-way and that the synapse is the site of communication betweeen nerve cells.

To study connections between neuronal groups that are far apart, observations in normal material are not sufficient. Experimental methods were developed on the basis of the fact that when an axon is cut, characteristic structural changes occur in the perikaryon and in the parts of the axon distal to the cut (Fig. 3.1). The perikaryon first swells and thereafter shrinks and disappears, undergoing *retrograde degeneration.* By making restricted experimental lesions and looking in the microscope for signs of retrograde degeneration, the main features of

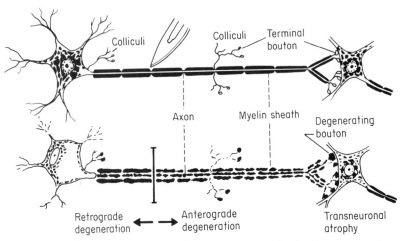

Fig. 3.1. *Transection of an axon in the central nervous system.* The distal part of the axon dis-
integrates and is finally removed. The perikaryon exhibits a characteristic, *chromatolytic* reaction.

the central nervous system's connections were clarified. The axonal changes distal to the cut are called *anterograde degeneration.* The first method that visualized axons undergoing anterograde degeneration was the Marchi method, which stains degenerational products of myelin. By destroying the perikarya of a nucleus, it was possible to follow the course and, to some extent, the termination of their axons. Since, however, many axons are unmyelinated, either along their full course or just before they end, the Marchi method cannot visualize all fiber tracts or even for the myelinated ones, their exact sites of termination.

If a neuronal group is destroyed, the target neurons on which they form synapses sometimes also show signs of degeneration. The neurons may shrink and eventually disappear by this *transneuronal degeneration,* which may give valuable information about connectivity. For example, connections from the retina to the thalamus were described in detail on the basis of this method. The transneuronal degeneration is presumably caused by the lack of a trophic substance normally delivered by the presynaptic neuron to the postsynaptic one, but lack of activity also appears to play a role.

In the 1950s, methods were developed that enabled vastly improved precision in the determination of neuronal connectivity. These methods were based on the impregnation of degenerating axons by silver salts, the *silver impregnation methods* (the Nauta method and the Fink and Heimer method have been used most widely). With such methods the axons can in some cases be followed even to their boutons. In about 20 years these methods brought a wealth of new information and improved considerably our understanding of how the nervous system is organized.

By the end of the past century, when neurohistological techniques provided new insight into the internal structure of the nervous system, physiological studies based on the electrical nature of the nerve impulse were also in rapid progress. Increasingly sensitive methods were developed to record the activity of nerve cells and to stimulate well-defined parts of the nervous system. From initially being able to record only the activity of large neuronal assemblies, it became possible to record the activity of single neurons.

Modern Methods for Tracing of Neuronal Connections

Another great leap forward in the investigation of neuronal connections was made at the end of the 1960s with the introduction of methods using *axonal transport* of tracer substances. In contrast to degeneration methods, they take advantage of the normal processes of the cells and avoid damaging the neurons under study. This eliminates several of the sources of error of the degeneration methods. In addition, the axonal transport methods are more sensitive than the degeneration methods, and in a short time many "new" connections were described. Our concepts of how neurons are interconnected had to be partly revised on the basis of these new findings.

Axonal transport is directed both *anterogradely* and *retrogradely,* as described in Chapter 1. The first method to be utilized was *anterograde transport of radioactively labeled amino acids.* Amino acids are normally taken up by the perikarya and used for protein synthesis. Many of these proteins are transported anterogradely to the boutons. After injection of (most often) tritium-labeled leucine or proline, the transported material can be visualized in tissue sections by autoradiography. This method can also be used for electron microscopy and then enables definite conclusions about synaptic relations. For *retrograde transport* especially, the enzyme *horseradish peroxidase* (HRP) has been widely used, either alone (free HRP) or conjugated to another molecule (wheat germ agglutinin [WGA]) that is taken up more readily by the nerve cells than free HRP. A small amount (for example, 0.1 μl) of a solution of the tracer is injected and is then taken up by the nerve terminals in the injected area and transported retrogradely

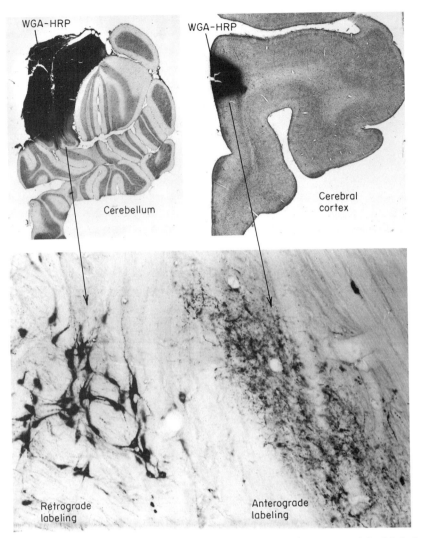

Fig. 3.2. *Retrograde and anterograde axonal transport.* A cat received injections of HRP–WGA in the cerebellum and in the cerebral cortex (0.2 μl in each). The extension of the tracer at the injection site is seen in the sections by the black reaction product obtained after incubation of the sections with tetramethylbenzidine (TMB). The tracer is transported retrogradely from the cerebellum to the pontine nuclei in the brain stem. The retrogradely labeled cells are black in the section from the pontine nuclei shown below. From the injection site in the cerebral cortex, the tracer is transported anterogradely to the pontine nuclei. The terminal ramifications and the boutons of the axons are seen as black dust in the section of the pontine nuclei. Magnifications, ×8 (upper photomicrographs) and ×150.

to the cell bodies (Figs. 3.2 and 9.3). HRP is, however, also transported anterogradely after perikaryal uptake. Thus, the method can also be used to demonstrate the terminal sites of specific neuronal groups. HRP can be visualized in tissue sections by utilizing its peroxidase activity to form a colored reaction product from a colorless substrate (diaminobenzidine, tetramethylbenzidine, and others). The uptake of HRP takes place by endocytosis, and the enzyme is subsequently internalized in lysosomelike bodies.

Several other substances are also used for axonal transport; some of these are transported only anterogradely, others only retrogradely. Substances that have no enzyme activity to help their visualization may be demonstrated by immunocytochemical techniques using antibodies raised against the transported molecule. This is the case for the plant lectin *Phaseolus vulgaris leukoagglutinin* (PHAL), which is only transported anterogradely. This lectin has the advantage of an extremely small and well circumscribed injection site, yet the transport is good and the labeled terminal fibers are shown in very fine detail in the sections.

Small-molecular, fluorescent substances that are subject to axonal transport have proved very valuable for tracing neuronal connections. Their advantage is that several tracers that fluoresce at different wavelengths of ultraviolet light can be injected in the same animal. This makes it possible to decide, for example, whether a cell group sends axonal collaterals to more than one target. In such *double-labeling experiments,* two fluorescent tracers are injected (each in a different place) and the region of interest is examined under the fluorescence microscope to look for perikarya that fluoresce under both wavelengths. Axonal transport of fluorescent tracers can also be combined with immunocytochemical methods to show the transmitter candidates of the labeled neurons.

It is also possible to label a transmitter molecule radioactively, and then inject it into the tissue. Only neurons that use this particular transmitter have specific uptake mechanisms for it. After uptake, the transmitter is transported anterogradely and can be subsequently localized in the tissue by autoradiography. Thus connections of transmitter-specific neuronal populations can be determined.

Neuronal connections can also be traced by electrophysiological methods. A cell group of nucleus is stimulated electrically, and the subsequent change of neuronal activity in other regions—caused by synaptic influence from the stimulated cell group—is recorded (orthodromic stimulation). By measuring the time from the stimulus to the response, it is usually possible to determine whether connections between two cell groups are monosynaptic or polysynaptic. Stimulation of axons within a fiber tract or their terminal ramifications can be used to determine the location of their parent cell bodies. In this instance the action potentials set up in the axons travel retrogradely toward the cell body (antidromic stimulation).

Electron Microscopic Examination of Nervous Tissue

Toward the end of the 1950s, electron microscopic techniques made it possible to characterize the structure of the subcellular elements of nerve cells in detail (Figs. 1.5, 1.8, 1.10, and 1.11). Of particular importance was the demonstration of the fine structure of the synapse, which enabled correlations to be made with physiological, biochemical, and pharmacological data pertaining to synaptic processes. Electron microscopy also made it possible to describe the various types of filaments involved in axonal tranpsort. Another example is the clarification of the structure of myelin.

Because boutons undergoing degenerative changes after destruction of the perikaryon show characteristic alterations in the electron microscope, the synaptic relations of specific sets of afferents to a nucleus could be determined. Moreover, some axonally transported tracer substances can be identified in the electron microscope. Likewise, the exact subcellular localization of tissue antigens (transmitters, transmitter-related enzymes, and other substances of functional interest) can be identified electron microscopically after immunocytochemical treatment.

Determination of Neuronal Content of Neurotransmitters and Distribution of Receptors

To understand the functions of a nerve cell, it is necessary to know the transmitters it uses. With biochemical methods, the content of transmitters in parts of the brain and

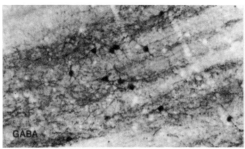
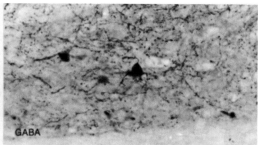

Fig. 3.3. *Immunocytochemical demonstration of neurotransmitters.* An antibody binding to a GABA-protein complex in the section. The darkly stained perikarya, showing GABA-like immunoreactivity, are interneurons in a brain stem nucleus (monkey). The darkly stained fibers are partly dendrites, partly axons and boutons.

in subcellular fractions can be determined. To obtain further knowledge, however, it is also necessary to link the transmitters to specific neurons with known connections and physiological properties.

The first possibilities of studying the anatomy of neurons with known transmitters arose in the 1960s, when it was discovered that monamine-containing neurons can be made fluorescent by a special treatment with formaldehyde. This marked the beginning of intense investigations, with other methods as well, of characterizing neurons with regard to connections and at the same time with regard to their transmitters. It became evident that neurons with a certain transmitter may not be restricted to cytoarchitectonically homogeneous nuclei and, vice versa, that neurons within one cytoarchitectonically defined nucleus may use different transmitters.

The introduction of immunological methods, such as *immunocytochemistry,* to localize substances in nervous tissue has been of particular importance during recent years. By purifying a potentially interesting substance present in nervous tissue, antibodies may be raised against it (either polyclonal antibodies raised in animals, or monoclonal antibodies produced in cell cultures). The antibodies bind to their antigens at the site where they are exposed in the tissue sections, and the antibodies can be visualized subsequently with the use of secondary antibodies. The secondary antibodies may be labeled with a fluorescent molecule, or they

may be identified in other ways. Such methods have been widely used to demonstrate the localization of enzymes that are critical for synthesis or degradation of certain transmitters, such a tyrosine hydroxylase, which is necessary for the synthesis of dopamine and norepinephrine (Fig. 10.9), choline acetyltransferase (ChAT) for synthesis of actylcholine (Fig. 16.9), and glutamic acid decarboxylase (GAD) for GABA. Even transmitter molecules that are themselves too small to serve as antigens can be specifically identified in tissue sections with immunocytochemical methods when conjugated to tissue proteins with glutaraldehyde. This is the case for GABA (Fig. 3.3), glutamate, and glycine. Immunocytochemical methods can also be applied to ultrastructural analysis, in order to determine the transmitter accumulated at specific synapses and also whether the transmitter is localized to certain organelles, such as presynaptic vesicles. Figures 3.4 and 3.5 show examples of demonstrating glycine in the spinal cord and GABA in the cerebellum, using secondary antibodies that are labeled with small gold particles (immuno-gold method). Since the gold particles are electron-dense, they appear as black dots in the electron micrographs. Such methods can also be used quantitatively in studies of relations between transmitters and different functional states and to determine whether diseases are related to alterations in specific transmitters.

Combination of axonal transport methods and immunocytochemical procedures

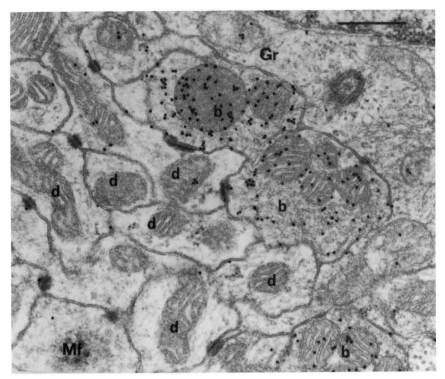

Fig. 3.4. *Electron microscopic, immunocyto-chemical demonstration of neurotransmitters.* The small black dots represent gold particles bound in the tissue where GABA is present. The gold particles are conjugated to an antibody directed against a GABA-protein complex. The gold particles are concentrated over a particular kind of bouton (b), whereas dendrites (d) and part of a perikaryon (Gr) are not labeled. Another kind of bouton (Mf) is also unlabeled and most likely contains a neurotransmitter other than GABA. Rat cerebellum. Courtesy of Dr. O. P. Ottersen.

makes it possible to determine both the connections as well as the transmitter candidates and other neuroactive substances of specific neuronal groups.

Even though the determination of the transmitter candidates present in a neuron is of great importance, it is not always possible to know whether the substance has been synthesized in the cell or whether it has merely been taken up. Furthermore, the concentration of transmitter in parts of a neuron may be so low that it cannot be reliably detected with immunocytochemical methods. The use of *in situ hybridization techniques* helps to overcome this kind of problem. By these methods, it is not the neuroactive peptides or enzymes related to transmitter metabolism that are demonstrated but the presence of the corresponding mRNA.

Immunocytochemical techniques are also used to study the distribution of molecules other than those assumed to function as transmitters, such as proteins and peptides that may play specific roles during development of the nervous system and molecules that may serve as markers to differentiate types of glial cells.

Techniques of molecular biology have also been instrumental in the localization and characterization of *receptors* and *ion channel proteins*. Receptors, for example, can be localized by binding to specific agonists or antagonists that are radioactively labeled, and their distribution can then be correlated with what is known of connections and distribution of transmitters for the cell groups under study. Specific binding of ligands to receptors also makes it possible to purify the receptor molecules of subsequent

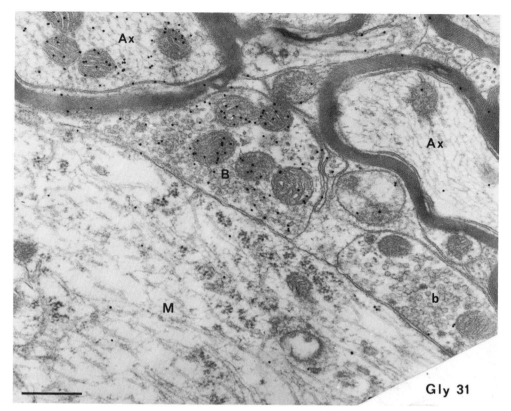

Fig. 3.5. *Electron microscopic, immunocyto-chemical demonstration of neurotransmitters.* Experimental procedures corresponding to those in Figure 3.4, except that the antibody gold particle conjugate binds to a glycine protein complex in the tissue. M is part of a spinal motoneu-ron; B is a labeled bouton forming an axosomatic synapse; and b is an unlabeled bouton. A labeled and an unlabeled axon (Ax) are also seen. Glycine is an inhibitory neurotransmitter. The bar represents 1 μm. Courtesy of Dr. O. P. Ottersen.

determination of their amino acid sequence. It is also possible to study changes in the receptor density after experimental manipulations. Receptor studies can also be carried out postmortally on the human brain—for example, to ascertain whether certain neurological and psychiatric diseases are associated with alterations of specific transmitters and their receptors.

Lesion and Stimulation Experiments Are Used to Determine the Functions of Cell Groups

A fundamental approach to the study of the function of specific parts of the nervous system is to make circumscribed *lesions* and to observe the functional disturbances that

ensue. Such a lesion may constitute interruption of fiber tracts, destruction of neurons within a nucleus, or removal of large parts, such as a whole lobe of the cerebral hemisphere. It is also possible to cool circumscribed regions reversibly, so that neurons are "silenced" only temporarily. Corresponding reversible effects can be obtained with the use of local anesthetics. To study the functional and behavioral changes, highly sophisticated test methods may be necessary. Also, control experiments with lesions of other parts are usually crucial.

Examples of lesion experiments in animals and observations in humans with brain damage are mentioned throughout in this book. The interpretation of the association between the normal function of the structures and the symptoms that ensue after lesions is often far from straightforward, however. For example, a lesion may destroy not only a certain group of neurons but also fibers passing through the area. The symptoms may in such cases be caused by dysfunction of neuronal groups distant from the lesion. The interpretation is generally least problematic when lesions are confined to large, well-delimited tracts, whereas symptoms after lesions of the cerebral cortex may be much more difficult to interpret. A fundamental problem remains, however, in all such experiments: To what extent can normal function of a part of the brain be deduced from the deficits and disturbances resulting from its removal? In many instances the symptoms occurring are for the most part a consequence of dysfunction and compensations of cell groups not damaged by the lesion.

Electrical stimulation of tracts and specific cell groups can be used to study their function, assuming that the physiological and behavioral effects are closely related to their normal function. One example is electrical stimulation of the motor cortex in the precentral gyrus, which elicits more or less isolated muscle contractions in the opposite side of the body. This example also illustrates the limitations of such methods: The experiments tell us that the motor cortex is of importance for the start of movements but tell us very little about how the complicated pattern of activity in many muscles, which is so characteristic of our voluntary movements, comes about. The difficulties of interpretation become much greater, however, when regions with multifarious connections with other parts of the brain are stimulated (this may be particularly obvious for stimulation experiments of the so-called limbic system; see Chapter 16).

Since stimulation experiments often have to be performed on anesthetized animals, this further limits the conclusions about normal function. Many cell groups are much less excitable during general anesthesia. This problem can be overcome to some extent by the use of *chronically implanted electrodes*,

which enable stimulation to be carried out in conscious animals. Such electrodes are inserted in the brain under general anesthesia and are fixed to the skull to remain in place (the electrodes cause no pain because the nervous tissue is devoid of nociceptors). The behavioral effects of stimulation of specific parts can then be observed repeatedly. After the experiments, the exact location of the electrode can be verified histologically. Such experiments also entail problems of interpretation. After all, the evoked activity is artificial, and one usually cannot know whether identical patterns of activity occur naturally.

With the use of autoradiography, it is possible to map the metabolic activity of various brain regions in relation to specific stimuli or behaviors. *Radioactively labeled 2-deoxyglucose* is given intravenously and is taken up by the neurons. Unlike glucose, however, deoxyglucose is not metabolized by the neurons and therefore accumulates. The neuronal uptake of glucose is closely related to the level of activity. After autoradiography of tissue sections, neuronal groups with high levels of deoxyglucose can be identified. These have most likely been particularly active just before the death of the animal and are therefore presumably related to whatever specific activities were going on at that time.

Recording of Single-Cell Activity

Microelectrodes, with tips less than 1 μm thick, can be used to record the activity of single neurons and their processes (single units) intracellularly. Among other things, this has made it possible to study in detail the electrical events at the synapses and how they are influenced by various experimental manipulations. The effects of different concentrations of ions intra- and extracellularly have been studied, as have the synaptic effects of various transmitter candidates and drugs. Thin implanted extracellular electrodes can be used to record the activity of single neurons in relation to specific stimuli or behavioral tasks. This method has, for example, provided new insight into functional specializations within various areas of the cerebral cortex.

The *voltage clamp* technique, which permits manipulation of the membrane potential, has been instrumental to our understanding of the properties of synapses and the basic mechanisms underlying their operations. Likewise, great progress has been made with the newly developed *patch clamp* technique, making possible measurements of ion currents limited to even single ion channels. The study of the properties of ion channels and membrane receptors is today highly interdisciplinary.

By combining anatomic and physiological techniques, it has been possible to determine the functional properties of structurally defined cell types. After intracellular recording has been made from a neuronal cell body or its axon, it can be filled with a tracer substance, such as HRP, through the same pipette. Afterwards, the neuron with all its processes can be visualized in sections. This has been done, for example, for several neuronal types in the dorsal horn of the spinal cord. Thus, the types of sensory receptors acting on the neuron can be identified before filling the neuron. In general, such techniques have provided important contributions to the correlation of structure and function in the nervous system.

The Living Human Brain Can Be Studied with Computer-Based Imaging Techniques

New techniques for computer-based image analysis of the living human brain has revolutionized the possibilities for localizing disease processes in the brain and for studying normal structure and function. With *computer tomography* (CT), we can see pictures of thin slices through the brain, on the basis of X rays. The plane of sectioning may be chosen by the examiner. This enables much more precise visualization of the structures than conventional X-ray examination, by

which all tissue between the X-ray tube and the film is included in the picture. The method also provides good visualization of the ventricular system.

A further technical development is represented by *magnetic resonance imaging* (MRI). This technique is based not on X rays but on signals emitted by protons when they are placed in a magnetic field. Depending on the proton concentration in different tissue components, the pictures may show clearly, for example, the contrast between gray and white matter (Figs. 2.2, 2.28, and 2.31). The bone of the skull gives very little or no signal and is seen as black in the pictures. With this technique, the brain can be visualized in slices with a resolution not far from that of a corresponding section through a fixed brain. Areas with changes in the tissue—for example, infarction, bleeding, or tumor—can be identified. Apart from the diagnostic advantages, the MRI technique also improves the correlation of the functional disturbances with the actual damage of the brain. MRI can also be used to study dynamic processes in the brain.

The last technique we will cover is *positron emission tomography* (PET). With this method, images are produced that visualize the distribution of an inhaled or injected radioactively labeled substance. The picture shows the distribution at a certain time. By labeling substances of biological interest, their distribution can be determined. The flow of blood through specific parts of the brain can, for example, be correlated with certain stimuli or activities. Also, the regional metabolism can be examined after injection of radioactively labeled deoxyglucose. The metabolic activity or the blood flow can be examined in the cerebral cortex at rest and during specific sensory, motor, or mental activities. Substances known to bind specifically to certain receptor types can also be labeled radioactively and injected. Thus, the normal distribution of such receptors can be determined, as well as possible changes in neurological and psychiatric diseases.

II

Sensory Systems

Sensory impulses from nearly all parts of the body are transmitted to the central nervous system, bringing information about conditions in the various tissues and organs and in our surroundings. The structures where sensory impulses originate are called sense organs or *receptors*. There are several kinds of sensory receptors, and their classification, together with their common basic properties, will be described before we discuss the various types and the pathways leading from them.

In this part of the book we will deal with the somatosensory system, which is primarily concerned with sensory information from the skin, joints, and muscles; the optic system (vision); the auditory system (hearing); and the olfactory system (smell). For practical reasons, the senses of equilibrium and taste are treated in Chapter 13 (The Cranial Nerves), and sensory information from the internal organs (viscera) is dealt with in Chapter 14 (Peripheral Parts of the Autonomic Nervous System).

SENSORY RECEPTORS IN GENERAL
AND THEIR CLASSIFICATION

The task of the receptors is to respond to stimuli of various kinds. Regardless of the nature of the stimulus, the receptor "translates" the stimulus to the language spoken by the nervous system—that is, electrical impulses in the form of action potentials. Most receptors are built to respond only or preferably to one kind of stimulus energy (mechanical, chemical, thermal, and so forth). The kind of stimulus to which the receptor responds most easily—that is, with the lowest threshold—is called the *adequate stimulus* for the receptor. We also say that the receptor is *specific* for this kind of stimuli.

When a particular kind of receptor is stimulated with sufficient intensity to cause a consciously perceived sensation, we always get the same kind of *modality*[1] of sensory experience (for example, light, touch, pressure, warmth, pain, sound). This does not imply, however, that the receptor necessarily has been subjected to its adequate stimulus. Thus, most receptors can respond also to stimuli of other kinds (inadequate stimuli), although the threshold then is much higher for evoking a response. As an example, we can mention the perception of light upon a blow to the eye (mechanical stimulus of the receptors rather than the normal light stimulus), and perception of sound upon chemical, rather than the normal mechanical, irritation of the receptors for hearing. *The kind of perceived sensation—the quality or modality of sensation—is thus characteristic for each type of receptor* (the "law of specific nerve energies" of Müller). Irritation of the axon leading from the receptor will also evoke the same sensory modality as when the receptor is stimulated by its adequate stimulus.

Receptors differ not only with regard to their adequate stimulus or specificity. Many receptors send action potentials only when a stimulus starts (or stops). If the stimulus is continuous, this kind of receptor ceases to respond and thus provides information about changes in stimulation only. Such receptors are called *rapidly adapting*. When after a short time we cease noticing that something touches the skin, this is partly because so many of the receptors in the skin are of the rapidly adapting type. Other receptors, however, go on responding (and thus sending action potentials) as long as the stimulus continues. Such receptors are called *slowly adapting*. One example of slowly adapting receptors is those that are responsible for the sensation of pain. It would not be appropriate if the body were to adapt to painful stimuli since these usually signal danger and threat of tissue damage. Receptors signaling the position of the body in space and the position of our bodily parts in relation to each other must also be slowly adapting; if not, we would lose this kind of information after a few seconds if no movement took place. Adaptation is a property of the receptors themselves, and not (only) of processing within the central nervous system, as can be verified by recording the action potentials from sensory fibers supplying various kinds of receptors. For example, afferent fibers from receptors excited by warming of the skin stop sending impulses if the same stimulus is maintained for some time, whereas afferent nerve fibers from sense organs in a muscle continue to send impulses as long as the muscle is held in a stretched position.

Classification of Receptors on the Basis of the Origin of the Adequate Stimulus

This system for classification of receptors is convenient and functionally meaningful. We usually distinguish between *exteroceptors, proprioceptors,* and *enteroceptors. Exteroceptive* impulses reach the body from the outside, from our environment. Most exteroceptors are located in the skin, whereas the receptors in the eye and the internal ear represent important special kinds of exteroceptors responding to *teleceptive* impulses. *Proprioceptive* impulses originate in the body itself. The term is mostly restricted, however, to impulses arising in the musculoskeletal system, including the joints. *Enteroceptive* impulses arise from the internal (visceral) organs.

Classification of Receptors on the Basis of the Kind of Adequate Stimulus

Receptors can be further characterized and classified in accordance with the nature of their adequate stimulus. A large group of receptors, the *mechanoreceptors,* responds primarily to distortion of the tissue in which they lie and thus informs the central nervous system about mechanical stimuli. Such receptors are numerous among exteroceptors, proprioceptors, and enteroceptors. Many mechanoreceptors have a low threshold and send impulses even on the slightest touch of the skin or a just barely perceptible movement of a joint. Other mechanoreceptors require very strong stimulation to respond; such stimuli are usually perceived as painful. Depending on their location, mechanoreceptors may give information of very different events (even though all are mechanical): A low-threshold mechanoreceptor in the wall of the urinary bladder provides information about its degree of distension, and mechanoreceptors in the inner ear inform us about sound (movement of air molecules), whereas mechanoreceptors around the root of a hair respond to the slightest bending of the hair.

Another large group of receptors, *chemoreceptors,* responds primarily to certain chemical substances in the interstitial fluid surrounding the receptor. Many chemoreceptors respond to substances produced by or released from cells as a result of tissue damage and inflammation, regardless of the cause (mechanical trauma, burns, infection, and so forth). Other kinds of chemoreceptors are the receptors for taste and smell.

Receptors in the retina responding (with an extremely low threshold) to visible light are called *photoreceptors. Thermoreceptors* respond most easily to warming or cooling of the tissue in which they lie.

Classification of Receptors on the Basis of
Subjective Sensory Experience

Although more problematic than the above kinds of classification, receptors are also commonly classified by the conscious sensory experience they are believed to evoke. Thus, we use the term *nociceptors* to describe receptors that, when stimulated, produce pain. Stimulation of *cold receptors* causes a feeling of coldness, stimulation of *warm receptors* gives a feeling of warmth, and so on. Only exceptionally is it possible, however, to know whether a sensory experience is caused by one receptor type only, or by the simultaneous activation of several kinds. Since only human beings can inform the observer directly of what they feel, animal experiments alone cannot resolve the question of the relation between receptors and conscious sensations. On the other hand, the very same receptors examined physiologically cannot be examined anatomically in human beings. Important insight has nevertheless emerged from correlation of observations obtained in animals with psychophysical observation in humans (see also "Microneurography" in Chapter 4).

Not all impulses reaching the central nervous system from the receptors are consciously perceived. In particular, enteroceptive impulses are mostly processed only at a subconscious level. For impulses from all kinds of receptors, however, a considerable selection and suppression of signals take place at all levels of the sensory pathways in the spinal cord and the brain, to leave out "irrelevant" information. At the same time, "relevant" signals may be enhanced in the central nervous system—for example, to increase the contrasts in a visual scene.

We cannot explain how it happens that action potentials, which are of the same kind in all nerve fibers, evoke entirely different conscious sensations depending on where the stimulus arises. In general, we can say that the receptors function as *analyzers* by recording different kinds of external and internal events influencing the body. The *integration* of the various bits of information takes place in the central nervous system and forms a necessary basis for our conscious, subjective sensations.

NOTE

1. The words *modality* and *quality* are both used to describe aspects of sensation but unfortunately somewhat differently by various authors. *Quality* is used here to describe further the nature of a sensory modality–for example, pain is a sensory modality that may have a burning quality.

4

The Somatosensory System

The term *somatosensory* includes, strictly speaking, all sensations pertaining to the body (soma). It is therefore more comprehensive than the significance commonly assigned to it—namely, sensory information from skin, joints, and muscles only.

EXTEROCEPTORS: CUTANEOUS SENSATION

The skin and the subcutaneous tissue contain receptors that respond to stimuli from our surroundings. Among the almost indefinitely varied sensory experiences that can be evoked from the skin, we usually distinguish only a few, regarded as the basic modalities: *touch, pressure, heat, cold, and pain.* There is indirect evidence that each of these sensations can be evoked by stimulation of one receptor type. Yet it is important to realize that terms such as pain, cold, and touch refer to the quality of our subjective sensory experience evoked by certain kinds of stimuli. Thus, a classification of sensations on this basis does not enable us to conclude that for each subjective quality of sensation there exists one particular kind of receptor. Sensations such as itch, tickle, dampness, or dryness, the texture of surfaces, and the firmness or softness of objects are thought to arise from the simultaneous stimulation of several kinds of receptors in the skin and also in deeper tissues. As mentioned earlier, our conscious sensory experience is the result of a synthesis in the brain of information from a multitude of receptors.

Functionally, skin receptors can be classified by their adequate stimulus as *mechanoreceptors, thermoreceptors,* and *nociceptors.*

The Structure of the Skin

The skin consists of two layers (Fig. 4.1). The upper layer, the *epidermis,* consists of stratified squamous epithelium. Like all epithelia, the epidermis lacks vessels and is nourished by capillaries in the underlying *dermis.* This is built of relatively dense connective tissue with numerous collagen fibers. The dermis sends small projections, *dermal papillae,* upward into the epidermis. In the dermis and partly in the loose connective tissue beneath it—the *subcutaneous layer*—there are sweat glands and sebaceous glands. The *hairs,* obliquely oriented to the surface of the skin, have their roots in the upper parts of the subcutaneous layer. A tiny smooth muscle runs obliquely from the root of the hair upward to the upper part of the dermis (the arrector pili muscle). Contraction of this muscle straightens the hair so that it stands more perpendicular to the surface of the skin.

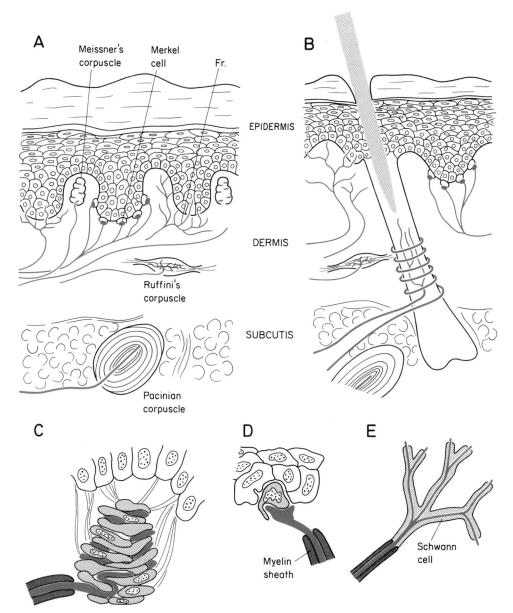

Fig. 4.1. *Cutaneous receptors.* Schematic drawing of receptors as they appear in sections through the skin. Sensory nerve fibers and receptors in (**A**) glabrous skin (palms of the hands and soles of the feet) and (**B**) hairy skin. Nerve endings in hairy skin wind around the hair follicles and are activated by the slightest bending of the hair. **C.** Meissner corpuscle (from glabrous skin). The axon (red) follows a tortuous course between flat, specialized connective tissue cells. The whole sense organ is anchored to the epidermis with thin collagen fibers. **D.** A disk of Merkel (present in both glabrous and hairy skin). The axonal terminal is closely apposed to a Merkel cell in the epidermal cell layer. **E.** Free nerve endings are covered by Schwann cells except at their tips, where, presumably, the receptor properties reside.

Free and Encapsulated Receptors

Receptors in the skin (and also in deep tissues) are conveniently subdivided on a structural basis into free and encapsulated, although there are numerous transitional forms. In *encapsulated receptors,* the terminal ramifications of the sensory axon are surrounded by a specialized capsulelike structure of connective tissue cells, whereas such a structure is lacking around the *free receptors* or endings (Fig. 4.1E). The axonal ramifications of the free receptors are covered by Schwann cells, except at their tips, where their receptor properties presumably reside. Free receptors are the most numerous and widespread, being present in virtually all parts of the body. In the skin they are particularly numerous in the upper parts of the dermis, and they also extend for a short distance between the cells of the deeper layers of the epidermis.

Nociceptors

Nociceptors in the skin and as far as we know, in all other tissues from which painful sensations can be evoked, are free receptors. It is characteristic that most stimuli we experience as painful are *so intense that they produce tissue damage or will do so if the stimulus is continued.* Functionally, skin nociceptors are of two main kinds: One responds to intense mechanical stimulation only (such as pinching, cutting, stretching) and is therefore termed *high-threshold mechanoreceptor.* The other kind is also activated by intense mechanical stimuli but, in addition, by intense warming of the skin (above 40°C) and by chemical substances that are liberated by tissue damage and inflammation. Because they can be activated by different sensory modalities, such receptors are termed *polymodal nociceptors.* Recent studies indicate that there are in addition many nociceptors that are purely sensitive to chemical substances.

A characteristic feature of nociceptors is their tendency to be *sensitized* by prolonged stimulation. This partly explains why even normally nonnoxious stimuli (such as touching the skin) may be felt as painful when the skin is inflamed (inflammation acitvates a large number of nociceptors). This condition of lowered threshold for evoking pain is called *hyperalgesia.*

Not All Nociceptors May Signal Tissue Damage

Although the properties described above for nociceptors pertain to most nociceptors in the skin, in muscles, and around joints, nociceptors in visceral organs often have quite different properties. Some stimuli that are tissue damaging (such as cutting or perforating a hollow organ) do not evoke pain, whereas other stimuli that are not necessarily tissue damaging (such as distension of a hollow organ) may be intensely painful. Also, the pain arising from visceral organs in many cases can hardly serve a protective role, which is the obvious function of many nociceptors in, for example, the skin.

A large number of nociceptors (presumably the majority) respond only to the slow buildup of certain substances in inflamed tissue (subsequent to trauma or infection). In the urinary bladder, for example, only a small percentage of the sensory units innervating it respond to even painful distension, whereas many more respond when the bladder wall is inflamed by injection of an irritating substance. Also, the joints and the skin appear to be innervated by many sensory units that respond neither to mechanical stimuli nor to noxious heat, but only to chemical irritants liberated during inflammation. It is possible that this kind of nociceptor does not function primarily as a warning system for impending tissue damage but rather "plays a more general long-term role in evaluating and signalling the status of the microenvironment in peripheral tissue," as suggested by the British neurophysiologist McMahon.

Thermoreceptors

It was previously believed that cold and warm stimuli were mediated by two kinds of encapsulated receptors (the Krause and Ruffini corpuscles, respectively). This cannot be the case, however, since sensations of both cold and heat can be perceived from regions of the skin containing only free receptors. Combined physiological and histological analysis has also strengthened the view that free endings are responsible for the perception of heat and cold.

The *adequate stimulus* for thermoreceptors is the temperature of the tissue surrounding them or, rather, *changes in the temperature*. The receptors send action potentials with a relatively low frequency at a steady temperature, whereas a small change in the temperature elicits a marked change in the firing frequency. A heat receptor, for example, may at constant room temperature fire with a low frequency, but if the skin is warmed even slightly, there is a marked increase in the firing rate. The response is particularly brisk if the warming happens rapidly (thus, lukewarm water may be perceived as hot if the hand is cold when put into it). A change in skin temperature of 0.2°C is sufficient to cause a marked change in firing rate from a thermoreceptor. Thus, the thermoreceptors do not give an objective measure of the actual skin temperature but rather signal changes that may be of significance for our adjustment to the environment.

Mechanoreceptors of the Skin Have Been Thoroughly Studied

The study of receptors for pain and temperature sensation is more difficult than the study of low-threshold mechanoreceptors. There are several kinds of mechanoreceptors in the skin, ranging from free receptors to those with an elaborate capsule. Some adapt slowly or not at all; others adapt very rapidly. An example of rapidly adapting receptors is those found close to the roots of hairs (Fig. 4.1B). They are stimulated by even the slightest bending of a hair, as can be easily verified by touching the hairs on the back of one's own hand. If the hair is held still in the new position, however, the sensation disappears immediately.

The thick, *glabrous skin* on the palm of the hand and on the sole of the foot lacks hair. Elaborate encapsulated receptors are,

however, particularly abundant at these locations. They are obviously related to the superior sensory abilities of these parts, the fingers in particular. One such receptor is the *Meissner corpuscle,* mediating information about touch (Fig. 4.1C). These are small oval bodies located in the dermal papillae just beneath the epidermis (in fact, as close to the surface of the skin as possible without being directly exposed). Several axons approach the corpuscle and follow a tortuous course inside the capsule, between the lamellae formed by connective tissue cells. The Meissner corpuscles respond by sending action potentials even when the skin overlying the receptor is pressed down only a few micrometers. If the skin is kept in this position, however, the receptor stops sending action potentials, whereas a few action potentials are elicited on release of the pressure. The Meissner corpuscle is thus *rapidly adapting,* and it also obviously has a *low threshold* for its adequate stimulus. It is presumably well suited, among other things, to signal direction and velocity of objects moving on the skin.

The *Ruffini corpuscles* are also low-threshold mechanoreceptors and are most likely *slowly adapting*. They consist of a bundle of collagen fibrils with a sensory axon branching between the fibrils (Fig. 4.1A). The collagen fibrils are connected with those in the dermis, and stretching of the skin in the direction of the fibrils is the adequate stimulus for the receptor. This tightens the fibrils, which in turn leads to deformation and depolarization of the axonal ramifications, thus producing action potentials in the afferent fiber. It is therefore assumed that the Ruffini corpuscle functions as a *low-threshold stretch receptor* of the skin, informing us about the magnitude and direction of stretch.

Another kind of *slowly adapting,* low-threshold mechanoreceptor in the skin is the *Merkel's disk* (Fig. 4.1A and D), present particularly on the distal parts of the extremities, on the lips, and the external genitals. An axon ends in close contact with a large epithelial cell in the basal layer of the epidermis. Even after several minutes of constant pressure on the skin overlying the receptors, they continue to send action potentials at about the same rate.

Finally, a fourth type of low-threshold mechanoreceptor, the *Pacinian corpuscle* (Fig. 4.1A), is found at the junction between the dermis and the subcutaneous layer (it is also present at other locations, such as in the mesenteries, vessel walls, joint capsules, and in the periosteum). These are large (up to several millimeters long) ovoid bodies, which can be seen macroscopically at dissection. A thick, unbranched axon is surrounded by numerous lamellae formed by a special kind of connective tissue cell. Between the cellular lamellae there are fluid-filled spaces. The Pacininan corpuscle is very rapidly adapting, eliciting only one or two action potentials in the afferent fiber at the onset of indentation of the skin. The adequate stimulus is therefore extremely rapid indentation of the skin. In practice, this is achieved by vibration with a frequency of 100—400 Hz. If a vibrating probe is put in contact with the skin, the frequency of action potentials in the afferent fiber follows closely the frequency of vibration. Vibration with a frequency below 100 Hz appears to be signaled by the Meissner corpuscles.

What Information Is Signaled by Low-Threshold Cutaneous Mechanoreceptors?

Together the four types of low-threshold mechanoreceptors described above are thought to mediate the different qualities of our sense of touch and pressure, which are so well developed in glabrous skin (fingers, toes, and lips). One important aspect is the ability to judge the speed and direction of a moving object in contact with the skin, as well as the friction between them. Thus, we may perceive quickly that an object is slipping from our grip and also judge from the friction the force needed to stop the movement. Two of the receptor types, the Merkel's disks and the Ruffini corpuscles, are slowly adapting and, as long as the stimulus

lasts, continue to provide information about slight pressure and strectching of the skin, respectively. The two others, the Meissner and the Pacinian corpuscles, are rapidly adapting and signal only the start and stop of stimuli. It seems likely that the Meissner corpuscles would be particularly well suited to signal the direction and speed of a moving stimulus (see "Microneurography," below).

Free Receptors May Have Different Functional Properties

It was previously thought that each sensory modality has a corresponding morphologically distinct receptor. This simplistic view cannot be upheld, however. In particular, there are numerous examples of free receptors that are structurally indistinguishable but have quite different adequate sitmuli.

There is good evidence that all *nociceptors* are free endings of thin myelinated and unmyelinaed axons, even though there are at least two subgroups of nociceptors (high-threshold and polymodal). Furthermore, low-threshold mechanoreceptors for touch are not always of the encapsulated type described above (Meissner, Ruffini, and others) but may also be of the free-ending type. Cold and heat receptors are also structurally free endings of axons, as mentioned above.

The differences in adequate stimulus among structurally identical sensory receptors are presumably due to differences in the membrane properties at the exposed ("naked") tip of the free endings (Fig. 4.1E)—for example, different ion channels and membrane receptors.

Punctate Localization of Cutaneous Sensation: Receptive Fields

A sensory neuron—which in the somatosensory system is a pseudounipolar ganglion cell—with all its axonal ramifications constitutes a *sensory unit*. The region of the skin from which a sensory unit may be activated is called the *receptive field* of the unit (Fig. 4.2). The size of the receptive field depends on the area of the skin receiving axonal

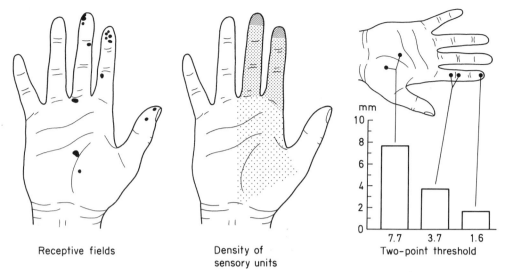

Receptive fields   Density of   Two-point threshold
                          sensory units

Fig. 4.2. *Receptive fields.* **A.** Size and location of the receptive fields of 15 sensory units, determined by recording from the median nerve. All of these sensory units were rapidly adapting and were most likely conducting from Meissner corpuscles. Within each receptive field there are many Meissner corpuscles, all supplied by the same axon. **B.** Relative density of sensory units conducting from Meissner corpuscles (that is, number of sensory units supplying 1 cm²). Note that the density increases distally and is highest at the volar aspect of the fingertips. **C.** Two-point discrimination. The numbers give the shortest distance between two points touching the skin that can be identified by the experimental subject as two (reducing the distance further makes the person experience only one point touching the skin). Average of 10 subjects. Based on microneurographic studies by Vallbo and Johansson (1978).

branches from the sensory neuron. In general, the *density of sensory units*—that is, the number of units innervating, for example, 1 cm² of the skin—is highest in distal parts of the body (fingers, toes, and lips) (Fig. 4.2), and the receptive fields are smaller distally than proximally. This explains why the stimulus threshold is lower and the ability to localize a stimulus is more precise in the palm of the hand than at, for example, the upper arm.

Microneurography

Studies with techniques that enable recording from and stimulation of peripheral nerves in conscious human beings have provided important information with regard to the functional properties of receptors (Fig. 4.2). This technique was pioneered by the Swedish neurophysiologists Hagbarth, Vallbo, Johansson, and others. With the use of very thin needle electrodes, it has been possible to record the activity of single sensory axons within a nerve, such as the median nerve at the forearm. Thus, it is possible to determine the receptive field of this particular sensory unit, and also its adequate stimulus. In glabrous skin of the fingers and palms, four types of low-threshold mechanoreceptors have been charaterized. Most likely, they correspond to the four encapsulated types described above. Thus, there are *two types of rapidly adapting sensory units,* one with a small receptive field (most likely the Meissner corpuscle) and the other with a large and indistinct receptive field (Pacinian corpuscle). The *two* other types of sensory units are *slowly adapting,* and again one has a small receptive field (Merkel's disk) and the other a large but direction-specific receptive field (most likely the Ruffini corpuscle).

Stimulation of the axons of the sensory units that have just been recorded from enables correlations to be made between the conscious sensory experience evoked by stimulation of only one sensory unit. Stimulation of single sensory units most likely ending in Meissner corpuscles produces a feeling of light touch, like a tap on the skin with the point of a pencil. As a rule, the person localizes the feeling to exactly the point on the skin previously found to be the receptive field of the sensory unit. Activating a sensory unit that presumably leads off from Merkel's disks evokes a sensation of light, steady pressure (as long as the stimulus lasts). Stimulating axons that appear to end in Pacinian corpuscles gives a feeling of vibration. For unknown reasons, no conscious sensation has so far been evoked by stimulating slowly adapting, stretch-sensitive sensory units of the skin (presumably Ruffini corpuscles).

It has been known for a long time that cutaneous sensation is *punctate;* that is, there are distinct tiny spots on the skin that are sensitive to different sensory modalities. We therefore use the terms *cold, warm, touch,* and *pain spots.* Cold spots are most easily demonstrated. Between the spots sensitive to cooling of the skin, there are others where contact with a cold object is felt only as pressure. The same can be found, however, for pain spots at relatively proximal body parts (for example, this can easily be observed by pricking with a needle at different sites on the trunk).

The punctate arrangement of the cutaneous sensation is of importance for *our ability to localize stimuli.* Being able to determine that the skin is touched by two pointed objects (like the legs of a compass) rather than one must mean that the two spots are innervated by separate units. The distance between two points on the skin that, when touched, can be identified as two is not surprisingly shortest where the density of sensory units is highest, and the receptive fields are smallest—that is, on the fingertips (Fig. 4.2). Determining this distance gives a measure of what is called *two-point discrimination* and is often used clinically. Another useful test for this kind of *discriminative sensation* is the writing of letters or figures on the skin (with the subject's eyes closed). The figures that can be interpreted are quite small on the fingertips, somewhat larger on the palms, much larger on the upper arm, and even larger on the trunk. The pathways conducting the sensory impulses from the spots on the skin are, as one might expect, arranged topographically so that impulses from different parts of the skin are kept separate at all levels up to the cerebral cortex.

PROPRIOCEPTORS: DEEP SENSATION

As mentioned above, the term *proprioceptive* is used of sensations pertaining to the *musculoskeletal system*—that is, muscles, tendons, joint capsules, and ligaments.

There are many similarities in structure and basic properties between proprioceptors and cutaneous receptors. There are, for example, numerous free receptors (belonging to thin myelinated and unmyelinated axons) in the muscles, the muscle fascia, and in the dense connective tissue of joint capsules and ligaments. Many of these are *nociceptors* as in the skin. Here, however, we are going to deal with specialized, encapsulated sense organs in muscles and around joints. These are all *low-threshold mechanoreceptors,* and the signals from them are conducted centrally in thick, myelinated axons. The *adequate stimulus* of these receptors is *stretching of the tissue in which they lie.* Whether located in a muscle or in a joint capsule, joint movement is the natural stimulus that leads to activation of such receptors. We will first discuss the special encapsulated sense organs present in muscles, the *muscle spindle,* and the *tendon organ.*

The Structure of the Muscle Spindle

The name *muscle spindle* is derived from the oblong shape of this sense organ. The muscle spindles are located within the muscle, among the striated muscle cells, and consist of a few (2–12) specialized muscle cells enclosed in a connective tissue capsule. The capsule is approximately 0.2 mm in diameter and 1–5 mm long. The muscle fibers (or muscle cells) of the spindle are called *intrafusal* and are much thinner than the ordinary, *extrafusal,* muscle fibers. In contrast to the extrafusal muscle fibers, the intrasfusal fibers show cross-striation only at their ends. This means that they are able to contract only these parts and not their middle portions. There are two main types of intrafusal fibers. One type is called the *nuclear bag fiber* because the nuclei are all collected in the

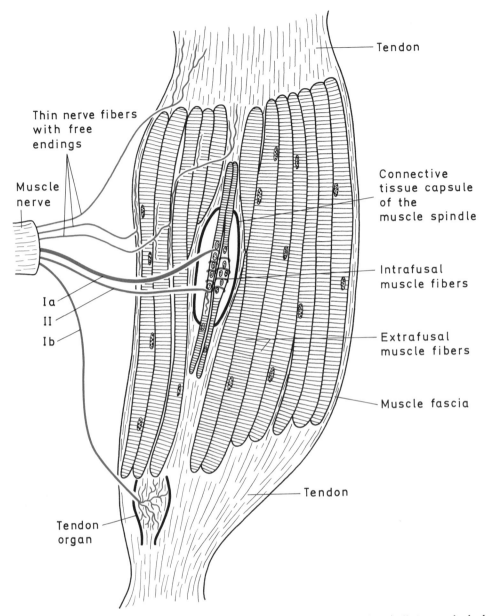

Fig. 4.3. *Sensory innervation of skeletal muscles.* The size of the receptors relative to the muscle is exaggerated. Note that the muscle spindle is attached via connective tissue fibers to the tendons. Thus, the muscle spindle is stretched whenever the whole muscle is stretched. Many of the free nerve endings are nociceptors.

middle part of the fiber (Fig. 4.4). In the other type, the *nuclear chain fiber,* the nuclei are evenly distributed along the fiber.

The number and density of muscle spindles vary from muscle to muscle, *the density being highest in muscles used for precision movements,* such as the extraocular muscles, the intrinsic muscles of the hand, and the small muscles around the joints of the neck. In large muscles like the latissimus dorsi, although the density is low, the total number of muscle spindles is about 400, whereas the small abductor pollicis brevis with a much higher density contains about 80.

The nerve supply of the muscle spindles is

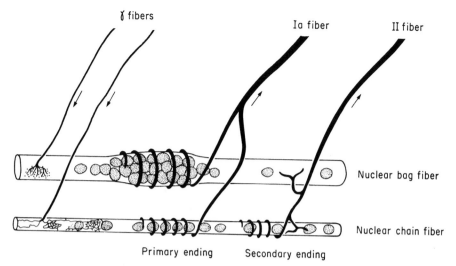

Fig. 4.4. *The muscle spindle.* Schematic representation of the two kinds of intrafusal muscle fibers and their innervation. Slightly changed from Matthews (1964).

highly complex, and only the main features will be treated here (Figs. 4.3 and 4.4). A thick afferent fiber ends with a spiraling course around the middle portion of the nuclear bag and nuclear chain fibers, forming the *primary sensory ending* of the muscle spindle. In addition, a thinner afferent fiber ends in relation to the nuclear chain fibers only, forming the *secondary sensory ending.* Afferent nerve fibers from muscles are classified with regard to thickness (and thus to conduction velocity) in groups I–IV, with group fibers comprising thick myelinated axons, and group IV unmyelinated ones. Group I is further divided into Ia and Ib, the former being the thickest. The primary sensory ending belongs to a *group Ia afferent fiber,* whereas the secondary sensory ending originates from a *group II afferent fiber.* Both types of sensory neuron have their perikarya in the spinal ganglia.

The *adequate stimulus* for the primary and secondary sensory endings is *stretching of the intrafusal muscle fibers.* This deforms the spiraling axonal branches and thus elicits depolarization and (if the depolarization is strong enough) action potentials in the group Ia and II sensory fibers.

The muscle spindle is also supplied with *motor axons,* called *fusimotor or γ fibers,* from γ *motoneurons* located in the ventral horn. The γ fibers end in the distal cross-stri-

ated parts of the intrafusal fibers and make them contract. This contraction leads to stretching of the noncontractile middle part of the intrafusal fibers, where the sensory endings are located. It should be emphasized that because the intrafusal fibers are so few and thin, their contraction does not contribute to the tension or shortening of the whole muscle.

The Properties of the Muscle Spindle

To understand how the muscle spindle functions, one must know that it is *arranged in parallel with the extrafusal muscle fibers.* Thus, both ends of the spindle are attached to the connective tissue within the muscle and are thereby indirectly anchored to the muscle tendons (Fig. 4.3). From this structure one many deduce that *when the whole muscle shortens as a result of contraction of the extrafusal fibers, the intrafusal fibers will be shortened passively. Conversely, stretching of the whole muscle will stretch the intrafusal muscle fibers.* The rate of shortening or lengthening will be the same for the muscle spindle as for the whole muscle.

Action potential can be recorded from single group Ia and II muscle afferent fibers in the dorsal roots of anesthetized animals (most often cats). It is then possible to study how the primary and secondary sensory

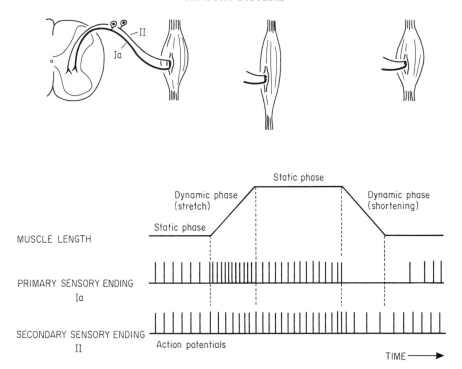

Fig. 4.5. *The functional properties of the muscle spindle.* The diagram shows how both the primary and the secondary sensory endings signal the static length of the muscle (static sensitivity), whereas only the primary ending signals the length changes (movements) and their velocity (dynamic sensitivity). The diagram is based on recordings from single dorsal root fibers of anesthetized cats. The change of firing frequency of endings behave in response to various stimuli. As expected from the anatomic facts described above, both types of afferent fibers increase their firing rate (that is, the frequency of action potentials) as the length of the muscle increases (Fig. 4.5). If the muscle shortens, the firing rate decreases (if the muscle is sufficently shortened, no action potentials can be recorded; see Fig. 4.6). When the length of the muscle is kept constant, the firing rate is also constant (static phase in Fig. 4.5)—the muscle spindle afferents are thus slowly adapting. This property of the muscle spindle is called *static sensitivity.* Since the firing rate of both the group Ia and the group II fiber depends on the length of the muscle, they both inform the central nervous system about the *length of the muscle* at any time (or the static length).

group Ia and group II fibers can then be related to static muscle length (static phase) and to stretch and shortening of the muscle (dynamic phases). The frequency of action potentials in the dorsal root fibers is indicated by the density of the vertical lines on the two lower rows. (The muscle spindle is not under the influence of γ motoneurons in this experiment.)

During the phase in which the *muscle length is changed,* however, the group Ia and group II afferent fibers behave differently (dynamic phase in Fig. 4.5). The firing rate of the group Ia fiber is much higher during the stretching than when the length is kept stationary in the stretched position, whereas the group II fiber does not show a similar change in firing rate. During the shortening phase, the Ia fiber becomes completely "silent." Although not shown in Figure 4.5, the firing rate of the group Ia fiber also depends on the velocity of the length change. Thus, the *Ia fiber signals that the length of the muscle is changing and the velocity with which it is occurring.* This property is called *dynamic sensitivity.*

These facts indicate that the *primary sensory ending* of the muscle spindle has both

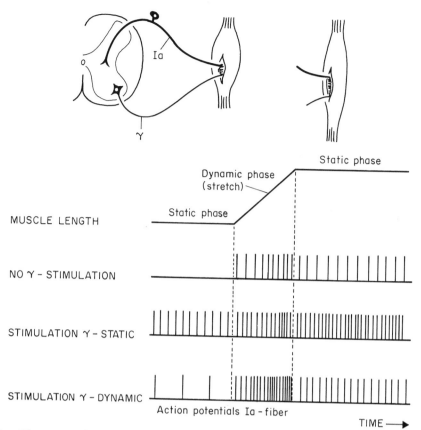

Fig. 4.6. *The action of γ motoneurons on the muscle spindle.* The experimental setup is as in Figure 4.5, except that in addition to recording the activity of group Ia fibers in the dorsal root, γ axons are isolated in the ventral roots so they can be electrically stimulated. In this example, there is no firing of the Ia fiber at the resting length of the muscle when the γ fibers are not stimulated. Stimulation of a static γ fiber (innervating the same spindle that the Ia fiber conducts from) makes the Ia fiber fire even at the static resting length, and stretching the muscle to a new static length increases the firing frequency to a new stable level. Stimulation of a dynamic γ fiber increases the firing frequency of the Ia fiber mainly during the stretching phase.

static and dynamic sensitivity: It should be capable of informing about the actual length of the muscle (position of a joint), whether the length is constant or changing (joint movement), and the velocity of change (velocity of the movement). Since the *secondary sensory ending* almost totally lacks dynamic sensitivity, it should be able to inform primarily of the static length of the muscle.

That the primary and secondary sensory endings (and their afferent nerve fibers) have different properties is most likely due to differences in viscoelastic properties of the nuclear bag and nuclear chain intrafusal muscle fibers. There is much evidence to suggest that *the nuclear bag fibers are responsible for*

the dynamic sensitivity of the primary sensory ending, whereas the nuclear chain fibers are responsible for the static sensitivity of both the primary and secondary sensory endings.[1]

Effects of Gamma Innervation on the Properties of the Muscle Spindle

What is described above of the properties of the muscle spindle derives from experiments in which there was no impulse traffic in the fusimotor (γ) axons (because the ventral roots were cut before recording from the dorsal roots). Impulses in γ fibers elicit contraction of the distal, cross-striated parts of the intrafusal muscle fibers, as mentioned above. This stretches the midportion of the intrafusal fibers with the sensory endings (Fig. 4.3). In addition, it also alters the stiffness of the intrafusal fibers so that their reaction to stretch is altered. In general, *the γ motoneurons and their γ fibers enable the brain to control the sensitivity of the muscle spindle to length and changes in length.*

In animal experiments (particularly in anesthetized cats), single γ fibers in the ventral roots have been stimulated while at the same time the activity of group Ia and group II afferent fibers in the dorsal roots were recorded. It has thus been shown that there are *two types of γ motoneurons* (Fig. 4.6). One type *increases the dynamic sensitivity of the muscle spindle* and is therefore called γ_D (gamma dynamic). Upon a fairly rapid stretch of the muscle, the firing rate of a group Ia fiber increases more when the muscle spindle receives impulses from γ_D motoneurons than without such influence. The firing rate during static length is, however, not significantly altered (Fig. 4.6). The muscle spindle's increased sensitivity to stretch enables the central nervous system to react more rapidly and forcefully to any unwanted change in muscle length (imposed, for example, by external forces upsetting body balance or ongoing movements).

Impulses from the other type of γ motoneurons *increase the static sensitivity of the muscle spindle,* and are therefore called γ_S (gamma static). The activity of γ_S motoneurons increases the firing rate of muscle spindle afferent fibers during constant length, as compared with a situation without γ activity. Although not shown in Figure 4.6, the firing rate of both group Ia and group II afferents increases. This influence of the γ system may be of importance to prevent the muscle spindles from becoming "silent"— that is, sending no action potentials—during the shortening of the muscle. In other words, the *length sensitivity* of the muscle spindle increases. Thus, the muscle spindle may signal the length of the muscle in its entire range of movements, which would seem important for precise movement control.[2]

Since the bag fibers appear to be solely responsible for the dynamic sensitivity of the muscle spindle, it has been assumed that dynamic γ fibers end on bag fibers and static γ fibers end on chain fibers. This is not fully clarified, however.

Even though the above description of the properties of muscle spindles is based on experiments in animals, there is evidence that it applies to the human muscle spindle. However, results from anesthetized animals, often with the spinal cord isolated from the rest of the brain, do not enable us to draw final conclusions as to the functions of the muscle spindle in intact organisms—for example, in human voluntary movements.

Microneurography and Muscle Spindles in Man

The activity of group Ia efferent fibers in the nerves of the arm and the leg has been recorded in conscious human subjects by microneurographic techniques. It appears (unexpectedly, on the basis of animal experiments) that in a resting muscle there is very little or no impulse traffic from the muscle spindle. Indirectly, this shows that there is no fusimotor (γ) activity either. If, however, the muscle contracts isometrically (that is, without change of length) there is a sharp increase of the firing frequency of Ia fibers. This must be caused by increased fusimotor activity, occurring simultaneously with the increase in α motoneuron activity (which evokes the contraction of the extrafusal fibers). This phenomenon of simultaneous activation of α and γ motoneurons is called *α–γ coactivation.* This ensures that the sensitivity of the muscle spindle is increased whenever the muscle is being used. In fact, the firing rate of the Ia fiber is upheld or increased even if the muscle is shortened during active contraction. This must mean that the fusimotor activity (firing rate of the γ motoneurons) *increases* during active shortening of the muscle.

The above example of α–γ coactivation does not mean that the γ motoneurons are activated *only* in conjunction with the α motoneurons, even though direct proof of separate activation is lacking. There are situations in which it would be desirable to have increased sensitivity of the muscle spindle without simultaneous muscle contraction. It is also difficult to understand why the elaborate γ system has developed if its activity were always to reflect that of the α system.

There are, in fact, some collaterals of α axons, so-called β *(beta) axons,* that innervate some intra-fusal muscle fibers, and in submammalian species (for example, in the frog) there are only β fibers. During evolution, the γ system appeared first in mammals.

The Tendon Organ

The other kind of proprioceptive receptor we will describe is the *tendon organ,* also called the *Golgi tendon organ.* It is built more simply than the muscle spindle and consists of a sensory nerve fiber that follows a convoluted course among collagen fibrils of the tendon, close to the musculotendi-nous junction (Fig. 4.3). The number of ten-don organs in a muscle appears to be only slightly lower than the number of muscle spindles. The afferent fiber leading from the tendon organ belongs to group I and is called a *group Ib fiber* because it is somewhat thin-ner than the group Ia fiber forming the pri-mary sensory ending of the muscle spindle. There is *no efferent innervation of the ten-don organ* (in contrast to the muscle spin-dle)—its sensitivity cannot be controlled from the central nervous system.

The *adequate stimulus* of the tendon organ is stretching of the part of the tendon in which it lies. Stretching tightens the col-lagen fibers, and thus the axonal branches between them are compressed. This depolar-izes the receptor and, if the stimulus is of suf-ficient intensity, evokes action potentials in the afferent Ib fiber. Recording of the activ-ity of Ib fibers shows that the receptor is *slowly adapting.* It is important to realize that *the tendon organ, in contrast to the muscle spindle, is coupled in series with the extrafusal muscle fibers.* Both passive stretch and active contraction of the muscle in-crease the tension of the tendon and thus ac-tivate the tendon organ receptor. The ten-don organ, consequently, can inform the central nervous system about the *muscle ten-sion.* In contrast, the activity of the muscle spindle depends on the muscle length and not on the tension.

Recording from single group Ib fibers in the dorsal root of anesthetized cats (Fig. 4.7) confirms what was expected on the basis of the structure of the tendon organ. In addi-tion, however, such experiments have shown that *the tendon organ is much more sensitive to tension produced by active con-traction than to that produced by passive stretch.* The tendon organ therefore appears to be primarily concerned with signaling how hard the muscle is contracting, rather than with how hard it is passively stretched.

Why Tendon Organs Are More Sensitive to Contraction Than to Passive Stretch

Structural details may explain why the tendon organ is more sensitive to active contraction than to passive stretch. Each tendon organ is directly attached to a small bundle of extrafusal muscle fibers. If one or a few of these contract, the ten-sion set up in this particular small part of the ten-don is very high compared with the tension mea-sured for the whole muscle. To obtain the same tension in this particular tendon organ by passive stretch, much higher overall tension of the mus-cle would have to be produced. The muscle fibers attached to one tendon organ appear to belong to several motor units (see Chapter 8). Each tendon organ probably monitors the tension produced by only a few motor units. Thus the central ner-vous system is informed not only of the overall tension produced by the muscle but also of how the workload is distributed among the different motor units.

Joint Receptors

Not only is information from muscle spin-dles and tendon organs of importance for our awareness of movements and for motor control—receptors in the connective tissue around the joints also bring relevant infor-mation. The relative importance of infor-mation from joint and muscle receptors is not yet clear, however, and the view of the functional role of the joint receptors has changed considerably during the past 30 years.

Many sensory nerve fibers end in the joint capsules and in the ligaments around the joints (Fig. 4.8). Many are free-ending recep-tors; others are encapsulated endings corre-

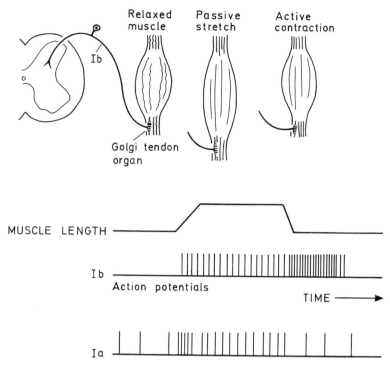

Fig. 4.7. *Functional properties of the tendon organ.* Action potentials are recorded from isolated Ib fibers in the dorsal roots. The firing frequency is indicated by vertical lines on the lower rows. Both passive stretching and active contrac- tion of the muscle increases the firing frequency of the Ib fiber, but active contraction produces the greatest increase. The firing frequency of a Ia fiber during the same experiment is shown for comparison.

sponding anatomically and with regard to response properties to encapsulated recep- tors in glabrous skin. The encapsulated joint receptors are *low-threshold mechanorecep- tors* and have been divided into four groups. The *type 1 joint receptor* resembles the *Ruf- fini corpuscle* in the dermis (Fig. 4.1). A mye- linate axon ramifies among collagen fibrils, within a thin connective tissue capsule. They are found almost exclusively in the fi- brous part of the joint capsules. The *ade- quate stimulus* of these Ruffini-like receptors is *increased tension* in the part of the capsule in which they lie. The higher the capsular tension, the higher the firing rate in the af- ferent sensory fiber from the receptor. Like the Ruffini corpuscle in the skin, this joint receptor is *slowly adapting*. Because the ten- sion in various parts of the capsule depends on the joint position, type 1 receptors would appear suited to signal the position of the joint. For example, receptors in the posterior

part of the elbow joint capsule would be highly active in a flexed position of the joint, which stretches the capsule, and less active in an extended position, which relaxes the capsule. The receptor also has dynamic sen- sitivity, giving a stronger response (higher firing rate) to a rapid movement than to a slow one. *The type 1 or Ruffini-like receptor thus seems capable of signaling static joint position, joint movements, and direction and speed of movements.* As will be discussed later, however, the ability of the type 1 re- ceptor to signal static joint position appears to be limited.

The *type 2 joint receptor* resembles struc- turally and functionally the Pacinian cor- puscle but is considerably smaller (it is also called *Paciniform receptor*). Type 2 recep- tors are present only in the fibrous part of the joint capsules. They are *rapidly adapt- ing*, and their *adequate stimulus is stretching of the part of the capsule in which they lie*.

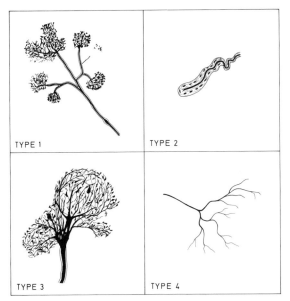

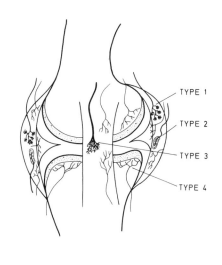

Fig. 4.8. *Joint innervation.* A knee joint, showing the distribution of the various kinds of joint receptors. To the **left,** the morphology of the four main receptor types is shown in more detail. From Brodal (1981).

Owing to their rapid adaptation, they can inform only of joint movements, not of static position. They appear particularly suited to signal movement velocity and have also been called "acceleration receptors."

A third kind of encapsulated receptor (type 3) resembles the tendon organ and is present in ligaments only. It is slowly adapting (like the tendon organ), but its functional role is unknown. A protective role in signaling overstretching of joints has been proposed but has not gained experiment support.

The fibrous part of the joint capsule and the ligaments are richly supplied with thin axons (myelinated and unmyelinated) ending in *free receptors*. These have been termed *type 4 joint receptors.* Many of these, like free endings in other tissues, are *nociceptors*. Others appear to play a role in circulatory and respiratory reflexes that are known to be elicited by passive joint movements.

Whether the *synovial membrane* of the joints receives sensory nerve fibers has been a matter of dispute. Recent immunocytochemical studies in man show, however, that there are thin fibers ending freely in the synovial membrane, and that such fibers contain peptides such as substance P (SP) and calcitonin gene-related peptide (CGRP), which are known to be present in many primary sensory neurons. In addition, there is a rich efferent (autonomic) innervation of the synovial vessels.

Kinesthesia

The term *kinesthesia* (sometimes used synonymously with *joint sensation*) is commonly, and also here, used to refer to *the perception of joint position, joint movements, and the direction and velocity of joint movements.* Strictly speaking, however, the word kinesthesia (Greek: kinesis = movement) encompasses only the dynamic and not the static aspect of sensation. The term joint sensation is not a good alternative, however, since it may give the false impression that kinesthesia depends *only* on joint receptors.

Our ability to judge the position of a joint (without seeing it), even after a long period without movement, is usually fairly precise, as can be verified by trying to match the position of the joint to be tested with the joint of the other side (for example, finger or elbow joints). This is the static part of kinesthesia. Nevertheless, the precision of our judgment is increased considerably if movements are allowed, particularly active movements.

The *static aspect of kinesthesia* depends on slowly adapting receptors that change their firing rate with changing joint position. The *dynamic aspect of kinesthesia*—that is, the ability to perceive that a movement is taking place and to judge the direction and velocity of the movement—depends on receptors with dynamic sensitivity, many of them rapidly adapting. Receptors with such properties, which are influenced by joint movements, are found in the skin, muscles, and around the joints. The accumulated evidence today indicates that *muscle spindles, joint receptors, and skin receptors all contribute to kinesthesia*. Muscle spindles appear to provide their most important contribution to kinesthesia with regard to large joints, such as the hip and knee joints, whereas joint receptors and skin receptors may provide more significant contributions with regard to finger and toe joints.

Changing Views of the Significance of Various Receptors for Kinesthesia

The views on which receptor types are responsible for kinesthesia have undergone considerable changes. At the beginning of this century, the newly discovered muscle spindle was held responsible for all aspects. Investigations during the 1950s and early 1960s, however, indicated that joint receptors had the necessary properties to signal all information needed for kinesthesia. It was also argued that the muscle spindle cannot give the necessary information, since the firing rate of its afferent nerve fibers depends not only on the actual position and movements of a joint but also on whether the γ motoneurons are active. It was also commonly held that impulses from the muscle spindles do not reach consciousness. Later, however, it was convincingly dem-

onstrated that signals from the muscle spindles *can* reach consciousness, and that they contribute to our kinesthetic sense. A simple demonstration to this effect was performed by vibrating the muscle belly or the tendon of the biceps muscle in a normal subject. Vibration is known to be a powerful way to stimulate the primary sensory endings of muscle spindles (the stimulus consists of brief stretches of the muscle). The subject, who is blindfolded, feels that the forearm is moving downward even though no such movement is occurring—that is, there is an illusory extensory movement at the elbow joint. This corresponds to a *lengthening* of the biceps muscle, and under normal circumstances, of course, this would be the normal cause of an increased firing rate in muscle spindle afferents.

Reexamination of the properties of joint receptors showed a striking paucity of slowly adapting joint receptors (type 1) that are active in midrange positions of the joint—that is, the range in which the precision of kinesthesia is best. Most type 1 receptors appear to reach their maximal firing rate only toward extreme joint positions. Thus, it seems unlikely that joint receptors alone can give all the necessary information.

Furthermore, examination of patients with artificial joints who lack joint capsules (and thus presumably most of their joint receptors) show that their kinesthesia is only slightly reduced—at least with regard to the hip joint and the metacarpophalangeal joints. Presumably, muscle spindles (not tendon organs) are responsible for the remaining kinesthesia in such cases, even though skin receptors may contribute as well (particularly for the metacarpophalangeal joints). For the knee joint, however, elimination of presumably all afferent signals from the joint capsule and the overlying skin by local anesthesia did not impair kinesthesia appreciably. Local anesthesia of finger joint capsules and the skin of the fingers gives more marked reduction of kinesthesia, but not even in such cases is the loss of kinesthesia complete.

THE SENSORY FIBERS AND THE DORSAL ROOTS

Afferent (sensory) fibers from the receptors follow the peripheral nerves toward the central nervous system. Close to the spinal cord, the sensory fibers are collected in the dorsal roots and enter the cord through these. The sensory fibers of the spinal nerves have their perikarya in the dorsal root ganglia (Figs. 2.1 and 2.13). Likewise, the sensory fibers in the cranial nerves have their perikarya in ganglia close to the brain stem (Chapter 13).

As mentioned, the spinal ganglion cells are pseudounipolar and send one long process peripherally, ending freely or in encapsulated sense organs. Functionally and structurally, both the peripheral and the central processes are axons. The central process enters the cord and then divides into an ascending and a descending branch (Fig. 4.9). These branches give off several collaterals ventrally to the gray matter of the cord. One sensory neuron, entering the cord through one dorsal root, can therefore influ-

ence spinal neurons at several segmental levels of the cord.

Are There Sensory Fibers in the Ventral Roots?

An old controversy concerning the question of whether there are afferent fibers in the ventral roots seems to have been settled recently. Electron microscopic investigations have demonstrated the presence of a large number of unmyelinated fibers in the ventral roots of several species, including man. Some of these are efferent, preganglionic autonomic fibers, but physiological data indicate that many are sensory and react to stimulation of nociceptors. Studies with retrograde axonal transport have furthermore shown that these sensory fibers have their perikarya in the dorsal root ganglia. Most pass only for a short distance in the ventral root, however, and either innervate the pia mater or curve back to enter the cord through the dorsal roots. Few,

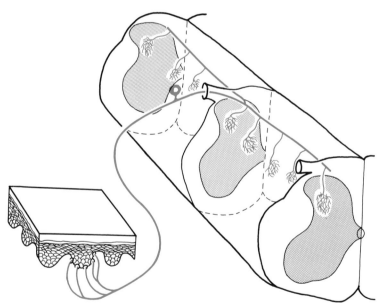

Fig. 4.9. *Terminal pattern of a dorsal root fiber.* A dorsal root fiber (in this case conducting from disks of Merkel) divides into an ascending and a descending branch after entering the cord. These branches give off several collaterals ending in the dorsal horn. The piece of the cord shown is about 1 cm long, but the axon continues be-

yond this in both directions. Corresponding reconstructions have been made for sensory units leading from several other kinds of receptors, and each sensory unit has a characteristic terminal pattern in the dorsal horn. Based on Brown (1981).

if any, appear to enter the cord through the ventral roots. The functional significance of these peculiar arrangements is unknown.

Classification of Dorsal Root Fibers in Accordance with Their Thickness

The dorsal root fibers vary in thickness, from the thickest myelinated ones, with a diameter of 20 μm and conduction velocity of 120 m/sec, to the thinnest unmyelinated fibers, with a diameter of less than 1 μm and conduction velocity of less than 1 m/sec. The thick fibers belong to the ganglion cells with large perikarya, and the thin fibers belong to those with small perikarya. We have previously mentioned classification of sensory axons from muscle mechanoreceptors by their thickness (conduction velocity) into groups I and II. Another classification of sensory neurons, on the basis of their conduction velocity, is also used (mainly for cutaneous afferents). *Myelinated fibers* fall within *group A*, and *group C* contains the *unmyelinated fibers*. In the A group, the fastest conducting (thickest) fibers are termed Aα, somewhat slower conducting fibers are Aβ, and the thinnest of the myelinated fibers are called Aδ.

The different kinds of sensory receptors are supplied with axons of characteristic thickness. Impulses from low-threshold mechanoreceptors are, for example, conducted in thick myelinated fibers (Aα and Aβ). Impulses from cold receptors are conducted in thin myelinated fibers (Aδ), whereas unmyelinated (C) fibers conduct from heat receptors. Impulses from nociceptors are conducted in Aδ and C fibers. In the spinal cord, the terminations of the Aδ and C fibers are almost completely separated from those of the Aα and Aβ fibers (Fig. 4.10).

Fibers from Different Receptors End in Different Parts of the Dorsal Horn

Early physiological experiments showed that impulses from different receptor types activate neurons in somewhat different parts of the spinal gray matter. For example, neurons particularly

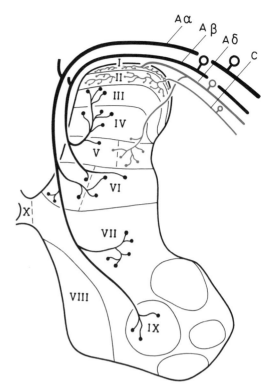

Fig. 4.10. *The terminal regions of the dorsal root fibers in the cord.* The thickest myelinated fibers (Aα, from muscle spindles and tendon organs) end in the deep parts of the dorsal horn and partly also in the ventral horn. Thick, myelinated fibers from cutaneous mechanoreceptors (Aβ) end in laminae III–VI. The thinnest myelinated and unmyelinated dorsal root fibers (Aδ and C)—many of them leading from nociceptors—end in laminae I, II, and parts of V. Based on experiments with axonal transport of tracer substances.

in Rexed's lamina VI are activated by joint movements, whereas impulses from cutaneous low-threshold mechanoreceptors activate mostly neurons in laminae III to V. That afferent fibers from low-threshold mechanoreceptors—that is, Aα and Aβ fibers—end in deep layers of the dorsal horn has been verified with combined physiological and anatomic techniques (intra-axonal tracer injections after physiological characterization). Such experiments have also made it possible to study in detail the pattern of the spinal termination of individual sensory units. Figure 9.4 gives an example of this. Single axons in the dorsal root have been penetrated with thin glass microelectrodes (pipette). After determination of the receptive field and adequate stimulus of the sensory unit, the same pipette is used to inject HRP intra-axonally. The axon and its ramifications can subsequently be followed in sections of the spinal cord. A remarkable degree of specificity has been shown in the pattern of termination of fibers belonging to functionally different receptors.

Thin Aδ and C fibers conducting impulses from nociceptors have been shown to end almost exclusively in the dorsalmost parts of the dorsal horn—that is, laminae I and II (substantia gelatinosa). The Aδ fibers, however, to some extent also terminate in lamina V.

Whereas the thin afferent fibers (many coming from nociceptors) from the skin end in laminae I, II, and V, corresponding fibers from the viscera have been shown to end almost exclusively in laminae I and V, thus avoiding the substantia gelatinosa. Thin muscle afferents appear to terminate in the same parts of the dorsal horn as the fibers from viscera. It is a common experience that pain of visceral origin, and also that arising in muscle, has different qualities than pain evoked from the skin—being much more diffuse and difficult to localize. Presumably, the anatomic arrangements in the dorsal horn may be partly responsible for such differences.

Fiber Categories and Conscious Sensations

Relations between impulses conducted in sensory fibers of various calibers and conscious sensations have been investigated primarily by graded electrical stimulation of peripheral nerves and selective block of axonal conduction. By *electrical stimulation* of peripheral nerves, the weakest stimulation evokes activity only in the thickest myelinated fibers, and with increasing intensity the thinner fibers are recruited progressively. Thus, the thickest fibers have the lowest electrical threshold for activation. In human subjects, pain is evoked by such stimulation only if the stimulus is strong enough to activate Aδ fibers. The person then typically reports that the pain is of a sharp, pricking quality. If the stimulus strength is increased to recruit C fibers as well, the person experiences an intense, often burning pain that

continues after the stimulus stops. These experiments are in agreement with the common experience that one usually can distinguish two phases of pain after an acute injury: The first phase, or *fast pain,* is experienced immediately after the stimulus, is well localized, and not very intense; the second phase, or *slow pain,* occurs with a longer latency and is more unpleasant, is not well localized, and usually continues after the end of the stimulus. The slow pain is delayed because it is dependent on being conducted in C fibers with a conduction velocity of less than 1 m/sec.

Injection of *local anesthetics* around a peripheral nerve blocks the thinnest (C) fibers first and the thickest myelinated ones last. Accordingly, with local anesthetics the pain disappears first, whereas the tactile sensation is conserved considerably longer, and some may remain throughout the period of anesthesia. When peripheral nerves are subjected to *pressure,* conduction in thick fibers is blocked first, and, accordingly, there first occurs a reduction of the ability to perceive light touch and to judge the position of joints, whereas pain perception is still present.

The difference in conduction velocity between fibers giving rise to fast and slow pain is most easily observed when something painful hits the foot (for example, when a toe is bumped into a hard object), because the pathway from the toe to the cerebral cortex is longer than from any other part of the body, so the time lag between the impulses conducted in thick and thin fibers is greatest. The very first sensation is in fact only that something touched the foot, due to activation of low-threshold mechanoreceptors. Almost simultaneously, the sharp and well-localized fast pain is perceived, and we then know that the pain will soon be worse—the diffuse, burning, and intensely unpleasant slow pain continuing for some time.

Primary Sensory Fibers and Neurotransmitters

Probably all primary sensory neurons release a classical transmitter with fast synaptic actions in the spinal cord. Among other evidence, this is based on the observation that boutons originating from dorsal root afferents contain small, clear vesicles, which have been shown in other parts of the nervous system to contain this kind of neurotransmitter. The most likely candidate for dorsal root neurons is the excitatory amino acid *glutamate*. There is also indirect evidence that some primary sensory fibers release the nucleotide *ATP*, shown in other parts of the nervous system to exert fast, excitatory synaptic actions.

Several neuropeptides have been demonstrated in the central and peripheral terminals and in the perikarya of spinal ganglion cells with immunocytochemical techniques. These include substance P (SP) vasoactive intestinal polypeptide (VIP), cholecystokinin (CCK), somatostatin, calcitonin gene-related peptide (CGRP), galanin, and others. The functions of these peptides are largely unknown, but they presumably mediate slow, modulatory synaptic actions in the dorsal horn. Coexistence of classical transmitters and neuropeptides is probably the rule for spinal ganglion cells, as for many central neurons. Most of the peptides are, however, found only in small ganglion cells, which have thin axons. Together with the demonstration that SP is released from dorsal root fibers in the dorsal horn on nociceptor activation, this has led to the assumption that SP is a neurotransmitter for nociceptive sensory neurons. A clear correlation between the adequate stimulus for single ganglion cells and the kind of neuropeptide they contain, however, has not emerged from studies combining physiological and immunocytochemical characterization of single spinal ganglion cells.

Even less is understood about the function of neuropeptides present in the peripheral ramifications of primary sensory neurons than about those in the central terminals. Several of these peptides, when liberated in the tissues, have profound effects on vessels, as shown in the skin and mucous membranes. SP and VIP both produce vasodilatation and thereby increased blood flow, and also increased extravasation of fluid from the capillaries and edema. It is not known, however, whether these peptides are released under normal circumstances and take part in the normal control of blood flow. Inhalation of irritating gases may provoke release of SP from peripheral sensory fibers in the airways, and the same takes place in the skin upon strong mechanical stimulation, such as scratching. The liberation of SP in such cases is probably due to an *axon reflex* (see

p. 366), because afferent signals from the receptors are transmitted not only toward the spinal cord but also distally in branches of the sensory fibers (that is, distally in the branches that were not stimulated).

The Segmental Innervation: The Dermatomes

The ventral branches (rami) of the spinal nerves form plexuses supplying the arms (Fig. 8.1) and the legs. Each of the nerves emerging from these plexuses contains sensory and motor fibers coming from several segments. In the peripheral distribution of the fibers, however, the segmental origin of the fibers is retained. Thus, sensory fibers of one spinal segment—that is, of one dorsal root—supply a distinct part of the skin. *The area of the skin supplied with sensory fibers from one spinal segment is called a dermatome.* In the thorax and abdomen, these dermatomes are shaped like circular belts. In the extremities, however, conditions are more complicated (Figs. 4.11 and 4.12). Knowledge of the segmental innervation of the skin (and also of the segmental innervation of muscles and viscera, dealt with in Chapter 8 and 14) is of great practical value in clinical neurology. For example, if a dorsal root is interrupted, the skin sensation is reduced or abolished in the corresponding dermatome.

Because the dermatomes overlap, each spot on the skin is innervated by sensory fibers from at least two dorsal roots. Interruption of a single dorsal root therefore may not produce a clear-cut sensory deficit. Nevertheless, careful examination usually shows a narrow zone (centrally in the dermatome) where the cutaneous sensation to touch is slightly reduced and that for pain is abolished (analgesia). The usually more marked reduction in pain than in touch sensation is due to less extensive overlap of fibers coming from nociceptors than of fibers coming from low-threshold mechanoreceptors.

When a dorsal root is subjected to irritation, as may happen by compression or

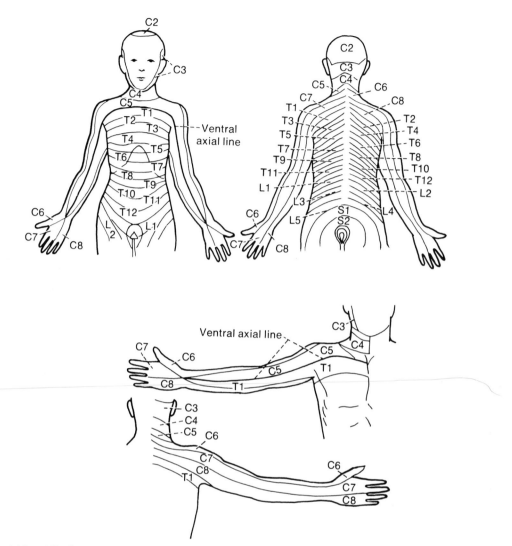

Fig. 4.11. *The dermatomes of the trunk and the upper extremity.* Dermatomes not supplied by neighboring spinal segments meet at the ventral axial line (C_5 and T_1). From Keegan and Garrett (1948).

stretching in connection with growth of an intraspinal tumor or protrusion of an intervertebral disk, this causes pain and other sensory phenomena (numbness, pricking, tingling, and so forth) in the territory of the dermatome. Often the symptoms are felt only in smaller parts of the dermatome. With a protruding (herniated) intervertebral disk in the lumbar spine, for example, most often the roots of the fifth lumbar or first sacral nerves are affected (Fig. 4.12), and the pain is felt in the leg (sciatica).

How the Dermatomes Have Been Determined

The oldest method for determining the dermatome was to follow the distribution of the nerves by dissection. To follow the course of fibers from a root through the plexuses is, of course, far from easy. Certain diseases may affect single dorsal roots and produce changes restricted to the dermatome. Shingles (herpes zoster), for example, is a viral infection of the spinal ganglion cells that produces skin eruptions in the dermatome of the affected dorsal roots. Examination of many patients with this disease served as a basis for maps

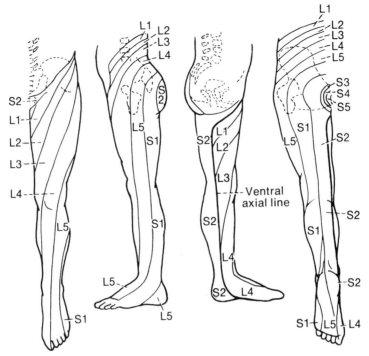

Fig. 4.12. *The dermatomes of the lower extremity.* From Keegan and Garrett (1948).

showing the dermatome (Head). Electrical stimulation of dorsal roots during operations (Foerster) and comparison of observations during operations for herniated intervertebral disks with the information given previously by the patient of where the pain and sensory loss were localized also helped to determine the location of dermatomes. Local anesthesia of single or several dorsal roots in healthy volunteers has also been of value. The best method is to eliminate impulse conduction in several dorsal roots on each side of one that is left intact. This can only be performed systematically in animals, as was done by Sherrington in monkeys, and the results are not directly applicable to humans.

The dermatomal map presented here (Figs. 4.11 and 4.12, reproduced from Keegan and Garrett) is based on observations of a large number of patients with root compressions (usually due to a herniated intervertebral disk) and, in addition, on examination of the distribution of reduced sensation in volunteers subjected to local anesthesia of dorsal roots. The skin regions with reduced sensation (hypesthesia) were carefully mapped out before operation, and during operation it was determined which root was affected.

Local anesthesia also produces a sensory loss much less extensive than the total distribution of sensory fibers of one dorsal root. Thus, the borders between dermatomes as presented in Figures 4.11 and 4.12 are imaginary. They ignore, for example, the great overlap between neighboring dermatomes, and on the other hand, that the dermatomes are much wider than the zones of hypesthesia occurring after damage to one dorsal root.

It should be kept in mind that all dermatomal maps are composites of many single observations—in no single person have more than one or a few dermatomes been determined. For this reason, all maps showing dermatomes for the whole body can only be regarded as approximations, not taking into account, for example, the considerable individual variations that exist. This, together with the fact that different methods have been used, probably explains why the dermatomal maps of different authors vary so much. For the student the main emphasis should therefore be on learning certain main features of the dermatomal distribution rather than the artificial (and falsely accurate) borders indicated on the maps.

Sensory Fibers Are Links in Reflex Arcs: Spinal Interneurons

Sensory information reaching the spinal cord through the dorsal roots is further conveyed to higher levels of the central nervous system, as will be described later. In addition, however, it should be observed that many of the spinal neurons that are contacted by dorsal root fibers are not links in ascending sensory pathways but have axons that ramify within the cord—that is, they are *spinal interneurons*. The axons of these interneurons establish synaptic contacts with other spinal neurons, among them motoneurons and neurons in the intermediolateral cell column, giving origin to efferent fibers to smooth muscles and glands (sympathetic preganglionic fibers). In this manner, *reflex arcs* for several important somatic (skeletal muscle) and autonomic (visceral) reflexes are established. Most, if not all, spinal interneurons also establish connections between neurons at different segmental levels (propriospinal fibers). Each spinal interneuron thus establishes synaptic contacts with a very large number of other neurons in the spinal cord. *Impulses entering the cord through one dorsal root may influence neurons at several segmental levels* both via their own ascending and descending collaterals and via their influence on interneurons with propriospinal collaterals (Figs. 4.9 and 8.9). How far the impulses from one dorsal root fiber are propagated from interneuron to interneuron depends on what other synaptic influences these interneurons are subjected to. For example, higher levels of the central nervous system, such as the brain stem and the cerebral cortex, can selectively facilitate or inhibit spinal interneurons. This enables the impulse traffic from dorsal root fibers to be directed so that certain reflex arcs are used, whereas other are "turned off," in accordance with the need of the organism as a whole.

Spinal reflexes are treated in more detail in Chapter 8.

CENTRAL PARTS OF THE SOMATOSENSORY SYSTEM

So far in this chapter we have dealt with the peripheral parts of the somatosensory system—the receptors and the primary sensory neurons. We now turn to the tracts and nuclei conveying and processing somatosensory information within the central nervous system. The term somatosensory pathways is not entirely appropriate, however, because these pathways transmit signals not only from somatic structures, such as skin, muscles, and joints, but also from visceral organs. Most impulses from visceral organs are not consciously perceived, and visceral sensory processes have been less intensively investigated than somatosensory ones.

Main Features of the Organization of the Somatosensory Pathways

There are several parallel somatosensory pathways, but most *consist of three neurons forming a chain from the receptors to the cerebral cortex.* The first, the *primary sensory neuron,* has its perikaryon in a spinal ganglion or a cranial nerve ganglion; the next, the *secondary sensory neuron,* has its perikaryon in the gray matter of the spinal cord or in the brain stem; and the third, the *tertiary sensory neuron,* has its perikaryon in the thalamus (Figs. 4.13 and 4.14). *All of the somatosensory pathways are crossed,* so that signals from one side of the body are brought to the cerebral hemisphere of the other side. The actual crossing over takes place at different levels for the various pathways, however. Another important point is that the pathways are *somatotopically organized,* which implies that neurons that conduct impulses from different parts of the body are kept separate. The pathways are also organized so that, to a large extent, neurons conveying signals related to different sensory modalities are kept separate.

Whereas axons of different thicknesses conducting from different kinds of receptors lie intermingled in the peripheral nerves and

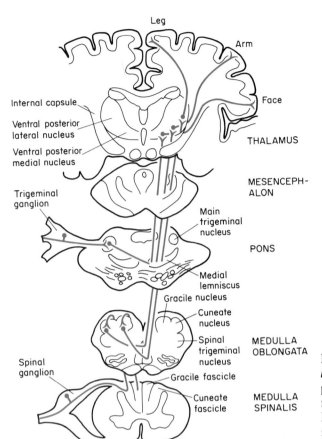

Fig. 4.13. *The dorsal column–medial lemniscus pathway.* This is the main pathway for transmission of signals from low-threshold mechanoreceptors. Fibers leading impulses from mechanoreceptors in the face join the medial lemniscus in the brain stem.

the dorsal roots, they are grouped in accordance with their thickness as soon as they enter the spinal cord. *The thick dorsal root fibers pass medially, whereas the thin ones follow a more lateral course into the dorsal horn* (Fig. 4.10). Their further course is also different: The medially located, thick dorsal root fibers continue without synaptic interruption rostrally in the dorsal funiculus, as part of the *dorsal column–medial lemniscus pathway* (Fig. 4.13). The perikarya of the secondary neurons in this pathway are located in the medulla oblongata, and the crossing of the pathway also takes place at the medullary level. Since the thickest dorsal root axons mainly conduct impulses from *low-threshold mechanoreceptors,* one might expect that the dorsal column–medial lemniscus pathway is of importance for perception of *touch, pressure, vibration,* and *kinesthesia.* As will be discussed below, this is

largely correct. It should be emphasized, however, that the pathway is of primary importance for discriminatory aspects of sensation—that is, the ability to distinguish differently located and different kinds of stimuli. The pathway appears not to be necessary for the mere perception of, for example, light touch or movement of a joint.

The pathway followed by impulses conducted in the *thin dorsal root fibers* is different. The thin (Aδ and C) primary afferent fibers end in the gray matter of the dorsal horn, where most of the secondary sensory neurons of this pathway are located. The axons of the secondary neurons cross to the other side of the spinal cord and form the *spinothalamic tract* (Fig. 4.14). As the name implies, the fibers of this tract terminate in the thalamus. The spinothalamic tract is of primary importance for the *perception of pain and temperature,* which is consistent

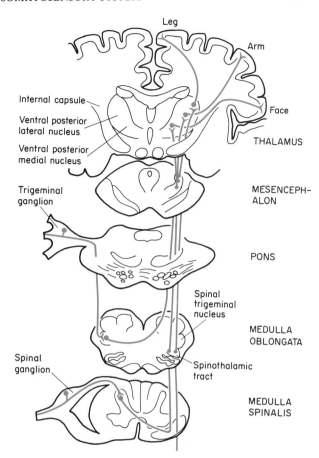

Fig. 4.14. *The spinothalamic tract.* This is the main pathway for transmission of signals from nociceptors and thermoreceptors.

with the observation that it primarily transmits information from Aδ and C dorsal root afferents. (There are also some other, less important, pathways capable of transmitting somatosensory information.)

Before we describe the two major somatosensory pathways in more depth, a few basic features of the thalamus need to be emphasized.

The Thalamus—Relay Station for Sensory Pathways

Almost all pathways conducting sensory information from the receptors to the cerebral cortex—the somatosensory pathways among them—are synaptically interrupted in the thalamus. In addition, the thalamus has a decisive influence on the general level of neuronal activity of the cerebral cortex and thus on the level of consciousness. The macroscopic appearance of the thalamus was described and illustrated in Chapter 2 (Figs. 2.23, 2.25, and 4.19). Three major subdivisions, delimited by the Y-shaped *internal medullary lamina,* can be identified macroscopically (Figs. 2.25 and 2.28): the *anterior, medial, and lateral nuclear groups.* The lateral nucleus is usually divided into a dorsal and a ventral part (each consisting of several subnuclei; see also Figs. 4.19 and 17.7). Within and close to the internal medullary lamina are several less clearly defined groups of neurons, the *intralaminar thalamic nuclei.* These are of particular interest because of their relation to the thalamic influence on consciousness and sleep (this is further described in Chapters 12 and 17). The intralaminar nuclei are probably also of importance for the perception of pain.

Each of the three major thalamic subdivisions (the anterior, medial, and lateral nuclei) can be further subdivided into smaller parts on the basis of cytoarchitectonics. These are also called the *specific thalamic nuclei,* because most of them are relays in precisely organized, major pathways reaching certain parts of the cerebral cortex only.[3] The various specific nuclei have different functional tasks, and they receive fiber connections from the somatosensory nuclei, the retina, the nuclei of the auditory pathways, the cerebellum, the basal ganglia, and some other cell groups. Each nucleus as a rule receives afferents from only one of these sources.

The somatosensory pathways terminate in a subdivision of the lateral thalamic nucleus, as will be dealt with in more detail later in this chapter.

The Dorsal Columns and the Medial Lemniscus

The thick, myelinated fibers in the medial portion of the dorsal roots curve rostrally within the dorsal columns just after entering the cord. Many of these fibers ascend to the *dorsal column nuclei* in the medulla, where they terminate and establish synaptic contacts (Fig. 4.13). As the fibers ascend in the dorsal columns, they send off collaterals ventrally to the spinal gray matter (Fig. 4.9). Most of these collaterals establish snyaptic

contact with interneurons, but some reach as far as the ventral horn and contact α motoneurons.

The fibers occupying the medial part of the dorsal columns, the *gracile fascicle* (fasciculus gracilis), conduct impulses from the lower part of the trunk and the legs (Figs. 4.13 and 4.15). These fibers end in the *gracile nucleus* (nucleus gracilis). Impulses from the upper part of the trunk and the arms are conducted in the lateral part of the dorsal columns, the *cuneate fascicle* (fasciculus cuneatus). The fibers of the cuneate fascicle terminate in the *cuneate nucleus* (nucleus cuneatus). Why the longest fibers of the dorsal columns are situated most medially is explained by the simple fact that they enter the cord at the lowermost level, where no other long ascending fibers are present. At higher levels, fibers entering from the dorsal root occupy positions lateral to those that have entered at more caudal levels. Initially the fibers of the dorsal columns are arranged *segmentally* (Fig. 4.15), but as they ascend, the fibers rearrange themselves so that they are organized *somatotopically* (Fig. 4.16)—that is, fibers conducting from the hand lie together, separated from those of the forearm, and so on (compare with the dermatomal map in Fig. 4.11). Thus, fibers from different dorsal roots are mixed at higher levels of the dorsal columns.

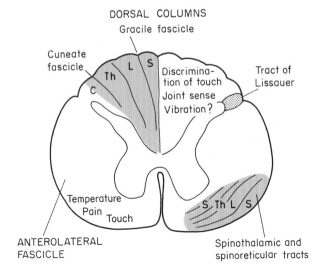

Fig. 4.15. *Somatosensory pathways.* Position and segmental arrangement in the spinal cord white matter.

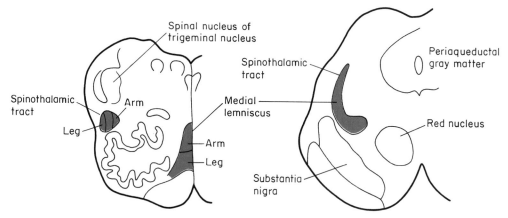

Fig. 4.16. *Somatosensory pathways.* Position and somatotopic arrangement in the medulla and the mesencephalon.

The primary afferent fibers ascending in the dorsal columns end in a particular cytoarchitectonic subdivision of the dorsal column nuclei. The morphology and arrangement of the neurons in these "cluster regions" ensure a particularly precise topographic arrangement of the afferent and efferent connections. The neurons of the "cluster regions" of the dorsal column nuclei send their axons rostrally to the thalamus, forming the *medial lemniscus.* The fibers first course anteriorly and cross the midline to occupy a position just dorsal to the pyramid (Figs. 2.17 and 4.16). In the

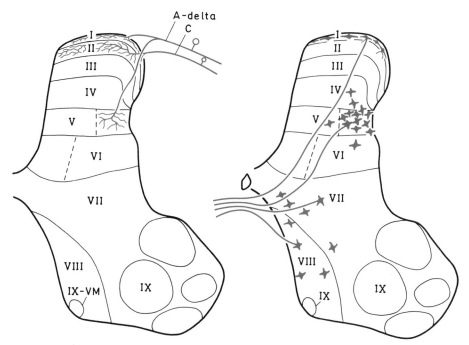

Fig. 4.17. *Signal transmission from nociceptors in the spinal cord.* The terminal region of thin dorsal root fibers leading from nociceptors, and the position of cells sending their axons to the opposite thalamus (spinothalamic neurons). Note that lamina II (the substantia gelatinosa) receives many C fibers, but the neurons of this lamina do not send their axons to the thalamus.

pons and the mesencephalon, the medial lemniscus is placed more laterally (Figs. 2.19 and 4.16).

The medial lemniscus ends in the *ventral posterolateral nucleus (VPL)* (nucleus ventralis posterior lateralis) (Figs. 4.13 and 4.19). The fibers of the medial lemniscus are somatotopically organized,[4] and this pattern is maintained as the fibers terminate in the VPL. Fibers from the gracile nucleus (sensory impulses from the leg) terminate most laterally, with fibers from the cuneate nucleus (arm) terminating more medially. Most medially, in a separate nucleus, the *ventral posteromedial nucleus (VPM),* ends the fibers from the sensory trigeminal nucleus (relaying impulses from the face).

The neurons of the VPL and the VPM send their axons into the internal capsule (Figs. 2.28 and 4.13) and further through this to the *postcentral gyrus*. This part of the cortex, made up of cytoarchitectonic fields 3, 1, and 2 (after Brodmann; see Fig. 17.3), constitutes the *primary somatosensory area (SI)* (Figs. 4.13, 4.19, and 4.20). In addition, some fibers from the VPL and the VPM end in the *secondary somatosensory area, SII,* situated in the upper wall of the lateral cerebral fissure (Fig. 4.20).

On electrical stimulation of SI or SII, human subjects (during operations with local anesthesia) report that they experience sensory phenomena (tingling, itching, numbness, and other). Just as the somatosensory pathways are somatotopically organized, this is also the case within SI and SII (Figs. 4.13 and 4.20). Fibers conducting impulses from the leg end most medially within the postcentral gyrus, then follow fibers conveying impulses from the trunk, arm, and face successively in the lateral direction. The parts of SI receiving sensory impulses from the feet, hands, and face are much larger than those receiving impulses from other parts of the body (Fig. 4.21). Also, the region devoted to the thumb is larger than that devoted to the palm of the hand, which in turn is larger than that devoted to the forearm, and so on. This is mainly a reflection of the much higher density of sensory units that supply the skin at distal parts of the extremities (and parts of the face) than more proximal parts of the trunk. To utilize this very detailed information from the most densely innervated parts of the body, a large volume of cortical gray matter—that is, many neurons—has to be available for information processing.

Certain Kinds of Epilepsy Demonstrate the Cortical Somatotopic Pattern

On irritation of the cortex within the postcentral gyrus—for example, by a chip of bone from a skull fracture—the patient may experience fits of abnormal sensations. In the same person, the fits have the same characteristic pattern each time: The sensations are felt in one particular part of the body and then spread gradually to other parts. The spreading follows the known somatotopic pattern within SI (Fig. 4.21). For example, the patient may first experience a tingling sensation in the thumb, then it moves to the index finger and the other fingers, then to the forearm, upper arm, shoulder, and even further. Such epileptic seizures are called *Jacksonian fits* (after a famous British neurologist, Hughlings Jackson). They signify the presence of a local disease process of the brain, and the starting point of the abnormal sensations indicates the focus of the disease. Often the sensory phenomena are followed by muscle spasms (convulsions) due to spreading of the abnormal cortical electrical activity to the motor cortex of the precentral gyrus.

The Function of the Dorsal Column–Medial Lemniscus System

Two types of investigations usually form the basis for our conclusions about the function of a particular tract or pathway in the central nervous system. One kind of data derives from the recording of the activity of the neurons of the pathway, to determine the factors that influence their activity. Most of our knowledge of the properties of single neurons in the somatosensory pathways thus derives from experiments in animals, even though recordings have sometimes been done in humans during brain surgery. The other type of investigation is to study the functional deficits that follow disruption of the tract of interest. In humans, diseases and injuries seldom affect one tract or pathway alone (for example only the dorsal columns), and furthermore, it is often not possible to determine the exact site of the damage.

With regard to the two major somatosensory pathways, there is agreement on most points that pertain to the adequate stimulus for single neurons at different levels of the central nervous system. When it comes to the deficits caused by their interruption, however, findings are partly conflicting. This is particularly true of the dorsal column–medial lemniscus system.

Why Similar Experiments May Produce Very Different Sensory Deficits

It may be difficult to understand why apparently identical experimental lesions of sensory tracts in the same species are in one laboratory reported to produce marked disturbances of movements and sensation, whereas in another laboratory hardly any deficits are observed. One explanation may be that, in spite of histological control of the lesions, they may have been of different magnitude and may have either included more than the tract under study or not interrupted all the fibers of the tract. Thus, experiments in cats have shown that sparing as little as 10% of the fibers of the dorsal columns may markedly reduce the sensory deficits with regard to, for example, the discrimination of surfaces with different roughness (as compared with a lesion comprising all fibers). Another reason for different results may be that sometimes the acute effects and the long-term effects of a lesion are not clearly distinguished. As a rule, the acute deficits—that is, those occurring immediately after a tract is cut—are much more severe than those present after some weeks or months.

As mentioned above, the *dorsal columns contain primarily fibers coming from low-threshold mechanoreceptors in the skin, muscles, and joints.* Recording the activity of single units in the dorsal columns has confirmed this and has also shown that there is a predominance of rapidly adapting sensory units—relatively few are slowly adapting. Recordings from neurons in the cluster regions of the dorsal column nuclei show that many neurons are activated only by one kind of receptor and that they have small receptive fields, mostly at the distal parts of the extremities. Some are activated only by joint movement, others only by light touch of the skin, others only by vibration and so on. Such neurons are called *modality-specific* (because they react only to one kind of stimulus) and *place-specific* (because they are activated only from one restricted part of the body). Neurons in the VPL and SI also have the same characteristic response properties as those described for the neurons of the dorsal column nuclei, even though there is an increasing number of neurons that are activated by more than one kind of receptor. Also, the receptive field tends to be somewhat larger for neurons in SI than, for example, in the dorsal column nuclei.

The Dorsal Columns Do Not Only Contain Primary Afferent Fibers

The fiber composition of the dorsal columns is more heterogeneous than was previously believed. Thus, some of the ascending axons that synapse in the dorsal column nuclei do not belong to spinal ganglion cells but to neurons with their perikarya in the dorsal horn (so-called postsynaptic dorsal column neurons). The functional properties of these are different from those of the primary sensory neurons with fibers in the dorsal columns. Thus, the postsynaptic units are often activated from several types of receptors. Some have a high stimulus threshold, suggesting that they are activated from nociceptors. The functional role of the postsynaptic dorsal column fibers is so far unknown. Such fibers terminate in other parts of the dorsal column nuclei than do the primary afferent fibers (that is, not in the cluster regions), and it is possible that their signals are not relayed further in the medial lemniscus to the VPL. There is no convincing evidence that the dorsal columns are of importance for pain perception.

Many of the primary afferent fibers in the dorsal columns do not reach the dorsal column nuclei, even though they may pass for many segments—for example, from the lumbar to the cervical levels. In addition, the dorsal columns contain a large number of propriospinal axons (that is, from neurons located in the spinal gray matter).

Finally, at least in experimental animals, the dorsal columns also contain some descending axons coming from neurons in parts of the dorsal column nuclei and making synaptic contacts in the dorsal horn. Thus, the dorsal column nuclei may be able to influence the processing of sensory information at the spinal level.

The axons at all levels of the dorsal column–medial lemniscus system are thick and rapidly conducting. This, together with the data from single-unit recordings briefly mentioned above, enable us to conclude that *the dorsal column–medial lemniscus system is particularly well suited to bring fast and precise information from the skin and musculoskeletal system about the type of stimulus, the exact site of the stimulus, and when it starts and stops.* Thus, it informs about the sensory quality and the spatial and temporal characteristics of any stimulus of low intensity ("what," "where," and "when").

Experiments with cutting of the dorsal columns in monkeys and observations in humans with damage more or less limited to the dorsal columns indicate that the dorsal column–medial lemniscus system is not necessary for all aspects of cutaneous sensation and kinesthesia. First of all, temperature and pain perception appear to be unaltered by lesioning the dorsal columns. Secondly, light touch of the skin can easily be felt, as can passive joint movements. Two-point discrimination may not be appreciably reduced, and some reports even indicate that the ability to recognize objects by manipulation may be retained (clinical observations do not support the latter point, however). What appears to be consistently impaired is the ability to solve tasks that require spatially and, in particular, *temporally* very accurate sensory information. Thus, a coin pressed into the palm of the hand may perhaps be recognized, but the patient is unable to decide which is the larger of two coins. The patient may also correctly identify that something is moving on the skin, but not the direction of the movement. To ask the patient to identify figures written on the skin is, for example, one sensitive test of the function of the dorsal column–medial lemniscus system. Some careful clinical observations furthermore indicate that the perception of

joint position and movement is abnormal after lesions of the dorsal columns.[5]

All that the above-described sensory deficits occurring after lesions of the dorsal columns have in common is that they concern *spatial and temporal comparisons of stimuli,* that is, what we call *discriminative sensation.* Such sensory information is of crucial importance for the performance of many voluntary movements and, indeed, *disturbances of voluntary movements are characteristic of lesions affecting the dorsal column–medial lemniscus system.* Most studies (with some exceptions) indicate that in monkeys, as in humans, acute damage to the dorsal columns produces severe *ataxia* (insecure and incoordinated movements), which recedes partly or completely within weeks to months after the damage. In some patients, the ataxia may be so severe that they cannot walk without support. After the acute phase, the movement deficits concern first and foremost movements that require fast and reliable feedback information from the moving parts. For example, the ability to adjust the grip when an object is slipping is clearly reduced. Delicate movements, such as writing and buttoning, are performed only with difficulty after lesions of the dorsal columns. It is not possible to throw an object accurately or to perform a precise jump, presumably because such activities require feedback information from skin receptors to judge the pressure exerted on the hand by the object or by the ground against the sole of the foot.

Many of the deficits that occur after damage to the dorsal column–medial lemniscus system may not be revealed by a routine neurological examination but may nevertheless render the patient severely handicapped in daily life. One example from a thorough clinical study by the British neurologist Nathan may serve to illustrate this point: A patient with damage to the dorsal columns was aware of a toe being passively moved by the examiner; nevertheless, his shoe would easily slip off his foot without him noticing, and he was unable to roll over in bed because he did not realize that one leg was hanging off the bed.

The Spinothalamic Tract

As mentioned, the fibers in the lateral portion of the dorsal roots are predominantly thin (Aδ and C fibers). Immediately after entering the cord, such fibers divide into short ascending and descending branches—passing only for one or two segments in each direction. The collaterals and terminal branches of these fibers pass ventrally to end in the gray substance of the dorsal horn (Figs. 4.10 and 4.17), where they establish synaptic contacts with other neurons. The thinnest (largely C fibers) among the ascending and descending branches of the dorsal root fibers form a small bundle immediately dorsal to the dorsal horn, called the *tract of Lissauer* or the *dorsolateral fasciculus* (Figs. 2.12 and 4.15).[6]

Many neurons in the dorsal horn have long ascending axons. Most of these first course almost horizontally and somewhat ventrally across the midline through the gray substance. After having entered the lateral funiculus on the opposite side, the fibers curve sharply in the rostral direction (Figs. 4.14 and 4.17). As mentioned, some of these fibers ascend without interruption as far as the thalamus, thus forming the *spinothalamic tract*. The fibers of this tract are located anteriorly within the lateral funiculus (anterolateral fascicle) (Fig. 4.15). The spinothalamic fibers are intermingled in the anterolateral fascicle with other fibers that, for example, terminate in lower parts of the brain stem and numerous propriospinal fibers. In the brain stem, the spinothalamic tract is situated laterally and fairly superficially (Fig. 4.16).

The use of axonal transport methods in experimental animals has made it possible to determine the location of the perikarya of the neurons that give rise to the spinothalamic tract (Fig. 4.17). Such methods combined with physiological studies of the adequate stimuli and response characteristics of spinothalamic cells have provided new insight in recent years. Particularly, conditions in monkeys may be expected to correspond closely to those in humans (there are differences with regard to the organization of the spinothalamic tract among, for example, the rat, cat, and monkey). *Many spinothalamic cells are located in lamina I.* When we recall that many thin dorsal root afferents establish synapses in lamina I (Fig. 4.17), the relation between the spinothalamic tract and perception of pain becomes understandable. Another major group of spinothalamic cells is located in lamina V and particularly in those parts that receive Aδ fibers from the dorsal roots. In addition, scattered spinothalamic cells are found more ventrally in laminae VII and VIII (Fig. 4.17). It may appear surprising, however, that hardly any of the neurons in lamina II (substantia gelatinosa) send fibers into the spinothalamic tract, since most of the dorsal root C fibers terminate in this lamina.

The anatomic data indicate that *most thin dorsal root fibers do not synapse directly (monosynaptically) onto the spinothalamic cells but rather influence them indirectly via spinal interneurons.* The numerous small neurons in lamina II, which are contacted by dorsal root C fibers, send their axons in part dorsally into lamina I—where spinothalamic cells can be influenced—and in part ventrally in the dorsal horn to contact other interneurons, which in their turn form synapses on spinothalamic cells in laminae V, VII, and VIII. In addition, many of the neurons in lamina II send axon collaterals to spinal segments above and below their own (passing in the tract of Lissauer).

The synaptic arrangements underlying further transfer of signals transmitted in thin dorsal root afferents—many coming from nociceptors—must be very complicated. The large number of very small interneurons and the numerous neuroactive substances (for example, numerous neuropeptides) in the dorsal horn make it a difficult task to clarify how the impulses from nociceptors are processed in the spinal cord, and it is understandable that much remains in this respect. Generally, however, we can at least say the the *interneurons of the dorsal horn, especially those of the substantia gelatinosa, have a decisive influence on whether the signals from nociceptors will be transmitted to higher levels of the nervous system.*

These interneurons can both inhibit and facilitate the impulse traffic that will ascend in the spinothalamic tract. Thus, they will determine to a large extent how intense the experience of pain will be on a certain stimulation of nociceptors. As we will discuss later in this chapter, the central nervous system can control impulse transmission from receptors in general to our consciousness by, among other things, descending fibers acting on the dorsal horn interneurons.

The *thalamic termination site* of the spinothalamic tract is more extensive than that of the medial lemniscus. Many of the fibers end in the VPL with a somatotopic pattern (Fig. 4.14), but not in exactly the same parts as the fibers of the medial lemniscus. The terminal ramifications are also different for the two pathways, reflecting their functional differences. In addition, fibers of the spinothalamic tract end in more posterior parts of the thalamus (in the so-called posterior complex, PO) and in some of the *intralaminar nuclei* (among them, the central lateral nucleus, CL, and the nucleus submedius). These three thalamic regions may possibly be related to somewhat different aspects of pain perception (see below).

The further transmission of impulses from the thalamus takes place—as for the dorsal column–medial lemniscus system—in thalamocortical fibers passing to the primary and secondary somatosensory areas (SI and SII). Recordings of single-unit activity in monkey SI indicate that neurons activated by high intensity—presumably noxious—cutaneous stimuli are concentrated in a narrow zone at the transition between Brodmann's areas 3 and 1. This may primarily concern impulses relayed through the VPL, whereas impulses from other parts of the thalamus receiving spinothalamic fibers may directly and indirectly influence other cortical areas as well.

The Function of the Spinothalamic Tract

As mentioned above, perception of pain and temperature are particularly dependent on the spinothalamic tract. A relatively crude sense of touch and pressure can also be mediated by this pathway, as witnessed by clinical observations. These conclusions fit well with physiological studies of single spinothalamic cells and of thalamic cells in the terminal regions of spinothalamic fibers. It also is in accord with the physiological observation that spinothalamic cells are preferentially activated from thin (Aδ and C) dorsal root fibers.

The spinothalamic cells in the cord can be classified by their response properties: (1) *low threshold units*—cells that react only to light mechanical stimuli (for example, light touch of the skin); (2) *wide dynamic range units* (WDR)—cells that react to stimuli of high intensity (activating nociceptors) and to light stimuli. The impulse frequency of these cells increases with increasing stimulus intensity; (3) *high-threshold units* (HT)—cells that respond only to stimuli of an intensity sufficient to activate nociceptors; and (4) *thermosensitive units*—cells that respond only to either warming or cooling of the skin, indicating that they are activated by thermoreceptors.

These properties of spinothalamic cells, which have been determined in animal experiments, agree well with clinical observations in patients who have been subjected to therapeutic interruption of the anterolateral funiculus (containing the spinothalamic tract and other fibers). This operation, called *chordotomy,* is sometimes applied to alleviate intense pain that cannot be overcome in any other way (particularly pain caused by cancer of the lower abdominal and pelvic viscera). After such an operation, sensations of pain and temperature are almost totally abolished in the opposite side of the body in the parts supplied by sensory fibers from the spinal segments below the level of interruption.[7] Observations in patients with spinal injuries that leave only the anterolateral fascicle intact for the central transmission of sensory signals also indicate that some sensations of touch and kinesthesia remain.

Single-unit recordings in the three main thalamic terminal regions of the spinothalamic tract have suggested that there are certain functional differences among them. Schematically, the fibers ending most posteriorly (in PO) may be responsible for the immediate awareness of something painful ("ouch!"); those ending in the VPL signal *where* exactly the painful stimulus is ("my finger!"), whereas fibers ending in the intralaminar nuclei may be responsible for the intense discomfort and obligatory emotional aspects of pain sensation ("it hurts so—help me!"). So far, however, too little is known to enable this to be viewed as more than an interesting hypothesis. In particular, properties of neurons in the intralaminar nuclei are still insufficiently known.

Spinothalamic Cells Receive Impulses from Both Somatic and Visceral Structures: Referred Pain

Recording from spinothalamic cells in the spinal cord has shown that many can be activated by nociceptive stimuli applied to visceral organs and to the skin. Impulses from the skin and viscera *converge* onto the same neuron, which then conveys the information to the thalamus. Nociceptive impulses from muscles and skin can also converge onto the same spinothalamic neuron. *Sensory convergence of this kind pertains to regions of the skin and deep tissues and to visceral organs that receive sensory innervation from the same segments of the cord.* The primary sensory fibers can activate the spinothalamic cells monosynaptically or via one or more interneurons (polysynaptically). In any case, presumably it will not be possible for higher levels of the central nervous system to decide whether the impulses arriving from a particular spinothalamic cell (receiving convergent inputs) originate in the skin or in a visceral organ. But because nociceptors in the skin are stimulated often during daily life, whereas those in, for example, the heart are only activated when the organ is diseased, we assume that the brain gets used to interpreting the signals as always coming from the skin. When signals arise for the first time in the heart, they are misinterpreted as coming from the skin. The pain is felt in the skin and perhaps deep structures, even though it arises elsewhere. This phenomenon, commonly experienced with diseases of visceral organs, is called *referred pain*. Infarction of the heart, for example, is usually accompanied by pain localized to the left arm, diseases of the gall-

bladder may manifest themselves with pain below the right shoulder blade, irritation of the diaphragm produces pain at the top of the shoulder, and so forth. Convergence on spinothalamic cells may also explain the phenomenon of *hyperesthesia*—that is, a region of skin becomes abnormally sensitive, such that even light touch may provoke pain. This is commonly observed with diseases of visceral organs, and careful examination to search for hyperesthetic skin regions may provide valuable diagnostic information. Thus, impulses from the visceral organ excite the spinothalamic cell so that less excitation from the skin is necessary to fire the cell (recall that many spinothalamic cells receive inputs from both low-threshold and high-threshold receptors—the wide dynamic range neurons).

Furthermore, it has been found that the peripheral nerve fiber of at least *some spinal ganglion cells divides, with one branch going to the skin and another going to a visceral organ* or a muscle. This may also serve to explain the phenomenon of referred pain. Cutaneous hyperesthesia may in such instances be caused by a so-called *axon reflex* (see "The Axonal Reflex" in Chapter 14), since sensory impulses from the visceral organ are conducted not only into the cord but also peripherally in the branch to the skin. There neuropeptides, such as SP and VPI, may be liberated from the sensory fibers and cause changes of blood flow in the hyperesthetic area of the skin.

Alterations of autonomically regulated processes of the skin, such as blood flow and sweat secretion, may also be mediated by spinal reflexes. Thus, impulses from visceral nociceptors may activate sympathetic (preganglionic) neurons in the cord, which influence vessels and sweat glands. Again, the skin manifestations are localized to dermatome that are supplied from the same spinal segments as the diseased visceral organ.

Nociceptors and the Perception of Pain

It should be emphasized at this point that activation of nociceptors—provoked by noxious stimuli—and the conscious experience of pain may occur independently of each other. The usual definition of a *nociceptor* is purely physiological: *A receptor that is activated by stimuli that produce tissue damage, or would do so if the stimulus continued.*

On the other hand, *pain* is a subjective experience with a psychological definition: *An unpleasant sensory and emotional experience, which occurs together with actual or threatening tissue damage, or is described as if it were caused by tissue damage.* Usually, of course, the pain we feel is caused by nociceptor activation by noxious stimuli, and when we feel pain we more or less automatically put it in conjunction with something that harms our body. Nevertheless, there are many examples of persons exposed to massive nociceptor stimulation who feel no pain, and, vice versa, a person may suffer the most intense pain, yet there may be no evidence of nociceptor stimulation. Examples of the first situation are seen in serious accidents in which the injured person may experience no pain immediately afterward, in spite of considerable tissue damage. This is most likely explained by mechanisms of the brain preventing signals from nociceptors from reaching consciousness (further considered below). The experience of pain without any signals from nociceptors is perhaps most dramatically exemplified in patients with injuries in which the dorsal roots are literally torn out of the cord. Even though no sensory signals at all can enter the cord, the patient often feels excruciating pain in the denervated parts of the body (called *deafferentation pain*). The so-called phantom pain that sometimes occurs after amputations is another example: In this case, the pain is felt in a part of the body that no longer exists. Thalamic lesions may sometimes be accompanied by the experience of severe pain, which is completely independent of what is going on in the painful part of the body (thalamic pain). There are also many examples from clinical practice of pain that continues or even gets more severe long after the injury that initially caused the pain is completely healed. In such cases we must assume that alterations have occurred in the central nervous system itself—for example, in the dorsal horn or in the thalamus—that perpetuate without any external stimuli the neuronal activity in regions of the brain related to the experience of pain.

Stimulation of intralaminar thalamic nuclei in some patients undergoing brain surgery for movement disorders (that is, without chronic pain) are reported not to produce pain (or any other sensation), whereas stimulation of corresponding sites in patients suffering from pain of the deafferentation type can provoke or intensify their usual type of pain.

Clinical experience and animal experiments indicate that many parts of the brain (among them, parts of the so-called limbic system) are of importance for our perception of pain and how we cope with it. After large lesions of the frontal lobes, for example, a peculiar indifference to pain may occur. The patient feels the pain, but the emotional coloring—which makes us describe pain more vividly than other sensations—is lacking. But in healthy persons, too, as most of us have experienced, the intensity of pain may vary considerably with our state of mind. For example, anxiety makes the pain much worse. If we do not know the cause and fear that it may be caused by a dangerous disease, the pain may be felt as intolerable. As soon as we are told that the cause is innocent and that the pain will soon pass, it feels less intense.

Additional Pathways for Transmission of Somatosensory Information: The Spinocervicothalamic and the Spinoreticulothalamic Tracts

In animals such as cats and monkeys, pathways for somatosensory signals have been discovered in addition to the two major ones described above. One pathway is interrupted in a small cell group located in the lateral funiculus at cervical levels of the cord, the *lateral cervical nucleus*. The afferents to this nucleus come from neurons in the dorsal horn, located particularly in lamina IV. The neurons of the lateral cervical nucleus send their axons to end—after crossing the midline—in the VPL of the thalamus. This spinocervicothalamic pathway has been most intensively investigated in the cat, in which it conducts impulses both from nociceptors and from cutaneous low-threshold mechanoreceptors. The functional role of this pathway is not clear, however, and it is not established with certainty that it is present in man.

Another pathway, of particular interest with regard to transmission of impulses from nociceptors, perhaps deserves more attention. Intermingled with the spinothalamic fibers of the anterolateral fascicle lie numerous fibers that terminate in the reticular formation of the brain stem. The perikarya of these *spinoreticular neurons* are located mainly in laminae VII and VIII. As mentioned, some spinothalamic neurons also have their perikarya in these lamina (Fig. 4.17), and it was not unexpected when it was found that a small proportion of the spinoreticular fibers are collaterals of spinothalamic ones. Recordings from spinoreticular neurons have shown that some of them are activated by nociceptors. Many of the neurons in the reticular formation send their axons to the thalamus (see Chapter 12). Of special interest with regard to pain perception is that these fibers terminate preferentially in the intralaminar thalamic nuclei (as do some of the spinothalamic fibers). Thus, there is a *spinoreticulothalamic pathway*. Whereas the spinothalamic pathway is predominantly crossed, the spinoreticulothalamic one is bilateral, so that the thalamus (and cerebral cortex) of both sides may be influenced from one side of the body. The pathway lacks a precise somatotopic organization and can therefore hardly contribute to our localization of painful stimuli. Rather it has been assumed that it is of particular importance for the emotional, affective aspects of pain perception. It has also been suggested that the spinoreticulothalamic pathway plays no role in normal pain sensation but contributes under certain pathologic conditions. The respective functional roles of the spinothalamic and the spinoreticulothalamic pathways for pain sensation are, however, far from easy to ascertain, mainly because of the spinothalamic and spinoreticular fibers lie intermingled and therefore cannot be lesioned in isolation. Chrodotomy, mentioned above, and similar lesions in animals must interrupt both pathways. It should also be emphasized that many spinoreticular neurons—most likely the majority—do not take part in transmission of sensory signals destined for the thalamus (see Chapter 12).

The Transmission of Sensory Impulses Can Be Controlled from the Brain

It has been known that there are descending fiber connections from the cerebral cortex and the brain stem ending in the various relay nuclei of the somatosensory pathways. One important group of such connections arises in the *primary somatosensory area (SI) and terminates in the thalamus (VPL and other nuclei), the dorsal column nuclei, the sensory trigeminal nucleus, and the dorsal horn of the cord.* These connections are somatotopically organized and enable selective control of sensory signal transmission from particular parts of the body and from particular receptor types (the fibers ending in the dorsal horn of the spinal cord constitute part of the pyramidal tract; see Chapter 9). Physiological studies indicate that descending connections from the SI sometimes can facilitate impulse transmission through the sensory relay nuclei, but inhibitory effects appear to be most common. The latter effects are most likely mediated via inhibitory interneurons. Recordings from single units of the medial lemniscus in conscious monkeys have shown reduced impulse traffic from cutaneous receptors immediately before a voluntary movement. There is indirect evidence of the same phenomenon in man: The threshold for perceiving a vibratory stimulus is elevated immediately before a voluntary movement. Perhaps this happens because proprioceptive signals are of greater importance than cutaneous ones in this particular situation. We know from daily life that we have the ability to leave out sensory signals that are irrelevant at the moment. Without such filtering mechanisms, we would be flooded by sensory information. *The sensory information finally reaching the cerebral cortex is therefore "censored" and distorted compared with the stimuli received by the receptors.*

Central Control of Transmission from Nociceptors and Pain Sensation

Among the various aspects of central control of sensory impulse transmission, those related to pain in particular have received much attention in recent years. A dramatic observation by Reynolds in the late 1960s was the starting point for much later research. He showed that by electrical stimulation of a mesencephalic region, the *peri-aqueductal gray matter* (PAG) (substantia grisea centralis) (Figs. 2.21 and 4.16), conscious rats could be subjected to major surgery without apparently feeling any pain (as judged from their behavior and other observations). The stimulation produced *analgesia* (no experience of pain on noxious stimuli). In humans, too, electrical stimulation of regions close to the PAG has been tried, to treat patients with severe chronic pain, with some good results. Subsequent research with anatomic, physiological, and pharmacological methods indicates that the effect of PAG stimulation can be explained, at least in part, by activation of descending fiber connections to the dorsal horn. Although a sparse direct pathway from the PAG to the spinal cord exists, the main pathway appears to be synaptically interrupted in cell groups in the medulla, especially the *raphe magnus nucleus* (NRM) (Figs. 12.1 and 12.5) and other nearby cell groups in the medullary reticular formation (see Chapter 12). The descending fibers from these nuclei (raphespinal fibers) lie in the dorsal part of the lateral funiculus (dorsolateral fascicle) (Fig. 4.18), and cutting the latter abolishes the effects of PAG stimulation almost completely. Electrical stimulation of NRM inhibits spi-

nothalamic cells so that they are less readily activated by impulses from nociceptors. We do not know in detail the neuronal interconnections in the spinal cord mediating these effects from the brain stem, but it is of interest that fibers from the NRM establish synapses in the dorsalmost part of the dorsal horn (laminae I and II), which receives most dorsal root fibers conveying impulses from nociceptors. Many of the NRM neurons contain *serotonin,* and this is apparently a transmitter at synapses established by the boutons of the raphespinal fibers in the cord.[8] The actions of serotonin are complex—so far, seven different kinds of serotonin receptors have been discovered in the brain. Not surprisingly, the actions of serotonin in the dorsal horn are not fully understood, but experiments with microinjections of serotonin indicate that it has an inhibitory effect on nociceptive spinothalamic cells. Probably, the inhibitory effects are mediated partly by direct synapses on spinothalamic cells of raphespinal fibers and partly by synapses on dorsal horn interneurons (Fig. 4.18).

Some of the dorsal horn interneurons contain *opioid peptides.* These neuropeptides, found in many parts of the brain, got their name because they have actions that resem-

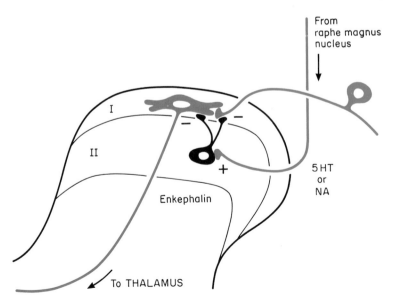

Fig. 4.18. *The substantia gelatinosa.* One of several possible wiring patterns in the substantia

gelatinosa, which can contribute to inhibition of spinothalamic cells.

ble closely those of the opiate-type drugs (such as morphine). The naturally occurring (endogenous) peptides of this kind are also called *endorphins*—that is, endogenous morphine. Opioids, when injected locally in the dorsal horn, have inhibitory effects on spinothalamic cells, but it is not known whether this is caused by a direct action or is mediated by interneurons (or both). Three main groups of endorphins have so far been discovered, each with its characteristic distribution in the brain and spinal cord. Best characterized are *β endorphin,* two varieties of *enkephalin,* and *dynorphin.* Whereas *β* endorphin is restricted to one neuronal group in the hypothalamus (the arcuate nucleus), the enkephalins and dynorphin are present in interneurons in many parts of the central nervous system (among them, parts that are not concerned with aspects of pain sensation).

The effects of PAG stimulation on pain sensation are probably not only mediated by descending connections to the cord. There are also ascending connections from the PAG, which may influence impulse transmission at the thalamic level or in other cell groups related to pain sensation.

We may conclude so far that the brain contains groups of neurons and fiber connections that, under appropriate circumstances, can effectively suppress the experience of pain (produce analgesia) or, in the case of animal experiments, suppress behavior that is normally linked with experience of pain. There is nevertheless much to be learned before we know the anatomic organization of the pain-suppressing systems and, in particular, the interactions between the numerous transmitters and neuropeptides involved. We furthermore do not understand the functional role of these systems and under which conditions they are activated normally. It is reasonable to assume, however, that they are active in situations with severe injuries and little or no experience of pain (as, for example, in war and major civil accidents). Suppression of pain may in such situations enable continuation of intense physical activity for a while, which may be of vital importance. Also, in more peaceful vigorous physical activities, such as sport competitions, it is obvious that pain sensitivity may be markedly reduced. Animal experiments further indicate that analgesia may be produced in certain stressful situations, characterized by the inability of the animal to escape a threatening or unpleasant situation ("stress-induced analgesia"). It has been suggested that *suppression of pain sensation is just one among several adjustments of the body, controlled by the nervous system, to certain kinds of extraordinary physical demands or stress.* Thus, the distribution in the brain of the opioid peptides shows that they are of importance for functions of the autonomic system, with, for example, marked effects on circulatory and respiratory control.

Analgesia Can Be Produced by Drugs, Nerve Stimulation, or Stress

That morphine and other opiates can alleviate severe pain has been known for hundreds of years. Today we know that there are receptors in the brain to which opiates can bind and exert their effects. These receptors are actually receptors for the endorphins, and at least five different receptors, each with affinity for a certain subgroup of endorphins, have so far been identified. Opiate receptors (binding morphine) are present in, among other places, the periaqueductal gray (PAG), the raphe magnus nucleus (NRM), and parts of the spinal dorsal horn (especially laminae I, II, and V; compare with Fig. 4.17). Microinjection of morphine in the PAG can produce analgesia in experimental animals that depend at least partly on connections from the NRM to the spinal cord. The actions of morphine appear thus to be exerted both in the spinal cord and in the PAG. In the cord, binding of morphine to opiate receptors on inhibitory interneurons in the substantia gelatinosa and, presumably, on primary afferent terminals leads to inhibition of spinothalamic cells. The action in the PAG occurs most likely by activation of the descending pathway from NRM and probably also by activation of ascending connections from the PAG acting on higher levels of the central nervous system. Binding of morphine in other parts of the brain, such as nuclei of the limbic system, is probably also of importance to explain the actions of morphine.

Conditions are indeed complex, as witnessed by experiments indicating that stimulation of the PAG may produce analgesia by two different mechanisms. Stimulation of the ventral part of the PAG in rats produced analgesia that appeared to be mediated by opioids (endorphins), because the effect could be abolished by injections of naloxone (which prevents binding of some opioids to their receptors). Stimulation of dorsal parts of the PAG, on the other hand, produced an analgesia that could not be reversed by naloxone, suggesting that transmitters other than endorphins were responsible for the analgesia.

Analgesia may also be produced by *stimulation of peripheral nerves*. When done with surface electrodes, the procedure is called *transcutaneous nerve stimulation* (TNS). One kind of analgesia occurs immediately and is mediated by activity of thick myelinated fibers in the stimulated nerves (that is, fibers leading from low-threshold mechanoreceptors). Selective stimulation of such fibers is elicited by electrical stimulation with high frequency and low intensity or by natural stimuli such as vibration, light touch, or pressure. The analgesia is restricted to parts of the body innervated by the peripheral nerves, and it usually disappears when the stimulation stops. This kind of analgesia is thought to be mediated by activity in collaterals of the thick dorsal root fibers that can inhibit impulse transmission from the thin (Aδ and C) fibers in the dorsal horn (most likely via inhibitory interneurons). This mechanism is presumably the basis of the everyday observation that it helps to blow at a finger that hurts, that it may help to move the part that has received an acute injury, that the pains of labor may be alleviated by rubbing over the lower back, and so forth.

Another kind of stimulation-induced analgesia requires that thin sensory fibers be activated. This can be achieved by electrical stimulation of low frequency with relative high intensity. Classical *acupuncture* probably obtains the same effect by rotation of thin needles in the tissue. The analgesia produced by this kind of stimulation occurs with a latency after the stimulation has started, and it may last for hours after termination of the stimulation. If analgesia occurs (it does not always happen), it is not limited to the parts of the body that were stimulated. This kind of stimulation-induced analgesia is most likely due to, at least in part, activation of the descending connections from the brain stem described above. This may happen by way of collaterals from spinothalamic and spinoreticular cells to the PAG and adjacent parts of the reticular formation, assuming that activation of thin dorsal root afferents first activate spinothalamic cells in the cord. The analgesia has been reported to be reversed or prevented by intravenous injection of naloxone, and in animal experiments it has been blocked by sectioning the dorsolateral fascicle. The results of such control experiments are, however, in part contradictory and indicate that not all aspects of stimulation-induced analgesia can be explained by liberation of endorphins.

Various kinds of *stressful situations can also produce analgesia* in experimental animals (rats in particular have been used for this kind of research). Depending on the nature of the stress, the analgesia may be mediated by liberation of endorphins or by apparently endorphin-independent mechanisms. There is also evidence to suggest that the emotional state of the animal is of importance for whether analgesia is produced or not. Thus, if the animal is frightened instead of calm and relaxed at the start of the period of stress (which may constitute vibration, mild electrical shocks, and so forth), hyperalgesia (increased pain sensitivity) rather than analgesia may occur. Thus, the same stimulus may produce either hyperalgesia or analgesia depending on the state of the animal. It is perhaps of relevance to compare with the well-known effects of anxiety on pain perception in humans.

The Somatosensory Cortical Regions

As mentioned, the sensory impulses conducted in the medial lemniscus and the spinothalamic tract finally reach the two somatosensory areas, SI and SII. Both of these cortical regions receive somatotopically organized projections from the VPL and VPM (Figs. 4.19 and 4.20). Somatosensory impulses also reach other cortical regions, however, such as the motor cortex (MI) in the precentral gyrus. Not unexpectedly, primarily signals from proprioceptors are conveyed to the motor cortex.

SI in particular has been the subject of intense anatomic and physiological investigations. The subdivision of SI into different cytoarchitectonic areas—3, 1, and 2 of Brodmann—corresponds to functional differences. These areas extend as narrow strips from the midline laterally along the postcentral gyrus—that is, perpendicular to the somatotopic arrangement (Figs. 4.19 and 17.3). Animal experiments, particularly by the American neurophysiologist Mountcas-

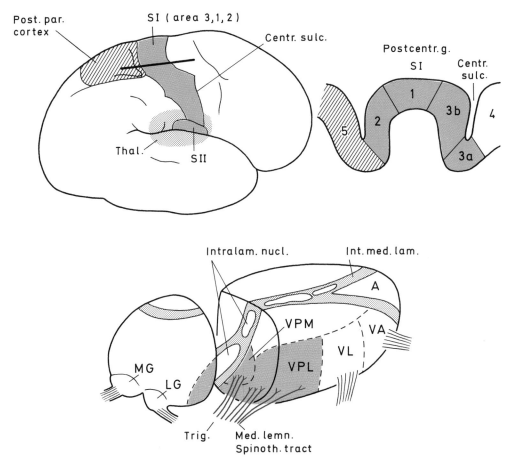

Fig. 4.19. *The somatosensory cortex and its thalamic afferent nucleus.* **Upper left** drawing shows the location of the SI and SII and parts of the posterior parietal cortex in the human brain. The extension of the various cytoarchitectonic areas of the central region is shown in the **top right** drawing. **Below,** the VPL—supplying the SI and SII with somatosensory signals—is marked on a schematic drawing of the right thalamus. The main afferent pathways to the VPL are also indicated. A = anterior thalamic nucleus; LG = lateral geniculate body; MG = medical geniculate body; VA = ventral anterior nucleus; VL = ventral lateral nucleus.

tle, show that the cytoarchitectonic subdivisions differ with regard to the kinds of receptor from which they receive information. Area 3a, on the transition to the motor cortex[9] (Fig. 9.3), receives sensory signals from muscle spindles in particular. Neurons in area 3b are first and foremost activated by stimulation of cutaneous receptors (predominantly by low-threshold mechanoreceptors). Neurons receiving information from rapidly adapting receptors appear to be separated from those receiving from slowly adapting receptors. Area 2 is influenced by proprioceptors to a larger extent than area

3b—for example, many neurons are most easily activated by bending of a joint. Within each of the cytoarchitectonic subdivisions it appears that the whole body has its representation; thus there are probably three body maps within SI. The map in Figure 4.20 therefore gives a somewhat misleadingly simplified presentation.

Even though many neurons in SI are activated only or most easily from one receptor type—that is, they are *modality-specific*—there are also neurons in SI with more complex properties. Many neurons have, for example, large receptive fields, indicating

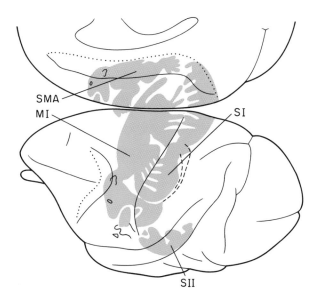

Fig. 4.20. *The somatosensory regions SI and SII and their somatotopic organization* (monkey). Motor areas are also shown. Redrawn from Woolsey (1964).

that they receive convergent inputs from many primary sensory neurons. Even though many neurons are activated by movement of just one joint in one direction, others are activated by several joints. Some neurons in SI require specific combinations of receptor inputs to be activated. Thus, some processing of the "raw" sensory infor-

mation takes place already in SI—it is not merely a simple receiver of sensory information.

The number of *neurons in SI activated from nociceptors* has been found in animal experiments to be surprisingly low, considering that no other area appears to contain more of them than SI. Although pain sensa-

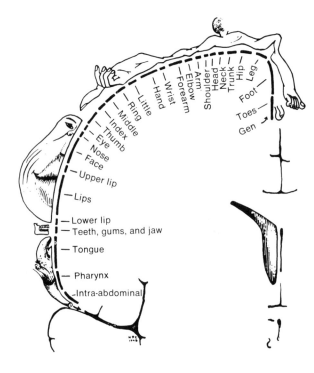

Fig. 4.21. *Relative size of the cortical regions representing various body parts.* Schematic section through the postcentral gyrus (SI) of the human brain. Based on electrical stimulation during brain surgery under local anesthesia. From Penfield and Rasmussen (1950).

tions have been elicited by electrical stimulation of SI in humans, this is an infrequent effect of such stimulation. Ablations of SI do not necessarily reduce pain perception, and only occasionally has it been reported to relieve chronic pain. It is fair to say that *the central processing of signals from nociceptors is far less understood than the processing of signals from other kinds of receptors.*

Lesions of SI in humans entail reduced sensation in the opposite half of the body. A localized destruction of the SI, or of the fibers reaching it from the thalamus, may produce loss of sensation in a restricted area (corresponding to the somatotopic localization within SI). Not all sensory qualities are affected equally, however. Discriminative cutaneous sensation and kinesthesia are particularly disturbed; much less reduced (if at all) is pain sensation. As is the case with lesions of the dorsal columns, the sensory deficits gradually diminish after the time of the lesion. The least improvement is seen, however, in the discriminative aspects of sensation, and is the most pronounced for pain. This can perhaps be explained by the fact that the pathways for signals from nociceptors are to a larger extent bilateral than the pathways from low-threshold mechanoreceptors, or perhaps pain sensation is less dependent on cortical processing than other sensory modalities.

Further Processing of Sensory Information: The Posterior Parietal Cortex

Even though some processing takes place already in SI, clinical and experimental observations show that the cortex posterior to SI is necessary for comprehensive utilization of the sensory information reaching the cerebral cortex. The *posterior parietal cortex comprises areas 5 and 7* (Figs. 4.19 and 17.12) and belongs to the so-called association areas of the cerebral cortex, which will be treated in Chapter 17. Areas 5 and 7 do not receive direct sensory information from the large somatosensory pathways but via numerous association fibers from SI and SII.

They also receive numerous connections from other parts of the cortex.

Neurons in area 5, for example, often have large receptive fields and respond only to complex combinations of stimuli, as shown in monkeys. Their activity may depend not only on what is occurring in the periphery but also on whether the attention of the monkey is directed toward the actual stimulus. Some neurons are only active in conjunction with the monkey stretching its arm toward something it wants. Broadly speaking, in areas 5 and 7 the bits of information reaching SI are put together and compared with other inputs (such as visual information, and information about the mental state of the animal).

NOTES

1. In reality, the conditions are even more complex. There are, among other things, two types of nuclear bag fibers differing ultrastructurally and histochemically, and only one of them, called bag_1, appears to be responsible for the dynamic sensitivity of the primary sensory ending. The other type, called bag_2, behaves more like a nuclear chain fiber and contributes presumably only to the static sensitivity.

2. Figure 4.6 shows that stimulation of γ_s in fact *reduces* the dynamic sensitivity of the primary sensory ending, since there is no extra increase in firing rate of the Ia fiber during the stretch phase. Under the influence of γ_s, the primary sensory ending behaves more like a secondary one.

3. The intralaminar thalamic nuclei were formerly often called the *unspecific thalamic nuclei,* because their connections with the cerebral cortex were thought to be diffusely distributed, in contrast to the connections of the specific thalamic nuclei. More recent studies have, however, questioned the unspecific nature of the intralaminar nuclei.

4. That fibers carrying impulses from the leg are located more anteriorly within the medial lemniscus than those related to the arm (Fig. 4.13) is simply because the gracile nucleus is situated more caudally than the cuneate nucleus. When fibers from the cuneate nucleus join those from the gracile nucleus, the most anterior position is already occupied.

5. Fibers conveying impulses from slowly adapt-

ing low-threshold mechanoreceptors in muscles and joints are found only in the cuneate fasciculus and not in the gracile fasciculus, at least in the monkey. Primary afferent fibers with such impulses from the legs leave the gracile fasciculus at the low thoracic level and enter the dorsal horn, where they synapse on second-order sensory neurons. The axons of the latter continue in the dorsal part of the lateral funiculus. Since slowly adapting receptors are responsible for static aspects of kinesthesia, it makes sense that in monkeys no defect of static joint sense is observed in the legs after lesions of the dorsal columns at thoracic or cervical levels. Whether this pertains also to humans is not known, however.

6. There has been a long-standing controversy with regard to the fiber composition of the tract of Lissauer, largely because of difficulties in tracing unmyelinated fibers. Recent investigations with improved methods indicate that about 80% of the fibers of the tract of Lissauer are primary afferent (dorsal root) fibers. The other fibers are propriospinal fibers ensuring cooperation between neighboring segments. This concerns in particular Rexed's laminae I and II, which also receive most of the synapses formed by the thin primary afferent fibers.

7. Usually, however, the pain returns during some months to a year after chordotomy. The reason for this is so far unknown, but possibly other pathways that under normal conditions are not of importance for transmission of painful stimuli take over.

8. Transmitters other than serotonin, such as *norepinephrine,* apparently also contribute to the effects on pain transmission obtained by stimulation of NRM and nearby structures. Conditions are complex, with several brain stem cell groups that can, in their own way, influence the transfer of nociceptive impulses to spinothalamic cells. Many of the NRM neurons contain one or more neuropeptides in addition to serotonin.

9. Some have argued that area 3a should be considered a part of the motor cortex rather than of SI. In certain respects, anatomically and physiologically, it represents at least a transitional zone.

The Visual System

Vision is the most important of the special senses of humans. There are approximately 1 million axons in the optic nerve, constituting almost 40% of the total number of axons in the cranial nerves. A correspondingly large part of the cerebral cortex is devoted to the analysis of visual information. The receptors for sight, *photoreceptors*, are the *rods* and *cones* of the *retina*. Their adequate stimulus is electromagnetic waves with a wavelength between 400 and 700 nm. The photoreceptors do not react to light with shorter (ultraviolet light) or longer (infrared light) wavelengths.

In this chapter we will deal with the pathways for visual impulses from the eye to various parts of the central nervous system and also with how visual parts of the central nervous system and also with how visual information is processed at various levels of the visual pathways. To understand the visual system, it is not sufficient to know the *conscious use of visual information;* the many *reflex effects* elicited by visual stimuli must also be taken into account. Among the reflex effects are those ensuring that our gaze is fixed on the object we want to examine and follows it if it moves, and those ensuring that the visual images formed at the retina are always in focus. Such visual reflexes,

however, are only briefly mentioned in this chapter. They are discussed more thoroughly in Chapter 13 in relation to the innervation of the eye muscles and the vestibular apparatus.

STRUCTURE OF THE EYE

The Eye and a Camera Have Certain Features in Common

The eyeball (bulbus oculi) (Figs. 5.1 and 5.2) has a firm outer wall of dense connective tissue covered on the inside by the light-sensitive retina. Between these two layers is a vascular layer the *choroid*, which is highly pigmented, thus ensuring that light enters the eye only through the pupil and also preventing reflection of light (compare with the dull black inside a camera). The diameter of the pupil (the shutter) controls the amount of light allowed into the eye. Refraction of the light takes place on its way through the cornea and the lens. The curvature of the lens can be varied by the use of the ciliary muscles, so that the retinal image is always sharply focused (in a camera, the focusing is brought about by varying the distance between the lens and the light-sensitive film). External eye muscles (extraocular muscles)

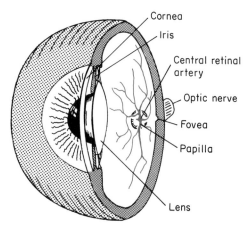

Fig. 5.1. *The left eye.* The eye is divided in two along the optic axis.

are attached to the eyeballs and can move them to coordinate their positions, so that the visual images are formed at *corresponding points* of the two retinas (Fig. 5.3). This is a prerequisite for our perception of one image, and not two (two slightly different images are formed in the eyes).

Main Structural Features of the Eye

The wall of the eye consists of three layers. Outermost is the *sclera*; then follows the *choroid*, and the *retina* is the innermost layer. The eye keeps its spherical shape because the sclera has a certain stiffness, but mainly because the pressure inside the eye is higher than outside (15 cm H_2O).

Anteriorly, the sclera has a circular opening, in which the transparent *cornea* sits like a glass of a wristwatch. The cornea consists of a special kind of connective tissue with densely packed collagen fibrils arranged strictly geometrically. This arrangement is a prerequisite for the transparency of the cornea, as is also its lack of blood vessels. The cornea is nourished by the tear fluid and by the fluid inside the eye. The cornea contains numerous unmyelinated sensory nerve fibers, providing information about even the slightest touch to the cornea. The cornea is covered on the outside by stratified squamous epithelium that is only a few cells thick.

The *choroid* (the vascular coat) is rich in vessels that nourish the cells of the outer parts of the retina. In addition, the connective tissue of the choroid contains numerous highly pigmented cells.

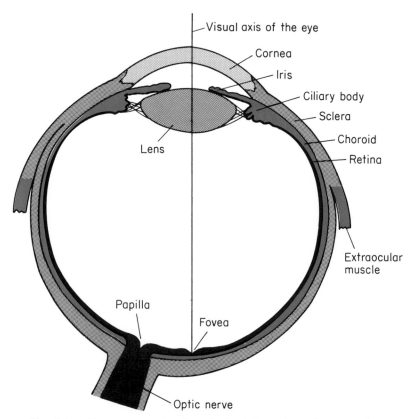

Fig. 5.2. *Transverse section through the right eye* (seen from above).

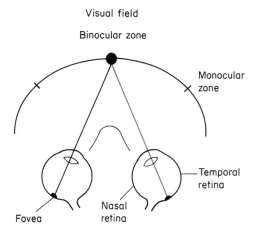

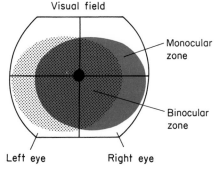

Fig. 5.3. *The visual field.* The positions of the eyes ensure that the images fall on corresponding parts of the two retinae **(top)**. The **lower** figure shows the visual fields of both eyes when the gaze is directed straight ahead.

Anteriorly, close to the opening in the sclera, the choroid is thickened and forms a ring (Figs. 5.1 and 5.2) called the *ciliary body* (corpus ciliare). This contains smooth musculature, the *ciliary muscle,* which controls the curvature of the lens. From the anterior edge of the ciliary body, approximately at the junction between the sclera and the cornea, the choroid continues as the *iris.* This is a circular disk with a central opening, the *pupil.* The iris contains smooth musculature that serves to regulate the size of the pupil. Muscle fibers arranged circularly form the *pupillary sphincter muscle* (m. sphincter pupillae), which, when it contracts, makes the pupil smaller so that less light enters the interior of the eye. Muscle fibers that are arranged radially in the iris widen the pupil when they contract: the *pupillary dilatator muscle* (m. dilatator pupillae).

The space inside the eye in front of the lens and the iris is called the *anterior chamber* (camera anterior). It is filled with a clear watery fluid

that is produced by small processes of the ciliary body. The space behind the lens, the *posterior chamber,* is filled with a clear jellylike substance called the *vitreous body* (corpus vitreum).

The eyeball is moved inside the orbit by six small striated muscles, the *extraocular muscles* (Fig. 13.24). The muscles originate in the wall of the orbit, and their tendons insert in the sclera. The muscles cooperate very precisely to produce the movements of the eyes that are necessary to ensure that the images of the objects we look at always fall on corresponding parts of the retina and to rapidly change our point of visual fixation. The extraocular muscles are discussed more comprehensively in Chapter 13 in connection with the cranial nerves innervating them (the third, fourth, and sixth cranial nerves).

The Visual Field

The visual field is the part of our surroundings from which the eyes can perceive light (without movement of the eyes or the head). Together the two eyes cover a large area (Fig. 5.3). Light from a particular point in the visual field falls on a particular point on the retina. Because of the refraction of the light when it passes the optic media of the eye, the image on the retina is upside down. The retina and the visual field can be conveniently divided vertically in two halves: the *temporal* parts—that is, lateral parts, toward the temple—and the *nasal parts.* The nasal halves of the retina receive light from the temporal halves of the visual field, and the temporal halves of the retina from the nasal visual field. The situation is of course the same for the upper and lower halves of the retina and the corresponding parts of the visual field. Thus, light from the lower half of the visual field reaches the upper half of the retina.

The Lens and the Far and Near Points of the Eye: Accommodation

The lens is transparent and built of a special kind of cell forming long fibers. It is elastic and, when loosened from the ciliary body to which it is attached with thin threads (see Fig. 5.2), it becomes rounder. Contraction of the ciliary muscle reduces the diameter of the ring formed by the ciliary body. This slackens the lens threads and enables the lens to become rounder; that is, its curvature (convexity) and thus also the refraction of the light increase. Contraction of the ciliary muscle is required to see sharply objects that are closer to the eye than approximately 6 m. This distance is called the *far point of the eye.* When viewing objects at distances greater than about 6 m, the lens maintains the same convexity, and yet the image is always focused on the retina. This is because the light rays entering the eye from points at such distances are all virtually parallel and are therefore collected in the plane of the retina (like a camera focused at infinite distance). The closer an object comes within the far point of the eye, the more the convexity of the lens must be increased by contraction of the ciliary muscle. Such adjustment of the lens for near sight is called *accommodation.* The closest distance from the eye at which we can see an object sharply is called the *near point of the eye.* One's own near point can be easily determined by fixing the eyes on an object (for example, a finger) that is gradually moved closer to the eye, until it no longer can be viewed sharply.

Whereas the far point of the eye depends on the curvature of the lens in its "relaxed" state—that is, with no contraction of the ciliary muscle—and remains stable throughout life, the near point depends on the ability of the lens to increase its curvature and moves gradually away from the eye from birth until about the age of 60. This happens because the lens becomes gradually stiffer and less elastic, so that the ability to increase its convexity is reduced. At the age of 45 the accommodative ability is so much reduced—or, in other words, the near point is so far away—that it is difficult to read fine print. This condition, called *presbyopia,* can be corrected by the use of convex (+) glasses of appropriate strength.

THE RETINA

The retina forms the innermost layer of the eye (Fig. 5.2). The outer part of the retina, which adjoins the choroid, is called the *pigmented epithelium* and consists of one layer of cuboid cells with large amounts of pigmented granules in their cytoplasm. Internal to the pigmented eipthelium follows a layer with *photoreceptors,* and then two further layers with neurons (Fig. 5.4). The processes

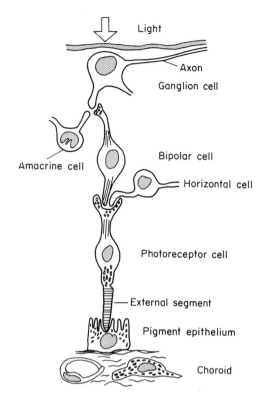

Fig. 5.4. *The retina.* The main cell types and their interconnections (highly simplified).

of the photoreceptors contact the *bipolar cells,* which in their turn transmit signals to the *retinal ganglion cells.* The axons of the ganglion cells leave the eye in the *optic nerve* to end in various nuclei in the diencephalon and the mesencephalon. The retinal layer with pigmented epithelium extends forward to the edge of the pupil (Fig. 5.2), whereas the photoreceptors, bipolars, and ganglion cells are present only in parts of the retina posterior to the ciliary body (pars nervosa retinae).

Unlike many other receptors, the photoreceptors are not of peripheral origin but belong to the central nervous system. The retina is formed in embryonic life as an evagination of the diencephalon (Fig. 2.4). Strictly speaking, the term retinal ganglion cell is not correct, but it is nevertheless maintained.

Since the photoreceptors are located external to the two other neuronal layers, the light has to pass the latter to reach the photoreceptors. Because there are no myelinated axons in the retina, however, the layers internal to the photoreceptors are sufficiently translucent.

In addition to the neuronal types mentioned above, the retina also contains many *interneurons* (Fig. 5.4). Altogether more processing of sensory information takes place in the retina than in any other sense organ. Thus, the visual information transmitted to higher centers of the brain from the retina is already "distorted" by enhancement of the contrast between light and darkness and by preference for signals caused by light from moving objects.

The Retina Has a Layered Structure

Under the microscope, several distinct layers of the retina can be identified in sections cut perpendicular to its surface (Figs. 5.5 and 5.8). Externally, toward the pigmented epi-

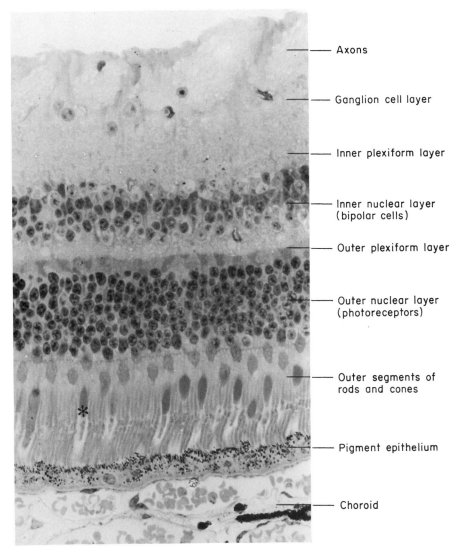

— Axons

— Ganglion cell layer

— Inner plexiform layer

— Inner nuclear layer (bipolar cells)

— Outer plexiform layer

— Outer nuclear layer (photoreceptors)

— Outer segments of rods and cones

— Pigment epithelium

— Choroid

Fig. 5.5. *The retina.* Photomicrograph of a microscopic section showing the various layers (monkey). The section is from the peripheral part of the retina (this explains the low density of ganglion cells as compared with Fig. 5.8). The outer segment of a cone is marked with an asterisk. Magnification, ×175.

thelium, lie the light-sensitive parts of the photoreceptors—their *external segments*. The two types of photoreceptors, the *rods* and the *cones,* can be distinguished because the external segments of the cones are thicker and usually somewhat shorter than those of the rods. Internal to the layer of the external segments, there are three distinct layers with cell nuclei. The *outer nuclear layer* consists of the nuclei of the photoreceptors. The *inner nuclear layer* is formed by the nuclei of the bipolar cells (and many of the interneurons). The innermost layer of nuclei belongs to the ganglion cells—the *ganglion cell layer.* Between the nuclear layers are found the processes of the neurons and their synapses, consequently termed the *outer and inner synaptic layers* (or plexiform layers). In the outer synaptic layer, the processes of the bipolar cells end in depressions in the processes of the photoreceptors (Fig. 5.4). The photoreceptor processes contain synaptic vesicles close to the presynaptic membrane.

A special kind of glial cell—*the Müller cells*—extends through the retina from the pigmented epithelium to the vitreous body. They are most likely a form of astrocyte.

Photoreceptors and the Photopigment

Electron microscopically, the external segments of the rods and cones can be seen to be packed with folded membrane. Thereby a large surface containing the light-sensitive photopigment is formed. In the rods, the folds of membrane lie mostly intracellularly, whereas in the cones they are partly invaginations of the surface membrane. The folds of membrane are constantly removed and resynthesized.

The kind of photopigment in the rods and the cones differs. The *rods* contain *rhodopsin,* whereas the *cones* contain three different varieties of photopigment (iodopsin and two other opsins). Rhodopsin has been the most studied, and consists of a protein part (opsin) and retinene, which is an aldehyde of the vitamin A molecule. Retinene is light-ab-

sorbing and is changed by light. At the same time the opsin part is changed, and via intermediaries this produces alteration of the membrane potential of the photoreceptor. This affects the bipolar cells and retinal interneurons, which are synaptically connected with the photoreceptors, and eventually the frequency of action potentials conducted from the retinal ganglion cells in the optic nerve to the visual centers of the brain is altered.

Dark Adaptation

When looking into the eye (for example, through an ophthalmoscope), the color of the retina is a deep purple because of the content of rhodopsin. The color bleaches quickly on illumination of the retina, but it returns slowly in the dark. The rhodopsin has been broken down by the light, and some time is needed to resynthesize it. The time taken for this process of *dark adaptation* can be experienced when entering a dark room from strong sunlight. In the beginning we can hardly see anything, but gradually the ability to see returns. This happens in two stages; first, there is a rapid stage of improvement of about 10 min and thereafter a slower stage of almost 1 h until full light sensitivity has been restored (if the initial illumination was very intense).

Rods and Cones Have Different Properties

The rods are much more sensitive to light than the cones and react to extremely small amounts of light, whereas the cones need fairly strong light to react. This is partly because the outer (external) segment of the rod is longer and contains more photopigment than that of the cone. *The rods are thus responsible for vision when the light is dim— night vision.* (That vitamin A is necessary for the synthesis of rhodopsin explains why vitamin A deficiency causes night blindness.) The distribution of light sensitivity for different wavelengths of light is the same for all the rods; hence they cannot help us discriminate between light of different wavelengths, a prerequisite for color vision. The cones, on the other hand, are of three kinds, each with a particular variety of photopigment with maximal light sensitivity to different wavelengths. They can therefore inform us about colors. One kind of cone responds best to light with wavelengths in the blue part of the spectrum, another in the red part, and the third kind in the green part. By comparing the degree of activation of the different kinds of cones, the neurons receiving signals from them can extract information about the distribution of wavelengths in the light falling on the retina. *The cones are thus responsible for color vision.* As mentioned above, however, they are not very sensitive to light; from daily experience we know that we need fairly strong light to perceive the color of objects. In poor light, everything appears as a variation of gray.

Other important differences between rods and cones concern their connections with other neurons in the retina. For example, many rods are connected to one bipolar cell—that is, there is a high degree of *convergence*. For the cones, on the other hand, there is typically much less convergence, with a few cones connected to one bipolar cell. This means that the cones provide information with a higher *spatial resolution* than the rods—that is, two points must be farther apart to be perceived as two and not one when the rods are responsible for transmitting the information than when the cones are responsible (compare with our inability to perceive visual details, such as small letters, in dim light). *Thus, the cones are also responsible for our ability to perceive visual details.*

The different degrees of convergence also help us understand why less light is required to convey signals through the optic nerve from the rods than from the cones.

Photoreceptors Are Hyperpolarized by Light

The photoreceptors do not behave like other receptors when exposed to their adequate stimulus: They are *hyperpolarized* instead of depolarized. How hyperpolarization of the receptors can elicit action potentials in the neurons conducting the signals to the brain will be briefly discussed. One important point is that the photoreceptors are unusual also in another respect: They are in a depolarized state in the dark with a membrane potential around -30 mV. This is probably caused by Na^+ channels that are open under such conditions. Like other receptors, the photoreceptors (and the bipolar cells) do not produce action potentials but only graded changes of the membrane potential. Because the distance is very short from the outer segment—where the membrane potential changes are produced—to the synapses between the photoreceptors and the bipolar cells, even small fluctuations of the membrane potential cause alterations of the transmitter release from the photoreceptors. (There is thus no need for the production of action potentials, which are important when signals are to be propagated over long distances.) Light falling on the retina most likely causes closure of the Na^+ channels of the photoreceptors via degradation of the photopigment and cyclic GMP. Closing of Na^+ channels hyperpolarizes the cell. Transmitter release from the photoreceptors (as from other neurons) is caused by membrane depolarization without any definite threshold that has to be exceeded. Thus, in the dark the photoreceptors release transmitter continuously, whereas the release is reduced by light (as if darkness were the adequate stimulus). Recording from bipolar cells has shown that they are of two kinds: One is depolarized by light and the other is hyperpolarized.

Glutamate—which most likely is the transmitter of the photoreceptors—has a depolarizing (and therefore excitatory) effect on neurons in other parts of the central nervous system. With regard to the bipolars, however, one kind appears to be *hyperpolarized by glutamate,* and another depolarized. This is presumably due to the existence of two different kinds of postsynaptic glutamate receptor. When light hyperpolarizes the photoreceptors, the release of glutamate is reduced, as mentioned above. This leads to less hyperpolarization—which is the same as depolarization—of one kind of bipolar. Thus, some of the bipolars are depolarized and therefore increase their own transmitter release. This is an example of *disinhibition.* The opposite happens with the other kind of bipolar cell, which is hyperpolarized (receives less depolarization) and therefore reduces its transmitter release. The bipolar cells have depolarizing (excitatory) effects on the retinal ganglion cells (and on amacrine cells), and we can then understand why there are also *two kinds of ganglion cells: one that is ex-*

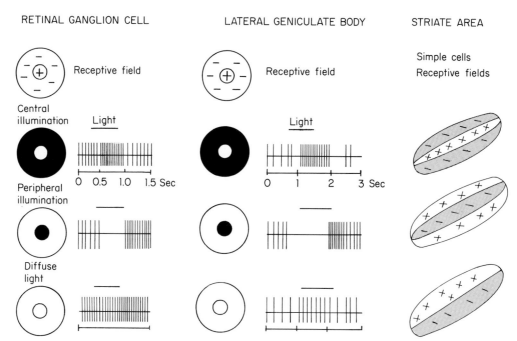

RETINAL GANGLION CELL   LATERAL GENICULATE BODY   STRIATE AREA

Fig. 5.6. *Receptive fields of cells at various levels of the visual pathways.* Retinal ganglion cells and cells of the lateral geniculate body have similar receptive fields. The firing frequencies of the neurons when subjected to different kinds of light stimuli are also shown. Only cells that are excited by shining light on the central part of the receptive field are shown here (on-center field), but cells with the opposite properties—that is, inhibition from the central field and excitation from the periphery—also exist (off-center field). The receptive fields of simple cells of the area striata are typically oblong with an excitatory and an inhibitory zone. The cells are called orientation-specific because they respond preferentially to a stripe of light with a specific orientation. The figure shows only one orientation of the receptive fields, but all orientations are represented among cells of the striate area. Based on Kuffler et al. (1984).

cited, and one that is inhibited by light hitting the photoreceptors to which they are coupled.

Receptive Fields of Retinal Ganglion Cells

Most retinal ganglion cells have in common that they are excited most effectively by shining light on small circular spots on the retina. These are the *receptive fields* of the ganglion cells and can be defined as *the area of the retina from which a ganglion cell can be influenced.* The receptive field can of course be determined not only for ganglion cells but for neurons at all levels of the visual pathways. The ganglion cells are typically excited from a small central circle and inhibited from a peripheral circular zone, or vice versa (Fig. 5.6). This was first demonstrated by the American neurophysiologist Kuffler in the early 1950s. He introduced the terms *on-center* and *off-center* for ganglion cells that are activated and inhibited, respectively, by light hitting the central zone of the receptive field.

Illumination of a small spot on the retina can lead to increased activity in one chain of neurons—forming, as it were, a channel for signal transmission to the higher visual centers—and reduced activity in another. (The arrangement of a central excitatory field and a peripheral inhibitory zone is unique to neurons of the visual pathways but is found also in the somatosensory system.) For receptive fields of the retinal ganglion cells, the central excitatory or inhibitory part of the receptive field may be explained by direct coupling from photoreceptors to bipolars and further to ganglion cells, whereas the peripheral zone with opposite effects must involve retinal interneurons. As expected, illumination of the whole receptive field—the central and peripheral zones simultaneously—gives a much weaker response from the ganglion cells than illumination of only the central zone (Fig. 5.6). *In conclusion, each ganglion cell brings information to higher visual centers about a particular small, round area in a definite position on the retina, and thus in the visual field.*

Together, the receptive fields of all ganglion cells cover the whole visual field with the same type of concentrically arranged receptive fields. Ganglion cells that lie side by side in the retina have overlapping, but not identical, receptive fields.

It should be emphasized that the retinal ganglion cells do not give information about *absolute light intensity,* as appears from recording of ganglion cell activity under different lighting conditions. Rather, their activity depends on the *contrast* of intensity between the light falling on the central and the peripheral parts of the receptive field. For example, for an on-center cell, maximal firing frequency would be achieved by a narrow beam of strong light hitting precisely the center of the receptive field while the peripheral zone is in darkness.

This preference of the visual system for contrast in light intensity can be demonstrated, for example, by looking at a gray circular spot surrounded by black. Exchanging the black surrounding with white makes the gray spot appear darker (even though the amount of light the eye receives from the gray area is unchanged).

Interneurons in the Retina

As mentioned, the retina contains interneurons in addition to the photoreceptors, bipolars, and the ganglion cells (Fig. 5.4). The *horizontal cells* send their processes in the plane of the retina— that is, perpendicular to the orientation of the photoreceptors and the bipolars. The horizontal cell processes establish contact with the inner segments of the photoreceptors and with the den-

drites of the bipolars. There are apparently several kinds of horizontal cells, as witnessed by their varied content of transmitter candidates. Morphologically, at least two kinds can be distinguished. One important action of the horizontal cells is most likely to inhibit transmission from photoreceptors around those that are illuminated; that is, they produce *lateral inhibition,* which is common in sensory systems. They thus function to increase the contrast between the illuminated and nonilluminated parts of the retina.

The other kind of retinal interneuron, the *amacrine cell,* is located with its perikaryon in the inner nuclear layer and establishes contact both with the axons of the bipolar cells and with the dendrites of the ganglion cells. They are thus intercalated between bipolar cells and the ganglion cells, and many bipolar cells exert their effect on ganglion cells only or mainly via amacrine cells. This is, for example, the rule for bipolar cells that are connected with rods (rod bipolars). Some of the processes of the amacrine cells also extend horizontally for considerable distances. The actions of the amacrine cells are varied and complex, and there are numerous morphological varieties. They are also heterogeneous with regard to their content of transmitter candidates. One subgroup of amacrines contains, for example, GABA; others contain acetylcholine or dopamine. At least seven different neuropeptides have been associated with amacrine cells. The amacrines play an important role in influencing the activity of many ganglion cells, the properties of which cannot be explained by transmission lines going directly from bipolars to ganglion cells.

The Size of Receptive Fields Is Different in Different Parts of the Retina: Visual Acuity

We know from everyday experience that, in order to perceive visual details, the eyes have to be directed toward the object we are looking at. The visual axes have to be oriented so that light from the object falls on a small region of the retina in the back of the eye, the *macula lutea,* corresponding to a small depression, the *fovea centralis* (Figs. 5.1–5.3, and 5.7). Here the *visual acuity* is maximal, and it decreases steeply when moving peripherally on the retina. The visual acuity can be expressed as the distance (in degrees)

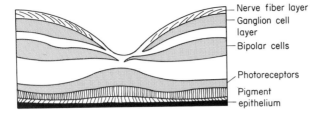

Nerve fiber layer
Ganglion cell layer
Bipolar cells
Photoreceptors
Pigment epithelium

Fig. 5.7. *The fovea centralis.* Schematized drawing of microscopic section through the posterior pole of the eye. Note how the bipolar and the ganglion cells are "pushed" aside in the most central part of the fovea (the foveola), whereas the density of photoreceptors is at its highest.

two points in the visual field have to be apart to be perceived as two and not one. In clinical work, visual acuity is usually determined by viewing letters of different sizes at a fixed distance (at the far point of the eye). The macula is about 2 mm in diameter, and has a yellowish color when viewed through an ophthalmoscope, distinguishing it from the purple color of the surrounding retina. The central depression at the fovea exists because the bipolars and the ganglion cells are "pushed" aside, to enable maximal access for light to the photoreceptors. The small region is also devoid of capillaries. *In the central part of the macula, only cones are present,* and only in the macular part of the retina is the visual acuity sufficient to enable us to read ordinary print (for example, a newspaper). The farther we move peripherally from the macula, the lower the visual acuity. One can demonstrate this easily by trying to determine how far out in the visual field one can recognize a face. *Closely linked with these differences in visual acuity are dif-*

ferences in the size of the receptive fields of ganglion cells in the central and peripheral parts of the retina.

What is the basis for such striking differences in the size of the receptive fields of ganglion cells? One important factor is that the *degree of convergence* varies dramatically. There are about 100 million photoreceptors in the human retina and only 1 million ganglion cells; on the average, 100 photoreceptors must be connected to 1 ganglion cell. In peripheral parts of the retina, however, the convergence is much greater than 100:1, whereas it is much smaller in central parts (Fig. 5.8). In the central parts of the macula (foveola, Fig. 5.7) there are even 1:1 connections—that is, one photoreceptor connects to one bipolar, which is connected to only one ganglion cell. As mentioned, the rods show a greater convergence than the cones, which is in accordance with the distribution of the rods and cones: In the macula it is almost cones only, whereas in the most peripheral parts it is almost rods only. The rel-

Central retina

Peripheral retina

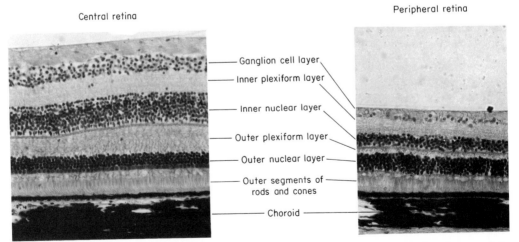

Ganglion cell layer
Inner plexiform layer
Inner nuclear layer
Outer plexiform layer
Outer nuclear layer
Outer segments of rods and cones
Choroid

Fig. 5.8. *Central and peripheral parts of the retina.* Photomicrographs illustrating how the various retinal layers differ in thickness wher moving from central to peripheral parts of the retina. Note especially the difference in the density of ganglion cells.

ative absence of cones in the peripheral parts of the retina (receiving light from peripheral parts of the visual field) can be demonstrated by how far out in the visual field the color of an object can be perceived. It then appears that the visual field for color is considerably smaller than that within which we can perceive a moving object.

Another factor that contributes to the higher visual acuity in the central parts of retina—particularly in the region of the fovea—is that the *density of photoreceptors* is higher there than more peripherally. Figure 5.10 illustrates a third contributing factor: The *dendritic arborizations of the ganglion cells* are more restricted in central than in peripheral parts of the retina, which is also of importance for the degree of convergence on each ganglion cell. Finally, differences between the retinal interneurons in central and peripheral parts of the retina also play an important role.

Where the optic nerve leaves the eye, there is a circular area devoid of photoreceptors, appropriately called the *blind spot* (Figs. 5.1, 5.2, and 5.9). We do not notice

these blind areas of the two retinae, however, because they are not located at corresponding points (Fig. 5.3).

There Are Two Main Types of Retinal Ganglion Cells

Anatomic studies showed many years ago that the retinal ganglion cells differ greatly in size. One tendency, mentioned above, is that the dendrites of the ganglion cells are longer peripherally than centrally (Fig. 5.10). This is related to differences in the size of their receptive fields. But ganglion cells with the same placement with regard to eccentricity on the retina also vary in size. It is now customary to recognize two main kinds of retinal ganglion cells, together constituting about 90% of all—the *M cells and the P cells*. As seen in Figure 5.10, the P cells are tiny compared with the M cells, but both types are much smaller centrally than peripherally. Physiological studies of their properties indicate that *the M cells primarily signal movement and contrasts of illumination, whereas the P cells are responsible for*

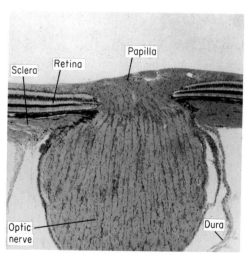

Fig. 5.9. *The optic nerve and the optic papillae.* Photomicrograph of section through the posterior pole of the eye at the exit of the optic nerve (the blind spot). The optic nerve swells immediately outside the eye because the axons become myelinated (the ganglion cell axons are unmyelinated as long as they course through the innermost layer of the retina).

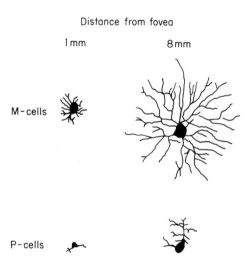

Fig. 5.10. *Two main kinds of retinal ganglion cells* (monkey). Note how both types increase in size in the peripheral direction (distance from the fovea). The extension of the dendritic tree is related to the size of the receptive fields of the ganglion cells. The cells have been visualized by intracellular injection of HRP. Based on Shapley and Perry (1986).

*providing information about fine features
(high visual acuity) and color.*

In the following part of this chapter, we
will discuss the organization of the pathways followed by the signals from the retina,
and we will see that information from the
two main types of ganglion cells is kept separate—at least to some extent—up to the
cortical level.

More about Retinal Ganglion Cells

The functional properties of the two main morphological types of ganglion cells have been clarified by intracellular staining of cells that first
have been characterized by their response to various kinds of light stimuli. Particularly the cat's
but also to some extent the monkey's retinal ganglion cells have been studied in depth. Even
though cat and monkey (and presumably human)
ganglion cells have several features in common—
for example, with regard to the organization of
their receptive fields—there are also important
differences. This concerns both properties of the
ganglion cells and the pathways conducting their
signals to the visual cortex. One reason for such
differences is that the cat has practically no ability to differentiate colors (that is, it is color-
blind). Another difference concerns the visual
acuity of the central parts of the retina, which is
much higher in the monkey (and man) than in
the cat (the cat has no macula). The subdivision
of X, Y, and W retinal ganglion cells of the cat
can therefore hardly be used without modifications for man. The monkey visual system is much
more like the human in several respects, notably
with regard to both color vision and visual acuity. Recent studies in the monkey indicate that
the M cells described above correspond functionally to both the X and Y cells in the cat, whereas
the P cells are not found in the cat (or in a very
small number). What follows here is based on
findings in the monkey.

The *M cells* (called A cells by some authors)
have a large perikaryon and a fairly extensive
dendritic tree (Fig. 5.10). The axon is relatively
thick. The *P cells* (= B cells) have smaller perikarya, a less extensive dendritic tree, and a thinner axon than the M cells. The P cells are most
numerous and probably constitute about 80% of
all of the ganglion cells. The anatomic differences
fit well with the M cells' having larger receptive
fields than the P cells and with the fact that their
signal is conducted faster to the higher visual centers. A major difference is that many of the P cells

respond preferentially to light with a particular
wavelength—that is, they are color-specific—
whereas M cells do not have such specificity. The
M cells, however, are more sensitive than the P
cells to contrasts in intensity of illumination. A
third difference is that the M cells appear to respond better than the P cells to moving stimuli.
Thus, in general the M cells tend to respond especially when a stimulus starts and stops,
whereas the P cells tend to give a signal as long
as the stimulus lasts.

A third kind of retinal ganglion cell does not
fit into the two groups described so far. In the
monkey, they constitute about 10% of all ganglion cells. Both anatomically and physiologically this group is heterogeneous, but the cells are
predominantly smaller than the P cells and have
thinner axons. The common feature of this
group is that the cells send their axons to the
mesencephalon rather than to the thalamus, like
the M and P cells. A small fraction of the M cells
sends an axon (most likely a collateral of the
axon going to the thalamus) to the mesencephalon. It gives one some insight into the development of the visual system to compare the proportion of retinal ganglion cells that sends axons
to the mesencephalon in various species. Thus, in
the cat, about 50% of the axons in the optic
nerve pass to the mesencephalon, and the proportion is most likely higher in lower mammals
like the rat. In humans, there is reason to believe
that even less than 10% pass to the mesencephalon. With increasing development of the cerebral cortex, more and more of the analysis of visual information takes place at the cortical level
rather than in the brain stem visual centers.

ORGANIZATION OF THE
VISUAL PATHWAYS

The axons of the retinal ganglion cells constitute the first link in the central visual
pathways. All ganglion cell axons run toward the posterior pole of the eye, where
they pass through the wall of the eyeball at
the *papilla* (papilla nervi optici) (Fig. 5.9).
They then form the *optic nerve,* which
passes through the orbit and enters the cranial cavity. Here the two optic nerves unite
to form the *optic chiasm* (Figs. 2.14 and
5.11). In the optic chiasm some of the axons
cross, and crossed and uncrossed fibers continue in the *optic tract,* which curves around

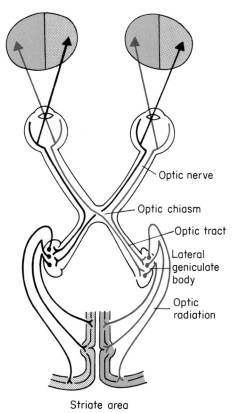

Fig. 5.11. *The visual pathways.* For didactic reasons, the visual field of each eye is shown separately (cf. Fig. 5.3).

the crus cerebri to end in the *lateral geniculate body* (corpus geniculatum laterale) of the thalamus (Figs. 2.22, 2.23, 5.12–5.14). Here the axon terminals of the retinal ganglion cells establish synaptic contact with neurons that send their axons posteriorly into the occipital lobe. These efferent fibers of the lateral geniculate body form the *optic radiation* (radiatio optica) (Fig. 5.12). The optic radiation curves anteriorly and laterally to the posterior horn of the lateral ventricle and ends in the *primary visual cortical area,* situated around the *calcarine fissure* (Figs. 2.27 and 5.16). Some of the fibers of the optic radiation lie in the posterior part of the internal capsule, where they can be damaged together with the fibers of the pyramidal tract—for example, by bleeding or infarction—producing a combination of weakness (paresis) of the muscles of the opposite side of the body and blind areas in the op-

posite visual hemifield. The primary visual area is *area 17* of Brodmann, which is also called the *striate area* (area striata). The latter name (which we will use here) refers to a white stripe in the cortex running parallel to the cortical surface. The stripe is made up of myelinated fibers and is therefore white in a freshly cut brain, whereas it appears dark in microscopic sections stained to show myelin (Fig. 5.15).

Not all fibers of the optic nerve terminate in the lateral geniculate body. Some (about 10% in the monkey) terminate in certain *mesencephalic nuclei* (the superior colliculus and the pretectal nuclei). These fibers are of importance primarily for reflex adjustments of the position of the head and the eyes (this will be discussed in Chapter 13).

Axons from the Two Main Types of Ganglion Cells Terminate in Different Layers of the Lateral Geniculate Body

The human lateral geniculate body (and that of other primates, like monkeys) consists of six cell layers (Figs. 5.13 and 5.14). The two ventralmost laminae (1 and 2) are composed of large cells and are therefore called the *magnocellular layers,* whereas the dorsal four are composed of small cells and are called the *parvocellular layers.* Anatomic and physiological studies have shown that the large retinal ganglion cells (M or A cells) send their axons to the magnocellular layers of the lateral geniculate body, whereas the small ganglion cells (P or B cells) send their axons (at least preferentially) to the parvocellular layers (Fig. 5.13). There is thus a division of the lateral geniculate body corresponding largely to the functional division among retinal ganglion cells. The significance of this will be discussed in connection with the visual cortex.

Visual Impulses from One Side of the Visual Field Reach the Hemisphere of the Other Side

Figure 5.11 shows how the fibers are arranged in the optic chiasm. The fibers com-

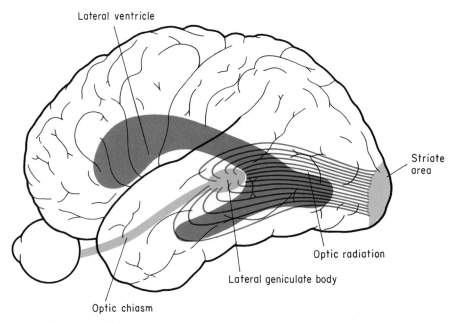

Lateral ventricle

Striate area

Optic radiation

Lateral geniculate body

Optic chiasm

Fig. 5.12. *The optic radiation.* The course of the fibers from the lateral geniculate body to the striate area. Note how the fibers bend around the

lateral ventricle and extend partly into the temporal lobe. Redrawn from Brodal (1981).

ing from the nasal halves of the two retinae cross, whereas the fibers from the temporal halves pass without crossing. In this way the left lateral geniculate body receives fibers from the temporal retina of the left eye and from the nasal retina of the right eye. *The lateral geniculate body thus receives light from the contralateral half of the visual field.* In functional terms, the crossing of signals

corresponds to that taking place in the somatosensory system.

Optic nerve fibers from the two eyes are kept separate at the level of the lateral geniculate body, since three of the six layers receive fibers from the ipsilateral eye, and the three others from the contralateral eye (Fig. 5.14). After cutting one optic nerve, almost all cells in three of the layers degenerate

Lateral geniculate body

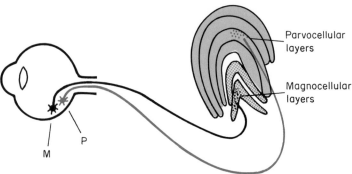

Parvocellular layers

Magnocellular layers

P

M

Fig. 5.13. *The lateral geniculate body.* The two main kinds of retinal ganglion cells end in differ-

ent layers of the lateral geniculate. Based on Shapley and Perry (1986).

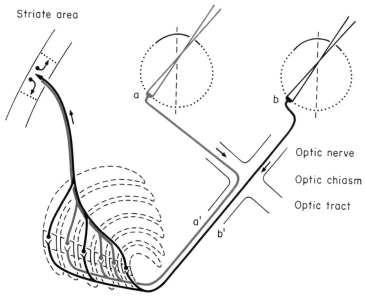

Fig. 5.14. *Fusion of the visual images.* The impulses from corresponding points on the two retinae end in different layers of the geniculate— that is, impulses from the two eyes are kept separate at this level. The convergence of impulses takes place in the striate area.

(transneuronal degeneration), whereas the other three layers remain normal. Physiological experiments also show that neurons within each layer of the lateral geniculate body are influenced from one eye only—the cells are *monocular*. We first encounter cells that are influenced from both eyes—*binocular cells*—at the level of the striate area.

The Visual Pathways Are Retinotopically Organized

The arrangement of the visual pathways described above concerns merely retinal halves—that is, a crude *retinotopic localization* ensuring that signals from different parts of the visual field are kept separate

Fig. 5.15. *The striate area.* Photomicrograph of a myelin-stained section through the human striate area, showing the characteristic dark stripe in layer 4 (the line of Gennari). The arrows mark the border between the striate area and neighboring extrastriate areas. (See also Fig. 17.4 for a thionine-stained section from the striate area.)

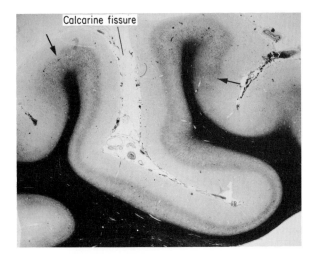

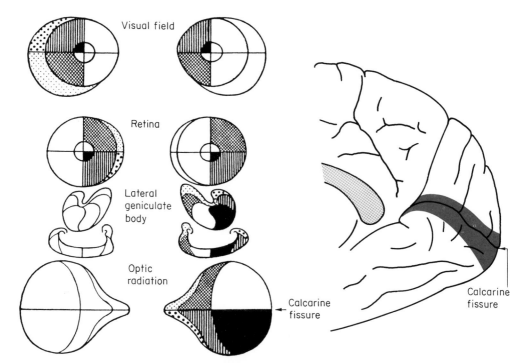

Fig. 5.16. *Retinotopic localization of the visual pathways.* The striate area has been unfolded. Note that information from the upper half of the visual field reaches the part of the striate area below the calcarine fissure, whereas the lower visual field projects above. Central parts of the visual field are represented most posteriorly and pe-

ripheral parts most anteriorly in the striate area. The **right** drawing illustrates the extension of the striate area on the surface of the occipital lobe; most of it is buried in the calcarine fissure. The striate area is similarly oriented in the **left** and the **right** figures.

(compare with somatotopic localization within the somatosensory pathways). The retinotopic localization is, however, much more fine-grained than what appears in Figure 5.16. Although many fiber systems of the brain are topographically organized, no one is as sharply localized as the visual pathways—they show a true point-to-point localization.

In the *lateral geniculate body,* fibers from differently placed tiny parts of the retina end differently. Each small spot in the retina— and thus in the visual field—is "represented" in its own part of the lateral geniculate (Fig. 5.14). The retinotopic localization in the lateral geniculate is such that neurons influenced from the same part of the visual field—that is, from corresponding points on the retina—lie stacked in a col-

umn perpendicular to the layers. This has been demonstrated with various anatomic techniques, and physiologically by inserting microelectrodes perpendicular to the layers and determining the receptive fields of the cells that are encountered.

The connections from the lateral geniculate body to the striate area are also organized with a precise retinotopic arrangement. This has been demonstrated, for example, by injection of small amount of HRP in the striate area: Retrogradely labeled cells are then confined to a narrow column extending through all six layers of the lateral geniculate. That all links of the visual pathways are retinotopically organized can be verified by shining light on a small spot on the retina. This evokes increased neuronal activity in a small region of the striate area, and when the light is shone on other parts of the retina, the evoked cortical activity changes position systematically. This kind of experiment has clarified how the visual field is represented in the cerebral cortex of animals. Careful examination of patients with circumscribed cortical lesions (often gunshot wounds) provides the basis for maps of the human visual cortex, as shown in Figure 5.16. Electrical stimulation of the human occipital lobe confirms the retinotopic arrangement within the striate area. Stimulation with a needle electrode usually evokes the sensation of a flash of light in a certain part of the visual field. When the electrode is placed close to the occipital pole of the cerebral hemisphere, the person reports that the flash is located straight ahead, in agreement with the fact that fibers carrying signals from the macula end near the occipital pole. As the electrode is moved forward along the calcarine fissure, the light flash is perceived as occurring progressively more peripherally in the visual field (at the opposite side of the stimulated hemisphere). If the electrode is placed above (dorsal to) the calcarine fissure, the light occurs in the lower visual field, whereas stimulation below the calcarine fissure elicits a sensation of light in the upper visual field.

Disease processes (for example, a tumor) involving the visual cortex may also sometimes elicit sensations of light because the neurons are abnormally irritated. Epileptic seizures originating in the visual cortex often start with a "visual aura"—that is, the muscular convulsions are preceded by bizarre patterns of light in the visual field opposite the diseased hemisphere.

Central Parts of the Visual Field Are Overrepresented in the Visual Pathways and in the Visual Cortex

In addition to the extremely precise retinotopic arrangement of the visual pathways, another important feature must be mentioned. We have described above that the density of retinal ganglion cells is consider-ably higher in central than in peripheral parts of the retina (particularly high in the macula). This corresponds to conditions in the somatosensory system, where the density of receptors is highest at the fingertips ("the somatosensory macula"). Figure 5.16 illustrates that axons from central parts of the retina end in a disproportionally large part of the lateral geniculate body and that this *overrepresentation* of the central parts of the retina becomes even more marked in the striate area. Again, conditions are similar to those in the somatosensory system (Fig. 4.21). Thus, *the parts of the body and the visual field in which we have the best somatosensory and visual abilities are provided with a higher density of receptors than other parts, and, furthermore, a much larger number of neurons at higher levels are devoted to the analysis of information from these parts.*

The Lateral Geniculate Body Is More Than a Simple Relay Station

Although the receptive fields of neurons in the lateral geniculate body are closely similar to those of retinal ganglion cells, the lateral geniculate is not merely a simple relay station. Anatomic and physiological studies indicate that signals from the retina are subject to modification before being forwarded to the striate area. There are, for example, a large number of *GABA-containing interneurons.* This presumably enables neurons with somewhat different receptive fields to influence each other. There are also complex synaptic arrangements and numerous dendro-dendritic synapses, indicating that substantial interactions take place between neurons of the lateral geniculate.

In addition to its afferents from the retina, the lateral geniculate body also receives strong, retinotopically organized projections from the visual cortex itself. These connections most likely can control the impulse traffic through the lateral geniculate and have been shown physiologically to influence the properties of the neurons. Descending connections from the visual cortex may contribute to the suppression of vision of one eye in patients who are cross-eyed (strabismus). This has the obvious advantage of avoiding double vision.

Finally, the lateral geniculate also receives fibers from other sources, notably from *cholinergic cell groups* of the pontine reticular formation.

These connections probably regulate the signal transmission through the lateral geniculate to the striate area in accordance with the level of consciousness and attention.

THE VISUAL CORTEX

The retinotopic localization within the visual pathways may make it appear that a copy of the two retinal images is formed in the striate area. Indeed, the striate area was formerly sometimes called "the cortical retina." We now know, however, that such a view represents too much of an oversimplification; considerable processing and integration of the visual information takes place in the striate area. Thus, most neurons have properties that are different from those encountered at lower levels of the visual pathways. It should also be emphasized that, when using the term visual images, we do not mean images or pictures in the usual sense, either in the retina or in the visual cortex. Rather, there are temporally and spatially specific patterns of neuronal activity that represent the patterns of light falling on the retina. So far, however, we have only vague ideas about how the activityy of the neuronal populations engaged in visual processing at the cortical level is related to our subjective visual experiences.

We will now look at certain fundamental features of the functional organization of the striate area and also mention the regions surrounding the striate area, the so-called *extrastriate visual areas*. These take part in the further processing of visual information. Thus, the visual cortex consists of much more than just the *primary visual cortex* (V1), the striate area, even though most of the fibers from the lateral geniculate body terminate there. There is anatomic, physiological, and clinical evidence that different aspects of visual processing such as analysis of color, form, and movement take place in partly different subdivisions of the extrastriate areas. Schematically, the signals from the retina first reach the striate area and are then forwarded to other cortical areas, each specialized to take care of only certain aspects of the information arriving from the retina. It is not clear, however, how far this specialization goes.

Extrastriate Visual Areas

As mentioned, several areas around the striate area take part in visual processing. These are collectively called the extrastriate visual areas and consist mainly of *Brodmann's areas 18 and 19*, which in the monkey each consist of several subdivisions. Whereas V1 is often used for area 17 (the striate area), parts of the extrastriate areas are termed V2–V5. Other parts have specific names. In total, about 20 visual areas have been characterized so far in the monkey, each with a more or less complete representation of the visual field. Most of them are also retinotopically organized, although with different degrees of precision.

It is not immediately clear why the cerebral cortex is organized so that the visual field is represented repeatedly in different parts. It may perhaps be a result of the adoption of novel functions by the visual cortex during evolution; this probably occurs more easily by adding new areas (or duplicating an old one) than by already existing areas taking up new functions. It is presumably also a simpler solution to have several separate areas than one large area with regard to arrangement of the necessary fiber connections.

Properties of Nerve Cells in the Striate Area

The retinal ganglion cells and cells of the lateral geniculate body have relatively simple, round receptive fields with a central zone that elicits excitation or inhibition when illuminated and a peripheral zone with the opposite effect (Fig. 5.6). But round spots of light are not an effective stimulus for the neurons of the visual cortex. What constituted the adequate stimulus for the cortical cells remained a mystery for a long time. Diffuse light was not found to be effective, and neither was the kind of stimulus that so effectively affected the cells of the lateral geniculate. In 1962, however, the Nobel laureates (1981) Hubel and Wiesel from the United States were able to show that *many cells in the striate area respond briskly to elongated fields of light or elongated con-*

trasts between light and darkness. It was furthermore striking that many cells required that the light stimulus be oriented in a specific direction—turning a bar of light some degrees reduced the response markedly. This property was termed *orientation selectivity.* Some cells required a bar of light or a straight light/darkness transition of a specific orientation in a specific part of the visual field to respond, whereas other cells responded to a properly oriented stimulus within a larger area. Such cells thus appear to detect contours with a certain orientation regardless of their position within a larger part of the visual field. Hubel and Wiesel called the first type *simple cells* and the latter type *complex cells* (within each group there are several subtypes according to details of their properties). Why the properties of the complex cells are more complex than those of the simple ones may not be obvious, but presumably the terms were used because Hubel and Wiesel assumed that the properties of the complex cells could be explained by several simple cells acting on one complex cell. The properties of the simple cells, Hubel and Wiesel suggested, could be explained if several neurons in the lateral geniculate with round receptive fields in a row (together forming a stripe) converge on one cortical cell. It is, however, not entirely clear which neuronal interconnections underlie the properties of cells in the striate cortex.

Hubel and Wiesel also discovered other fundamental properties of cells in the striate area. Among other things, *cells generally respond much better to a moving than to a stationary stimulus.* Many cells respond preferentially to a line or contour that is moving in a specific direction. Such *direction-selective cells* thus can detect not only the orientation of a contour but also in which direction it is moving. Other kinds of specificities have also been described for cells in the striate area.

In addition to single cells being specific or selective with regard to their adequate stimulus, there is also a *strong tendency for cells with similar properties in this respect to be located together,* more or less clearly separated from cells with other properties. This is called *modular organization* and concerns properties such as orientation selectivity, wavelength (color) selectivity, and ocular dominance (that is, which eye has the strongest influence). Such segregation of neurons in the striate area requires that fibers carrying different aspects of visual information from the lateral geniculate end at least to some extent differentially in the cortex. In agreement with this, fibers from the parvocellular layers of the lateral geniculate (Fig. 5.13) terminate deeper in lamina 4 than fibers from the magnocellular layers.

Modular Organization of the Visual Cortex

The first example of modular organization discovered by Hubel and Wiesel was the tendency for cells with similar *orientation selectivity* to be grouped together in columns perpendicular to the cortical surface. If we imagine, however, that the striate area is unfolded and we are viewing it from above, the groups of cells with similar orientation selectivity are located in an irregular pattern of curving bands. This has been demonstrated with the deoxyglucose method (see Chapter 3), which demonstrates the neurons that are most active at a certain time. When an experimental animal is exposed for some time to parallel stripes of light, increased glucose uptake takes place in cells distributed in bands in the striate area.

Another modular organization concerns *ocular dominance.* As mentioned, many cells in the striate area respond to light from corresponding points in the two retinas, but for most cells the influence is strongest from one of the eyes. The use of various tracer techniques and the deoxyglucose method has shown that neurons sharing ocular dominance are also distributed in bands within the striate area. Such *ocular dominance columns* can also be demonstrated in animals with monocular blindness (Fig. 5.17).

A final example of modular organization concerns cells that are *color-specific.* They are not aggregated in bands but rather in clumps or *blobs* in laminae 2–3 of the striate area of monkeys. For some unknown reason, these blobs have a higher cytochrome oxidase activity than the surrounding tissue and can thus be easily identified in sections with a simple histochemical procedure (Fig. 5.18).

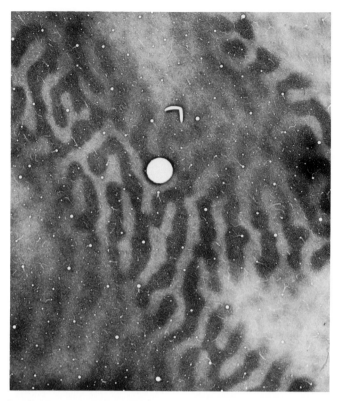

Fig. 5.17. *Ocular dominance columns.* Photomicrograph of a section cut tangentially to the cortical surface of the striate area and stained to reveal differences in cytochrome–oxidase activity. The section is from a monkey that was blind in one eye, causing reduced cytochrome–oxidase activity in the regions (light stripes) of the striate area connected mainly with the blind eye. The dark stripes receive their main input from the normal eye. Magnification, ×25. Courtesy of Dr. J. G. Bjaalie.

Further Processing of Visual Information Outside the Striate Area

The properties of single neurons in the striate area suggest that these neurons together are the basis for the cortical analysis of form, depth, movement, and color. Their properties, for example, fit predictions made on the basis of psychophysical experiments in humans, such as the preference for contours and for moving stimuli. Nevertheless, what is taking place in the striate area appears to be mainly a first analysis and sorting of raw data, which must be further processed elsewhere to form the basis for our conscious visual experiences. For example, at some stage in the processing, different features of the visual image (such as form, color, movement, and location in the visual field) must be brought together and integrated. We will return to this below. It is, however, mainly the question of separate treatment of the various features of visual images that has been intensely investigated recently. We will mention here only a few examples.

It has been proposed that one stream of information concerning *object identification* ("what") passes downward from the occipital lobe to the temporal lobe, whereas another stream concerned with *spatial features and movement* ("where") passes upward to the parietal lobe (Fig. 17.10). This concept is partly based on results from experiments in monkeys with lesions restricted to "visual" parts of either the temporal lobe or the pos-

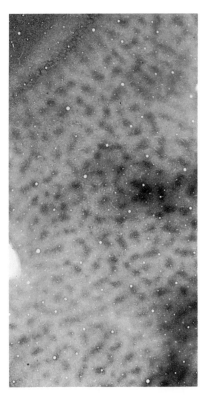

Fig. 5.18. *Color-specific "blobs" in the striate area.* Photomicrograph of a section cut tangential to the surface of the striate area of a normal monkey stained to show differences in cytochrome–oxidase activity. The section passes through laminae 2–3 and shows numerous small, darkly stained patches or blobs, which correspond to regions with color-specific neurons. Magnification, ×25. Courtesy of Dr. J. G. Bjaalie.

terior parietal cortex. Monkeys with *bilateral lesions of temporal visual areas have reduced ability to identify objects.* They can, for example, no longer distinguish between a pyramid and a cube. On the other hand, *lesions of visual parts of the posterior parietal cortex reduce the ability to localize an object in space and in relation to other objects.* It suffices with a unilateral lesion of the parietal lobe to produce deficits in the contralateral half of the visual field. This resembles the symptoms occurring in humans after damage to the posterior parietal cortex (see Chapter 17). The pathways taken by the impulses from the striate area to the temporal

and posterior parietal visual regions are not known in detail, but several visual areas are intercalated in the pathways.

Clinical observations indicate that separate processing of different aspects of visual information also occurs in humans. Thus, after restricted cortical lesions, several selective visual deficits have been described, for example, with regard to object identification. A patient may be unable to recognize faces, another may have no problem with faces but cannot recognize fingers (finger agnosia), and so on. Selective loss of color vision after lesions restricted to a region below the calcarine fissure (in the lingual gyrus) has been convincingly documented. Patients with unilateral lesions in this region are reported to see everything in the opposite half of the visual field in black and white, whereas the other half has normal colors. Other aspects of vision (such as visual acuity and depth perception) appear to be completely normal.

Are There Three Functionally Different "Routes" Out of Area Striata?

A striking feature of the projections from the striate area to other visual areas is that the fibers terminate in patches and bands. Closer examination of such patterns and correlation with the physiological properties of cells within the patches and bands indicate that three functionally different pathways out of the striate area may exist. One pathway comes from cells in the striate area that are predominantly influenced by the magnocellular layers of the lateral geniculate. The properties of these striate cells indicate that they signal movement and depth cues. Another pathway comes from cells that appear to be influenced by the parvocellular layers of the lateral geniculate. Accordingly, these striate cells have small receptive fields and are orientation-selective, and the pathway presumably signals forms and patterns and would seem particularly important for our ability to discern visual details. A third pathway originates in striate neurons also influenced by the parvocellular layers, but these neurons are, at least to a large extent, color-specific.

These three pathways from the striate area appear to be kept separate, at least partly, also at the next station—that is, in area V2, which is adjacent to the striate area. From V2, information about movement appears to be channeled to area V5 (also called MT, the middle temporal visual area), whereas information about color is channeled primarily to area V4. The major outflow from V5 has been traced to the posterior parietal cortex. How far the specialization goes within each of these areas is not known, however. Single neurons in area V5, for example, are sensitive not only to movement but also to certain other visual features. Similarly, neurons in area V4 are not purely color-specific.

Where Are Data from Different Visual Areas Integrated?

The fact that there is much evidence of separate processing in the visual cortex of different aspects of visual information must not make us forget that at some level a synthesis has to occur. Information about form, position, movement, and color must in some way be linked together. After all, the color "belongs" to a certain object, with a certain form and position, and speed and direction of movement. How early synthesis occurs in the several synaptic steps out from the striate area is not fully known. It certainly appears in parts of the frontal lobe, receiving afferents from both the posterior parietal cortex and the temporal visual areas (Fig. 17.13). It may happen earlier as well. Thus, when studies of a particular visual area focus on its involvement in a particular aspect of visual processing, its participation in other aspects may be overlooked. Also, the numerous two-way interconnections between the visual areas indicate that they do not operate as isolated functional units within a hierarchical system.

Visual Information Can Reach the Cortex via the Superior Colliculus and the Pulvinar

Not all fibers in the optic nerve end in the lateral geniculate body, as mentioned above. About 10% (in the monkey) leave the optic tract to terminate in the *pretectal nuclei* and in the *superior colliculus* (Figs. 2.21 and 13.27). Some fibers end in the *pulvinar* (Figs. 2.22 and 2.23), and this nucleus (and another thalamic nucleus, LP, Fig. 17.7) receives afferents from the superior colliculus. Like other thalamic nuclei, these send their

efferents to the cortex, notably to the extrastriate visual areas (among other regions). Thus visual information may reach the cortex (through several links) even when the optic radiation or the striate area is damaged. Even though these visual pathways—circumventing the lateral geniculate body—are retinotopically organized, they are apparently capable of giving only very crude information about movement in the visual field. After bilateral damage of the striate area in monkeys, the animals react easily to moving stimuli, even though in other respects they behave as if they were blind. Studies of patients with damage at various levels of the visual pathways and of the visual cortex (localized with the use of MRI) indicate that, as long as parts of the extrastriate visual areas on the convexity are intact, the patients retain some capacity to recognize movements in the visual field. When sitting in front of a large screen with a random pattern of moving dots, patients with damage of the striate area (and surrounding areas on the medial aspect of the hemisphere) reacted with movements of the eyes, apparently following the moving objects. They reported that they felt something moving in front of them, and they had some ability to identify the movement direction. They had no feeling of *seeing* anything, however, and when tested with perimetry, they were completely blind.

The visual connections of the superior colliculus are primarily concerned with reflex movements of the eyes and the head, as already mentioned. Thus, most of the efferent connections from the superior colliculus pass to nuclei in the brain stem concerned with control of such movements. The pretectal nuclei constitute a link in the pathway for the light reflex (Fig. 13.27).

Fusion of Visual Images and Strabismus

Normally, we perceive one image of the objects we look at, even though two (slightly different) images are formed on the retina. The two images fuse into one, and the phenomenon is called *fusion*. Fusion requires that the optic axes of the two eyes be properly aligned, so that the images fall on *corresponding points* on the retina (Fig. 5.3). The two maculae are obviously corresponding points, and the images fall on them when we fix the gaze on a point to see it as sharply as possible. As mentioned, the signals from the two eyes are kept separate in the lateral geniculate body, but at the cortical level many cells are influenced from both eyes—that is, they are *binocular* (Fig.

5.14). Convergence in the cortex of signals from corresponding points in the two eyes is a prerequisite for fusion. Fusion is not present from birth but develops gradually from about the age of 3 to 7 months. During this period, the movements of the eyes become coordinated, so that all movements are *conjugated* and the images fall on corresponding points when the gaze is fixed.

Strabismus (cross-eyed) means that the optic axes of the eyes are not properly aligned, and, accordingly, the images do not fall on corresponding points. The lack of fusion in such cases leads to underdevelopment or suppression of vision for the eye not used for fixation. In this manner, bothersome double vision is avoided, but even a relatively brief period of strabismus in early childhood may lead to permanently reduced visual acuity. It has been shown in monkeys that strabismus (produced experimentally) leads to a reduced number of cells in the striate area that is influenced by both eyes. In one kind of squint, the two eyes are used alternatively for fixation, and in such patients the visual acuity is usually conserved for both eyes.

There may be causes for a lack of normal vision development other than a squint. If, for example, the eye does not receive proper stimulation because errors of refraction produce a retinal image that is out of focus or because light for some reason does not reach the retina, vision is not developed normally. In humans, the first 2–3 years (in particular the first year) are critical in

this respect; lack of meaningful use of the eye even for a short period may then give permanently reduced visual acuity, as mentioned above. Animal experiments furthermore show that vision is better preserved if both eyes are covered for a period than if only one is covered. This is so because the two eyes "compete" during the early development of the visual system. If only one eye is used, it gets an advantage and takes over neurons in the visual cortex that normally would have been utilized by the other eye.

Interruption of the Visual Pathways

Partial damage to the visual pathways produces symptoms that confirm the arrangement of the cells and fibers at various levels of the optic system (Fig. 5.19).

Interruption of the *optic nerve* prevents any visual signals from reaching the brain from that eye. On the other hand, if only the crossing fibers are damaged at the level of the *optic chiasm*, signals from the two nasal halves of the retinae are interrupted. The patient is blind in the temporal parts of the visual field on both sides (bitemporal hemianopsia). The patient may not notice this, however, because the blind part of the visual field is not experienced as darkness but rather as "nothing." The visual defect may

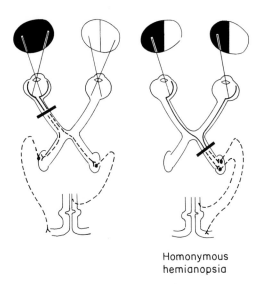

Homonymous
hemianopsia

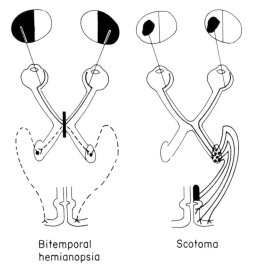

Bitemporal
hemianopsia

Scotoma

Fig. 5.19. *Visual field defects after lesions of the visual pathways.* The black areas indicate the blind parts of the visual field. The visual fields of

the two eyes are shown separately for didactic reasons (cf. Figs. 5.11 and 5.16).

be discovered incidentally by a tendency to bump into objects located a little to the side and perhaps by being hit by a car coming from the side when driving. This kind of visual defect may be caused by a tumor of the pituitary (located just below the optic chiasm). When the tumor grows, it has to expand upward since it is located in a bony excavation (the sella turcica) and thus first compresses the middle part of the chiasm. Damage to the *optic tract* produces a different clinical picture. If the damage is on the right side, visual signals from the temporal half of the right retina and the nasal half of the left retina are prevented from reaching the cortex—that is, the patient is blind in the left half of the visual field (homonymous hemianopsia). The same visual defect occurs when the optic radiation—or the striate area—is totally destroyed. More frequently, there are incomplete lesions of the optic radiation (note its position in the posterior part of the internal capsule) or of the striate area, producing blind spots or *scotoma* in the opposite visual field (at corresponding points). Because of the accurate retinotopic arrangement within the visual pathways (Fig. 5.16), mapping of such blind spots enables a precise determination of the site of the lesion.

6

The Auditory System

The sense of hearing is of great importance in higher animals—not least in humans, for whom speech is the most important means of communication. The adequate stimulus for the auditory receptors is sound waves with frequencies between 20 and about 20,000 Hz. The sensitivity is greatest, however, between 1000 and 4000 Hz and declines steeply toward the highest and the lowest frequencies; that is, a tone of 15,000 Hz must be much stronger than a sound of 1000 Hz to be perceived. The range of frequencies to which the ear is most sensitive corresponds fairly well to the range of frequencies for human speech. The frequency of sound waves determines the pitch, whereas the amplitude of the waves determines the intensity.[1] Many animals can perceive sound over a much wider range of frequencies than humans. For example, dogs can hear a whistle hardly noticed by humans, and bats use extremely high-pitched sounds for echolocation.

Sound waves pass through the air to the tympanic membrane, which transmits them via a chain of three tiny bones to the *cochlea*. The sensory cells of the cochlea are *low-threshold mechanoreceptors* sensitive to the bending of stereocilia on their surface. From the cochlea the signals are conducted to the

brain stem through the eighth cranial nerve, the *vestibulocochlear nerve*. This nerve also carries signals from the sense organ for equilibrium—the vestibular apparatus—which anatomically and evolutionarily is closely related to the cochlea. Functionally, however, these two parts have little in common, and we will describe the sense of equilibrium together with other aspects of vestibular function in Chapter 13.

THE COCHLEA
The Cochlea Is Part of the Labyrinth

The labyrinth consists of an outer bony part surrounding an irregular canal in the temporal bone, and an inner membranous part following and partly filling the canal (Figs. 6.1 and 6.2). The membranous canal is filled with a fluid called the *endolymph* (Fig. 6.7). Between the membranous and the bony parts is a space filled with a fluid called the *perilymph*.[2]

The labyrinth has two main parts. One is the cochlea and the other is the vestibular apparatus consisting of three semicircular ducts and two round dilatations (Fig. 6.2).

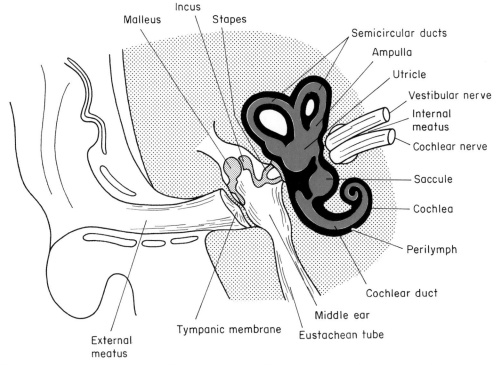

Fig. 6.1. *The ear.* Note the middle ear with the three ear ossicles and the inner ear with the membranous labyrinth (located in the temporal bone). The eustachian tube connects the middle ear with the pharynx.

Here we will consider only the organ of hearing, the cochlea.

The membranous part of the cochlea—the *cochlear duct*—forms a thin-walled tube with a triangular shape (in cross section), surrounded by the bony part of the cochlea.

The duct forms a spiral with two and a half to three turns (Figs. 6.2 and 6.3). The lowermost wall of the cochlear duct is formed by the *basilar membrane* (membrana basilaris), which is suspended between the two facing sides of the bony canal (Fig. 6.4). At

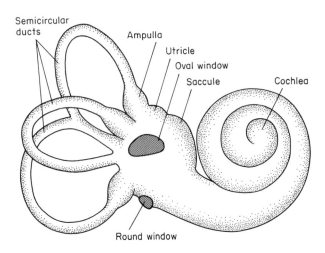

Fig. 6.2. *The membranous labyrinth* with its vestibular part (the semicircular ducts, the saccule, and the utricle) and the auditory part (the cochlea). The stapes is attached in the oval window.

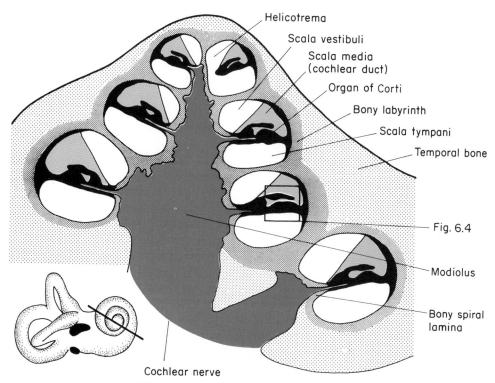

Fig. 6.3. *Section through the cochlea.*

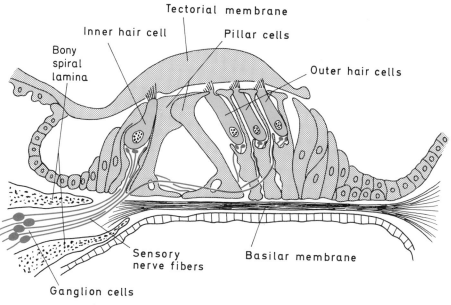

Fig. 6.4. *The organ of Corti.* Compare with Figure 6.3.

181

the inner side of the turns, the basilar membrane is attached to a bony prominence—the *bony spiral lamina* (lamina spiralis ossea), which follows the cochlea in its spiraling course (Figs. 6.3, 6.4, and 6.6). The sensory epithelium, forming the *organ of Corti,* rests on the basilar membrane (Figs. 6.3, 6.4, and 6.6). The length of the cochlear duct—and thus of the basilar membrane—is about 3 cm (Fig. 6.7). The upper wall of the cochlear duct is formed by the thin *vestibular membrane* (Fig. 6.6). The third, lateral or outer wall of the cochlear duct lies on the bony wall of the canal and is formed by a specialized, stratified epithelium. The room outside the cochlear duct is thus divided into two parallel canals. The one situated below the basilar membrane is called the *scala tympani;* the one above the vestibular membrane is called the *scala vestibuli* (Figs. 6.3 and 6.6). Both have openings or windows in the bone facing the middle ear (Figs. 6.2 and 6.7). The *oval window* (fenestra vestibuli) sits at the end of the scala vestibuli, whereas the *round window* (fenestra cochleae) sits at the end of the scala tympani. The windows are closed by the stapes and a thin membrane of connective tissue, respectively (Fig. 6.7).

How Sound Waves Are Transmitted to the Sensory Cells in the Cochlea

Conduction of sound waves from the air to the receptor cells in the cochlea occurs through the *external ear* (the auricle and the external auditory meatus) and the *middle ear* or *tympanic cavity* (Fig. 6.1). Sound waves hitting the skull can also be transmitted through the bone directly to the receptors. This kind of transmission, however, is very inefficient with regard to airborne sound waves and therefore plays no role in normal hearing (such bone conduction of sound waves is used for testing the function of the cochlea and also for certain hearing aid devices).

Sound waves hit the *eardrum* or *tympanic membrane* located at the bottom of the ex-

ternal meatus (Fig. 6.1). The eardrum consists of a thin, tense connective tissue membrane covered by a thin layer of epithelium on both sides (it is richly supplied with nociceptors, like the tight skin of the inner part of the external meatus). The three ossicles form a chain through the middle ear and connect the eardrum with the oval window (Figs. 6.1, 6.2, and 6.7). The *malleus* (the hammer) has a shaft that is attached to the inner side of the eardrum. The head of the malleus is connected to the *incus* (the anvil) by a joint, and the incus is further connected to the *stapes* (the stirrup) by a joint. The basal plate of the stapes is inserted in the oval window, thus closing the scala vestibuli (Fig. 6.7). The sound waves make the eardrum and the ossicles vibrate with the frequency of the waves, and thus the movement is transmitted to the fluid in the cochlea. Because the area of the eardrum is so much larger than that of the basal plate of the stapes, the pressure per square unit is increased 20 times. This *amplification mechanism* of course increases the sensitivity for sound dramatically, compared to a situation without the ossicles. Normally, even the slightest movement of the eardrum is sufficient to cause stimulation of the receptors in the cochlea. If the sound waves were to be transmitted directly from the air to the fluid in the cochlea, a large proportion would be reflected without acting on the cochlea. The sound would have to be much stronger to be perceived in such a situation. This is the case when diseases of the middle ear destroy the ossicles or stiffen their joints and thus eliminate the amplification mechanism. The ensuing hearing loss is called *conduction deafness.* A prerequisite for the free movement of the eardrum is that the pressure be equal on the two sides. This is ensured by the *Eustachian tube* (tuba auditiva), which connects the middle ear cavity with the pharynx (Fig. 6.1).

When the stapes is pressed (slightly) into the oval window, the pressure of the sound waves is transmitted directly to the fluid (the perilymph) in the scala vestibuli. Since water is incompressible, the sound waves can cause movement of the fluid only because the room can expand at some other point. Such expansion is allowed by the thin, compliant membrane covering the round window, which is pressed outward (into the middle ear) each time the stapes is pressed into the oval window. Movement of the perilymph in the scala vestibuli is immediately transmitted to the endolymph in the cochlear duct through the thin vestibular membrane. The movement is thus propagated to the basilar membrane, which is pressed slightly downward, and transmits the movement to the perilymph in the scala tympani. In short, *movements of the stapes in and out of the oval window in pace with the sound waves produce corresponding movements of the basilar membrane.* Movements of the basilar membrane stimulate the receptor cells.

We will now describe how the receptor cells are arranged in the organ of Corti and the mechanism by which movements of the basilar membrane lead to excitation of the receptors.

The Organ of Corti

The receptor cells in the cochlea are called *hair cells* because they are equipped with sensory hairs or *stereocilia* on their apical surface (Fig. 6.5). Along the basilar membrane there are two rows of receptor cells—one row formed by the *outer hair cells*, the other row by the *inner hair cells* (Fig. 6.4). The hair cells are surrounded by supporting cells. Two rows of especially large supporting cells, the *pillar cells*, separate the inner and outer hair cells and form the tunnel of Corti. Above the hair cells lies a thick plate, the *tectorial membrane*, which is indirectly attached to the bony wall of the cochlea. *Sensory (afferent) nerve fibers* of the eighth cranial nerve contact the basal parts of the hair cells (Fig. 6.4 and 6.5). The cell bodies of the sensory neurons are located in the *bony spiral lamina* (lamina spiralis ossea) close to the midportion of the cochlea (the modiolus, Figs. 6.3, 6.4, and 6.6). The hair cells are also

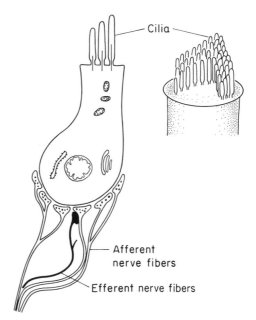

Fig. 6.5. *Inner hair cell.* Compare with Figure 6.4.

contacted by *efferent nerve fibers* (Fig. 6.5), which enable the central nervous system to control the sensitivity of the auditory receptors.

The mechanism by which the hair cells are stimulated most likely functions as follows: When the basilar membrane vibrates, the hair cells are displaced relative to the tectorial membrane, which is relatively immobile because it is anchored to the bony wall. The stereocilia, being embedded in the tectorial membrane, are thus moved back and forth in pace with the frequency of the sound waves. Bending of the cilia in one direction depolarizes the hair cell, whereas bending in the opposite direction hyperpolarizes it. Thus, the membrane potential of the hair cells oscillates in pace with the vibrations of the basilar membrane. Depolarization of the hair cells probably produces release of a neuroactive substance that transmits the signal to the sensory nerve endings. When sufficient amounts of the substance are released, action potentials are elicited in the sensory nerve fibers, and the signal is transmitted to the brain stem.

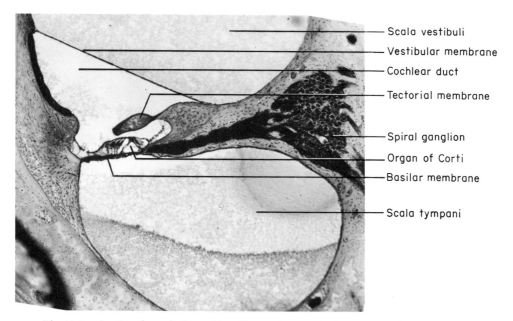

Scala vestibuli
Vestibular membrane
Cochlear duct
Tectorial membrane

Spiral ganglion
Organ of Corti
Basilar membrane

Scala tympani

Fig. 6.6.   *Section through the cochlea.* Photomicrograph. Compare with Figure 6.3.

Inner and Outer Hair Cells Have Different Properties

As mentioned, there are two rows of hair cells (Fig. 6.4). The inner row—closest to the bony spiral lamina—consists of a single row of *inner hair cells.* The outer row consists of three parallel rows of *outer hair cells.* There are approximately 3500 inner and 15,000 outer hair cells in the human cochlea. The two kinds of cells differ with regard to both morphology and innervation. Many more sensory nerve fibers contact the inner than the outer hair cells, whereas the situation is reversed with efferent innervation. It is now believed that *the inner hair cells are responsible for signaling sound, whereas the outer hair cells regulate the sensitivity of the sense organ.* The latter probably occurs by stiffening of the outer hair cells and their stereocilia (elicited by impulses from the efferent fibers). This is thought to lift the tectorial membrane a little away from the stereocilia of the inner hair cells.

Different Frequencies Are Registered at Different Sites along the Basilar Membrane: Tonotopic Localization

The ordered arrangement of neurons and nerve fibers signaling different pitches of sound (frequencies) is called *tonotopic local-ization* (compare with somatotopic localization in the somatosensory system and retinotopic localization in the visual system). As we will discuss later, the auditory pathways are tonotopically organized all the way from the cochlea to the cerebral cortex. The tonotopic localization in the cochlea has been demonstrated in several ways. After lesions restricted to a small part of the organ of Corti (which extends along the full length of the basilar membrane), experimental animals no longer react to sound in a certain, narrow range of frequencies (pitches), whereas they react normally to sounds of other frequencies. In humans, similar selective deafness may occur after prolonged exposure to noise—for example, in factories. Anatomic examination of the cochlea after death in such pesons has shown that the hair cells have disappeared in a restricted region on the basilar membrane, the position of the region differing with the frequency to which the person was deaf. The tonotopic localization has been determined in great detail by recording the response of single hair cells to sounds of different frequencies. Each hair cell is best activated by tones within a very narrow range of frequencies. Together, the

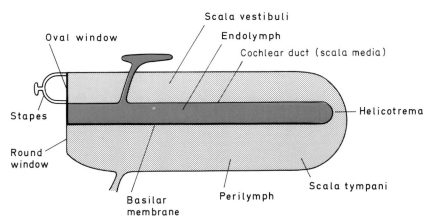

Fig. 6.7. *The cochlea.* The cochlear duct is pictured as if straightened. The oscillations of the stapes are transmitted to the fluid in the scala ves-tibuli and from there to the cochlear duct. Different tone frequencies set different parts of the basilar membrane in motion.

hair cells and the sensory fibers leading from them cover the total range of frequencies we can perceive.

The tonotopic localization is such that the *tones with the highest pitch (highest frequencies) are registered by the hair cells closest to the oval window—that is, on the basal part of the basilar membrane—whereas the lowest frequencies are registered at the top of the cochlea, that is, at the apical part of the basilar membrane.* This can be explained, at least partly, by the physical properties of the basilar membrane, as proposed by the German physicist Hermann Helmholtz in the nineteenth century. The basilar membrane is most narrow basally, and becomes progressively wider in the apical direction. The fibers of the basilar membrane are oriented transversely to the long axis of the basilar membrane (Fig. 6.4) and are therefore longer apically than basally. In analogy with the strings of an instrument (for example, a piano), basal parts would be expected to vibrate with a higher frequency than apical parts. This is the main basis of the resonance theory of Helmholtz, which postulates that each position along the basilar membrane corresponds to a certain frequency. Although later research has shown that even a pure tone makes large parts of the basilar membrane vibrate, the region in which the maximal amplitude occurs is very narrow.

In addition, there is evidence that the mechanical and electrical properties of the hair cells differ in accordance with their position on the basilar membrane, so that their thresholds are lower for certain frequencies than for others.

THE AUDITORY PATHWAYS

The anatomic organization of the central auditory pathways shows some unusual features, different from other sensory systems we have dealt with. More nuclei are intercalated in the auditory pathways and, furthermore, these nuclei have extensive and complicated interconnections. Finally, there are fibers crossing the midline at several levels of the auditory pathways. These features have made the auditory pathways more difficult to study than other sensory pathways. The crossing at several levels also renders hearing examinations of limited practical value for determining the site of lesions in the central nervous system.

The Cochlear Nerve and the Cochlear Nuclei

The part of the eighth cranial nerve conducting impulses from the cochlea is called the *cochlear nerve.* Most of the fibers are af-

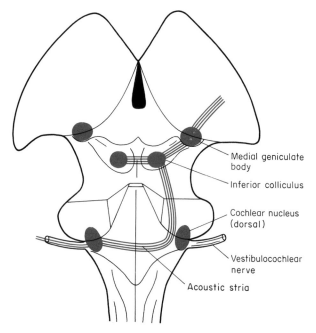

Medial geniculate body

Inferior colliculus

Cochlear nucleus (dorsal)

Vestibulocochlear nerve

Acoustic stria

Fig. 6.8. *Nuclei of the auditory pathways.* Impulses from the cochlea of one side reach the medial geniculate bodies of both sides (although not shown in the figure).

ferent and have their perikarya in the *spiral ganglion,* which is located in the bony spiral lamina (Figs. 6.3, 6.4, and 6.6). From the spiral ganglion the fibers pass through the midportion of the cochlea (the modiolus, Fig. 6.3) and through the internal acoustic meatus (internal auditory canal) to the cerebellopontine angle (Fig. 6.8). There the nerve enters the *cochlear nuclei,* which are two large nuclei (the dorsal and the ventral cochlear nuclei) located laterally on the medulla (Figs. 6.8, 6.9, and 13.2), external to the inferior cerebellar peduncle (Fig. 11.1). After entering the nuclei, the cochlear nerve fibers divide and end in precise tonotopic order in several parts of the nuclei. The tonotopic localization has been demonstrated, for example, with microelectrode recordings that make it possible to determine the response of single fibers and neurons to tones of different frequencies.

The *efferent fibers* of the cochlear nerve arise in the *superior olivary complex,* located in the rostral part of the medulla (Fig. 6.9). The fibers end, as mentioned, predominantly around the outer hair cells and enable the central nervous system to control the sensitivity of the inner hair cells.

Ascending Pathways from the Cochlear Nuclei

From the cochlear nuclei the auditory impulses are transmitted to the *inferior colliculus* (mainly of the opposite side). The pathway formed by the ascending fibers from the cochlear nuclei is called the *lateral lemniscus* (Figs. 6.8 and 6.9). Many of the fibers end, however, in other nuclei—such as the superior olivary complex—that send fibers to the inferior colliculus. Neurons in the inferior colliculus send their axons to the *medial geniculate body* of the thalamus (Figs. 2.20–2.23, 6.8, and 6.9). The fibers form an oblong elevation at the dorsal side of the mesencephalon, the *inferior collicular brachium* (brachium quadrigeminum inferius). The efferent fibers from the medial geniculate body end in the *auditory cortex* located in the temporal lobe (in the superior temporal gyrus, Figs. 6.9 and 6.10). The ascending fibers from the medial geniculate body are located in the posterior part of the internal capsule. At all levels, the auditory pathway is precisely organized, with cells responding to sounds of different frequencies arranged in parallel lamellae.

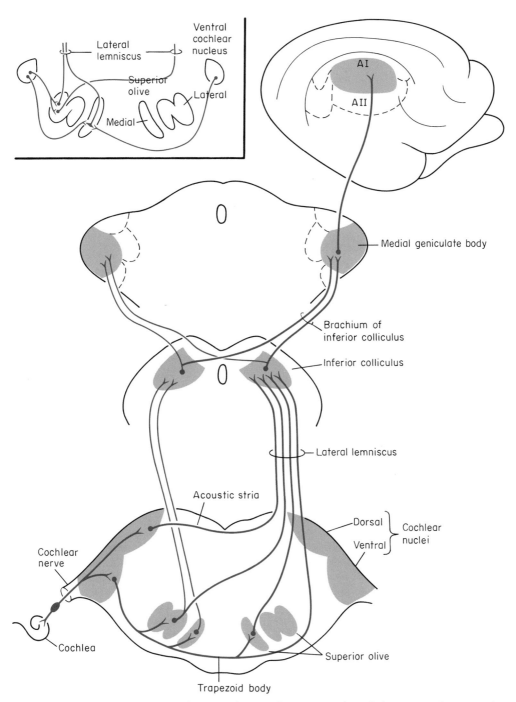

Fig. 6.9. *Ascending auditory pathways.* Schematic presentation based on experimental studies of the cat. Note that the connections are bilateral, so that AI on one side receives impulses from the cochleae of both sides. Inset: *Connections of the superior olive.* Only some main connections are shown. Note that impulses from both ears reach the medial part of the superior olive. This arrangement is believed to be of importance for localization of sound.

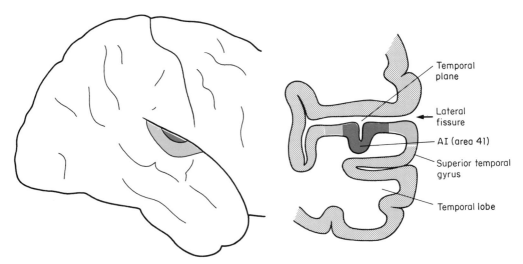

Fig. 6.10.   *The human auditory cortex.*

Even though the central auditory pathways are predominantly crossed, there is a significant uncrossed component. Therefore, unilateral damage to the pathways does not produce a clear-cut hearing deficit. The ability to localize from where a sound comes may be reduced, however.

The Auditory Pathways Consist of Functionally Different Components

Efferent fibers from the two cochlear nuclei take different routes (Fig. 6.9). Fibers from the *dorsal cochlear nucleus* pass in the *stria acusticae* dorsal to the inferior cerebellar peduncle and then cross through the reticular formation and join the lateral lemniscus. Most fibers from the *ventral nucleus,* on the other hand, pass ventrally and cross to the other side in the *trapezoid body* in the lowermost part of the pons. Some of these fibers end in the superior olivary complex of both sides, whereas others continue rostrally in the lateral lemniscus to the inferior colliculus. The functional significance of these parallel paths out of the cochlear nuclei is not fully understood, but animal experiments (especially in the cat) show that single cells in the dorsal and ventral nuclei have different properties. Schematically, many cells in the ventral nucleus respond to sound stimuli much like the primary afferent fibers of the cochlear nerve, whereas cells in the dorsal nucleus have more complex response properties. Cells in the dorsal nucleus are, for example, often

excited by sound with one particular frequency and inhibited by another frequency. It has been suggested that the dorsal nucleus forwards signals that are of importance for the direction of attention toward a sound, whereas information from the ventral nucleus is of importance for, among other things, localization of a sound.

Experimentally, two components of the ascending auditory pathways have been identified. One is called the *core projection* and is a pathway for auditory impulses only. It is precisely tonotopically localized at all levels and terminates in the primary auditory cortex, AI. The core projection is relayed through the central parts of the inferior colliculus and specific parts of the medial geniculate body. The other component is called the *belt projection*. It is relayed through peripheral parts of the inferior colliculus and terminates in the cortex surrounding the AI. The cells of this pathway are influenced by visual and somatosensory stimuli in addition to auditory ones. The belt projection is thought to be of importance for integration of auditory information with other kinds of sensory information.

Generalizations to conditions in humans on the basis of studies done in other species must, however, be made with particular caution for the auditory system. Species differences appear to be greater for the auditory system than for other sensory systems. This may be related presumably to the great differences that exist among species with how sound is used as a source of information. For example, certain nuclei that are large in the cat are very small in man, and vice versa.

The Superior Olive and Sound Localization

The superior olivary complex (superior olive) is located in the lower part of the pons, in the trapezoid body (Fig. 6.9). A striking feature is that most neurons are influenced from both ears, which led to the assumption that the superior olive is of particular importance for the ability to localize from where a sound comes. When a sound hits the head from the right side, it will reach the right ear slightly before it reaches the left, because the head is in the way. The sound will also be slightly weakened before reaching the left ear. Psychophysical experiments in humans indicate that side differences in both time and intensity are used by the auditory system to localize sounds. The time difference is most important for localizing sounds of low frequencies, whereas intensity differences are most important for sounds of higher frequencies (above 4000 Hz).

The superior olivary complex consists of several subdivisions. The *lateral part* receives afferents from the cochlear nuclei of both sides and projects bilaterally to the inferior colliculi. Most cells in the lateral part are excited by impulses from the ear of the same side and inhibited by impulses from the contralateral ear (via interneurons). The cells respond best when the sounds hitting the two ears are of different intensities. Consequently, the lateral part of the superior olive is assumed to use intensity differences for the analysis of sound localization.

The *medial part* of the superior olive appears to be of particular importance for localization of low-frequency sounds. It receives afferents from a particular subdivision of the ventral cochlear nucleus of both sides (Fig. 6.9A). Each cell has two long dendrites oriented transversely. One dendrite receives signals from the right ear, the other from the left. These cells are very sensitive to small time differences in synaptic inputs to the two dendrites and are most sensitive to sounds with low frequencies. The efferent fibers of the medial part pass to the central nucleus of the inferior colliculus on the same side.

Descending Control of the Auditory Pathways

There are descending fibers at all levels of the auditory pathways. There are numerous fibers passing from the auditory cortex to the medial geniculate body (like other thalamic nuclei) and to the inferior colliculus. There are also fibers descending from the inferior colliculus to nuclei at lower levels. As mentioned, there are also efferent fibers in the cochlear nerve ending in contact with the hair cells of the cochlea. Such fibers come from the superior olivary complex, and form the *olivocochlear bundle*. The descending connections are, at least in part, precisely organized and can therefore be expected to control selectively subgroups of neurons in the auditory pathways (for example, neurons transmitting information about a certain frequency).

There are many inhibitory interneurons in the nuclei of the auditory pathways, and both GABA and glycine appear to be used as transmitters for such interneurons. Physiological experiments show that the central transmission of auditory impulses can be inhibited, probably at all levels from the cochlea to the cerebral cortex. The censoring of the sensory information that is allowed to reach consciousness is perhaps even more pronounced in the auditory system than in other sensory systems. Selective suppression of auditory information is a necessity if we are to select the relevant sounds among numerous irrelevant ones. Such mechanisms are most likely at work when, for example, at a cocktail party with numerous voices we nevertheless are able to select and pay attention to only one of them.

Auditory Reflexes

The ascending auditory pathways convey signals that enable the conscious perception of sounds. Auditory information is, however, also used at a subconscious level to elicit reflex responses. The reticular formation receives collaterals from the ascending auditory pathways, and such connections mediate the sudden muscle activity provoked by a strong, unexpected sound—that is, a *startle response*. Other auditory impulses are transmitted to the nuclei of the facial and trigeminal nerves, which innervate two small muscles in the middle ear, the *stapedius and tensor tympani muscles*. Contraction of these muscles dampens the movements of the middle ear ossicles and thereby protects the cochlea against sounds of high intensity.

Other, more complex reflex arcs mediate automatic movements of the head and eyes, and even the body, in the direction of an unexpected sound. The reflex centers for such reflexes are probably located in the inferior and superior colliculi. The inferior colliculus sends fibers to the superior colliculus, which has connections with the relevant motor nuclei in the brain stem and spinal cord.

Interruption of the Auditory Pathways

Restricted lesions of the auditory pathways or the auditory cortex—*central lesions*—usually produce no clear-cut symptoms. As mentioned, this is because the connections from the cochlear nuclei to the cerebral cortex are bilateral (although with a contralateral preponderance). After destruction of the auditory cortex on one side, a person can still hear with both ears.

Destruction of the cochlear nerve (or the cochlea)—*peripheral lesions*—produces deafness of the ear on the same side (the same happens, of course, with a lesion of the cochlear nuclei). Destruction of the cochlear nerve may be caused by a tumor, called *acoustic neuroma,* in the internal auditory meatus (arising from the Schwann cells of the eighth cranial nerve). As the tumor grows, it compresses the cochlear, the vestibular, and the facial nerves (all passing through the internal meatus). Symptoms may therefore be caused by irritation (in the early phase) or destruction of all of these nerves. Thus, the first symptoms are usually due to irritation of the cochlear nerve, causing ringing in the ear (tinnitus), but gradually deafness develops. The cochlear nerve may also be compressed or torn by skull fractures passing through the temporal bone.

Peripheral leasions of the auditory system, in addition to unilateral deafness, also reduce or eliminate the ability to localize the source of a sound.

THE AUDITORY CORTEX

Each of the nuclei of the auditory pathways consists in reality of subdivisions that differ in morphology, connectivity, and functions. This concerns, as mentioned, the cochlear nuclei, the superior olive, the inferior colliculus, and the medial geniculate body. The highest level, the auditory cortex, also shows such parcellation. Fibers from the medial geniculate body end with precise tonotopic localization in the *primary auditory cortex, AI* (Figs. 6.9 and 6.10). This corresponds largely to the striate area of the visual system. Regions around the AI receive fibers from parts of the medial geniculate body other than from where AI receives fibers. The *second auditory area, AII,* appears to receive afferents that are not tonotopically organized, whereas other areas (in the cat at least four) receive connections with a less precise localization than AI. Thus, cells in AI respond to sounds within a narrower frequency range than cells in the other auditory areas. Many cells in AI, however, have complex properties. Some respond best to a sound when the frequency is increasing or decreasing. Many cells are influenced from both ears, but often such that they are excited by signals from one ear and inhibited from the other. The functions of the auditory areas surrounding AI are less well known than the functions of the corresponding areas in the visual cortex.

In humans, Brodmann's area 41 in the superior temporal gyrus (Fig. 6.10) is thought to correspond to area AI of monkeys and other animals. In humans (as in lower animals), the cortex around the primary auditory area most likely receives fibers from both the medial geniculate body and the AI. It is, furthermore, highly likely that these areas are of particular importance for the interpretation of auditory information. Patients with bilateral damage of the auditory cortex are reported to be able to perceive sounds and even discriminate tones with different pitches and intensities (even though not necessarily with normal speed and precision). This corresponds to findings made in monkeys. The ability to recognize and interpret tones in particular patterns, however, is reduced or abolished. Such patients are unable to recognize familiar sounds like laughter, a bell that tolls, sounds of various animals, and so forth. They are furthermore unable to understand the speech of other people, even though they can speak and read themselves. This is called *acoustic agnosia.*

NOTES

1. The most intense sound that the human ear can perceive is about 10^{12} times stronger than the weakest. A logarithmic scale is therefore used for sound intensity. One decibel (dB) represents the weakest perceptible sound and just below 130 dB represents the strongest (the pain threshold is at 130 dB). This scale gives *relative* measures of intensity, since the sensitivity of the ear differs for different frequencies.

2. The composition of the endolymph and of the perilymph differs: The concentrations of sodium and potassium ions in the perilymph are similar to those in the cerebrospinal fluid (that is, similar to those in the extracellular fluid), whereas the concentrations of these ions in the endolymph are like those found intracellularly. The protein concentration, however, is much higher in the perilymph than in the endolymph and the cerebrospinal fluid.

7

The Olfactory System

The sense of smell does not play the same important role for adult humans as the senses of hearing and vision. Going back in the evolution of the species, however, we find that smell is the most primitive of the senses. It is also the most important one at the lower stages of evolution. To understand the evolution of the brain, knowledge of the "olfactory brain" or *rhinencephalon* has been important because in primitive vertebrates almost the whole cerebrum is devoted to the processing of olfactory impulses. In higher vertebrates, new parts of the cerebrum emerge that gradually overshadow completely the phylogenetically old parts. The terms olfactory brain or rhinencephalon for these old parts are unfortunate, however. In higher vertebrates, large parts of the regions corresponding to the rhinencephalon in lower animals have nothing to do with the sense of smell but have taken on other important functions, the hippocampus (Chapter 16) being the most striking example. This is a common occurrence during evolution; structures that are no longer used for one function may form the basis for the development of new capacities.

RECEPTORS FOR SMELL

The special receptor cells for smell are located in the mucous membrane of the upper part of the nasal cavity, within an area of about 2 cm^2 (the olfactory epithelium). The receptor cells are equipped on their apical surface with microvilli, embedded in the layer of mucus covering the epithelium (Fig. 7.1). Any substance that is to influence the receptors must therefore be dissolved in the mucus. The olfactory epithelium probably contains about 100 million receptor cells in humans. These cells are constantly renewed even though they are in fact primitive neurons; they are therefore exceptions to the rule that neurons that die are not replaced.

Seven primary qualities of smell have been proposed—among the innumerable nuances we can perceive—on the basis of experiments with a large number of odorous substances. Molecules provoking the same primary quality seem to be of a common shape rather than being chemically related. *The stereochemical theory of smell* proposes that the receptor sites on the receptor cells have different shapes, and only molecules with a complementary shape fit into the receptor site. Not all observations support the existence of seven primary qualities, however. Binding of the odorous substance (the *odorant*) to the membrane receptor alters the membrane potential of the receptor cell, probably via intracellular signal molecules and perhaps also via direct action on ion channels.

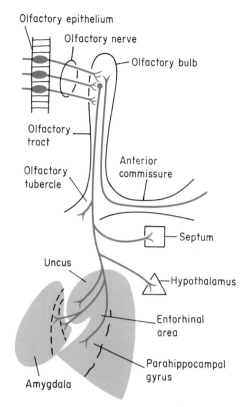

Olfactory epithelium
Olfactory nerve
Olfactory bulb
Olfactory tract
Anterior commissure
Olfactory tubercle
Septum
Uncus
Hypothalamus
Entorhinal area
Parahippocampal gyrus
Amygdala

Fig. 7.1. *The olfactory pathways.* Schematic illustration of some main connections. To the **upper left** are the olfactory receptors in the nasal mucosa, sending their central processes to the olfactory bulb. The neurons of the olfactory bulb send their axons to the cortex and various nuclei in the vicinity of the tip of the temporal lobe.

CENTRAL PATHWAYS FOR OLFACTORY IMPULSES

Like other sensory cells—for example, those in the inner ear and in the taste buds—the olfactory receptor cells are surrounded by supporting cells. In other respects, however, the olfactory receptor cells are different from other sensory receptors, showing a more primitive arrangement. Thus, the olfactory cells themselves send a process (an axon) centrally, whereas in the inner ear, for example, a peripheral process of a ganglion cell contacts the receptor cell. The axons of the olfactory cells form many small bundles, together constituting the *olfactory nerve* (the first cranial nerve; Fig. 7.1). The bundles

pass through the base of the skull close to the midline in the anterior cranial fossa (through the lamina cribrosa of the ethmoid bone). The olfactory nerve enters the *olfactory bulb* (Figs. 2.14 and 7.2), located just above the nasal cavity under the frontal lobe. In the olfactory bulb, the olfactory nerve fibers establish synaptic contacts with the *mitral cells,* which in their turn send axons to the brain through the *olfactory tract* (Figs. 2.14, 7.1, and 7.2). The fibers in the olfactory tract eventually take various directions, ending in different nuclei, most of which are located close to the tip of the temporal lobe.

The Olfactory Bulb

The structure of the olfactory bulb is complex. It is not a simple relay station but rather a small "brain" in itself, carrying out substantial processing of the sensory information reaching it. In this sense there are similarities with the retina—and both are parts of the central nervous system that have been moved outside the brain. There is some evidence that the olfactory bulb is of decisive importance for the *discriminative aspect of olfaction*—that is, the ability to distinguish different odors. Thus, lesions of nuclei in which the fibers from the olfactory bulb terminate have been reported not to impair seriously simple olfactory discrimination.

Different odors appear to be somewhat differently represented in the olfactory bulb—that is, there is an "odorotopical localization."

There are also efferent fibers in the olfactory tract, as shown with anatomic methods. Accordingly, electrical stimulation of the olfactory cortex can influence (primarily inhibit) the signal transmission through the olfactory bulb.

THE TERMINAL AREAS OF THE OLFACTORY TRACT

Most of the efferent fibers from the olfactory bulb end at the medial aspect of the temporal lobe, partly in the *cortex* and partly in the

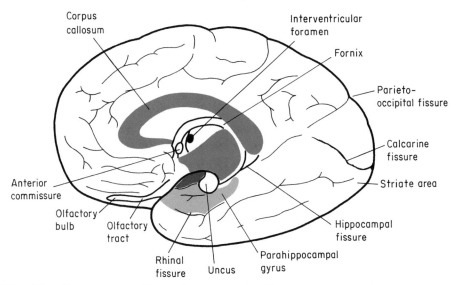

Fig. 7.2. *The olfactory cortex.* The medial aspect of the cerebral hemisphere. The primary olfactory cortex is located in the uncus (dark red). The olfactory cortex in humans most likely also encompasses parts of the entorhinal area (light red).

amygdaloid nucleus (Figs. 7.1 and 7.2). The latter is located just below the cortex in the tip of the temporal lobe (Fig. 16.1). In the cortex, fibers terminate both in the so-called *piriform cortex* in the uncus and in the adjoining parts of the entorhinal cortex (area 28). The fibers to the amygdaloid nucleus end only in the *corticomedial nucleus,* which sends efferent fibers to the hypothalamus (the amygdaloid nucleus will be discussed further in Chapter 16). The cortical regions in the temporal lobe that receive direct fibers from the olfactory bulb are called the *primary olfactory cortex.* It is believed that olfactory impulses come to consciousness in these and nearby cortical areas. Lesions affecting the uncus and the immediately surrounding cortex can be accompanied by subjective olfactory experiences (often unpleasant). Such sensations often occur as so-called *uncinate fits,* which frequently also include a peculiar feeling of experiencing the events in a dream (dreamy state). Often the patients feel that they have experienced the event before (*déjà vu*). Such uncinate fits may develop into an epileptic seizure, and the condition is regarded as a form of epilepsy.

Olfactory impulses reach not only the olfactory cortex and the amygdaloid nucleus but also other nuclei such as the *hypothalamus* and the *septal nuclei* (Chapters 15 and 16).

The olfactory nuclei on the two sides are interconnected by fibers running through the *anterior commissure.*

OLFACTORY IMPULSES AND REFLEXES

Olfactory connections to the hypothalamus—both direct and indirect ones via the amygdaloid nucleus—are of importance for eating and for behavior directed at acquiring food. Sexual reflexes and sexually related behavior are also influenced by olfactory impulses, although more so in lower mammals than in man. The structural basis for such reflexes and behavior is very complex and not known in detail. Olfactory connections to the amygdaloid nucleus are most likely of importance, not only because the amygdaloid nucleus acts on the hypothalamus but also because it acts on other parts of the so-called limbic system (see Chapter 16).

III

Motor Systems

The cell groups and tracts in the central nervous system that control the activity of the skeletal muscles compose the *motor systems*. We may also use the term *somatic motor systems* to distinguish them from systems controlling smooth muscles and glands.

The motor systems can be divided into several interconnected parts. First, the *peripheral motor neurons* (Chapter 8) and the *central motor pathways* (Chapter 9) are directly involved in mediating the commands from the motor centers to the muscles. These parts of the motor systems are necessary for the initiation of voluntary movements; paralysis ensues when they are damaged. Secondly, the *basal ganglia* (Chapter 10) and the *cerebellum* (Chapter 11) have their main connections with the central motor nuclei and are necessary for the proper execution of movements rather than for their initiation.

Motor and Sensory Systems Are Not Independent of Each Other

Although for didactic reasons we often treat the motor and sensory systems as independent entities, this is an oversimplification. For the motor systems to function, they must cooperate closely with the sensory systems. During most movements, the motor centers need constant information from receptors in muscles, around joints, and in the skin about whether the movement is progressing in accordance with the plan. Often visual information is also crucial for the proper execution of movements. Such sensory feedback information enables the central nervous system to adjust and correct the command signals issued to the muscles—either during the movement or the next time the movement is performed.

In addition, impulses from many other parts of the brain are necessary for movement—for example, those involved in the early stages of the movement planning and in the mediation of motivated behavior. Thus, large parts of the central nervous system may be considered motoric in the sense that they contribute to the activity of the more narrowly defined motor systems. On the other hand, such regions may also be considered sensory since they also take part in the processing of sensory information. At the higher levels of the central nervous system it becomes meaningless to classify regions as sensory or motoric—these concepts are much too narrow "pigeon holes" to encompass the complex tasks undertaken by large parts of the cerebral cortex and many related subcortical nuclei.

Classification of Movements

Before we describe the motor systems, some comments on movements in general may be pertinent. First, muscle contraction may not necessarily elicit movement (that is, alter the position of one or more joints). Just as often, muscle activity is used to prevent movement: For example, muscles maintain our posture by counteracting the force of gravity. In the latter case, the muscles may be said to *stabilize* a joint (against external forces) and to have a *postural function.* Furthermore, movement in one part of the body—for example, in an arm—requires that muscles in other parts contract to prevent the body balance from being upset. A muscle in one situation may be used as a mover and in another situation as a stabilizer.

Whether or not a movement is to occur depends on the magnitude of the force produced by the muscle contraction and the external forces acting on the joint. When the external force is smaller than the muscle force, the muscle shortens and a movement occurs (isotonic contraction). When the external forces equal the force of the muscle contraction, no movement occurs (isometric contraction). When the external force is greater than the opposing force produced by the muscle contraction, the muscle lengthens. The latter is the case, for example, with the thigh muscles when we walk down a staircase.

Movements may be classified by the *speed* with which they are performed. *Ramp movements* are performed relatively slowly. The crucial point is that the movement is slow enough to enable sensory feedback information to influence the movement during its execution. *Ballistic movements* are very rapid, their characteristic feature being that they are too fast to enable feedback control (the name derives from analogy with a bullet shot out of a gun).

Movements may also be classified according to whether they are *voluntary* or *automatic,* the latter taking place without our conscious participation. This is in reality much too crude a distinction: There is a gradual transition from what Hughlings Jackson in the past century termed the *most automatic* to the *least automatic* movement. The most automatic movements are basic, simple reflexes like the retraction of the arm from a noxious stimulus. Locomotion is an example of a semiautomatic movement—that is, the basic pattern is automatic, whereas start and stop, and necessary adjustments, may require conscious (voluntary) control. The least automatic movements are precision grips with the fingers and delicate manipulatory or exploratory movements such as writing, drawing, playing an instrument, and so forth. Equally precise voluntary control exists for the muscles of the larynx, the tongue, and some of the facial muscles. We also know that the degree to which a movement is automatic changes with learning: In the beginning a new movement requires full voluntary control, whereas in the process of learning the movement becomes more automatic. When playing a well-rehearsed musical piece on the piano, for example, we do not need to pay attention to the fingers and their movements.

As a rule, the most automatic movements require only the use of relatively simple reflex arcs at the spinal level; participation of higher motor centers is not necessary. Somewhat less automatic and more complex movements such as ventilation, locomotion, and postural control depend in addition on the participation of neuronal groups in the brain stem. Such movements do not require our attention directed toward them but can also be subjected to voluntary control. The least automatic movements depend on the participation of the highest level—the cerebral cortex—to coordinate and control the activity of motor centers in the brain stem and spinal cord.

8

The Peripheral Motor Neurons

MOTONEURONS AND MUSCLES

The peripheral motor neurons are nerve cells that send their axons to skeletal muscles. Another term is *lower motor neurons.* These are the *motoneurons* in the ventral horn of the cord and in the somatic motor cranial nerve nuclei. As mentioned in Chapter 4, there are two kinds: The α *motoneurons* innervate the extrafusal muscle fibers, whereas the γ *motoneurons* innervate the intrafusal muscle fibers of the muscle spindle (Figs. 4.3 and 4.4).

The axons of the motoneurons leave the spinal cord through the ventral roots and continue into the ventral and dorsal branches (rami) of the spinal nerves (Figs. 2.7 and 2.9) to innervate skeletal muscles of the trunk and the extremities (Fig. 8.1). Correspondingly, the axons from the cranial nerve motor nuclei supply the muscles of the tongue, pharynx, palate, larynx, face, and the extraocular muscles. The axons of all the motoneurons located in one spinal segment leave the cord through one ventral root and continue into one spinal nerve. The ventral branches of the spinal nerves form *plexuses* so that the motor axons from one spinal segment are distributed to several peripheral nerves (Fig. 8.1).

Contraction of skeletal muscles can only be elicited by impulses conducted in the axons of motoneurons. If these axons are interrupted, the muscles become *paralyzed.* The peripheral motor neurons thus constitute the *final common path* for all signals from the central nervous system to skeletal muscles (the term final common path was introduced by the British neurophysiologist and Nobel laureate Sherrington). The motoneurons may be compared with the keys of a piano on which higher levels of the central nervous system can play. As we will describe later in this chapter, many parts of the central nervous system cooperate in determining the activity of the motoneurons and thus the contraction of our muscles.

Each motoneuron probably receives about 10,000 boutons—some forming excitatory synapses, others inhibitory; some with fast synaptic actions, others with slow modulatory ones. The sum of these influences determines whether and with what frequency the motoneurons will send action potentials to the muscles.

That we can perform such a wide variety of movements is due to the ability of the central nervous system to select precisely, by way of the motoneurons, the combinations of muscles to be used and to determine the

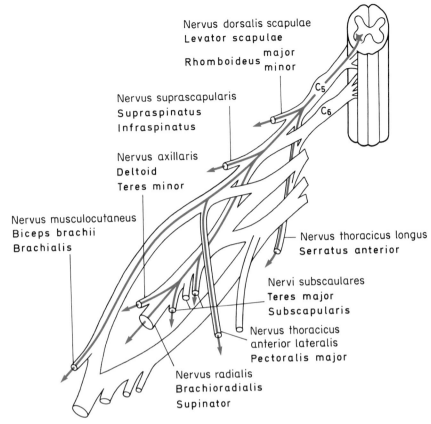

Nervus dorsalis scapulae
Levator scapulae
Rhomboideus major
            minor

C₅
C₆

Nervus suprascapularis
Supraspinatus
Infraspinatus

Nervus axillaris
Deltoid
Teres minor

Nervus musculocutaneus
Biceps brachii
Brachialis

Nervus thoracicus longus
Serratus anterior

Nervi subscaulares
Teres major
Subscapularis

Nervus thoracicus
anterior lateralis
Pectoralis major

Nervus radialis
Brachioradialis
Supinator

Fig. 8.1.   *The brachial plexus.* Note that axons of motoneurons in one spinal segment (C_5 is used as an example) are distributed to several peripheral nerves supplying various muscles of the arm. Each muscle also receives motor fibers from other segments, although not shown here. Based on Haymaker and Woodhall (1945).

speed and force with which they are to contract.

It is well-established that the motoneurons use *acetylcholine* as transmitter substance, and the synthesizing enzyme choline acetyltransferase can be demonstrated with immunohistochemical techniques in the motoneurons and in their terminals. Motoneurons also contain the neuropeptide calcitonin gene-related peptide (CGRP).[1]

The Motoneurons Are Somatotopically Organized

The motoneurons of the ventral horn and in the cranial nerve nuclei are easily recognized in microscopic sections because of their large size and the big clumps of rER (Nissl bodies)

in the cytoplasm of their perikarya (Fig. 1.2). The rich content of rER indicates that the neurons have a high protein synthesis. These proteins are, for example, enzymes for transmitter synthesis and metabolism, and various kinds of membrane proteins (the vast surface of the motoneurons with their large dendritic tree and long axons presumably explains why motoneurons contain more rER than most other neuronal types).

The motoneurons are collected in groups, which form Rexed's lamina IX in the spinal cord (Fig. 8.2). *The dendrites of the motoneurons do not respect the boundaries of lamina IX,* however, and extend far in the transverse and in the rostrocaudal directions—for example, into lamina VII, where many interneurons are located (Fig. 2.13).

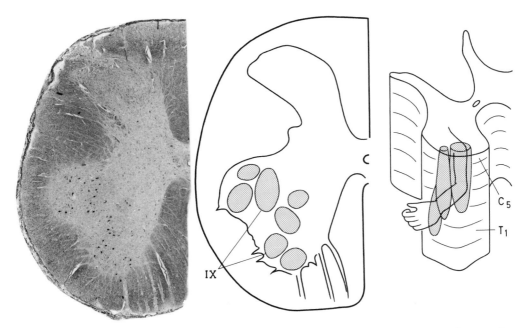

Fig. 8.2. *Motoneurons.* To the **left**, a photomicrograph and a drawing of a transverse section of the (lumbar) spinal cord. The motoneurons are collected in groups (columns) together forming the lamina IX of Rexed. To the **right**, schematic drawing of the somatotopic localization of the motoneuronal groups innervating the arm, located in the spinal segments C_5–T_1. Motoneurons supplying the intrinsic muscles of the hand are located most caudally (C_8–T_1) and most dorsally in the ventral horn.

The rostrocaudal (longitudinal) extension of the dendrites enables dorsal root fibers from several segments to act on each motoneuron. The dendritic tree increases the surface of the motoneurons enormously, and, not surprisingly, the vast majority of the boutons contacting motoneurons do so on the dendrites (forming axodendritic synapses).

When viewed three-dimensionally, the motoneurons are seen to be collected in *longitudinally oriented columns* (Fig. 8.2). Each column contains the α and γ motoneurons to one muscle (or a few functionally similar muscles). Within a column supplying more than one muscle, the motoneurons to each muscle are at least partly segregated. *Each column as a rule extends through more than one segment of the cord.* Consequently, each muscle receives motor fibers through more than one ventral root and spinal nerve. Destruction of one root or spinal nerve only— for example, by disk protrusion in sciatica or by a tumor growing in the spinal canal—

will not produce paralysis of a muscle but only a more or less pronounced weakness (paresis).

The anatomic organization of motoneurons has been studied in part by transection of muscle nerves in experimental animals. A retrograde reaction, which is easily seen in the microscope, occurs in the perikarya of the motoneurons. Modern methods with retrograde transport of tracer substances such as HRP have detailed the picture considerably. Study of patients with poliomyelitis has provided information about conditions in the human cord (the poliovirus infects and kills motoneurons). Because the distribution of paralyzed muscles usually has been determined before death, it can be compared with the distribution of cell loss among the motoneuronal groups in the cord and brain stem.

Groups of motoneurons that supply axial muscles—that is, muscles of the back, neck, abdomen, and pelvis—are located most me-

dially within the ventral horn, whereas motoneurons supplying muscles of the extremities are located more laterally. This explains
why the ventral horn is broader (extends
more laterally) in the segments of the cord
that send fibers to the extremities (i.e., C_5–T_1
and L_1–S_2; compare Figs. 2.10, 2.12, and
8.2). There is also a further somatotopic organization: Motoneurons supplying proximal muscles of the extremities (the shoulder
and hip) are located more ventrally than
those supplying the distal muscles (the hand
and foot). This is shown in Figure 8.2, which
also shows that the proximal muscles are
supplied from motoneurons located more
rostrally than those supplying the distal
muscles. For example, the shoulder muscles
are mainly innervated by the upper parts of
the brachial plexus (C_5–C_6), whereas the intrinsic muscles of the hand are innervated by
the lowermost segments (C_8–T_1).

Motoneurons Are of Functionally Different Kinds

As mentioned, the α and γ motoneurons
supplying one muscle lie together within
one column in the ventral horn. In a microscopic section of the cord it can be seen that
the motoneuronal perikarya vary in size
(Fig. 1.2). As in other parts of the nervous
system, the neurons with the largest perikarya have the thickest (and thus fastest-
conducting) axons. The smallest within a
group are the γ motoneurons, whereas the
size varies considerably among the α motoneurons. Such size differences among the α
motoneurons are related to differences
among the muscle cells supplied by the motoneurons. Briefly stated, the smallest α motoneurons control delicate movements with
little force, whereas the largest motoneurons
come into play only when a movement requires great force. The large α motoneurons
also have a much higher maximal firing frequency than the small ones. On the other
hand, the large ones tend to fire in brief
bursts with a high frequency, whereas the
small α motoneurons tend to go on firing for
a long time with a low frequency. These differences in firing pattern reflect that the

large motoneurons are used for forceful,
rapid movements of short duration, whereas
the small motoneurons can uphold a moderate muscular tension for a long time. For
these reasons, we apply the term *phasic α
motoneurons* to the large one, and *tonic α
motoneurons* to the small ones. The properties of the α motoneurons will be discussed
further when dealing with the motor units.

The Motor End Plate

After entering the muscle, the axon of a motoneuron divides into many thin branches or
collaterals. Each of these end or terminal
branches contacts one muscle cell only. *Each
muscle cell is thus contacted only by one
branch from one α motoneuron.* Such a
branch ends on the muscle cell approximately midway between its ends, forming
the *motor end plate,* where the signal transfer from nerve to muscle takes place (Figs.
8.3 and 8.4). Within the end-plate region,
the axonal branch divides further and forms
up to about 50 boutons, each establishing
synaptic contact with the muscle cell. The
postsynaptic side at this *neuromuscular
junction* is somewhat special compared with
synapses in the central nervous system, since
so-called junctional folds and a thin basal
lamina are intercalated between the presynaptic and postsynaptic membranes (Fig.
8.4B). The boutons contain *acetylcholine,*
and the postsynaptic membrane contains
acetylcholine receptors of the nicotinic type.
The density of acetylcholine receptors is
much higher in the end-plate region than
elsewhere on the muscle cell surface (this is
appropriate since only at the end plate is the
muscle cell normally exposed to acetylcholine).[2]

An action potential propagated along the
axon of the motoneuron depolarizes all the
boutons and elicits release of acetylcholine.
The transmitter binds to the acetylcholine
receptors, and—as at other excitatory synapses—this depolarizes the postsynaptic
membrane. This change in the membrane
potential is called the *end-plate potential.*
Normally, enough transmitter is released by
one action potential to depolarize the mus-

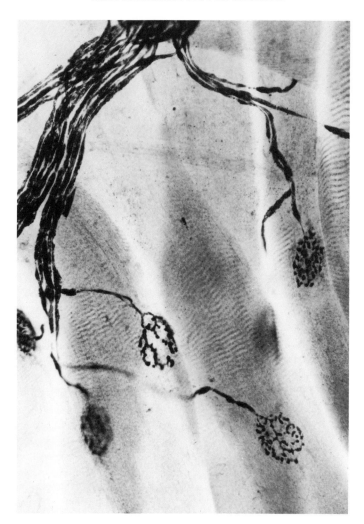

Fig. 8.3. *Motor end plates.* Photomicrograph of skeletal muscle cells and a small bundle of nerve fibers innervating the cells. The tissue is stained with gold chloride to darken the nerve fibers and their terminal boutons. Each motor end plate consists of numerous small boutons. Four end plates are seen in the photomicrograph. Magnification, ×600.

cle cell membrane to the threshold for an action potential. The action potential is propagated over the whole surface of the muscle cell and elicits a brief contraction. The action of acetylcholine is rapidly terminated by the enzyme *acetylcholine esterase* present in the junctional folds.

Neuromuscular Transmission Can Be Disturbed by Poison and Disease

Various drugs and naturally occurring poisonous substances can influence the signal transmission at the neuromuscular junction and produce involuntary muscle contractions or muscle paralysis. The South American Indian poison *curare* and similar synthetic substances paralyze the muscle cells by blocking the Ach receptors. Such drugs are often used during abdominal surgery to obtain sufficient muscle relaxation. Several kinds of snake poisons act by blocking Ach receptors so that the victim is paralyzed. The botulinum toxin (produced by a microorganism growing in certain kinds of spoiled food) paralyzes the muscles by preventing the release of Ach from the boutons at the motor end plate. A similar mechanism sometimes produces muscle weakness in patients with cancer; apparently, substances preventing release of Ach are produced in the body.

The disease *myasthenia gravis* is characterized

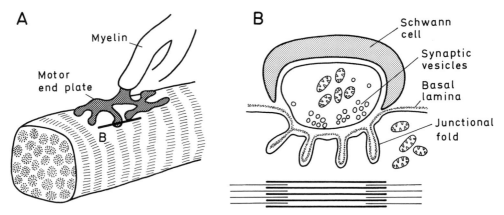

Fig. 8.4. *The motor end plate.* **A.** Schematic drawing showing how the myelinated nerve fiber loses the myelin sheath before it ramifies in the end-plate area, each terminal branch ending in a bouton. Each muscle cell has only one end plate. **B.** Drawing of a section through one of the boutons in **A**, based on electron microscopic observations. The synaptic cleft contains a thin basal lamina, and the postsynaptic membrane is thrown into deep folds (junctional folds).

by excessive fatigability of the striated muscle cells, which is caused by autoantibodies binding to the Ach receptors. Thus, there are fewer than normal Ach receptors available at the neuromuscular junction, and fewer ion channels are opened by release of Ach, leading to less than normal depolarization. The probability of evoking an action potential in the muscle cell membrane is consequently reduced. The symptoms may be lessened by drugs that inhibit the acetylcholine esterase. Thus, the transmitter gets a longer time to act, and the probability of evoking an action potential is increased.

The Force of Muscle Contraction Is Controlled by the Motoneurons

A single presynaptic action potential at the motor end plate elicits only a brief contraction, a *twitch,* of the muscle cell (Fig. 8.5). The twitch lasts only for about one-tenth of a second. If, however, another action potential follows shortly after the first one—that is, before the tension produced by the first twitch is over—the tension produced by the muscle may be sustained and, furthermore, increased considerably in magnitude. This is called *summation.* Up to a limit, the tension produced by the muscle cell increases with increasing frequency of action potentials; that is, *the force produced by the muscle cell is determined by the firing frequency of the*

motoneuron. Whereas the twitch is the response of the muscle cell to a single nerve impulse, *tetanic contraction* is the term used of the muscle response to a train of impulses with the highest frequency to which the muscle cell can respond (Fig. 8.5). The tetanic tension is thus the maximal force the muscle cell can produce. (One may, as shown in Fig. 8.5, differentiate between unfused tetanus at submaximal firing frequencies and fused or full tetanus at the maximal firing frequency. The term tetanus, as used above, refers to the fused tetanus.)

There Are Functionally Different Kinds of Striated Muscle Fiber Types

In both animals and humans, the skeletal muscles are composed of different kinds of muscle cells or muscle fibers (these terms are used interchangeably). The most clear-cut evidence is provided by the fact that in some species certain muscles have a fairly dark color ("red" muscles), whereas other muscles are light ("white" muscles)—for example, the almost white breast muscles and the dark leg muscles of the chicken. Such muscles are composed of muscle fibers of only one (or predominantly one) kind—and the muscle cells are classified as either white or red. The color difference is due to differences

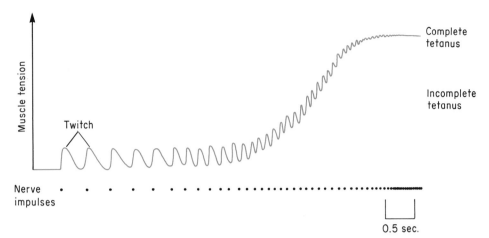

Fig. 8.5. *Muscle contraction.* The muscle tension increases with increasing firing frequency of the motoneurons innervating the muscle cell. Redrawn from Kandel and Schwarz (1985).

in the content of myoglobin, which is red (closely related to hemoglobin) and is of importance for oxygen transport within the muscle cell. Further study showed that white and red muscle cells differ with regard to *endurance*—that is, how long they can maintain tension. This is mainly due to differences in the capacity to take up oxygen and to oxidative phosphorylation (aerobic ATP production). As one would expect, the red muscles have the highest endurance. In addition to containing more myoglobin than the white muscle fibers (cells), the red ones also contain more mitochondria (which are responsible for the aerobic ATP production). There are also other important differences: The white muscle fibers contract more rapidly and develop greater force than the red fibers. With physiological methods, muscle cells can be classified as *fast twitch* (FT), corresponding largely to white fibers, and *slow twitch* (ST), corresponding to the red fibers. The differences with regard to contraction velocity and maximal force development are related to differences in the amount and type of myosin ATPase (enzymes cleaving ATP, thus providing the energy for the muscle contraction). With histochemical staining methods, muscle fibers can be classified in accordance with their ATPase activity (Fig. 8.6). On the basis of ATPase staining, human muscle fibers are

classified as *type 1,* corresponding largely to the red and the ST fibers mentioned above, and *type 2* fibers, corresponding largely to the white and FT fibers. The type 2 group is heterogeneous, however, and consists of type 2A fibers, which resemble the type 1 fibers in having a relatively high oxidative capacity, and the type 2B fibers, which are the most typical white fibers with low oxidative capacity. The central nervous system thus can select muscle fibers in accordance with the requirement of the task: One fiber type is best suited for contractions of moderate force that last for a long time, whereas the other type is used particularly for contractions with high force but short duration.

Human skeletal muscles are, with few exceptions, composed of a mixture of type 1 and type 2 muscle fibers. Histochemical examination of many different muscles in several individuals has indicated that the composition of fiber types is fairly constant when comparing muscles from one individual, whereas the interindividual differences are great. Thus, some persons have a high percentage of type 1 in most of their muscles, whereas others have a strong preponderance of type 2 fibers. Studies of fiber composition in successful athletes have shown that those engaged in endurance sports (such as marathons and cross-country skiing) usually have a high percentage of type 1 fibers, whereas a

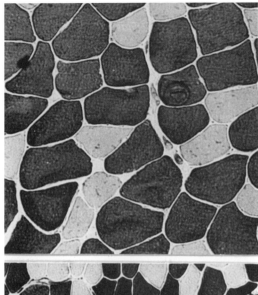

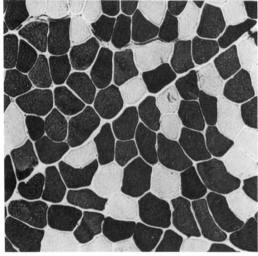

Fig. 8.6. *Muscle fiber types.* Photomicrograph of cross sections of skeletal muscle (human). The sections are treated so that the color intensity of the muscle fibers depend on their myosin–ATPase activity. With this particular treatment the type 1 fibers are light, and the type 2 fibers are dark. The **lower** photomicrograph is from a "normal" person, whereas the **upper** is from a weight lifter. Note the difference in muscle fiber thickness. Magnification, ×200. Courtesy of Prof. H. A. Dahl.

high percentage of type 2 fibers is found in those engaged in sports requiring explosive force (such as ice hockey and weight lifting).

Muscles Also Contain Connective Tissue

A muscle consists of a large number of muscle cells, stretching from tendon to tendon (usually at an angle to the longitudinal axis of the muscle). Bundles of muscle fibers are surrounded by connective tissue containing the vessels and nerves. The whole muscle is wrapped in a connective tissue sheath, the *muscle fascia*. In some muscles the fascia is thick and fairly tight; in others it is thin and loose. The connective tissue of the fascia and within the muscle is continuous with the tendons. Therefore, *the passive proper-*

ties of a muscle—that is, its consistency and resistance to being stretched—depend not only on the muscle cells but also on the amount and arrangement of the connective tissue.

Motor Units

As mentioned, the axon of the motoneuron divides into numerous branches when entering the muscle, and each terminal branch makes synaptic contact with one muscle cell. Furthermore, each muscle cell is innervated by one motoneuron only. *When an α motoneuron sends action potentials to a muscle, all muscle cells innervated by that*

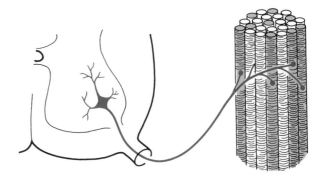

Fig. 8.7. *A motor unit.* Schematic drawing showing a motoneuron in the ventral horn and its axon, which branches to supply many muscle fibers. The muscle cells belonging to one unit (red) line intermingled with muscle cells belonging to other motor units.

motoneuron contract simultaneously. *An α motoneuron and all the muscle cells that it innervates* therefore in a sense constitute the smallest functional unit of the motor system and were called a *motor unit* by Sherrington (Fig. 8.7). (Compare with the term sensory unit, introduced in Chapter 4). *The size of a motor unit*—that is, the number of muscle cells supplied by one motoneuron—varies greatly. This has been studied by counting the axons in the muscle nerve (after destruction of the dorsal roots, to let the sensory axons degenerate) and counting the muscle cells. An average seems to be around 150 muscle cells per motoneuron, with a range of from less than 10 to more than 1000. As might be expected, the smallest motor units are found in muscles that are used for delicate movements, which we must be able to control very precisely. Examples are the intrinsic muscles of the hand, the muscles of the larynx, the facial muscles, and, as mentioned earlier, the extraocular muscles. The largest motor units are found in large muscles used for movements of considerable force and with less precise control, such as the muscles of the back, the abdomen, and the thigh. Within one muscle, however, the motor units also vary in size.

The force of muscular contraction can, as we all know, be finely graded within very wide limits, from a barely perceptible contraction to a tension high enough to tear the muscle loose from its insertion. This depends on the ability of the central nervous system to control the activity (the level of excitation) of the motoneurons. *There are two means by which the force of muscle contrac-*tion can be increased in a graded manner.* One consists of making more and more α motoneurons send action potentials to the muscle. This is called *recruitment,* because more and more motor units—and thus muscle fibers—are called into action. The other means is by increasing the *firing frequency of the α motoneurons* already recruited and thereby increasing the force developed by each motor unit. Thus, the force exerted by each motor unit (as by each muscle cell) can be graded from the small and brief tension produced by a single twitch to full tetanic tension (Fig. 8.5).

Muscle cells belonging to the same motor unit are all of the same fiber type. Thus, they not only contract simultaneously but also share properties with regard to contraction velocity, maximal force, and endurance. Furthermore, there is a relationship between the size of the motor units and the fiber type of which they are composed. The smallest motor units consist of type 1 fibers, whereas the largest ones consist of type 2B fibers. This further increases the difference between large and small motor units with regard to their maximal force; not only are there more muscle cells in the large units, but each cell also develops more force. Recruitment of one extra motor unit with type 1 fibers adds just a little extra to the total tension of the muscle, which thus can be graded finely (like an electrical switch with many small steps to vary the heat of a stove). Such motor units are, not unexpectedly, used for precisely controlled movements of small force. Recruitment of a large motor unit consisting of type 2 fibers, on the other hand, gives a comparatively large increase in the total tension of the muscle (the switch has large steps). Such motor units are recruited only when large force production is needed. Often this concerns fast movements because high acceleration requires a large force.[3]

There is also a *relationship between the size of a motor unit (in terms of number of muscle fibers) and the size of its motoneuron.* Thus, the largest motor units have the motoneurons with the largest perikarya and the thickest axons. This fits with the use of large motor units for fast and forceful movements: The large motoneurons have the highest maximal firing frequencies, and their axons conduct the impulses to the muscles with a minimal delay.

When a muscle contraction is initiated, the small motoneurons are always recruited first, and with increasing force the larger ones are recruited successively. This is called the *size principle of recruitment* and was demonstrated by the American neurophysiologist Henneman in the 1960s. The excitability of the motoneurons is inversely related to their size; thus, the small motoneurons are more easily excited to the threshold for initiation of action potentials than the large ones. This is presumably related to differences both in membrane properties of the motoneurons and in the density of excitatory synapses. The size principle ensures selection of the motor units that are best suited for a particular kind of movement.[4]

Muscle cells belonging to different motor units lie intermingled in the muscle, as is obvious in sections stained to identify fiber types (Fig. 8.6). Correspondingly, muscle cells belonging to one motor unit are spread over a considerable part of the total cross-sectional area of the muscle (Fig. 8.7).

Electromyography

As mentioned, muscle contraction is elicted by an action potential that is propagated along the muscle cell membrane. Like action potentials of nerve cells, the muscle cell action potential can be recorded with an electrode. This is called *electromyography* (EMG) and is performed either with

an electrode placed on the skin overlying the muscle, or with a thin needle electrode inserted into the muscle. The first method gives an impression of the total electrical activity of the muscle, whereas needle electrodes sample the activity of a small part of the muscle. It should be understood, however, that the EMG is a measure of the electrical activity and not of the *mechanical* activity of the muscle. It is therefore not well suited to measure muscle force production. In some instances of prolonged activity, the muscle force may be declining in spite of constant or even increasing EMG activity—the declining force being caused by changed conditions in the muscle itself, whereas muscle action potentials are evoked normally by the nerve to the muscle. When recording from a normal muscle at the start of a weak, very voluntary contraction, the EMG shows regular, single potentials—presumably caused by the activity of one motor unit only. As the force increases, more potentials occur in the EMG, reflecting the recruitment of more motor units. At a certain level of force, the potentials are so frequent that the picture becomes unclear—that is, it is impossible to recognize a further increase of the EMG activity. This occurs not only because of recruitment but also because the frequency of action potentials for each motor unit increases.

EMG is a valuable tool for studying the participation of various muscles in normal movements: for example, to determine the timing of contraction in muscles of the leg during walking. EMG also aids in the diagnosis of diseases of the peripheral motor neurons and of the muscles themselves. For example, it can be determined whether a disease affects the motoneurons or the muscle. If the motoneurons are put out of action, the EMG activity will be reduced or absent, whereas in a disease affecting the contractile apparatus of the muscle, the EMG may be normal. Also, in cases of injury to peripheral nerves, it can be ascertained whether the lesion is complete (no EMG activity) or incomplete (even though there may be no visible movements).

Injury of Peripheral Motor Neurons: Regeneration

When all motoneurons (or their axons) supplying a muscle are destroyed, the muscle cannot be made to contract: It is *paralyzed*. Both voluntary and reflex movements are abolished. If not all of the motoneurons (or their axons) supplying a muscle are destroyed, the muscle can still contract, although with less speed and force than normal. This is called a *partial paralysis* or *paresis.* Typically, the paretic muscle feels soft and *flaccid,* and there is a marked reduction in the muscle mass. This is called *muscular atrophy* and is more marked the more complete the destruction of the motoneurons. The muscle cells that no longer receive impulses from the motoneurons become thinner and eventually disappear if no reinnervation takes place (see below).

This kind of muscle weakness, caused by the loss of the α motoneurons or their axons (lower motor neurons), is called a *peripheral paralysis (paresis),* to distinguish it from a *central paralysis* caused by interruption of the central motor pathways (the upper motor neurons; this will be treated further in Chapter 9). *Characteristic of peripheral pareses—apart from the weakened or abolished voluntary contractions—is that the muscles are flaccid, reflex movements are weakened or abolished, and muscular atrophy progresses rapidly and becomes marked.* In cases of peripheral pareses, the distribution of affected muscles may tell us where the disease process is located. For example, the distribution will differ depending on whether the lesion is located in the cord, in the plexuses formed by the spinal nerves, or in the peripheral nerves more peripherally (Fig. 8.1).

When a peripheral nerve is injured so that the axons are interrupted, the distal parts of the axons degenerate and are gradually removed (by macrophages). The perikarya (of the motoneurons and the spinal ganglion cells) show retrograde changes and, even though some of the cells die, many survive. The proximal parts of the axons of the surviving neurons start to grow. When possible, the growing axons follow the canals in the nerve left by the degenerated axons. The Schwann cells do not die and form a lining of the canals for the growing axons. The axons grow 1–2 mm per day, although the growth gets slower the farther peripherally the axon grows.

The final outcome of this *regeneration* of the axons depends on several factors, among them the conditions at the site of injury and the age of the person. If the continuity of the nerve is not lost—as when the nerve is crushed or damaged by compression—the growing axons have a fair chance of finding the right track and reaching the target they innervated formerly. If the nerve is completely severed (for example, by tearing or a cut), many axons will follow a wrong path even though the cut ends are meticulously stitched together. Thus, motor axons may innervate different muscles than previously, and, likewise, sensory axons may innervate different regions of the skin than before the injury. For example, motoneurons formerly supplying an extensor muscle may after the regeneration supply a flexor; sensory nerve fibers formerly supplying the thumb may innervate the index finger; and so forth. The longer the distance an axon has to grow after the damage, the poorer the chances that it will reach its target. Thus, one cannot expect full functional recovery after suture of a cut peripheral nerve. The results are better in children than in adults, however. This may be because children have a greater regenerative capacity, but presumably also because their brains adapt more easily to a novel pattern of innervation in the periphery.

In cases of incomplete severance of a nerve, the remaining motor axons usually send out new branches within the muscle. This is called *collateral sprouting.* The sprouts grow into and make synaptic contacts at the "empty" motor end plates left by the degenerated axons. In this case, many of the muscle cells, which shortly after the injury were paralyzed, become reinnervated and some of the muscle power is regained. The remaining motor units of the muscle become larger, and therefore the control of the muscle may become less precise than before the injury.

REFLEXES

Reflexes in General

When a response to a stimulus is automatic (involuntary), and the response is mediated by the nervous system, we call it a *reflex.* There are numerous reflexes. Even though they differ in many respects, they nevertheless share some fundamental properties. Reflexes are stereotyped and constant because the same stimulus always gives the same kind of response. With increasing strength of the stimulus, however, the response usually also increases in strength or magnitude. The reflexes are inborn—we do not need to learn them from experience (an example illustrating the need for inborn motor behavior is the sucking reflex in the newborn child).[5] Many reflexes are found in large groups of animal species. All mammals, for example, have several reflexes in common. In general, the reflexes are appropriate and useful and ensure that the individual adapts to the environment. Reflexes are also fundamental for reproduction. Some reflexes are simple with regard to both the stimulus and the response, like the blink reflex (closing of the eye when something touches the cornea). Others are much more complex and require cooperation of many structures, like the swallowing reflex. Some reflexes involve lower parts of the central nervous system only (spinal cord, brain stem), whereas others involve the higher parts (even the cerebral cortex). Some reflexes are mediated by a chain of only two or three neurons, others by complicated and extensive pathways. Many of the tasks of the nervous system are carried out reflexly—that is, independent of our consciousness. This, of course, frees the higher levels of the brain from handling numerous trivial everyday tasks.

Even though reflexes are independent of our will, some of them can be *suppressed* voluntarily (for example, the reflexes for emptying the bladder and the rectum). Other reflexes take place without our being aware of them, and with no possibility of influencing them voluntarily (like most of the reflexes related to the control of visceral functions).

Reflexes involving skeletal muscles (those that participate in somatic motor control) have been most studied, and much of our knowledge of reflexes in general stems from such studies.

The structural basis of a reflex is a *reflex arc,* which consists of the following links:

1. A *receptor,* which records the stimulus and "translates" it to action potentials.
2. An *afferent link* (a primary sensory neuron), which conducts the action potentials to the central nervous system.
3. A *reflex center,* in which the signals from the receptor may be modified (increased or decreased) by signals from other receptors and other parts of the central nervous system, whereafter signals are issued to effectors.

4. An *efferent link* (neurons with axons passing out of the central nervous system), which conducts action potentials to the organ producing the response.
5. An *effector,* which may be skeletal (striated) muscle, cardiac muscle, smooth muscle (in the wall of vessels and visceral organs), or glands.

Some reflex *arcs* are simple; others are highly complex. Reflexes with their reflex center in the spinal cord are called *spinal reflexes. Brain stem* reflexes, as the name implies, have their center in the medulla, pons, or mesencephalon, whereas *cortical reflexes* have a reflex center that involves parts of the cerebral cortex.

We will now discuss two reflexes as examples, both of them with skeletal muscles as effectors, although in other respects quite different. The first one has the simplest possible reflex arc, with only one synapse intercalated in the reflex center. Such a reflex is called *monosynaptic.* The other reflex to be discussed involves several synapses (coupled in series) in the reflex center and is therefore called a *polysynaptic reflex.*

As an example of a monosynaptic reflex, we will use the *patellar reflex* (Fig. 8.8). The *stimulus* is a tap on the patellar ligament (the tendon of the quadriceps muscle). The *response* is a contraction of the quadriceps muscle, thus producing a brief extension movement at the knee joint. The reflex arc is shown schematically in Figure 8.8. The receptors are the muscle spindles in the muscle that is stretched; the afferent link is the Ia fiber, which ends in the spinal cord—notably with some collaterals ending directly (monosynaptically) on the α motoneurons supplying the quadriceps muscle. The axons of the α motoneurons constitute the efferent link, which at the motor end plate activates the extrafusal fibers of the quadriceps muscle (the effector).

Even a monosynaptic reflex is not quite as simple as Figure 8.8 indicates, however. Stretching of the muscle activates not one but presumably most of the muscle spindles of the muscle, and many motor units con-

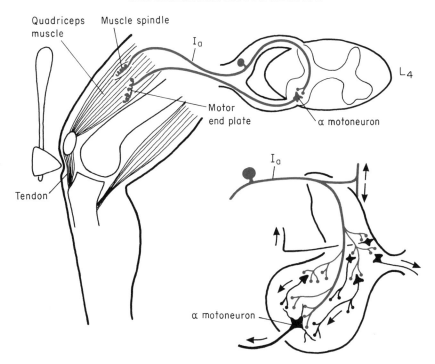

Fig. 8.8. *A monosynaptic reflex.* The patellar reflex is used here as an example of a reflex with only one synapse intercalated between the afferent and the efferent link of the reflex arc. The stimulus is a tap on the patellar ligament below the patella, which stretches the muscle. The response is a brief muscle contraction. The **inset** shows that the Ia fiber from the muscle spindle contacts the motorneurons monosynaptically but also that it contacts many interneurons. Some of these are excitatory, mediating a polysynaptic activation of some motoneurons; other interneurons are inhibitory, mediating inhibition of other motoneurons.

tribute to the response. The reflex center (the region with the coupling between the afferent and the efferent links) is not restricted to one spinal segment. Thus, α motoneurons supplying the quadriceps muscle are present in several lumbar segments (L_2–L_4). The motoneurons receive influences not only from the muscle spindle afferents but also from other kinds of receptors and higher levels of the central nervous system. This explains why the strength of the response—even when the stimulus is kept constant—may vary considerably from person to person and for one person depending on, for example, the level of anxiety.

Most reflexes have a more complex reflex arc than the patellar reflex. As an example of a *polysynaptic* reflex, we will discuss the *flexion reflex* (withdrawal reflex). In this case one or more interneurons are intercalated between the terminals of the afferent sensory fiber and the motoneurons producing the response. When, for example, a foot hits a sharp object while walking, the whole leg is immediately withdrawn away from the object. That this is a reflex is clear from, among other things, the fact that it may be elicited even when the spinal cord is transected above the reflex center. The flexion reflex disappears in deep unconsciousness. For surgery, anesthesia has to be sufficiently deep to abolish flexion reflexes.

The receptors for the flexion reflex are nociceptors of the skin. The stimulus in this case hits a tiny spot on the skin, whereas the response involves a complex array of muscles (such as extensors of the ankle, flexors of the knee and the hip). Contraction of the muscles in the leg that is withdrawn, however, is not sufficient. Muscles of the other

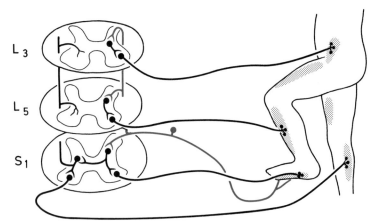

Fig. 8.9. *A polysynaptic reflex.* The flexion reflex is used as an example. The diagram is highly simplified. In this case there is more than one synapse intercalated between the afferent and the efferent links of the reflex arc. In this example nociceptors in the sole of the foot are activated (walking on a sharp object). The impulses are conducted centrally in a sensory fiber (red), which branches and activates via interneurons α motoneurons at several segmental levels of the cord. This in turn makes many muscles contract to produce lifting of the foot off the ground (away from the painful stimulus). At the same time, extensor muscles are activated in the other leg to maintain balance.

leg must also contract (primarily extensor muscles) to prevent loss of balance. Thus, the stimulus must be distributed to α motoneurons in many segments of the cord. This happens by way of ascending and descending collaterals of the primary sensory fibers, and spinal interneurons (Fig. 8.9). In response to a simple stimulus, a purposeful, harmonious movement occurs, requiring that all the muscles contract at the right time and with the right force. The synaptic couplings in the cord underlying this response must be both complex and precise.

The flexion reflex illustrates that even an apparently simple reflex may depend on rather complex neural networks. This means that the signal transmission through the reflex center is subject to modulation by impulses from other parts of the nervous system. As mentioned, this means that the strength of the response to a stimulus may vary. Because the excitability of the interneurons and motoneurons constituting the reflex center may vary, the extension of the reflex center may vary under different conditions. A reflex center should therefore not be imagined as a rigid set of interconnected neurons.

Some reflexes are present only during certain phases of development, such as the sucking reflex and the grasping reflex in infants. When the reflexes disappear, they are no longer needed and would only disturb voluntary movements. The reflex arcs do not disappear, but the reflex response is suppressed by higher levels of the central nervous system. That the nervous apparatus persists is witnessed by the persistence or reappearance of primitive reflexes in brain-damaged children and adults.

Stretch Reflexes

We will now discuss in more detail reflexes of particular importance for motor control. The activity of motoneurons is partly determined by inputs from receptors in the skin, muscles, and around the joints. Also, when a movement is started and controlled from higher levels, spinal reflexes contribute more or less to the final result. *Stretch reflexes*— an example of which was described above—

have been thoroughly investigated because of their importance for motor control. It has been shown that *muscle contraction occurring as a result of muscle stretching* is more complex than formerly believed. Thus, the contraction as recorded by EMG often consists of several distinct phases, each with a partly different neural substrate (the interval between the stimulus and the response is for all phases too short for any voluntary contribution). Thus, *there are different kinds of stretch reflexes.* Receptors for all stretch reflexes are the muscle spindles.

The Monosynaptic Stretch Reflex Is Phasic

The monosynaptic stretch reflex was described above (Fig. 8.8) To evoke a muscle contraction via this simple reflex arc, the muscle must be stretched rapidly—that is, by *phasic stretching.* The actual lengthening produced by the stimulus may be very little; the salient point is the velocity of stretching. Because both the stimulus and the response last only for a very short time, we also use the term *phasic stretch reflex.* This kind of stretch reflex can be elicited in most skeletal muscles but much more easily in some muscles than in others. There are also individual differences: In some healthy persons, phasic stretch reflexes cannot be elicited.

For the patellar reflex, the *latency* between the stimulus and the start of the contraction (as recorded with EMG) is about 30 msec, and a similar latency pertains to reflexes in the upper arm muscles (for example, the biceps reflex). The latency results from the conduction time from the muscle spindles to the spinal cord, the delay at the synapse between the Ia fibers and the α motoneurons, the conduction time from the motoneurons to the muscle, and, finally, the synaptic delay at the motor end plate. Measurement of the latency between the stimulus and the response makes it possible to decide whether a muscle contraction is the result of a monosynaptic stretch reflex, or whether other (polysynaptic) pathways are involved. Each intercalated synapse increases the latency.

The monosynaptic stretch reflex is more complex than what appears from the above description. Thus, while the impulses from the muscle spindle excite the α motoneurons of the muscle that is being stretched, the motoneurons of the antagonists are inhibited. This phenomenon is called *reciprocal inhibition,* and is obviously functionally appropriate: It prevents a stretch reflex from being elicited in the antagonists when they are stretched by the reflex contraction of the agonists (this, in turn, would elicit a new stretch reflex of the agonists, and so on). In the case of the patellar reflex, the motoneurons of the knee flexors are inhibited (Fig. 8.10). The reciprocal inhibition reduces unwanted oscillatory movements. The inhibition of the α motoneurons of the antagonist is mediated by inhibitory interneurons (Ia inhibitory interneurons), which are excited by Ia afferents from the agonist muscles.[6]

The Long Latency (Polysynaptic) Stretch Reflex

Stretching of a muscle may elicit reflex contraction via routes other than the monosynaptic reflex arc. The muscle spindle afferent fibers (Ia and II) contact not only α motoneurons but also many interneurons (Fig. 8.8; among them some that are inhibitory, as mentioned above). The British neurophysiologist Hammond showed already in 1956 that rapid stretching of the biceps muscle may elicit *two* reflex responses, as determined with EMG in human subjects. In addition to an early EMG activity with a latency of about 25 msec (the monosynaptic stretch reflex), another reflex contraction starts at about 50 msec—thus presumably mediated by a polysynaptic reflex pathway. This reflex response is called the *long-latency stretch reflex,* to distinguish it from the monosynaptic (short-latency) stretch reflex.[7]

A striking property of the long-latency stretch reflex is that the *strength of the response depends on whether the muscle is re-*

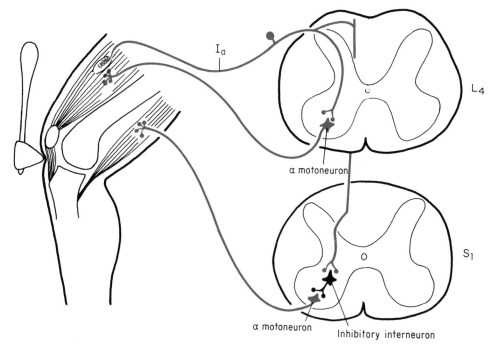

Fig. 8.10. *Reciprocal inhibition.* Schematic illustration of how the stretching of one muscle—producing a reflex contraction—elicits inhibition of the antagonistic muscles via inhibitory interneurons.

laxed or active at the time of stretching. If the muscle is relaxed or only slightly active when stretched, there is usually no long-latency reflex response at all. Furthermore, the strength of the response *depends on prior instruction to the subject* with regard to whether to resist the imposed stretch or to let go. When the person is asked to let go when an imposed movement (at an unpredictable time) stretches the muscle (for example, an imposed extension at the elbow that stretches the biceps muscle), the reflex response is much smaller than when the person is asked to resist the imposed movement. Thus, the magnitude of the reflex response can be adapted to what is functionally appropriate in a particular situation. It should be emphasized that this is not a voluntary response, since the earliest voluntary muscle contractions occur about 100 msec after the stretch (in the upper arm).

A further characteristic of the long-latency stretch reflex is that *the strength of the response may change during learning of a motor task.* Thus, by repeated trials, the reflex response becomes weaker in muscles in which a contraction in response to stretching is functionally inappropriate and stronger in muscles in which a contraction is appropriate. This learning effect or adaptation of the stretch reflex occurs only in connection with the particular learned movement; in connection with other movements, the reflex response of the muscle is unaltered.

Such adaptation of the stretch reflex response is presumably mediated by descending connections from higher levels of the central nervous system (for example, from the motor cortex) that determine how readily the motoneurons react to a certain input. This appears to be exerted mostly by a precise control of the excitability of specific sets of spinal interneurons, which are intercalated in particular reflex arcs. Thus, reflex arcs may be "opened" or "closed" in accordance with the need of the organism. It should be clear from the above that *stretching of a muscle does not necessarily elicit a reflex contraction.* Many factors influence whether there will be a response, such as the velocity of stretching, how long the stretch is, whether the muscle is active when being stretched, and whether a reflex contraction is functionally appropriate.

Motoneurons Can Inhibit Their Own Activity: Renshaw Cells

The numerous different neural inputs to the motoneurons together determine their level of excitability—that is, these inputs also determine the activity of the skeletal muscles. Besides the inhibition of motoneurons by primary afferent fibers (via interneurons) described above, the motoneurons can also inhibit their own activity. Thus, the α motoneuron axons send off collaterals before they leave the ventral horn (Fig. 8.11). Because they turn back, they are called *recurrent collaterals.* The recurrent collaterals end primarily on a group of inhibitory interneurons, the *Renshaw cells,* located ventromedially in the

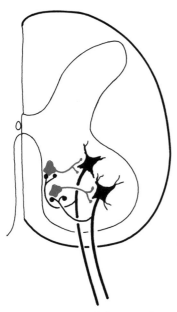

Fig. 8.11. *Recurrent inhibition.* The α motoneurons inhibit their own activity by sending recurrent collaterals ending on the inhibitory Renshaw cells. The Renshaw cells are also influenced by other cell groups in the cord and at higher levels, which determine how strongly they will respond to a certain input from the α motoneurons.

ventral horn. The axons of the Renshaw cells ramify extensively and contact primarily the α motoneurons (but also certain kinds of inhibitory interneurons). In this manner, the activity of the α motoneurons excites the Renshaw cells, which in turn inhibit the same α motoneurons and other α motoneurons that supply muscles with the same action (agonists). Furthermore, the Renshaw cells inhibit the inhibitory interneurons mediating the reciprocal inhibition (Fig. 8.10)—that is, the inhibition of the α motoneurons supplying the antagonists is reduced (disinhibition). In case of a stretch reflex, the activity of the Renshaw cells shortens the reflex contraction of the agonists and at the same time shortens the reciprocal inhibition of the antagonists. The Renshaw system seems important to prevent the α motoneurons from sending long trains of action potentials as a response to a brief stimulus. On the other hand, there are other situations, such as during voluntary movements, when prolonged motoneuronal activity is required. In such situations, descending connections from the brain stem and the cerebral cortex may inhibit the Renshaw cells supplying the working muscles. Thus, the activity of the Renshaw cells, as that of many other kinds of spinal interneurons, may be regulated in accordance with the overall plan for the movements being carried out.

The Long-Latency Stretch Reflex May Be Mediated via the Cerebral Cortex

In spite of much research, the exact central pathway followed by the impulses mediating the long-latency stretch reflex is still debated. That the receptor is the muscle spindle, however, is clear. Indirect data indicate that the reflex pathway may involve the motor cortex of the cerebral cortex. Therefore, the term *long-loop stretch reflex* is often used. In support of a transcortical route are the facts that the reflex is weakened or abolished by lesions of the descending motor pathways and by lesions of the dorsal columns (presumably carrying the signals from the muscle spindles to the cerebral cortex). Furthermore, the reflex is often weakened after lesions of the cerebellum. Such findings, however, may also be explained by a purely spinal reflex that is under strong supraspinal control. Indeed, some studies favor the view that the long latency of the reflex is caused by many spinal interneurons being intercalated between the primary afferent fibers and the motoneurons in the cord. Other data, although indirect, indicate that the afferent link may be the slowly conducting group II spindle afferent fibers (rather than the rapidly conducting Ia fibers). Thus, vibration of a muscle elicits a short-latency (monosynaptic) reflex contraction and not a long-latency reflex (or only a very weak one). Since vibration appears to stimulate fairly selectively the Ia afferents—that is, with no or negligible stimulation of the group II afferents—this would indicate that the Ia afferents cannot be responsible for the long-latency reflex. Other experiments, however, with cooling of peripheral nerves in humans show that the long latency cannot be explained by longer peripheral conduction time (cooling reduces the conduction velocity of the nerve fibers).

Some very recent findings in a few patients with a peculiar inborn abnormality of the pyramidal tract provide strong support for the transcortical route for the long-latency stretch reflex. These persons always perform mirror movements of the hands; asked to flex the index finger of the left hand, they invariably flex the right index finger as well (more proximal movements, for example, of the shoulders, are performed normally). This behavior appears from electrophysiological studies to be caused by branching of individual pyramidal tract axons to supply motoneurons of both sides of the cord. Thus, stimulation of the hand region of the motor cortex of one hemisphere causes symmetrical movements of both hands (unlike the normal situation, in which such stimulation always cause movements of the opposite hand only). When eliciting stretch reflexes in such patients, the monosynaptic reflex occurs only on the same side as the stretch is applied (as normal), whereas the long-latency stretch reflex occurs in both hands after a unilateral stimulus. The latter observation is hard to explain unless the reflex arc of the long-latency reflex involves the pyramidal tract.

The Function of Stretch Reflexes

One might perhaps think that the stretch reflexes, which after all are relatively simple, are well understood with regard to their functional roles. For example, the muscle spindles and the motoneurons are among the best characterized receptors and central neurons, respectively. Nevertheless, we still do not understand fully the role of the stretch reflexes in the control of voluntary movements and in the control of posture and muscle tone. We will discuss here only some possible functions.

One likely task of the stretch reflex is to *ensure that the length of a muscle is kept constant*. In many situations this is of obvious importance—for example, in the upright position when some external perturbation threatens the body balance. The sudden displacement of the center of gravity forward stretches the extensor muscles of the back and thus might elicit a stretch reflex tending to resume the former position. It is furthermore an obvious advantage that such a corrective contraction come as quickly as possible. Making such an adjustment dependent only on voluntary contraction would lengthen the latency fourfold, with the danger of the corrections coming too late. Also while walking, when external perturbations may disturb the programmed pattern of muscular activity, stretch reflexes may possible contribute to rapid adjustments. Nevertheless, it is not clear to what extent stretch reflexes really participate in such adjustments (see below).

Another situation in which stretch reflexes may be of importance is during slow, precise voluntary movements when the external opposing forces change unpredictably. Again, the advantage would be that the adjustment of muscle tension occurs much earlier than what can be achieved by voluntary action alone.

Stretch Reflexes May Correct for Change in External Resistance during Precision Movements

Studies of slow movements of the thumb by the British neurologist Marsden have shed light on the contribution of stretch reflexes during precision movements. The subject is asked to flex the thumb with a constant speed against an external opposing force of constant magnitude. The EMG of the flexor pollicis longus muscle is recorded continuously. The external force is then changed suddenly at unpredictable times during the movement—either increased or reduced. When the external force is increased, the movement is immediately slowed down. Because of the $\alpha-\gamma$ coactivation (see p. 124), the frequency of impulses from the muscle spindle increases.

The $\alpha-\gamma$ coactivation ensures that, as the muscle shortens owing to the activation of the α motoneurons, the spindle midportion is stretched. This upholds the firing of muscle spindle afferents in spite of the shortening, which otherwise would have led to reduced firing. To keep up with the steadily shortening muscle, the firing of the γ motoneurons must also increase steadily. When the movement is suddenly halted or slowed down, the firing frequency of the γ motoneurons continues increasing, in anticipation of further shortening of the muscle. Thus, for a moment, the firing of the muscle spindle afferents increases more than what is appropriate with regard to the actual length of the muscle. This increases the excitation of the motoneurons, and their firing increases, thus increasing the force of the muscle contraction. The result is that the increased external force is rapidly compensated for, and the original speed of the movement is resumed.

When the opposing external force is suddenly reduced, the opposite events take place. The speed of the flexion movement of the thumb increases, and the firing frequency of the spindle afferents decreases for a moment, thus reducing the firing of the α motoneurons and the force of contraction. The speed of movement is adjusted.

Probably, the stretch reflex functions in this manner especially during slow precision movements when we cannot predict accurately the external force at all times. The sensitivity of the muscle spindles is kept at a high level, so that they may record even the slightest perturbations and ensure that the activity of the α motoneurons is adjusted appropriately.

Automatic Adjustment of Muscle Contraction Is Not Only Due to Stretch Reflexes

Signals from receptors other than the muscle spindle can also influence the excitability of the motoneurons. When a reflex adjustment of muscle tension occurs (that is, the latency between the stimulus and the muscle contraction is too short for the contraction to be voluntary), we must therefore consider the possible contribution of signals from several kinds of receptors. Signals from the *tendon organ* (conducted in Ib afferent fibers) are known to influence the motoneurons via a

spinal reflex arc. In general, it appears that signals from the tendon organs inhibit (via spinal interneurons) the motoneurons of the muscle in which the receptors lie (autogenic inhibition). This has been shown in experimental animals, and we do not know the functional role of signals from tendon organs for reflex adjustments during natural movements in conscious human subjects.

We will now consider, as an example, a situation in which we know reflex adjustment of muscle tension occurs with possible contributions from several receptors. This situation occurs when the body balance in the upright position is disturbed. The contributions of various receptors have been studied in persons standing on a platform that can be tilted or moved forward or backward. When the platform is suddenly displaced backward (without tilting), the body first sways forward, with the movement primarily occurring at the ankle joints. The balance is regained mainly because the muscles at the back of the leg contract (the ankle flexors, primarily the triceps surae muscle; muscles of the hip, the back, and in the neck also contribute, however). The first part of the contraction of the leg muscles occurs so early after the perturbation that it must be mediated by a reflex. (Somewhat later there is also a voluntary contraction contributing to the final outcome of the postural adjustment). But what causes the reflex contraction of the leg muscles? We have to consider at least the following possibilities:

1. That the stretching of the leg muscles elicits a stretch reflex;
2. That the muscle contraction is caused by signals from receptors in the labyrinth (vestibular apparatus) stimulated by the movement of the head;
3. That the muscle contraction is produced by signals from the joint receptors of the ankle joint;
4. That stimulation of low-threshold mechanoreceptors in the skin on the sole of the foot produces the reflex contraction of the leg muscles;
5. That visual information (presumably re-

layed via the vestibular nuclei and their connections to the spinal cord) elicits appropriate automatic adjustments.

All of these kinds of information most likely contribute, and the muscle spindles are certainly not responsible alone. There is even evidence that normal subjects differ with regard to which kind of information is used primarily for the reflex adjustment. For optimal postural stability, however, all kinds of sensory information mentioned above seems to be necessary. Nevertheless, elimination of either vestibular or somatosensory information in human subjects does not impair seriously their ability to automatically adjust body balance after moderate perturbations. However, the movement strategy—that is, the joints in which the major compensatory movements occur—is altered when one of the sensory inputs is removed.

In other situations, such as when the platform is suddenly tilted backward, the muscles at the back of the leg are stretched, as in the former example. The center of gravity is now displaced backward instead of forward, and consequently a contraction of the posterior leg muscles in this situation would not help to regain the balance but would rather worsen the situation. To regain balance, the muscles at the front of the leg (for example, the anterior tibial muscle) have to contract as rapidly as possible, and these are, of course, shortened by the tilting of the platform. The contraction of the anterior leg muscles, which in fact takes place, cannot be caused by a stretch reflex. In this situation one also gets an impression of the adaptability of the stretch reflexes—how inappropriate reflex responses to stretch may be suppressed. Thus, the reflex contraction occurring in the posterior leg muscles when the platform is tilted backward becomes weaker as the perturbation is repeated, so that the person knows that at some (unpredictable) moment the platform will be tilted.

In summary, it is clear that *the reflex adjustments that occur in numerous muscles of the body on perturbations of the balance are caused by signals from several kinds of receptors.* The information from the various receptors is integrated at the brain stem and spinal level, to ensure a coordinated and purposeful pattern of muscle activity. If necessary, voluntary activity follows and supplements the automatic, reflex adjustments.

There are also situations in which *stimulation of low-threshold skin mechanoreceptors causes reflex muscular contraction.* For example, when during a precision grip with the fingers the object slips, a reflex increase of the grip force occurs. The latency from the start of the slip to the muscular response is only 60–80 msec—that is, too short to be mediated by a voluntary command. Examination of patients with reduced skin sensation but normal motor apparatus suggests that loss of such rapid, reflex adjustment of the grip force is partly responsible for their difficulties with precision movements.

MUSCLE TONE

The term *muscle tone* usually refers to the slight tension that can be felt in a relaxed muscle (a more precise term is therefore *resting tone*). In pathological conditions, the resting tone may be changed—either increased or decreased. The term muscle tone is not unambiguous, however, as witnessed by its use by various authors. (Some authors have suggested that the term is too imprecise and should therefore be abandoned.)

Muscle tone is usually determined by *palpation* (judging the consistency and stiffness of the tissue by pressing the muscle belly between the fingers) and by *stretching* (judging the resistance offered to passive stretch). Some authors use the term only about the tone as judged by stretching. Palpation and stretching do not test identical properties of the muscle. For example, after a stroke giving central pareses (capsular hemiplegia), the muscle tone is commonly reduced when judged by palpation (the consistency is reduced), whereas the resistance offered to passive stretching is increased. Examination of muscle tone is of importance for the diagnosis of diseases affecting the motor system. It is therefore regrettable that we do not have a clear understanding of the basis of normal muscle tone and of the mechanisms behind changes of muscle tone in disease states.

Muscle Tone Is an Expression of the Stiffness of the Tissue

The confusion about the exact meaning of the term muscle tone stems partly from the fact tht words like firmness, tension, stiffness, and elasticity are often used without definition. Different persons may therefore use them with different meanings. This is, unfortunately, often the case even when observations made by different examiners are compared. *Stiffness* and *tension* can, however, be defined in mathematical terms and can also be recorded and measured objectively. The definition of stiffness (K) is: $K = \Delta T/\Delta L$; that is, K expresses how much the muscles are stretched (ΔL) by a certain increase in tension (ΔT). The greater the stiffness, the higher the tension necessary to stretch the muscle. Note that this definition applies only to the component of muscle tension determined by passive stretching, and not to the consistency (firmness, elasticity) as judged by palpation. The latter can hardly be measured objectively and depends on the subjective assessment of the examiner.

Properties of the Muscle That May Contribute to Muscle Tone

From everyday experience we know that *contraction* of a muscle is the one factor that most markedly alters the muscle tone, as judged by both palpation and stretching. The purpose of the contraction, of course, is to increase the tension of the muscle. Under normal conditions, small contributions to the tension of the muscle stem from the passive viscoelastic properties of the muscle cells and the connective tissue of the muscle and its tendons. The elastic properties of the muscle explain why when the muscle is stretched passively beyond a certain length, the tension increases steeply (the slack is taken out of the elastic, as it were). This is experienced when a relaxed muscle becomes

firmer on palpation and offers increasing resistance to stretching toward extreme joint positions (therefore, such positions should be avoided when examining muscle tone).

Which of the two factors—active contraction and passive viscoelastic properties—is responsible for the normal resting tone? It was formerly assumed that even relaxed muscle was in a state of slight contractile activity (caused by impulses from α motoneurons) and that this activity was maintained by a steady flow of impulses from the muscle spindles. This was based primarily on observations in animals with transection of the brain stem (decerebration), in which the activity of the γ motoneurons is enhanced. This increases the impulse traffic from the muscle spindles, and thereby the muscles are in a state of tonic contraction. In accordance with these observations, muscle tone in normal human subjects was assumed to be upheld by the long-latency stretch reflex ("tonic stretch reflex"). This view can hardly be upheld in the light of more recent data, however. In the first place, several EMG studies show that in persons who are able to relax properly, there is no electrical activity in their muscles (and, therefore, no contractile activity). Furthermore, microneurographical studies have not confirmed that there is impulse traffic in muscle spindle afferents conducting from relaxed muscles in human subjects. In relaxed subjects, the resistance against even rapid passive stretching of a muscle is very low (except when the monosynaptic stretch reflex is elicited by a tendon tap). There is thus no evidence of a "reflex tone" in relaxed muscles. The tone felt in a relaxed muscle, which shows no EMG activity, probably depends on the passive viscoelastic properties of the muscle. However, many healthy persons are unable to relax their muscles completely, at least during an examination. Thus, EMG would show a modest electric activity when the muscles are handled by the examiner. Even in such cases, however, the contraction is probably not of a reflex nature but produced by voluntary commands (that is, by signals issued from the cerebral cortex). Thus, in such persons there is usually muscle activity also in muscles that are shortened passively as the examiner produces a joint movement (the person "helps" the examiner).

The individual differences that can be observed with regard to resting muscle tone in healthy persons may presumably be explained to a large extent by differences in the degree of relaxation. In addition, there are probably also individual differences with regard to the passive viscoelastic properties of the muscles. Thus, there is evidence that even in persons who are able to relax their muscles completely (as judged by EMG), the muscle tone (as judged by palpation) may vary.

Changes of Muscle Tone in Disease

Pathologically changed muscle tone is called *hypotonia* when it is lower than normal and *hypertonia* when higher than normal. To recognize abnormal muscle tone, one must by necessity first be able to decide what is normal. From the above discussion it should be clear, however, that "normal muscle tone" is not a precise, well-defined concept. The decision as to whether a muscle has a normal tone has to be based largely on the subjective judgment of the examiner. This judgment, of course, depends to a large extent on experience. Whereas hypertonus may be fairly easy to identify and even measure in semiquantitative terms by stretching the muscles, the decision as to whether a muscle has abnormally low tone (hypotonic) is more difficult. As mentioned, a normal, fully relaxed muscle will have a very low tension when tested by stretching. Some authors believe that when paretic or paralytic muscles feel softer and more flaccid than normal muscle, it is because of lack of voluntary contraction, which probably occurs to some extent during passive movements and palpation. Experiments measuring the resistance to passive stretching of normal and alleged hypotonic muscles did not show any consistent differences. The experiments were performed by measuring the falling time of the leg (passive flexion of the knee) in healthy persons with the ability to relax fully (EMG) and in patients with pareses of the quadriceps muscle (clinically judged as hypotonic). The individual differences in falling time—that is, muscle tone—among the normal subjects

were fairly large, presumably because of differences in the passive viscoelastic properties.

It should be kept in mind, however, that with peripheral pareses, rapid changes of the passive viscoelastic properties of the muscles may occur, which may help explain why the paretic muscles feel softer on palpation. After damage to peripheral motoneurons, the muscles atrophy rapidly, reducing the muscle volume to sometimes only 20–30% of normal in about 3 months. The metabolism of muscle cells is obviously dramatically altered by loss of contact between nerve and muscle.

Abnormally increased muscle tone, *hypertonus,* would imply that the muscles continuously have an increased tone, in spite of attempts to relax. As mentioned, many healthy persons are not able to relax completely, at least not in an examination situation, and the border between normal and pathologically increased muscle tone may not be easy to draw. In certain diseases of the central nervous system affecting the tracts and nuclei of the motor system, however, fairly characteristic disturbances of muscle tone occur. *Rigidity* is the term used to characterize the increased muscle tone occurring in Parkinson's disease (Chapter 10). Even with very slow, passive movements, an increased, "cogwheel"-like resistance is felt by the examiner. This may be caused by increased long-latency stretch reflexes that are elicited by abnormally slow movements.

The term *spasticity* is used in clinical neurology of a condition in which there is increased resistance only against *rapid stretching* of muscles. By palpation the muscles may feel normal or hypotonic, and there is no increased resistance against slow, passive movements. Spasticity occurs after damage to the descending motor pathways from the cerebral cortex to the motoneurons and is probably caused primarily by changed excitability of spinal interneurons. The increased resistance to rapid stretch is most likely caused by abnormally brisk monosynaptic stretch reflexes, whereas the long-latency stretch reflexes are weaker than normal.

Also with rigidity and spasticity, there is evidence of changed passive viscoelastic properties (in addition to the changed stretch reflexes). Thus, in patients with moderately severe Parkinson's disease, increased resistance to slow elbow extension was found, even though there was no EMG activity of the biceps muscle (which was being stretched). In some spastic patients, increased resistance even to slow stretching of relaxed leg muscles was present, but only when the spasticity had lasted for more than a year. Thus, it seems as though an altered pattern of impulses from the motoneurons—like those occurring in diseases with rigidity or spasticity—may change the passive, viscoelastic properties of the muscles (rigidity and spasticity will be further discussed in Chapters 9 and 10).

NOTES

1. The level of CGRP in the motoneurons is under the influence of descending connections from higher levels of the central nervous system; when such connections are transected, the level of CGRP drops. In vitro studies indicate that CGRP influences the synthesis of acetylcholine receptors of the muscle cells. Since CGRP is present in the motoneuron terminals (in addition to in the perikarya), it seems possible that CGRP also has such an effect in vivo.

2. During development—before the muscle cells have received their innervation—the acetylcholine receptors are evenly distributed all over the muscle membrane. Only when properly functioning synaptic contacts have been established are the receptors redistributed to attain the mature pattern. The neuropeptide *galanin* is expressed transiently during development of spinal motoneurons and may possibly be related to interactions between the motoneurons and the muscle cells at the time of synapse formation.

3. The fiber type used for a particular kind of movement has been studied by the so-called *glycogen depletion technique*. By prolonged use, all of the muscle fibers of a motor unit deplete their stores of glycogen, and this may be shown histochemically in frozen sections of a small piece of muscle tissue obtained by biopsy. The type 1 muscle fibers are depleted first when the force exerted is low—that is, no type 2 fibers are recruited. When the force is very high, however, the type 2 fibers are depleted first. In the latter case, type 1 fibers are also recruited, but because of their high endurance they are not depleted during the short period in which a maximal force can be maintained.

4. In spite of the general validity of the size principle for recruitment of motoneurons, motoneurons with similar size may have quite different firing rates and innervate muscle cells with different contractile properties (the latter is presumably a reflec-

tion of the fact that the firing rate of motoneurons influences the contractile properties of the muscle cells). Furthermore, experiments with the use of biofeedback (EMG) during voluntary movements indicate that humans can to some degree select among the low-threshold motor units. This must depend on the ability of higher motor centers to focus excitation among motoneurons with presumably the same size.

5. True reflexes should not be confused with another kind of automatic behavior, conditioned reflexes or, better, *conditioned responses*. In conditioned responses the stimulus evoking a true reflex response (the unconditioned stimulus) has been replaced—*by learning*—by another stimulus. This learning occurs when the unconditioned stimulus (for example, a puff of air on the cornea, eliciting a blink reflex) is regularly preceded by another kind of stimulus (for example, a tone; the conditioning stimulus). After some time, the conditioning stimulus will elicit the reflex response even when it is not followed by the unconditioned stimulus. The classical examples are the experiments of the Russian physiologist Pavlov, in which gastric secretion was produced by ringing a bell (conditioned stimulus). During the learning phase, the bell was always followed by food being presented (unconditioned stimulus).

6. Collaterals of the Ia afferents also contact other kinds of spinal interneurons. Thus, interneurons that inhibit the α motoneurons of the muscle being stretched are also contacted by Ia collaterals. This inhibitory effect is usually not evident when testing stretch reflexes—the excitatory, monosynaptic effect dominates. During natural movements, however, such autogenic inhibition may be of importance. Descending connections from higher levels of the central nervous system may direct transmission of the reflex arc, so that the excitatory or inhibitory effect dominates, depending on what is appropriate in the particular situation.

7. The long-latency stretch reflex has later been shown to consist of two distinct components. Thus, for the upper arm the first part occurs, as mentioned, with a latency of 50 msec and, in addition, a further response at about 80 msec (which is still too early to be a voluntary contraction). The two components cannot always be clearly distinguished in the EMG, however. If the reflex response is followed by a voluntary contraction, this is seen as increasing EMG activity with a latency of about 100 msec (for the upper arm).

9

Central Motor Pathways

Many parts of the brain are able to influence our movements because they send fibers that end in synaptic contact with the motoneurons (lower motor neurons) or with interneurons that in turn contact the motoneurons. These higher motor centers are neuronal groups (upper motor neurons) in the brain stem and in the cerebral cortex, which are highly interconnected. All of them participate (although to various extents) in most motor acts. The sharing of tasks among the higher motor centers is such that cell groups in the brain stem can by themselves control many automatic movements, whereas the participation of the cerebral cortex is necessary in less automatic movements. The importance of the cerebral cortex increases with the increasing degree of voluntary control of a movement.

Customarily, a division has been made between the pyramidal tract and all other nuclei and tracts more or less directly involved in motor control. The latter have often been collectively called the "extrapyramidal system." This term lacks a precise meaning, however, and can only be vaguely defined, a fact that has become more and more clear as our knowledge of the motor systems has improved. Thus, we will not use the term here. The pyramidal tract, however, is a well-de-

fined entity that can be described separately, even though it is just one of several motor pathways transmitting signals from higher levels to the motoneurons of the brain stem and the spinal cord. Figure 9.1 shows schematically the most important pathways descending from the cerebral cortex and the brain stem to the spinal cord. It should be noted, however, that such descending pathways not only serve motor tasks; some of them also participate in the control of signal transmission in the ascending sensory pathways (see Chapter 4).

THE PYRAMIDAL TRACT (THE CORTICOSPINAL TRACT)

The pyramidal tract is of crucial importance in our ability to perform precise, voluntary movements. The tract is formed by axons of neurons with their perikarya in the cerebral cortex, as indicated by its other name, the *corticospinal tract.* The axons descend through the internal capsule, the crus cerebri (cerebral peduncle), the pons, and the medulla (Figs. 9.2 and 9.5). Most of the fibers cross to the other side in the lowermost part of the medulla and continue downward in the lateral funiculus of the cord, to finally es-

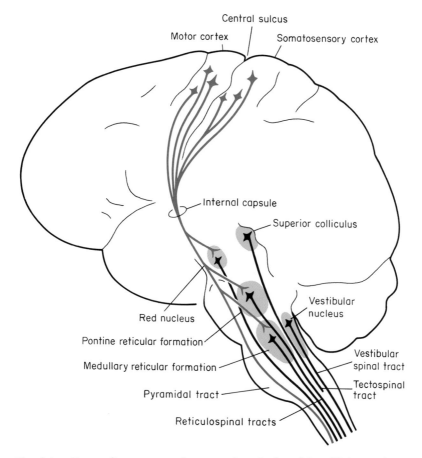

Fig. 9.1. *Descending motor pathways to the spinal cord.* In addition to the pyramidal tract, several tracts arise from brain stem nuclei.

tablish synaptic contacts in the spinal gray matter. *This is the only pathway that passes directly—that is, without synaptic interruption—from the cerebral cortex to the spinal cord.*

Fibers also leave the pyramidal tract on its way through the brain stem, to reach cranial nerve motor nuclei (Fig. 9.2). Such fibers form part of the *corticobulbar tract* (other corticobulbar fibers reach the red nucleus, the pontine nuclei, the recticular formation, the colliculi, the dorsal column nuclei, and other nuclei).

The pyramidal tract got its name from the pyramid of the medulla, which is formed by the fibers of the corticospinal tract (Figs. 2.16 and 2.17). Strictly speaking, therefore, the term *pyramidal tract* encompasses only the fibers destined for the spinal cord and

not those destined for the cranial nerve motor nuclei. Nevertheless, for practical reasons both groups are usually included in the term.

Origin and Course of the Pyramidal Tract

A large proportion of the fibers of the pyramidal tract comes from neurons with their perikarya in the precentral gyrus—that is, area 4 of Brodmann (Figs. 9.3, 9.4, and 17.3). This region is called the *primary motor area (cortex) (MI)*. In the last half of the nineteenth century, it was discovered in animal experiments that when the cerebral cortex was stimulated electrically, muscle contractions could most easily (with the weakest current) be elicted from area 4. Later, it was

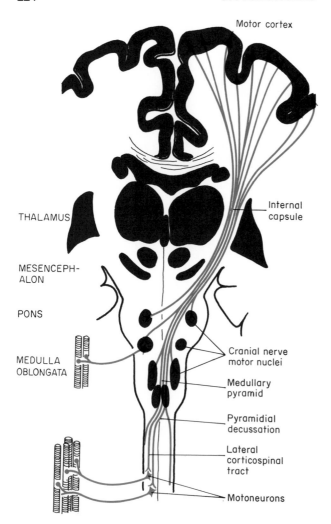

Fig. 9.2. *The course of the pyramidal tract.* Note that most of the fibers cross in the lower medulla.

verified that this region in humans is located in the precentral gyrus. It was originally thought that *all* fibers of the pyramidal tract came from area 4, and, furthermore, only from the cells with the largest perikarya, the giant cells of Betz. The number of Betz cells is, however, much too low to account for the number of axons in the pyramidal tract (about 1 million in humans).

Recent studies with retrograde transport of tracer substances have largely clarified the origin of the pyramidal tract in various animals (Fig. 9.3). Findings in the monkey are presumably most relevant for humans. In the monkey, *numerous cells in area 4, in addition to the Betz cells, contribute to the pyramidal tract, as do also many cells in areas*

outside area 4. With regard to the relative contribution from various areas, however, the results differ among authors: From less than half to three-fourths of the fibers of the pyramidal tract are reported to come from areas in front of the central sulcus—that is, MI (area 4) and area 6 (PMA and SMA in Fig. 9.7). The rest emanate from areas posterior to the central sulcus: SI (areas 3, 1, 2), SII, and parts of the posterior parietal cortex (area 5) (Figs. 4.19, 17.3, and 17.9). A fairly large proportion of the fibers from SI originate in area 3a (Fig. 9.3), which adjoins area 4 anteriorly (as mentioned in Chapter 4, area 3a is characterized by receiving sensory inputs from proprioceptors). The cell bodies of all neurons of the pyramidal tract lie in the

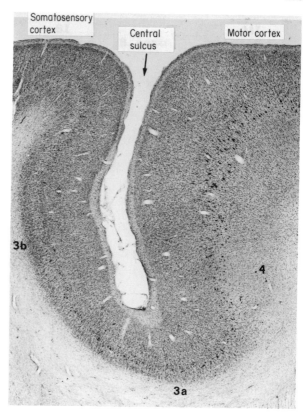

Fig. 9.3. *The central region with MI and SI.* Photomicrograph of a section perpendicular to the central sulcus (monkey). Note the difference in thickness between the MI and the SI. The dark dots in the deep parts of the cortex (in layer 5) are the perikarya of pyramidal tract cells that have been retrogradely labeled by an injection of HRP in the spinal cord. Note also that there are more labeled cells in the MI than in the SI.

cortical fifth layer (lamina 5; compare Figs. 9.3 and 17.2) and are called *pyramidal cells.* The name refers to the shape of the perikaryon (Figs. 1.1, 17.1, and 17.5). Muscle contractions can be elicited also from the areas outside MI, like SI, by electrical stimulation, but the stimulation has to be more intense than in area MI. This reflects that the pyramidal tract fibers from SI and the other regions outside area 4 have less direct access to the motoneurons than the neurons in area 4. The pyramidal tract fibers coming from SI and area 5 are probably more concerned with the control of sensory signal transmission than with the initiation of movements.

Electrical stimulation and localized lesions of the precentral gyrus (also in humans) have clarified the *somatotopic localization within MI* (Fig. 9.4). It corresponds closely to the localization in SI (Fig. 4.20).

As mentioned, the pyramidal tract passes downward through the *internal capsule,* where it occupies a posterior position (Fig. 9.5). It was formerly assumed that the pyramidal tract fibers were spread over a large part of the "posterior leg" of the internal capsule (as seen in cross section in Figs. 2.30 and 9.5). Observations after small lesions and stimulation during brain surgery of the internal capsule in humans point to the more restricted region shown in Figure 9.5. Within this region, fibers governing the muscles of the face are believed to lie most anteriorly.

The internal capsule contains many other fibers than those of the pyramidal tract; the latter constitute only a minority. There are, for example, sensory fibers ascending from the thalamus to the cortex and descending fibers from the cortex to the reticular formation and other cell groups of the brain stem. In the anterior part of the internal capsule lie the pallidothalamic fibers (related to motor functions of the basal ganglia), and posteriorly (in the lower part) the optic ra-

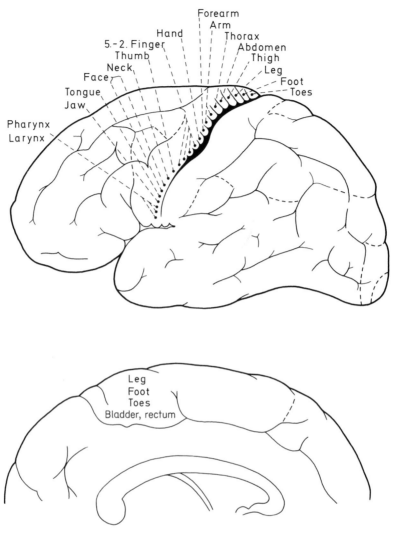

Fig. 9.4. *The somatotopic organization of the motor cortex.* The points indicate the sites from which muscle contraction in a particular body part was produced by weak electrical stimulation. Based on Foerster (1936).

diation passes through on its way to the occipital lobe. Therefore, damage of the internal capsule—such as an infarction caused by occlusion of an artery—may produce various kinds of sensory deficits in addition to pareses of the muscles of the opposite body half (capsular hemiplegia).

In the mesencephalon, the pyramidal tract fibers appear to be spread out over the middle two-thirds of the crus and to be mixed with other fibers (Fig. 9.5). As mentioned, all of the corticospinal fibers are collected within the pyramid at the ventral side of the medulla (Figs. 2.16, 2.18, and 9.5). At the caudalmost level of the medulla, most of the corticospinal fibers cross the midline and continue in the lateral funiculus of the cord as the *lateral corticospinal tract* (Fig. 9.2). A small contingent continues, without crossing, downward in the ventral funiculus as the *ventral corticospinal tract*. Some uncrossed fibers may also pass in the lateral funiculus (Fig. 9.6).[1] The pyramidal tract fibers that control the muscles of the head (the face, tongue, pharynx, and the larynx) leave the corticospinal fibers in the brain stem to

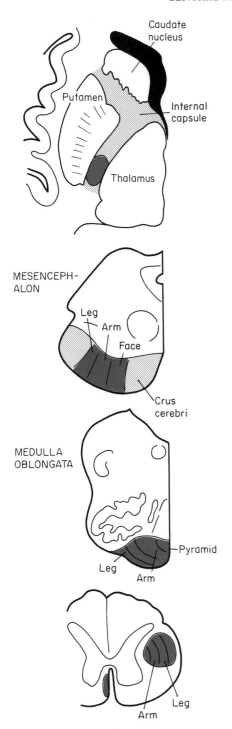

Fig. 9.5. *The pyramidal tract.* Its position and somatotopic pattern are illustrated in sections from various levels of the brain stem and the cord. The **upper** drawing is of a horizontal section (cf. Fig. 2.30), whereas the other drawings are of transverse sections.

end in or close to the motor and sensory cranial nerve nuclei (Fig. 9.2). Apart from most of the facial muscles, other muscles of the head as a rule receive both crossed and uncrossed pyramidal tract fibers. Thus, when the pyramidal tract fibers are interrupted in the internal capsule, there are seldom clearcut pareses of the muscles of the tongue, the pharynx, and the larynx, whereas the corner of the mouth hangs down on the opposite side of the lesion.

Termination of the Pyramidal Tract

The pyramidal tract fibers vary considerably in thickness, from the thickest myelinated kind to unmyelinated ones. Most are rather thin, with conduction velocities between 5 and 30 m/sec. In general, the thickest (and thus fastest conducting) fibers come from MI. In accordance with the somatotopic pattern within MI (Fig. 9.4), fibers from the medial parts of the precentral gyrus (leg representation) end in the lumbosacral part of the cord, whereas fibers from more lateral parts (arm representation) end in the cervical and upper thoracic cord.

Fibers from MI and SI also terminate differently in the cord (Fig. 9.6). Thus, fibers from SI end predominantly in the dorsal horn (laminae I–VI), whereas fibers from MI end more ventrally in laminae VII–IX. There are even differences with regard to the projections from individual cytoarchitectonic subdivisions within SI: area 3b—which receives primarily input from cutaneous low-threshold mechanoreceptors—sends fibers primarily to laminae III and IV, which receive the same kind of sensory input as area 3b. Fibers from area 3a end deeper in the dorsal horn, where primary afferents from proprioceptors end. Physiological experiments show that sensory cells in the dorsal horn are influenced from SI. Most often, neurons that are excited from low-threshold mechanoreceptors are inhibited from SI. It may be functionally important to be able to suppress selectively certain kinds of sensory information, for example, during movements.

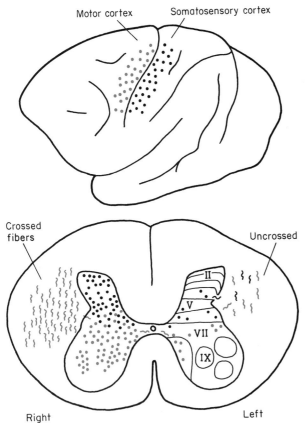

Fig. 9.6. *The terminal region of the pyramidal tract.* Based on experiments in monkeys with anterograde transport of radioactively labeled amino acids after injections in various parts of the MI and the SI. Note that corticospinal fibers from the MI end more anteriorly in the gray matter of the cord than those from the SI. The uncrossed fibers end predominantly medially in the ventral horn—that is, in contact with motoneurons supplying axial and proximal muscles. Based on Ralston and Ralston (1985).

Anatomic and physiological data show that *some of the pyramidal tract fibers coming from MI end monosynaptically on the motoneurons. This concerns primarily motoneuron groups that control the distal muscles of the extremities, in particular the intrinsic muscles of the hand.* During evolution the pyramidal tract has increased in size and also in the amount of monosynaptic connections with the motoneurons. This has taken place in parallel with increased versatility and precision of the movements of the hand, which are closely related to the increased size of the brain. In the rat and the rabbit, for example, the pyramidal tract is only slightly developed. It is more prominent in the cat, but there are no monosynaptic connections between pyramidal tract neurons in the motor cortex and motoneurons in the cord—all connections are with spinal inter-neurons. In monkeys, there is a modest proportion of monosynaptic connections, but the proportion is larger in the anthropoid apes (for example, the chimpanzee) and still larger in humans. The monosynaptic motoneuronal connections are of particular importance for the movements that require the highest degree of voluntary control (the least automatic movements) such as independent or fractionated finger movements. This relationship is witnessed by the fact that in certain lower mammals with an exceptional manual dexterity (and the ability to use the fingers individually), some monosynaptic motoneuronal connections are present.

The influence of the pyramidal tract on the muscles of the extremities is mediated almost exclusively by fibers that cross in the lower medulla. The small contingent of uncrossed (and doubly crossed) fibers mentioned above can influence only proximal and axial muscles—in particular, muscles of the back, the thorax, and the abdomen. This is in accordance with their termination medially in the ventral horn (Figs. 8.2 and 9.6).

The Pyramidal Tract Fibers May Open and Close Spinal Reflex Arcs

Even in humans, a large proportion of the pyramidal tract fibers end in synaptic contact with interneurons in laminae VII and VIII (Figs. 2.12 and 9.6). Many—perhaps most—of these interneurons make synaptic contacts either on motoneurons or on other interneurons, in their turn contacting motoneurons. In this manner, the pyramidal tract may mediate varied effects on the motoneurons. This concerns not only the α motoneurons but also the γ motoneurons, so that the pyramidal tract can control the sensitivity of the muscle spindle. Because many of the interneurons contacted by pyramidal tract fibers are intercalated in reflex arcs, *the motor cortex can ensure that the various spinal reflexes are adapted to the overall aim of the movements.* For example (as described in Chapter 8), the strength of the long-latency stretch reflex can be increased or decreased depending on what is appropriate during motor learning. The interneurons mediating reciprocal inhibition during stretch reflexes (Fig. 8.10) can also be controlled by the pyramidal tract. Likewise, the Renshaw cells (Fig. 8.11) are subject to supraspinal control, so that the strength of the recurrent inhibition can be increased or decreased selectively in various motoneuronal groups. A final example are interneurons mediating inhibition of motoneurons evoked by stimulation of tendon organs (in the same muscle as supplied by the motoneurons). This reflex arc can also be "opened" or "closed" by the pyramidal tract. Thus, this *autogenic inhibition* elicited by stimulation of tendon organs can be suppressed during voluntary contraction of the muscle, whereas at the same time the inhibition of other muscles may be enhanced.

The Terminal Ramifications and Boutons of Corticospinal Fibers

The terminal ramifications in the cord of single pyramidal tract axons have been visualized by intra-axonal injection of HRP. The injection is done after the axon has been identified physiologically as belonging to a neuron with its perikaryon in the motor cortex. The ramifications of a single pyramidal tract axon can be very widespread, thus contacting many motoneurons in different segments of the cord, supplying several different muscles. This may appear surprising in light of the very discrete and precise movements the pyramidal tract is capable of producing. However, as a rule the various muscles have similar actions—that is, they are synergists. Furthermore, the *strength* of the influence of one pyramidal tract cell probably varies greatly among the motoneurons it contacts, depending on the number and location of synaptic contacts. Thus, pyramidal tract boutons are found both on the cell soma and on the dendrites (even the thin distal parts of the dendrites), and the former exert a stronger influence than the latter on the excitability of the motoneuron. So each pyramidal tract neuron in the motor cortex probably has a powerful influence on some motoneurons but only a weak one on many others.

The *transmitter* used by the pyramidal tract neurons is most likely *glutamate* (with a fast excitatory action). This is indicated by immunocytochemical studies and by physiological experiments. Under the electron microscope, most boutons of the pyramidal tract axons contain round, clear vesicles typical of excitatory synapses. Some boutons, however, contain so-called pleomorphic vesicles, which usually are associated with inhibitory synapses.

The Function of the Pyramidal Tract

To clarify the role played by a nucleus or a tract in motor control, it is not sufficient to study the connections and properties of single cells, even though this information is important and necessary. One also needs to know the symptoms that ensue when the nucleus or tract is eliminated. In humans with lesions of the pyramidal tract, there is usually damage to other structures as well. As is well known, the fibers of the pyramidal tract are fairly isolated only in the pyramid.

In the internal capsule, the mesencephalon (crus), the pons, and in the cord, it is either mixed with or lies in close apposition to other tracts. In monkeys, however, it is possible to cut the pyramidal tract in the pyramid and to control the lesion microscopically later. Thus, the symptoms that occur when only the pyramidal tract is eliminated can be studied. It should be kept in mind, however, that the pyramidal tract is more developed in humans than in monkeys. Thus, the possibility cannot be excluded that symptoms would be somewhat more pronounced in humans after a corresponding lesion (as they are far more pronounced in a monkey than in a cat). Experiments in monkeys nevertheless provide good information about what the main tasks of the pyramidal tract are also in humans.

Shortly after unilateral transection of the pyramid, a monkey can move around apparently normally. Nevertheless, to use the hand to pick up a morsel of food, for example, is almost impossible for some time, even though the hand can be used effectively for climbing. Gradually, over some weeks, the ability to use the hand for grasping objects is regained, but the movements are clumsy and consist only of simultaneous flexion of all fingers (a sort of scraping movement). In the beginning, the fingers cannot be moved independently of the hand, but this improves over time. However, *the ability to move the fingers independently of each other—so-called fractionated movements—does not return* (even after 5 years). The precision grip, in which the thumb opposes the index finger, is permanently lost.

Monkeys in which the pyramid is cut shortly after birth never develop the precision grip. Thus, no other tracts can take over this task from the pyramidal tract. In humans with damage of the motor cortex or the pyramidal tract (often in the internal capsule), the most enduring symptom is difficulty with tasks requiring precise, fractionated finger movements, such as writing, tying shoelaces, buttoning a shirt, and picking up small objects (like a needle). Less precise movements involving larger muscle

groups are usually less severely affected. In addition, lesions of the internal capsule in humans produce characteristic changes of muscle tone and reflexes (spasticity), which do not occur in monkeys with lesions restricted to the pyramidal tract. We will return to the symptoms produced by lesions of the descending motor pathways in humans at the end of this chapter.

OTHER DESCENDING PATHWAYS TO THE SPINAL CORD

There are several pathways in addition to the pyramidal tract that mediate impulses from higher levels of the central nervous system to the motoneurons in the cranial nerve nuclei and the spinal cord. The nuclei giving origin to these other tracts are located in the brain stem, but several of them receive afferents from the cerebral cortex—in particular from the motor cortex (Fig. 9.1). Thus, several pathways that are synaptically interrupted in the brain stem transmit impulses from the cortex to the motoneurons. Other cell groups with descending connections to motoneurons are not controlled from the motor cortex and are primarily involved in control of automatic muscle contractions, such as those aiming at maintaining body balance and the movements of locomotion and of respiration.

Broadly speaking, the pyramidal tract is of importance primarily for the least automatic movements—that is, those requiring a high degree of conscious, voluntary attention—whereas the other pathways are important mostly for more automatic movements. This agrees with the fact that the pyramidal tract is of prime importance for the movements of the distal parts of the extremities, whereas the other pathways are more concerned with movements of the proximal parts of the extremities and of the trunk.

The Rubrospinal Tract

The *red nucleus* (nucleus ruber) in the mesencephalon (Figs. 2.21 and 2.22) sends fibers to the spinal cord, forming the *rubrospinal tract*. The tract crosses the midline just below the red nucleus and descends in the lateral funiculus, mixed with the fibers of the pyramidal tract. The rubrospinal tract is somatotopically organized. In the cat and the monkey, the fibers terminate in largely the same parts of the spinal gray matter as the pyramidal tract.

The red nucleus receives fibers from the motor cortex of the same side. A pathway is thus established from the cerebral cortex to the spinal motoneurons, which is synaptically interrupted in the red nucleus. The rubrospinal tract has been most studied in the cat and the monkey. It exerts its actions primarily on motoneurons supplying distal muscles, like the pyramidal tract. It may thus supplement the pyramidal tract in the control of voluntary movements. Whether the corticorubrospinal tract plays such a role in humans, however, is not certain. Thus, most rubrospinal fibers in monkeys (and presumably also humans) come from the caudal, large-celled or *magnocellular part* of the nucleus, which is very small in humans (it is smaller in monkeys than in cats, and even smaller in humans than in monkeys). This is a major reason why the existence of more than a rudimentary rubrospinal tract in man has been questioned.

The Red Nucleus Has Major Connections with the Cerebellum

Most of the red nucleus in monkeys and humans is made up of fairly small cells, forming the *parvocellular part*. This part receives its main afferents from the cerebellum (particularly the dentate nucleus). Many of the efferents from the parvocellular nucleus pass to the inferior olive, which is an important precerebellar nucleus— that is, it sends all its efferent axons to the contralateral cerebellum. Thus, it appears that the major part of the red nucleus is related to motor functions indirectly via its influence on the cerebellum. Efferents of the relevant parts of the cerebellum reach the thalamus and in particular the parts projecting to the motor cortical areas. The red nucleus may therefore possibly influence motor control via the effects of the cerebellum on the motor cortex.

The caudal, magnocellular part of the red nucleus receives many afferents from the anterior interpositus nucleus of the cerebellum and, as mentioned, projects to the spinal cord. Thus, the information sent to the spinal cord from the motor cortex via the red nucleus is modified by the cerebellum.

Reticulospinal Tracts

The *reticular formation* is an important source of descending fibers that can influence the motoneurons. The reticular formation is discussed more completely in Chapter 12 (its functions are not restricted to motor control). Reticulospinal fibers arise primarily from the reticular formation of the pons and the medulla (Figs. 9.1, 12.1, and 12.7). These areas also receive fibers from the cerebral cortex—*corticoreticular fibers*—in particular from the motor areas (areas 4 and 6). Thus, there is a *corticoreticulospinal pathway* that can mediate signals from the cortical motor areas to the spinal motoneurons (Fig. 12.7).

It is impossible to transect the reticulospinal tracts in the white matter of the cord without at the same time involving other tracts. This has made it difficult to clarify the role of the reticulospinal tracts in control of movements. Nevertheless, experiments with relatively selective lesions of the reticular formation indicate that *the reticulospinal tracts are of importance for maintaining the upright position (posture), for movements that orient the body toward external events, and for fairly crude, stereotyped voluntary movements of the extremities* (such as extending the arm toward an object). The first two kinds are mostly automatic, reflex movements—called postural reflexes—that are relatively independent of descending connections to the reticular formation from the cerebral cortex. We will return to the postural reflexes below. Relatively crude, voluntary (less automatic) movements of the extremities, on the other hand, are most likely mediated by pathways from the motor cortex via the reticular formation and the reticulospinal tracts (Fig. 12.7). At least in monkeys, the pyramidal tract is not indispensable for such movements, as described above.

More about Reticulospinal Pathways

The actions in the cord of the reticulospinal fibers are multifarious. In Chapter 4, we described reticulospinal fibers coming from the raphe nuclei (Fig. 12.5) and adjoining parts of the reticular formation in the medulla. These fibers descend in the dorsal part of the lateral funiculus and end in the dorsalmost part of the spinal gray matter (Fig. 4.18), with powerful effects on the central transmission of signals from nociceptors. The reticulospinal fibers that are of interest in relation to motor control terminate more ventrally in the spinal gray matter, with effects on the motoneurons—monosynaptic and polysynaptic via interneurons. These fibers descend in the ventral part of the lateral funiculus and in the ventral funiculus. They belong to at least two tracts with different sites of origin in the reticular formation and somewhat different sites of termination in the cord.

Thus, fibers from the pontine and medullary parts of the reticular formation (Figs. 12.1 and 12.7) run in different parts of the white matter: The pontine fibers are located in the ventral funiculus, whereas the medullary fibers are in the ventral part of the lateral funiculus. The medullary fibers terminate somewhat more laterally in the ventral horn (particularly in lamina VII but to some extent also in lamina IX) than the pontine fibers. The latter terminate mostly more medially in laminae VII and VIII. The medullary reticulospinal tract may thus be expected to have access to motoneurons innervating muscles of the extremities, whereas the pontine tract reaches mostly motoneurons of axial muscles (neck, back, and abdomen). Together, reticulospinal fibers terminate in large parts of the ventral horn but primarily in medial parts, where motoneurons to axial muscles and proximal muscles of the extremities are located. Connections are particularly ample to motoneurons innervating neck muscles, which are of importance for movements of the head.

Many of the reticulospinal fibers send collaterals to both cervical and lumbar segments of the cord and often to the ventral horns of both sides. Thus, such neurons are capable of influencing numerous muscles at the same time. This may be functionally meaningful in relation to adjustment of posture and body balance. Nevertheless,

there is also some degree of somatotopic organization among reticulospinal neurons, as demonstrated with retrograde axonal transport methods. Also, electrical stimulation of the reticular formation can elicit muscle contractions restricted to smaller parts of the body. Together, these data indicate that *the reticulospinal fibers can mediate both rather diffuse effects on large groups and muscles and more focused influences related to specific movements.*

Both excitatory and inhibitory effects on the motoneurons can be elicited by electrical stimulation of the reticular formation. Inhibition of reflex and voluntary movements can be produced by stimulation of a region in the lower part of the medulla (Fig. 12.10), whereas increased reflex movements and muscle tone can be elicited from a more rostral region. The reticulospinal fibers act on both the α and γ motoneurons. Thus, the reticular formation also controls the sensitivity of the muscle spindles, and in certain situations it is probable that it acts only on the γ motoneurons and not the α motoneurons. There is some evidence that the reticular formation may act selectively on either static or dynamic γ motoneurons.

The Tectospinal Tract

Several mesencephalic cell groups send axons to the spinal cord. A large number of fibers arises in the *superior colliculus* and forms the *tectospinal tract*. The descending fibers cross the midline shortly below the superior colliculus, and most terminate at cervical levels of the cord. The superior colliculus receives numerous fibers from the retina, the visual cortex, and also from the so-called frontal eye field (area 8, Fig. 13.31), which are of particular importance for control of conjugate eye movements. Efferent fibers from the superior colliculus act not only on the cord; motoneurons in the brain stem innervating extraocular muscles are also influenced (although indirectly via the reticular formation). In agreement with these anatomic data, electrical stimulation of the superior colliculus in experimental animals produces coordinated movements of the eyes and the head. The tectospinal tract is of particular importance for *movements of the head and the eyes as parts of optic reflexes—*

that is, the head and the eyes are directed toward something in the visual field. (Auditory impulses also reach the superior colliculus via the inferior colliculus and can thus elicit head movements.)

The superior colliculus receives afferents also from nonvisual parts of the cortex, like the SI and MI. Thus, a corticotectospinal pathway may also play a role in voluntary movements.

Vestibulospinal Tracts

Primary sensory fibers from the vestibular apparatus terminate in the vestibular nuclei, located in the pons and medulla (Fig. 13.16). Vestibular signals directly related to the position and movements of the head also indirectly provide information about the position of the body and about disturbances in balance. Two tracts, issued from the vestibular nuclei to the spinal cord, can contribute to the maintenance of body balance and posture. The largest is the *lateral vestibulospinal tract,* which comes from the lateral vestibular (Deiters) nucleus and reaches all levels of the cord. The tract lies in the ventral funiculus. The fibers exert an excitatory action on both α and γ motoneurons. Like the reticulospinal fibers, the vestibulospinal ones act primarily on motoneurons in the medial parts of the ventral horn—that is, axial muscles and proximal muscles of the extremities. Thus, the lateral vestibulospinal tract can adjust the contraction of muscles that oppose the force of gravity (antigravity muscles).

The other vestibulospinal tract is much smaller and reaches only the cervical and upper thoracic segments of the cord. This *medial vestibulospinal tract* is therefore primarily of importance for mediation of reflex head movements in response to vestibular stimuli. This conclusion is also supported by physiological experiments. Unlike the lateral vestibulospinal tract, many of the neurons of the medial tract are inhibitory (probably using glycine as transmitter).

In contrast to the other cell groups in the brain stem sending fibers to the cord, the vestibular nuclei do not receive afferents from the cerebral cortex. The vestibulospinal neurons are therefore more independent of the cerebral cortex than, for example, the reticulospinal neurons. The vestibular nuclei mediate primarily automatic, reflex movements and adjustments of muscle tone. Nevertheless, the activity of the vestibular nuclei may be influenced indirectly from the cortex, since they receive afferents from the reticular formation.

Monoaminergic Pathways from the Brain Stem to the Spinal Cord

Although often included among the reticulospinal pathways, descending monoaminergic fibers to the cord from the raphe nuclei (Fig. 12.5), the nucleus locus coeruleus (Fig. 12.6), and scattered cell groups in their vicinity will be treated separately. Such monoaminergic fibers terminate in the ventral horn (in addition to in the dorsal horn, as described in Chapter 4). Many of the raphespinal fibers contain *serotonin,* whereas the coeruleospinal fibers contain *norepinephrine.* In addition, several peptides coexist with the monoamines. Both these tracts are diffusely distributed in the cord and can hardly mediate information related to specific movements. More likely, they exert general, widespread facilitatory influences on the motoneurons, as judged from the effects on spinal motoneurons of microinjections of serotonin and norepinephrine. Thus, the excitability of most motoneurons may be enhanced, so that they react more vigorously to an input from pathways mediating specific motor commands (such as the pyramidal tract).

Possibly, these monoaminergic pathways may contribute to the effects of motivation on the performance of voluntary movements—the muscle contractions may occur with increased speed and force. At the same time the descending monoaminergic connections to the dorsal horn may prevent "disturbing" signals from nociceptors from reaching consciousness.

CONTROL OF AUTOMATIC MOVEMENTS

Postural Reflexes

As mentioned, the reticulospinal and vestibulospinal tracts mediate automatic, reflex muscle contractions that contribute to maintaining the upright position. We will now describe in more detail such reflexes, collectively called *postural reflexes.*

The tasks of these reflexes are to maintain an appropriate posture of the body, to help regain equilibrium when it is disturbed, and to ensure optimal starting positions for the execution of specific movements. Postural reflexes produce the automatic movements that help us to regain equilibrium quickly, for example, when slipping on ice. It is a common experience that these compensatory movements happen so rapidly that only afterwards are we aware of which movements we performed.

The most important *receptors* for postural reflexes are the vestibular receptors in the inner ear, proprioceptors close to the upper cervical joints, and vision.

The postural reflexes are difficult to study when the nervous system is functioning normally, and many parts from the cord to the cerebral cortex all cooperate in the production of movements. By transection of all descending tracts from higher levels (the cerebral cortex in particular) to the brain stem in animals, however, a condition with greatly exaggerated postural reflexes ensues. This is called *decerebrate rigidity* and is characterized by increased tone in the antigravity muscles—primarily extensors. In particular, two postural reflexes have been much studied, the *neck and labyrinthine reflexes,* which are elicited by stimulation of proprioceptors around the upper cervical joints and vestibular receptors, respectively.

Generally speaking, the labyrinthine reflexes serve to keep the position of the head constant. The neck reflexes, on the other hand, serve to keep the position of the body constant in relation to the head. The latter is a prerequisite for the labyrinthine reflexes to function properly; the vestibular apparatus can provide information only about the position of the head in space and not about its position relative to that of the body. Thus, the labyrinthine reflexes work on the assumption that the head has a constant position relative to the body; this is ensured by the neck reflexes.

As mentioned, in animals with an intact nervous system, many cell groups and tracts are of importance for the final muscle activity, and the postural reflexes are but one aspect of motor control. During voluntary movements, the postural reflexes—just like many other reflexes—can be suppressed or facilitated depending on what is appropriate for the task. After damage to higher levels of the central nervous system in humans, however, the postural reflexes may be seen in exaggerated forms.

Decerebrate Rigidity

In animals with transection of the brain stem just below the red nucleus (Figs. 2.21 and 9.1), the postural reflexes occur in an exaggerated and caricatured manner. As a result of loss of signals from higher levels, the animal persists in a state of increased extensor tone. Thus, such an animal—although deeply unconscious—can stand (with some support) with extended legs and the head and tail lifted. The animal is unable to walk, however, and, once fallen, it cannot get back on its feet. The animal does not die immediately from such *decerebration* because the control of respiration and circulation can be carried out by the lower brain stem independent of higher levels of the nervous system. The condition is called *decerebrate rigidity.* The name may seem misleading. There are no similarities to the condition called rigidity in clinical neurology, in which rigidity means the increased muscle tone in parkinsonism. There are, however, some similarities between decerebrate rigidity in animals and spasticity as occurring in humans after lesions of central motor pathways. In spasticity there may also be increased muscle tone in the extensor muscles of the legs (and in the flexor muscles of the arms, which in a sense may be regarded as postural muscles in humans).

The continuously increased muscle tension in decerebrate rigidity is caused by increased activity of motoneurons, but which nuclei and tracts are responsible? The *vestibular nuclei* and the *vestibulospinal tract* must contribute, since destruction of the lateral vestibular nucleus reduces the rigidity, whereas electrical stimulation of the nucleus increases it. In addition, the *reticular formation* and *reticulospinal* tracts play an important role. Since the corticobulbar and corticospinal neurons are excitatory, they must to a large extent influence neuronal groups in the brain stem that inhibit the vestibulospinal and reticulospinal neurons. The inhibitory region of the reticular formation in the lower medulla (Fig. 12.8) seems to be of particular importance in this connection. When this region loses its excitatory input from the cerebral cortex, the result is reduced inhibition of descending excitatory connections to the cord, producing increased α motoneuron firing. Since cutting the dorsal roots reduces or abolishes the decerebrate rigidity, the increased α motoneuron activity must also depend on increased muscle spindle afferent firing. This must be caused by increased firing of the γ motoneurons. Since increased activity of γ motoneurons plays a significant role, the decerebrate rigidity is also termed a γ rigidity (to distinguish it from α rigidity, in which there is no increased γ activity).

The cerebellum also influences the decerebrate rigidity in animals. Thus, electrical stimulation of the "spinal" parts of the cerebellum reduces the rigidity. This is because this part of the cerebellum sends inhibitory connections to the lateral vestibular nucleus.

Neck and Labyrinthine Reflexes

Studies of decerebrate animals have elucidated the postural reflexes, in particular the neck and labyrinthine reflexes. The latter reflexes, described below, may be either *tonic* or *phasic*. A phasic neck or labyrinthine reflex consists of a rapid, transient change of muscle tension in postural muscles as a response to a change of posture (usually a disturbance of the equilibrium). In a tonic reflex, the change of muscle tension lasts as long as the new position is maintained. Different receptors are responsible for evoking the neck and the labyrinthine reflexes.

In the *neck reflexes,* the response is a change of muscle tension—especially in the extremities—induced by a change in the position of the head relative to the body (such movements take place primarily in the upper cervical joints). To demonstrate clearly the neck reflexes in a decerebrate animal, the vestibular receptors must have been eliminated. When then the head is bent backward (extension of the neck), the muscle tension is increased in the extensor muscles of the fore-

limbs and decreased in the extensors of the hindlimbs. Forward bending of the head (flexion) induces the opposite pattern of changes (extension of the hindlimbs and flexion of the forelimbs). Tilting the head sideways increases the extensor tone on the same side and reduces it on the other side, as does turning the head sideways. These changes of the muscle tone aim at reestablishing the position of the body relative to the head. The receptors for these reflexes are located near the upper cervical joints, since they disappear after transection of the upper three cervical dorsal roots. Muscle spindles are the most likely candidates, but joint receptors may also contribute. The reflex center is located in the medulla, and the effects on the motoneurons are most likely mediated by both the reticulospinal and vestibulospinal tracts.

The functional role of the neck reflexes cannot be understood when observed in isolation; only in conjunction with the *labyrinthine reflexes* are their effects appropriate for the whole body. The labyrinthine reflexes are elicited by stimulation of the sensory receptors of the semicircular ducts and the utriculus of the labyrinth, which record the movements and the position of the head. To demonstrate clearly the labyrinthine reflexes, the neck reflexes must have been eliminated by cutting the upper dorsal roots (in a decerebrate animal). It then appears that *the effects produced by the labyrinthine reflexes are the opposite of those of the neck reflexes when the latter act alone.* Thus, bending the head backward elicits flexion of the forelimbs and extension of the hindlimbs, and vice versa when the head is bent forward. The purpose of these changes of muscle tone is to bring the head back to the position held before the movement—that is, to keep the position of the head in space constant. Provided the neck reflexes ensure that the body is kept in a constant position relative to the head, the labyrinthine reflexes will serve to maintain not only the position of the head in space but also the upright position of the whole body. The labyrinthine reflexes are shown clearly when the experimental animal stands on a platform that can be tilted in various directions. Tilting the platform forward increases the extensor tone in the forelimbs and decreases the tone in the hindlimbs. Tilting the platform sideways increases the muscle tone in the extensors on the side to which the tilt is directed. Both responses are obviously appropriate for the maintenance of body balance. When the platform is moved quickly in one direction and then back, the reflex response is transient (phasic reflex). When the platform is maintained in the new position, the altered muscle tone is upheld (tonic reflex). Vestibulospinal tracts are the most likely candidates for mediation of the labyrinthine reflexes (other reflexes are also elicited by stimulation of the labyrinth, as described in Chapter 13).

The neck reflexes are necessary because, as mentioned, the position of the head in space depends not only on the position of the body but also on the position of the head relative to the body. The vestibular receptors in the labyrinth can only inform about the position of the head in space, but since the neck receptors inform about the position of the head relative to the body, all necessary information is available to the central nervous system. When both reflexes work together in an intact organism, backward bending of the head, for example (with movement taking place only in the upper cervical joints and no change of body position), produces no change in muscle tension of the extremities. The tendency of the labyrinthine reflexes to produce forelimb flexion and hindlimb extension is canceled by the opposite tendency of the neck reflexes. On the other hand, when the same movement of the head is produced by a backward movement of the whole body (with no movement of the head relative to the body, like a horse that is rearing), the labyrinthine reflexes act alone to produce extension of the hindlimbs and flexion of the forelimbs. Another example is an animal standing on a platform tilting forward with no movement of the head taking place relative to the body. In that case the labyrinthine reflexes produce forelimb extension and hindlimb flexion. This is an appropriate response to maintain balance when standing on a downhill slope. If, on the other hand, the position of the head in space is kept constant and the body moved in relation to the head, the neck reflexes act alone. An example is a cat jumping down from a table: The neck is extended (keeping the head position fairly constant), producing extension of the forelimbs, which is appropriate for landing.

Other Postural Reflexes

We will now describe a few other reflexes that contribute to the maintenance of body equilibrium. An unexpected fall from some height elicits a contraction of the muscles of the leg as an appropriate preparation to the landing. The contraction begins about 75 msec after start of the fall and can therefore occur before landing (and thus before a stretch reflex can be elicited). The latency is also too short for the contraction to be voluntary. Animal experiments indicate that the receptors of this reflex are located in the labyrinth (probably in the macula sacculi, Figs. 13.10 and 13.11).

Visual impulses also contribute to adjustment of muscle tone with the purpose of maintaining the equilibrium of the body. Experiments with humans standing on a platform that can be moved unexpectedly indicate that the muscle contractions in response to a movement of the platform depend on whether the subject can see that the body moves in relation to the surroundings. If the experimental setup is such that it appears as though the surroundings do not move (that is, they are made to move in the same direction as the head), the earliest reflex contractions of the legs are weaker than when the sense of vision also informs about the movement. With monkeys also the earliest muscle response is much weaker when visual information about the unexpected movement is excluded. We do not know which pathways are used by the visual impulses that influence the postural reflexes, but vestibulospinal pathways are probably of importance.

The *grasp reflex* is usually regarded as one of the postural reflexes. It is normally expressed only in infants during the first few months and consists of the fingers firmly grasping an object that touches the palm. The purpose of this reflex is to ensure that the baby can cling to the mother, but whereas this is of vital importance for monkeys, the reflex has lost much of its importance in humans. After damage of the frontal lobes (presumably in particular the so-called supplementary motor area, SMA; Fig. 9.7), the reflex may reappear in adults. The strength of the grasp reflex depends on the position of the body.

Control of Locomotor Movements

The upright locomotion of man requires somewhat different movements than in animals walking on four legs. We should also keep in mind that the large size of the human brain has enabled many processes—which in lower animals are controlled from the spinal cord and the brain stem—to be controlled from the cerebral cortex. Nevertheless, with regard to basic mechanisms, the neural control of locomotion is probably very similar in humans and in other mammals. The following account is largely based on data obtained from animal experiments.

Fairly normal locomotion can be produced in animals (like cats) even when the spinal cord is isolated from the brain stem and the brain. This can be observed on a treadmill when the paws touch the moving ground (the animal has to be supported since there are no postural reflexes). *Central rhythm generators* must, therefore, exist in the cord, able to produce rhythmic, alternating leg movements in the absence of any command signals from higher levels. The rhythm generators consist of fairly complicated networks of interneurons with excitatory and inhibitory interconnections, eventually controlling the activity of the motoneurons. Some of the neurons within the network appear to have pacemaker properties; that is, they fire brief trains of action potentials with silent periods between, without receiving a rhythmically alternating input.

The rhythm generator is not dependent on sensory input from the moving parts to produce the motoneuron activity typical of locomotion. Thus, the rhythmic motoneuronal activity continues even after complete paralysis of the muscles (for example, after cutting of the ventral roots). This is called *fictive locomotion,* and the pattern of motoneuronal activity is strikingly similar to that observed during normal walking in intact animals.

This does not mean, however, that sensory inputs are without significance for locomotor control. The activity of the rhythm generators can indeed be modified by afferent signals from the peripheral receptors providing information about how the movements are proceeding. Inhibitory interneurons can contribute to the rhythmic pattern of activity by inhibiting the antagonists when the agonists have reached their maximal activity. Renshaw cells (Fig. 8.11) can probably also contribute by shortening impulse trains from the motoneurons and at the same time increasing the excitability of antagonist motoneurons.

There is probably one rhythm generator for each extremity. Long propriospinal fibers that interconnect the forelimb and hindlimb generators ensure that their activities are coordinated. The presence of rhythm generators in the human spinal cord is indicated by the occurrence of locomotionlike movements in anencephalic infants (born without most of the brain). In normal infants, walking movements of the legs can be elicited in the first few months (if the infant is held under the arms and the feet are made to touch the floor). This ability usually disappears, to reappear when the infant starts to crawl at about 8 months.

Several central cell groups contribute to the *control of the spinal rhythm generators.* Three regions have been identified physiologically in the brain stem: one in the so-called subthalamic region, one in the mesencephalic reticular formation, and one region in the pons. Continuous (nonrhythmic) stimulation of any of these regions can produce slow, walking movements in experimental animals. Most likely, the effects on spinal motoneurons from these regions are mediated by reticulospinal fibers, since they are abolished by cutting the ventral and ventrolateral funiculi. Furthermore, many reticulospinal neurons are rhythmically active in pace with walking movements. The connections of these locomotor regions, however, are not well known.

Connections from the cerebral cortex (especially the pyramidal tract) are of increasing importance for the control of locomotion as the ground becomes more uneven and unpredictable—that is, as each step has to be controlled individually. Thus, after destruction of the motor cortex, cats can still walk fairly normally on an even surface but are helpless when required to walk along a ladder or a narrow bar.

MOTOR CORTICAL AREAS AND THE CONTROL OF VOLUNTARY MOVEMENTS

As mentioned in the introduction to this chapter, there is no sharp division between the motor centers and other parts of the central nervous system. This is true also for the cerebral cortex. Improved methods have shown that large parts of the cortex are activated even in relation to a simple movement. When sensitive methods are used to record the electrical activity over the brain of a person asked to perform a simple flexion–extension movement of a finger, changes of activity over large parts of both hemispheres first occur. This is a slowly rising negative wave—a so-called *readiness potential*—starting about 850 msec before the movement. Approximately 60 msec before the movement, the activity is concentrated over the arm region of the motor cortex (on the side opposite the moving fingers).[2] The "motor program" appears to consist of information stored in many parts of the brain.

To decide whether a cytoarchitectonic cortical area (such as area 4) is "more motor" than other areas, we use various kinds of observations. First, we want to know the connections of the area in question. Are there more or less direct connections to cell groups known to be involved in motor control? Are the connections different from those of neighboring areas? Of particular importance is whether the area has efferent connections that can influence the motoneurons in the brain stem and in the spinal cord. Furthermore, electrical stimulation or destruction of the cortical areas gives valuable information, even though neither of these methods alone can disclose the normal functions of the area.

The American neurophysiologist Evarts made pioneer studies of the motor cortex in the 1960s and 1970s. He used microelectrode recordings in awake monkeys and correlated the activity of single neurons with movements that the monkey was trained to perform. This has become a very active field of research also with regard to other parts of the cortex. In man, the measurement of regional blood flow or other indicators of localized cortical metabolic activity can be correlated with various phases and aspects of movements. So far such methods have a fairly low resolution, so the activity can be only roughly related to specific cytoarchitectonic areas.

On the basis of the kinds of studies and data mentioned above, it is now customary to describe *three cortical motor areas* (Fig. 9.7). The *primary motor area (MI)*, which corresponds to area 4 in the precentral gyrus, has the most direct relation to movement control. Thus, most or all corticospinal fibers ending monosynaptically on the motoneurons have their perikarya in the MI. Accordingly, the threshold for eliciting movements by electrical stimulation is lower here than in any other part of the cortex. Furthermore, lesions of the MI produce clear-cut pareses, in contrast to other cortical regions. In addition to the MI, two other motor areas are found within area 6, just in front of area 4. The lateral part of area 6 is called the *premotor area (PMA)*, whereas the medial part (mostly located on the medial side of the hemisphere) is called the *sup-*

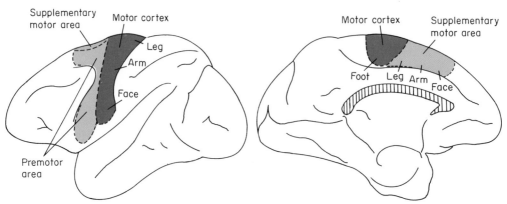

Fig. 9.7.   *The motor and the premotor areas.* The positions of MI, SMA, and PMA are shown in a drawing of the left hemisphere of a monkey.

plementary motor area (SMA). These latter areas are probably not at the same level as MI functionally. Rather, they are placed at a higher level in a hierarchy in which the PMA and SMA exert their motor control primarily by "playing" on the MI. In accordance with this, many of the efferent connections of area 6 are directed to area 4. The PMA and SMA have been termed *supramotor areas* to emphasize their higher level in the hierarchy. Assuming that area 6 of humans corresponds functionally to area 6 in monkeys, the supramotor areas have increased in size during evolution. Thus, areas 4 and 6 are of approximately the same size in monkeys (Fig. 9.7), whereas area 6 is much larger than area 4 in humans (Fig. 17.3).

In spite of many similarities, there are also functional differences between the PMA and SMA. The assumption that these areas are functionally related but not identical is strengthened by the fact that they differ with regard to connections. For example, they receive afferents from somewhat different parts of the lateral thalamus. Much is yet to be learned, however, before we have a full understanding of the roles of the PMA and SMA in motor control.

Even though the term "motor areas" is used only of areas 4 and 6 (that is, the MI, PMA, and SMA) in the frontal lobe, areas posterior to the SI—*areas 5 and 7*—and anterior to area 6—the *prefrontal cortex*—also contribute to certain aspects of motor control. Furthermore, the so-called limbic structures are important for (among other things) *motivation* and *attention,* which are crucial for motor performance. As a general rule, these various regions probably exert their effects on movements by directly and indirectly acting on the motor cortex and thus influencing the commands sent to the motoneurons.

The Primary Motor Area

As mentioned, the MI corresponds to area 4 in the precentral gyrus and is the part of the cortex from which movements are most eas-

ily produced by electrical stimulation. It is not clear, however, whether there is complete coincidence between the physiologically defined MI and the cytoarchitectonically defined area 4. Thus, some authors maintain that the MI extends anteriorly somewhat into area 6 with the representation of axial and proximal muscles.[3] It is well established that distal muscles are represented in the posterior part of area 4 (Fig. 4.20).

The MI receives main *afferents* from SI (areas 3, 1, 2), area 5, and area 6, in addition to afferents from "motor" parts of the thalamus (the ventrolateral nucleus, VL; Figs. 4.19 and 11.14). As mentioned, many of the *pyramidal tract* fibers originate in the MI. It should be realized, however, that not all effects produced by stimulation of the MI are mediated by the pyramidal tract. Thus, many *efferent fibers* from the MI reach other cortical areas and several subcortical nuclei involved in motor control, such as the *red nucleus, the reticular formation, the basal ganglia, and brain stem nuclei, which project to the cerebellum.* Nevertheless, the movements evoked by very weak electrical stimulation of the motor cortex are mediated by the pyramidal tract. Such movements occur in the opposite body half and can be limited to a few muscles in distal parts of the extremities and the face. With increasing stimulus strength, more muscles are recruited, and also more proximal ones. As with SI, a disproportionally large part of the MI is devoted to control of the hand (especially the thumb and the index finger) and the lips and the tongue (Fig. 9.8). In comparison, very small parts of the MI contain neurons controlling muscles of the back and the abdomen. How many cortical neurons are related to the motor control of a particular body part depends on the variety and precision of the movements rather than on the size of the part.[4]

Muscles that are often used simultaneously on both sides of the body, like the muscles of the back and the abdomen, can be relatively easily activated on both sides (bilaterally) by stimulation of the MI of one

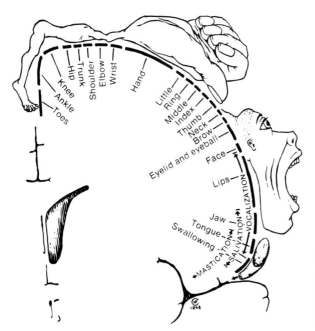

Fig. 9.8. *The relative size of the regions of the MI representing various body parts.* Based on electrical stimulation of the exposed human MI. From Penfield and Rasmussen (1950).

side. Movements of the fingers, however, can only be evoked on the opposite (contralateral) side by stimulation of the MI, which reflects that the fingers are used independently and usually differently on the two sides. The anatomic basis of this is the complete crossing of the pyramidal tract fibers controlling distal muscles, mentioned earlier. Similar conditions are found for the commissural fibers interconnecting the MI of the two hemispheres: Only parts of the MI representing the trunk and the proximal parts of the extremities are interconnected. The large areas representing the distal muscles are devoid of commissural connections, presumably as an expression of the independent use of the two hands (Fig. 17.11).

Many cells in the MI become active (or increase their firing frequency) immediately before a voluntary movement starts, as shown with microelectrode recordings. In contrast, most cells in the SI become active *after* movement onset, indicating that they are activated by sensory signals from the moving parts but do not contribute to the initiation of the movement. Some pyramidal tract neurons (corticospinal neurons) in-

crease their activity only in relation to the start of a movement, whereas others are active during the whole movement. The firing frequency of some neurons is related to the force of muscular contraction. In the MI of a relaxed monkey sitting quietly waiting for a signal to move, some corticospinal neurons fire continuously (that is, they are tonically active). This probably means that the motor cortex not only initiates and controls movements but also determines the "readiness" of selected motoneuronal groups by keeping them slightly depolarized (below the threshold for initiation of action potentials). This enables the motoneurons to respond more quickly to a "go" signal from the motor cortex, or from subcortical levels, such as the reticular formation, the vestibular nuclei, and sensory signals through the dorsal roots (for example, from muscle spindles).

It has been debated for many years whether the motor cortex is organized so that each muscle is controlled by a well-delimited, distinct group of corticospinal neurons, or whether it is organized in relation to movements rather than discrete muscles. Studies with microelectrodes and with intra-axonal transport of tracers have at least partly clarified the issue. Corticospinal neurons acting on the motoneurons of one particular muscle are usually not located in one small region of the cortex, but rather appear to be scattered over a wider area, intermingled with neurons controlling other muscles. (Nevertheless, all neurons controlling, for example, hand muscles are all confined to what has been determined as the hand region of the MI by means of less sensitive recording methods; compare with Fig. 4.20.) It has furthermore been shown anatomically and physiologically that one corticospinal neuron usually has collaterals acting on motoneurons to several muscles, although such muscles as a rule have synergistic actions. The strength of synaptic action differs among motoneurons of different muscles, so that each corticospinal neuron as a rule has strong effects on one muscle and weaker effects on several others. At the same time as a corticospinal neuron has excitatory effects on motoneurons of synergistic muscles, motoneurons of antagonistic muscles are inhibited (via inhibitory interneurons).

We do not fully understand how the appropriate corticospinal neurons are selected to produce a certain movement. We do know, however, that the selection has to involve afferent connections to the MI from other cortical areas and from the thalamus; the decision to initiate a particular movement is certainly not made in the MI. Several observations show that the selection of corticospinal neurons to be used can be extremely precise and varied. In the first place, one corticospinal neuron can be active when a certain hand muscle is used for a precision grip, whereas it is much less active or inactive when the muscle is used for a more crude grasping movement. Other corticospinal neurons must therefore be responsible for producing the required force from the muscle in the latter situation. Second, human subjects can quickly learn to recruit one specific motor unit among many others when allowed to see the EMG pattern of the muscle (biofeedback). This must be caused

by an almost incredible ability to focus excitation from the motor cortex on certain spinal motoneurons. Considering the precision of movements required of a violinist, a watchmaker, or a neurosurgeon, the above observations become perhaps less surprising.

The Supplementary Motor Area

Located in front of the MI on the medial side of the hemisphere (Fig. 9.7), the SMA sends fibers to both the spinal cord and the reticular formation. Thus, the SMA contributes to both direct and indirect corticospinal pathways. The SMA also, however, sends many fibers to the MI, and this pathway is probably most important for its influence on motor control. This assumption is primarily based on results obtained by microelectrode recordings in monkeys showing the properties of single cells and on measurements of blood flow and metabolic activity in the human cerebral cortex, which give indirect evidence of neuronal activity (with PET; see Chapter 3).

The neuronal activity in the SMA of humans appears to increase especially in relation to somewhat complex movements. When, for example, a person executes a series of simple flexion–extension movements of a finger, the activity is increased mainly in the MI hand area, not in the SMA. When the task is to perform a series of different movements in a specified sequence, however, there is also increased activity in the SMA. It appears that the activity increases first in the SMA and then in the MI. Increased activity in the SMA is not related to the movement itself, since it is sufficient that the person *imagines* the performance of a fairly complex movement. In such cases there is no increase of activity in the MI, which fits with the notion that the MI is instrumental in *initiating* the movement.

Damage of the SMA in monkeys produces striking difficulties with the simultaneous use of both hands to solve a task. When a piece of food is stuck in a hole in a Plexiglas plate, a normal monkey easily retrieves it by pushing with one finger from above and collecting the piece with the other hand from below. After damage to the SMA, both hands are used for pushing from above.

Recording of single-cell activity in the SMA has shown that many cells change their activity in relation to a sensory stimulus (light, passive movements, and so forth) that the animal knows is a signal to start a certain voluntary movement. SMA neurons respond to a visual stimulus, for example, only when the stimulus is connected with a movement response, and the SMA cells respond earlier than those in the MI.

Observations of the kinds discussed above have led to the suggestion that the SMA is *important for organizing and planning fairly complex movements and for mediating an appropriate motor response to sensory stimuli.* That the grasp reflex is disturbed (in adults it reappears) after damage to the SMA may possibly be explained by a disruption of normal integration of sensory stimuli and motor responses.

The Premotor Area

The PMA occupies the largest part of area 6 on the convexity of the hemisphere (Fig. 9.7). This region probably sends fewer fibers to the spinal cord than the SMA but has strong connections with the reticular formation, the red nucleus, the basal ganglia, and, indirectly, with the cerebellum. As with the SMA, however, the connections from the PMA to the MI are probably those most directly related to the motor functions of the PMA. Experiments in monkeys indicate that *the PMA is important for the control of visually guided movements,* such as the proper orientation of the hand and fingers when they approach an object to be grasped. Monkeys with lesions of the PMA also have difficulties with moving the hand around a transparent obstacle to reach an object: They persistently use the direct approach, bumping into the obstacle. After damage to the MI, the handling of an object is clumsy and insecure, but the ability to avoid an obstacle is not lost. Connections from the extrastriate areas in the occipital lobe to the PMA are necessary for the ability to perform such circumventive goal-directed movements.

In agreement with the above observations, *single-cell recordings* show that many cells in the PMA change their activity about 60 msec after a light signal that the monkey is trained to respond to with a certain movement. The activity of the PMA neurons continues until just before the movement starts, even when the monkey is trained to wait for many seconds after the signal before actually performing the movement.

Damage of the PMA often produces a peculiar tendency to continue a certain movement when first started, even though the movement is unsuccessful in achieving its goal. Thus, when the hand in one of the examples mentioned above bumps

into an obstacle (in this case a transparent plate), the monkey nevertheless repeats the same movement over and over. This phenomenon is called *perseveration* and can occur also in humans after damage to the frontal lobes.

The Posterior Parietal Cortex and Voluntary Movements

Area 5 is of particular importance for processing somatosensory information (received from SI), whereas area 7 also receives information from visual cortical areas (Figs. 17.9 and 17.10). Many neurons in these areas are active in relation to movements, as shown by Mountcastle and others. One kind of neuron is active before goal-directed, reaching movements, such as when a monkey stretches its hand toward a banana. Such neurons do not become active, however, in relation to a movement in the same direction but without a specific aim, or in relation to a passive movement. Other kinds of neurons increase their activity in relation to exploratory hand movements, such as when a monkey studies a foreign object. In area 7, some neurons increase their activity only when the monkey stretches the hand toward an object that it also looks at. Since there are ample connections from the posterior parietal cortex to the SMA and PMA (Fig. 17.12), it is likely that the behavior of cells in these motor areas is in part determined by the posterior parietal cortex. Indeed, damage to the posterior parietal cortex also produces motor disturbances. There are no pareses, however, but rather difficulties with the execution of more complex movements. Thus, in humans, lesions of the posterior parietal cortex may, for example, make them unable to open a door or to handle previously familiar tools like a screwdriver or a can opener. Such persons also have difficulties with proper orientation of the hand in relation to an object, and they easily miss an object even though they see it clearly. This kind of symptom is called *apraxia.* Interestingly, similar symptoms may occur after lesions of the frontal lobes in front of the MI in humans—presumably reflecting the intimate connections between the posterior parietal cortex and the frontal lobes.

SYMPTOMS CAUSED BY INTERRUPTION OF CENTRAL MOTOR PATHWAYS

The term *central pareses* is used of pareses that are caused by interruption of the central motor pathways conducting impulses from the cerebral cortex (especially the MI) to the motoneurons. Only the pyramidal tract goes directly; the other pathways are indirect, with synaptic interruption in the brain stem. We have discussed above that the various pathways take care of somewhat different aspects of motor control. The term *upper motor syndrome* is often used of the clinical picture resulting from interruption of the central motor pathways, to differentiate it from the *lower motor syndrome* (peripheral pareses) resulting from destruction of the motoneurons (including their axons). Even though central pareses can be produced by lesions located anywhere between the motor cortex and the motoneurons, the commonest cause is interruption of the descending fibers by bleeding or a thrombosis in the internal capsule (Figs. 2.28 and 10.1). The pareses then affect the muscles of the opposite half of the body (hemipareses, hemiplegia). The term *capsular hemiplegia* is commonly used of this condition.

The pareses in capsular hemiplegia are clearly different from peripheral pareses. Thus, the motoneurons are not put out of action and can still be activated by impulses through the dorsal roots from various receptors. They can also be influenced by fibers descending from cell groups in the brain stem, such as the reticular formation and the vestibular nuclei. Stretch reflexes may be consequently elicited, and there is not a marked wasting of the muscles. Immediately after the stroke causing the capsular hemiplegia, the stretch reflexes are weak or absent, but within weeks or months they increase in strength and become stronger on the paretic than on the normal side (hyperreflexia). Typically, the increased reflex response is primarily seen when muscles are stretched rapidly; usually there is no increased muscle tone when judged by slow stretching. In certain muscles, however, even the resting tone may be increased, with a characteristic distribution: In the arm the increased tone affects the flexors so that the arm is kept flexed at the elbow, whereas the extensors of the leg are affected (central pareses due to destruction in the spinal cord of motor pathways result in increased resting tone of flexors also in the leg). This condition with changed resting tone and increased phasic stretch reflexes is usually called *spasticity.* The most constant and characteristic feature of spasticity is the velocity-dependent increased strength of stretch reflexes, and some authors limit the definition of spasticity to this. Others use the term primarily of the characteristically increased resting tone in flexors of the arm and in extensors of the leg.

One important feature of central pareses, when compared with peripheral ones, is that *the velocity with which voluntary movements can be performed is more reduced than the isometric force* (that is, speed of movements is more reduced than strength). This phenomenon is called *retardation* of movements. It particularly concerns fine finger movements and movements of the lips and tongue, whereas larger movements are less severely affected. Writing, tying, buttoning, and similar movements may be impossible for a patient with capsular hemiplegia, or the movements are performed only very slowly and clumsily. The *fatigability* is also abnormally great—that is, the muscular force drops quickly when a voluntary movement is repeated several times. The patient also experiences a dramatic increase in the *mental effort* needed for voluntary movements: Movements that before the stroke required no mental effort can afterwards only be performed with the utmost concentration and strain.

Changes in the *contractile properties* of the paretic muscles have also been found in hemiplegic patients. Thus, in the intrinsic muscles of the hand the fatigability of type 1 muscle cells is increased, and the contraction velocity of the type 2 fibers is reduced. Such changes will presumably contribute to the retardation and increased fatigability in patients with central pareses.

Interruption of descending central motor pathways, as in capsular hemiplegia, also produces changes of reflexes other than the stretch reflexes. The so-called *plantar reflex,* elicited by stroking with a pointed object in a forward direction along the sole of the foot (especially the lateral margin), is *inverted*. Instead of the normal response, which is a flexion movement of the great toe (and the other toes), the great toe extends (moves upward).[5] This phenomenon, with extension instead of flexion of the great toe, is called the *sign of Babinski* and is a sensitive indicator of damage to the motor pathways leading from the cortex to the spinal cord. Thus, for example, increased intracranial pressure and unilateral herniation with compression of the descending motor fibers in the mesencephalon may invert the plantar reflex at a very early stage (this will occur with the foot contralateral to the herniation, owing to the crossing of the pyramidal tract in the lower medulla). An inverted plantar reflex may, however, also occur during general anesthesia and in other conditions with reduced cerebral activity.

Mechanisms Responsible for the Development of Spasticity

It is fair to say that the mechanisms underlying the development of spasticity are not fully understood. Conditions probably vary in different patients, even when the lesions appear to be similarly located. Studies of patients with central pareses (upper motor neuron syndromes) and spasticity indicate that the monosynaptic reflex response to stretch is enhanced, whereas the polysynaptic (long-latency) stretch reflex appears to be reduced in strength. This conclusion is based on EMG recordings in muscles subjected to accurately graded stretches and vibration.

It was formerly assumed that increased impulse traffic from the muscle spindles—as a result of increased γ motoneuron firing—explained the increased stretch reflex responses in spasticity. This has not been verified by microneurographic recordings, however, since the firing frequency of Ia afferent fibers was not increased. Only a few patients have been studied in this manner, however.

Several other factors may contribute to an increased α motoneuron excitability, so that they react with abnormal firing frequency and duration to a stimulus. Probably most important are changes in the spinal cord itself. Thus, the loss of descending corticospinal fibers most likely results in *decreased activity of inhibitory interneurons*. This has been studied for some types of inhibitory interneurons. There is some evidence, for example, of reduced activity in *inhibitory interneurons activated from tendon organs (Ib afferents)*; thus, the normal inhibition of certain α motoneurons from tendon organs when the muscular tension is increasing may be missing in spastic patients. There is also evidence of reduced activity of GABAergic interneurons mediating presynaptic inhibition of Ia afferent terminals. This would lead to a stronger excitatory effect than normal of muscle stretch (particularly rapid stretch) on the α motoneurons. Another possible factor may be *reduced recurrent inhibition of α motoneurons* in spastic patients. The Renshaw cells, mediating the recurrent inhibition (Fig. 8.11), are known to be under supraspinal control. Thus, Renshaw cells acting on the motoneurons of the antagonists of a working muscle are excited by corticospinal fibers. When, for example, ankle extensors contract, the motoneurons to the ankle flexors are inhibited by Renshaw cells so there is less chance of eliciting an unwanted stretch reflex in the flexors. Some studies indicate that the recurrent inhibition in such instances is reduced in spastic patients. This may perhaps contribute to the occurrence of repeated reflex contractions as a response to a single stretch in spastic patients. This phenomenon is called *clonus*. The interneurons mediating *reciprocal inhibition* (Fig. 8.10) are also excited by descending supraspinal pathways, and there is some evidence that the activity of such interneurons is reduced. This would also help to explain the occurrence of hyperreflexia and of clonus. Thus, for example, when the Achilles reflex is tested with a tap on the tendon, a monosynaptic stretch reflex is elicited in the calf muscles (ankle flexors). Normally, the reciprocal inhibition prevents a stretch reflex from being elicited also in the antagonists—that is, the ankle extensors. If, however, the reciprocal inhibition is reduced, a reflex contraction of the ankle extensors may occur, and this may in turn produce a new reflex contraction in the flexors, and so forth.

The "Pyramidal Tract Syndrome"

Formerly, all of the motor symptoms occurring in capsular hemiplegia were thought to be caused by damage to the pyramidal tract, and the term "pyramidal tract syndrome" is still widely used. Closer study indicates, however, that only some of the symptoms can be explained by damage to the pyramidal tract. Other symptoms must be assumed to arise from destruction of other corticofugal pathways descending in the internal capsule. This concerns especially the spasticity, which has not been produced by lesions restricted to the pyramidal tract in monkeys and in man (admittedly, very few human cases have been described in which there is sound reason to believe that only the pyramidal tract has been damaged). It seems likely that the spasticity is caused primarily by interruption of the corticoreticulospinal pathways. In monkeys, spasticity ensues after lesions of the motor and premotor cortex.

We should also keep in mind that a lesion of the internal capsule may interrupt many tracts of importance for motor control other than the corticospinal and corticoreticular ones. Thus, many fibers acting (directly or indirectly) on the cerebellum and on the basal ganglia will usually be destroyed, and this probably contributes to clumsiness of voluntary movements. Many patients with capsular hemiplegia have sensory symptoms in addition to the motor ones, because the thalamus itself may be partly affected, or the ascending fiber tracts conveying sensory signals from the thalamus to the cortex are interrupted. Reduced or altered cutaneous sensation and kinesthesia may also contribute to the motor symptoms.

For patients without any sensory symptoms, their difficulties with precise, voluntary movements—particularly of distal body parts—are most likely due largely or only to destruction of the pyramidal tract. When, as is often the case, movements of more proximal body parts are also affected, this is most likely caused mainly by destruction of descending fibers to the reticular formation.

NOTES

1. There are considerable individual variations in the percentage of the corticospinal fibers that are uncrossed, a matter of clinical importance. There are also individual variations with regard to the distribution of crossed and uncrossed fibers in the lateral and ventral funiculi. The uncrossed ventral component appears as a rule to be small, seldom reaching below the thoracic part of the cord. In monkeys, several studies with sensitive tracer techniques have failed to show a ventral corticospinal tract at lumbar levels. Some of the corticospinal fibers cross twice, first at the medullary level and then in the cord. Such fibers terminate medially in the ventral horn (Fig. 9.6).

2. Studies of monkeys with implanted microelectrodes have shown that not only the cerebral cortex is activated before a voluntary movement; there is also increased neuronal activity in the cerebellum, the basal ganglia, the thalamus, and parts of the limbic structures.

3. Such disagreement is probably caused by lack of clear-cut cytoarchitectonic changes when moving anteriorly from area 4 into area 6. Many cytoarchitectonic borders, as depicted so confidently in maps like that in Figure 17.3, are in reality seldom unequivocal. This is witnessed by the often great differences between maps published by different authors.

4. The so-called Jackson epileptic fits (described in Chapter 4) illustrate the somatotopic pattern within the MI. The abnormal discharges of the neurons start at one site in the MI and spread out in a regular manner. Thus, the muscular cramps start in one part of the body—for example, the foot—and spread to the lower leg, then to the thigh, the abdomen, the shoulder, and so forth. Nearly always, the fits start around the mouth, in the tongue, the thumb, or the big toe. This is best explained by the fact that cortical neurons controlling these parts occupy the largest volume of the MI, and also have the largest proportion of monosynaptic corticomotoneuronal connections.

5. The plantar reflex is normally extensor ("inverted") in infants and may be so for up to about 2 years. This correlates well with the myelination period of the human pyramidal tract and the concomitant development of fractionated movements of the fingers.

10

The Basal Ganglia

In the previous chapter, we discussed descending pathways from the cerebral cortex, which (directly and indirectly) influence the motoneurons and thereby are crucial for the initiation and control of movements. It was formerly believed that the basal ganglia also have ample connections to the spinal cord, and such connections were regarded as an important part of the so-called extrapyramidal system. That the basal ganglia are related to the control of movement has been known for a long time; diseases affecting primarily the basal ganglia lead to characteristic disturbances of movement and of the resting muscle tone. Improved methods for tracing fiber connections have shown, however, that the main efferent connections of the basal ganglia do not descend to motor nuclei in the brain stem and spinal cord but are rather directed "upstream" to the motor and other areas of the cerebral cortex. The fact that diseases of the basal ganglia do not produce pareses is in keeping with the fact that they play a different role in motor control than the descending central motor pathways.

Broadly speaking, *the basal ganglia are intercalated in a loop of fiber connections from the cerebral cortex and back to the cerebral cortex via the thalamus.* In this respect, the basal ganglia resemble the cerebellum. Infor-

mation from large parts of the cerebral cortex is processed in the basal ganglia (and in the cerebellum) before "answers" are sent back to, primarily, the motor areas of the cortex (Fig. 10.3). The nature of the processing that takes place in the basal ganglia is largely unknown, even though our knowledge about the internal "machinery" and the connections of the basal ganglia has increased enormously in the last few years.

The tasks of the basal ganglia are most likely not restricted to motor control, however. Even though the most obvious symptoms in diseases of the basal ganglia are related to the motor system, both clinical and experimental evidence indicates that the basal ganglia also play a role in higher mental functions. (This is another reminder that classification of parts of the brain into rigid functional categories such as "motor," "sensory," and "cognitive" must not be taken literally but rather as didactic oversimplifications.)

STRUCTURE AND CONNECTIONS OF THE BASAL GANGLIA

The term basal ganglia usually includes the *caudate nucleus, the putamen, and the globus pallidus* (Figs. 2.28, 2.30, 10.1, and

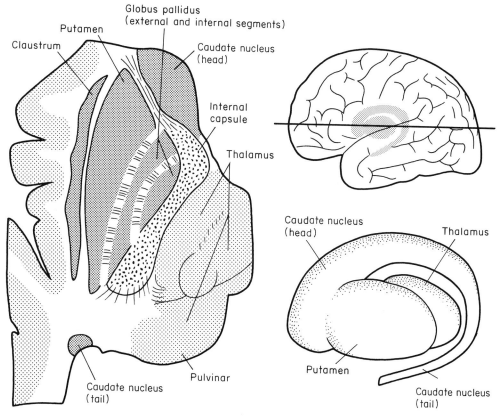

Fig. 10.1. *The shape and position of the basal ganglia.*

10.2).[1] Because of their macroscopic shape, the putamen and globus pallidus together are called the *lentiform nucleus*. The caudate nucleus and the putamen are similarly built, with predominantly small perikarya. They are also functionally related and are collectively termed the *striatum* or *neostriatum*. The neostriatum contains several neuronal types that differ with regard both to where they send their axons and which neurotransmitters they use (see below). Most of the neurons, however, send their axons out of the striatum (projection neurons), whereas a small group are interneurons with axons ramifying locally within the striatum. The presence of such neurons, among other things, indicates that the striatum is not simply a relay station but also performs considerable processing of information.

The globus pallidus has a different internal structure than the striatum, with larger, more "motoneuron"-like cells, and is also called the *paleostriatum* or *pallidum*. The term *corpus striatum* includes both the pallidum and the neostriatum. Phylogenetically, the caudate nucleus and the putamen developed together and are younger than the pallidum (thus the names neostriatum and paleostriatum). As we will see, these two main divisions of the basal ganglia differ also with regard to connections.

When the term basal ganglia (as in the present account) is used of a set of functionally related cell groups rather than in a strictly topographic sense, we should also include the *substantia nigra* and the *subthalamic nucleus* because both are intimately connected with the corpus striatum. Cell groups that join the corpus striatum ventrally without sharp transitions (such as the

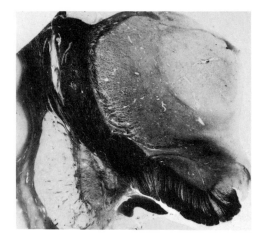

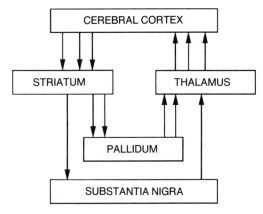

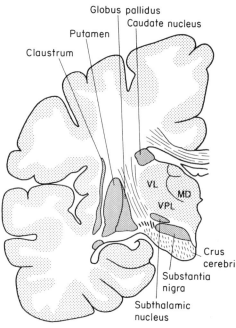

Fig. 10.2. *The basal ganglia in frontal sections.* The photomicrograph is of a myelin-stained section. The drawing **below** is from a slightly different anteroposterior level than the photomicrograph.

Afferent Connections of the Basal Ganglia

The striatum, which is largely the receiving part of the basal ganglia, is characterized by three sets of afferents from the *cerebral cortex,* the *intralaminar thalamic nuclei,* and *dopamine-containing cell groups in the mesencephalon* (Figs. 10.4 and 10.6).

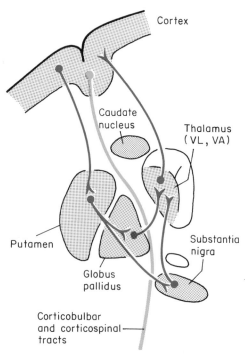

Fig. 10.3. *Main connections of the basal ganglia.* Note the pathway from the cortex, through the basal ganglia, and back to the cortex via the thalamus.

nucleus accumbens and the olfactory tubercle) often are now also included among the basal ganglia. These cell groups are collectively termed the *ventral striatum.*

Before going into detail about the connections of the basal ganglia, we may sum up the main features in the following diagram:

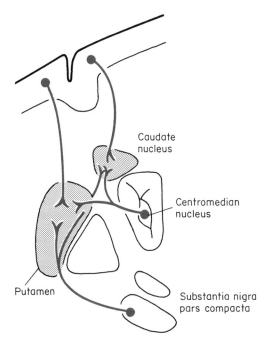

Fig. 10.4. *The main efferent connections of the striatum.*

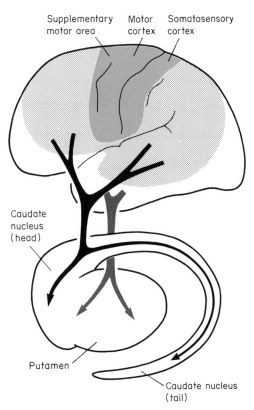

Fig. 10.5. *The putamen and the caudate nucleus* receive fibers from different parts of the cortex.

The largest contingent of afferents comes from the cerebral cortex. Almost all areas of the cortex send fibers to the striatum, but the caudate nucleus and the putamen receive from different parts of the cortex (Fig. 10.5). The putamen is dominated by somatotopically organized inputs from the SI and MI. The caudate nucleus, on the other hand, receives fibers predominantly from the association areas—that is, regions that perhaps are less directly concerned with motor control than with higher mental functions and emotions. Whereas the putamen receives relatively "raw," or unprocessed, information from sensory receptors via the SI and from motor cells in the MI, the caudate nucleus receives information that is a result of integration of signals from many sources. Such information reaching the caudate nucleus may, for example, concern earlier stages in the chains of neural events eventually leading to voluntary movements.[2]

In addition to cortical afferents, the striatum (including the ventral striatum) receives important connections from the *in-tralaminar thalamic nuclei* (Fig. 2.23), especially the *centromedian nucleus (CM)* (Fig. 10.4).

With regard to striatal afferents from *dopamine-containing cell groups in the mesencephalon,* the major contingent arises in the *substantia nigra.* More scattered dopaminergic cells outside the substantia nigra send their fibers primarily to the ventral striatum.[3]

Additional afferents to the striatum come from the *raphe nuclei* in the brain stem (serotonin), among other cell groups.

The Striatum Has a Complex Intrinsic Organization: Cell Types and Mosaic Arrangement

Anatomically, at least six different cell types have been observed in the striatum. Some of these have been characterized with regard to connections

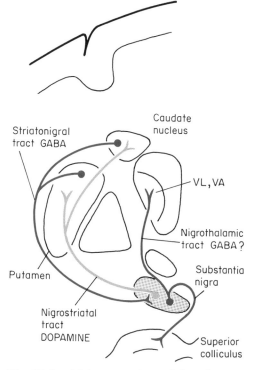

Fig. 10.6. *Main connections of the substantia nigra* (see also Fig. 10.10).

judged from electron microscopic cytochemical studies combined with HRP tracing. In agreement with this, both cell types express mRNA for dopamine receptors.

The various cell types, and in particular the neurotransmitters, are not evenly distributed throughout the striatum. Rather, different smaller compartments can be defined with regard to connections and cytochemistry. In microscopic sections, a mosaic pattern appears after staining to demonstrate acetylcholine esterase. Poorly stained patches called *striosomes* are embedded in a heavily stained *matrix*. Several neuropeptides, such as substance P, somatostatin, and enkephalin, are most abundant within the striosomes. GABAergic projection neurons are found within both the matrix and the striosomes. The two kinds of dopamine receptors are also differentially distributed (at least in the cat): D_1 receptors are reported to be 30%–50% more abundant in the striosomes than in the matrix, whereas the reverse situation exists with regard to D_2 receptors. Cholinergic interneurons appear to be present in both compartments. The connections of the striosomes and the matrix compartments also differ—for example, from which cortical areas they receive fibers, and even in which cortical layer the projecting cells are located.

It is fair to say that, in spite of a wealth of interesting data, the functional significance of the division of the striatum into numerous minor compartments is still a matter of speculation (and the interpretation of data is made more difficult by the existence of species differences). This should come as no surprise, considering the complexity of the striatum. To reveal for each neuronal type where it sends all its axonal branches and the cell types with which it establishes synaptic contacts, at the same time determine its content of transmitter candidates and other neuroactive substances, and furthermore correlate this with the distribution of receptors is a formidable task. It requires studies combining axonal tracing, Golgi impregnation of perikarya and dendrites, and immunocytochemistry (at the light and electron microscopic level). But this is not enough; we also need to know the physiological properties of the cell types, and this requires intracellular recording from single neurons, followed by intracellular staining. These kinds of data also have to be correlated in minute detail with the intricate patterns of afferent and efferent connections.

and content of neurotransmitters. More than 90% of the neurons have relatively small perikarya and dendrites with numerous spines (Fig. 10.11). This cell type contains GABA and sends its axon out of the striatum to the globus pallidus and the substantia nigra (called medium-sized, densely spiny neuron, or medium spiny neuron for short). There appear to exist two subtypes of this medium spiny neuron: One kind contains substance P in addition to GABA and projects primarily to the internal segment of the pallidum and to the substantia nigra; the other contains enkephalin in addition to GABA and projects mainly to the external segment of the pallidum. The other cell types are most likely interneurons—that is, their axonal arborizations remain within the striatum. One conspicuous kind of interneuron has a large perikaryon and smooth dendrites and contains *acetylcholine*. The action of acetylcholine in the striatum seems to be predominantly excitatory. Dopaminergic terminals of nigrostriatal neurons contact both projection neurons and the cholinergic interneurons, as

Efferent Connections of the Basal Ganglia

The effects exerted by the basal ganglia on other parts of the nervous system are mediated primarily by efferent fibers from the pallidum and the substantia nigra. These nuclei receive their main efferents from the striatum, as shown in the diagram on p. 248 (and Figs. 10.3 and 10.6). In this manner, information from the striatum is processed in the pallidum and nigra before being forwarded to the thalamus. The connections are topographically organized, so that subdivisions of the striatum are connected with specific parts of the pallidum and the nigra.

The *globus pallidus* consists of two parts, an *external* and an *internal segment* (Figs. 10.1, 10.2, and 10.7). Both receive their main afferents from the striatum. The main part of the efferents from the internal segment goes to the thalamus (Fig. 10.3).[4] Many of the fibers pass through the internal

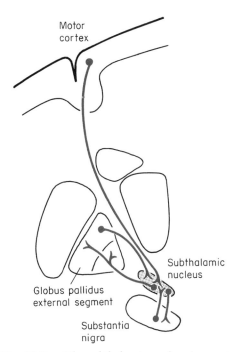

Fig. 10.7. *The subthalamic nucleus* has reciprocal connections with the pallidum and the substantia nigra.

capsule (Fig. 10.3) and can therefore be damaged by lesions in this region (this should be kept in mind when analyzing the symptoms occurring after the common infarctions in this region, as discussed in Chapter 9). In the thalamus the pallidal fibers end in the *ventral anterior nucleus (VA)* and in parts of the *ventral lateral nucleus (VL)* (Figs. 10.2, 10.3, 11.14, and 17.7). Some fibers also end in the *CM*. The VL and VA send their main efferents to the cerebral cortex (Fig. 11.14). The CM, on the other hand, as part of the intralaminar thalamic nuclei, sends its main efferent projection back to the striatum. This is one of several examples of subcortical "side loops" used by the basal ganglia, which in some way influence the messages that are sent to the cerebral cortex.

The VL and VA Are More Than Simple Relays

So far, we have considered the thalamic nuclei VL and VA as just relay stations in which impulses from the pallidum and nigra directed to the cerebral cortex are synaptically interrupted. Considerable processing of information takes place in these nuclei, however; what goes out is not a mirror image of what goes in. Thus, like other thalamic nuclei, the VL and VA receive afferents from sources other than the basal ganglia. They both receive ample connections from the parts of the cortex to which they project. (The VL receives connections from the cerebellum, but such fibers appear in the monkey to end in other parts of the VL than the pallidal fibers, making the possibility of interactions small.) The VA receives fibers also from the reticular formation and the intralaminar thalamic nuclei (especially the large CM). On the basis of anatomic and physiological evidence, the VA appears to be of special importance for the action of the reticular formation on the cerebral cortex and, thereby, probably on the level of consciousness (see Chapter 12).

The *substantia nigra* also sends fibers to the thalamus, ending in slightly different parts than the pallidal fibers.

The parts of the VL that receive fibers from the pallidum and the nigra project primarily to the *supplementary motor area*

(SMA), whereas the VA sends efferent fibers to the *premotor area* (PMA) and the *prefrontal cortex* (Fig. 11.14). Thus, *a large part of the impulse traffic from the basal ganglia is directed toward the motor cortical areas.* Physiological studies also indicate that the influence of the basal ganglia on motor control involves the corticospinal tract and indirect descending pathways from the cerebral cortex to the motoneurons (Fig. 10.3). It is worth noticing, however, that the caudate nucleus—which receives afferents mainly from association areas of the cortex—probably acts primarily on the prefrontal cortex, which is not directly involved in motor control but rather in *cognitive tasks.* Lesions of the caudate nucleus in monkeys produce symptoms similar to those seen after damage to the prefrontal cortex: Among other things, reduced performance in tests requiring spatial memory (such as to recall where an object is located when it is out of sight; this is discussed further in Chapter 17).

In addition to the massive connections from the basal ganglia to the thalamus, there are also efferents reaching the *reticular formation* (especially in the mesencephalon) and the *superior colliculus.* Connections to a part of the mesencephalic reticular formation called the *pedunculopontine nucleus (PPN)* has attracted special interest because this region may be coexistent with the mesencephalic locomotor region (electrical stimulation of this region elicits walking movements in cats). One may therefore speculate whether these connections are of relevance for the characteristic disturbances of locomotion seen in Parkinson's disease (in which there is marked cell loss in the substantia nigra). Connections from the substantia nigra to the superior colliculus (Fig. 10.6) are probably of importance for the control of coordinated head and eye movements.

The main efferent connections of the basal ganglia may be summarized as follows: *The internal segment of the globus pallidus and the substantia nigra send the final product of basal ganglia processing toward pre-* motor networks in the mesencephalic tegmentum, superior colliculus, and thalamus (Chevalier and Deniau).

Transmitters and Synaptic Actions of Neurons within the Cortex–Basal Ganglia–Cortex Loop: Disinhibition

To understand the processing going on within the basal ganglia and the effects of the ganglia on other parts of the brain, we need to know the transmitters and the synaptic actions of all the neurons involved. Hardly any other part of the brain has been as intensely investigated with regard to neurotransmitters and other neuroactive substances as the basal ganglia, and the conditions turn out to be extremely complex. More than 100 neuroactive substances have been found in the striatum so far, and more are undoubtedly still to be discovered. So far, however, only a few can be correlated with anatomic and physiological data (Figs. 10.6 and 10.11).

The *corticostriate* connections (Fig. 10.4) are excitatory, most likely due to release of glutamate (as is probably the case with all corticofugal fibers). The vast majority of the *striatopallidal and striatonigral* fibers (Figs. 10.3 and 10.6) are known to contain GABA and to have inhibitory effects. The *pallidothalamic* (and most likely also the nigrothalamic) fibers are also GABAergic and inhibitory. The *thalamocortical* fibers (from the VL and VA, as from other thalamic nuclei) are excitatory. Thus, the flow of information from the cerebral cortex through the basal ganglia and back is less straightforward than if all involved synapses were excitatory.

Theoretically, increased cortical input to the striatum would lead to decreased activity of the pallidal neurons (because excitation of striatal neurons produces increased inhibition in the pallidum). This in turn would increase the activity of thalamocortical neurons (because they would receive less inhibition from the pallidum). *Thus, excitatory impulses from the cortex would eventually produce disinhibition of the thal-*

amocortical neurons (and probably also of other "premotor" neurons in the reticular formation and the superior colliculus receiving fibers from the substantia nigra). Recordings of single-cell activity in the basal ganglia in awake monkeys are compatible with these considerations. At rest, most striatal neurons are "silent"—that is, they do not produce action potentials—whereas the pallidal neurons (and neurons in the pars reticulata of the substantia nigra) fire with a regular and high frequency. This would presumably keep the "premotor" neurons in the thalamus in a state of inhibition when the animal is not moving. Commands from the cortex to the basal ganglia in relation to the preparation or execution of movements would release the thalamocortical neurons from this inhibition. Indeed, electrophysiological experiments show that increased striatal activity reduces the activity of many pallidal and nigral neurons, followed by increased firing of thalamocortical neurons.

It has been proposed that the disinhibition of "premotor neurons" by the basal ganglia is a gating mechanism to control the access of other inputs (for example, sensory) to the motor cortex. Since the connections of the basal ganglia are topographically organized at all levels, this would be a specific and focused gating rather than a diffuse one, varying with the nature of the motor task.

The Actions of Dopamine in the Striatum Are Complex

The most studied basal ganglia connection is the *dopaminergic nigrostriatal pathway*, which is the most massive dopaminergic pathway in the central nervous system. Striatal neurons contain, not unexpectedly, dopamine receptors. The synaptic actions of dopamine in the striatum are nevertheless not fully understood. Possibly, dopamine has excitatory effects on certain striatal neuronal types and inhibitory effects on others. Thus, some studies indicate that dopamine has a weak excitatory effect on the GABAergic projection neurons of the striatum, whereas it has a strong inhibitory action on the cholinergic interneurons (Fig. 10.11). Recent studies suggest that the effects may be even more diverse: GABAergic striatal neurons (also containing substance P) pro-

jecting to the substantia nigra and the internal segment of the globus pallidus are excited by dopamine, whereas the GABAergic neurons (also containing enkephalin) projecting to the external segment of the globus pallidus are inhibited. This part of the globus pallidus sends fibers to the subthalamic nucleus with an inhibitory action. Furthermore, the effects of dopamine are probably not limited to actions on ion channels with subsequent brief depolarization or hyperpolarization.

With regard to *dopamine receptors,* both the D_1 and D_2 types are present in the striatum, but with somewhat different distributions within the striosomes and the matrix, as mentioned. Interestingly, in situ hybridization studies in the rat have shown that only about 50% of the medium spiny striatal neurons (that is, the neurons projecting out of the striatum) express mRNA for D_2 receptors. The effects of D_1 and D_2 receptor activation appear to be different: D_1 activates the enzyme adenyl cyclase, leading to increased intracellular level of cAMP, whereas D_2 inhibits adenyl cyclase activity. Such observations may perhaps explain why the synaptic effects on striatal neurons of dopamine are so varied and difficult to clarify.

The Subthalamic Nucleus Has Reciprocal Connections with the Pallidum and the Substantia Nigra

Whereas efferents of the internal pallidal segment primarily end in the thalamus, fibers from the external pallidal segment are directed toward the subthalamic nucleus (Fig. 10.7). Most of the efferents from the subthalamic nucleus go back to the pallidum and to the pars reticulata of the substantia nigra. The efferents of the subthalamic nucleus are topographically organized in the monkey, as shown with axonal transport methods. Thus, different neuronal populations project to the substantia nigra and the pallidum, and there are also differences with the regard to projections to minor parts of the pallidum.

Even though the subthalamic nucleus also receives some afferents from the motor cortex, it is primarily a part of side loops of the pallidum and the nigra—perhaps assisting them in certain computations. The violent involuntary movements of the opposite body half after destruction of the subthalamic nucleus (hemiballismus) are therefore presumably closely related to altered activity of neurons in the pallidum and nigra.

Contrary to previous findings, recent studies suggest that the subthalamic efferents use glutamate as a transmitter and have an excitatory effect on pallidal neurons (rather than GABA with inhibitory actions, as was the former view). Since neurons in the internal segment of the pallidum are known to inhibit thalamic neurons, the loss of subthalamic input would lead to *disinhibition* of the thalamic neurons (less inhibitory input from the pallidum). The thalamocortical neurons are excitatory, and thus the hemiballistic movements might perhaps be caused by hyperactivity among the thalamocortical neurons.

The Substantia Nigra

The substantia nigra and some of its connections have been mentioned several times, and we will

also return to it when dealing with Parkinson's disease, in which the nigra plays a crucial role. A collective treatment of the main features of the substantia nigra may therefore be pertinent at this stage. The substantia nigra can be divided anatomically into two parts, the *pars compacta* and the *pars reticulata* (Figs. 10.8 and 10.10). The compacta is richer in cells than the reticulata, whereas the latter (as the name implies) is dominated by dendritic arborizations. The reticulata also contains numerous neurons, however. The compacta neurons (Fig. 10.9) contain pigment (neuromelanin), which makes the nigra visible as a dark band in the freshly cut human mesencephalon. The pars reticulata, located ventral to the compacta, is lighter.

The *afferent* connections of the nigra (Figs. 10.6 and 10.7) arise in numerous cell groups, but quantitatively the most important input comes from the striatum. Even though most striatonigral fibers terminate in the pars reticulata, cells in the compacta can also be influenced because their long dendrites extend into the reticulata (Fig. 10.10). GABA is the most likely transmitter for the majority of the striatonigral fibers that exert an inhibitory effect on the cells in the nigra. Electrophysiological experiments show this inhibi-

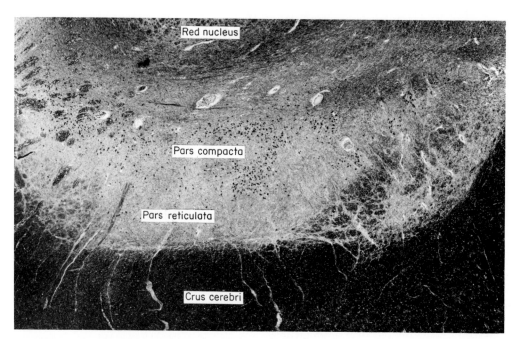

Fig. 10.8. *The substantia nigra.* Photomicrograph of transverse section through the mesencephalon (myelin stain). The cells of the pars compacta are clearly seen as dark dots. The dark color is due to their content of pigment. The photomicrograph is from the section shown in Figure 2.22.

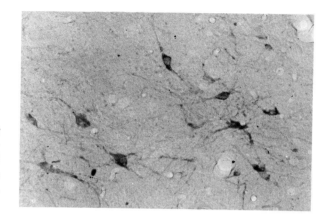

Fig. 10.9. *Dopaminergic cells in the substantia nigra.* Immunocytochemical demonstration of an enzyme used in the synthesis of dopamine (tyrosine hydroxylase). Magnification, ×180. Courtesy of Dr. J.-E. Aas.

tory effect, but, in addition, many nigral cells are excited by electrical stimulation of the striatum. This double action is not fully understood; it may perhaps be caused by release of substance P by a separate population of striatal efferent neurons (Fig. 10.11). Another possibility is that the efferent neurons of the pars reticulata, which are inhibited by the striatal input, send recurrent collaterals that inhibit other reticulata cells in their vicinity. Thus, these latter cells would be disinhibited and therefore increase their firing.

Other afferents to the substantia nigra arise in the *pallidum* (probably GABA), in the *subthalamic nucleus* (probably glutamate), the *nucleus locus coeruleus* (norepinephrine), and the *raphe nuclei* (serotonin).

The *efferent* connections of the substantia nigra (Figs. 10.3, 10.4, 10.7, and 10.10) pass primarily to the *striatum* and the *thalamus*, with smaller contingents to cell groups in the *reticular formation* and the *superior colliculus*, as mentioned above. The *dopaminergic nigrostriatal neurons* are located in the pars compacta (Fig. 10.9), whereas the *GABAergic nigrothalamic* neurons are located primarily in the pars reticulata. The nigral neurons sending their axons to the superior colliculus are also found in largely separate parts of the nigra. Furthermore, the nigral afferents from different parts of the striatum (such as the putamen and caudate nucleus) end differently. Thus, *the substantia nigra most likely consists of several functionally different parts*, differing both with regard to afferents and the cell groups on which they exert their action.

The Basal Ganglia Are Probably Arranged in Functionally Different, Parallel Circuits

Anatomic studies with the use of axonal transport methods have shown that the af-

Fig. 10.10. The *substantia nigra* consists of two parts, which differ structurally and with regard to connections. Note that afferent fibers to the pars reticulata contact the dendrites of the dopaminergic neurons in the pars compacta.

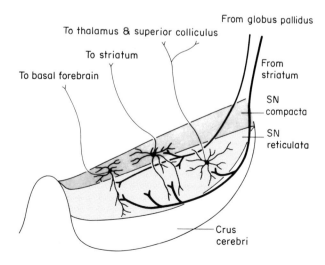

From globus pallidus

To thalamus & superior colliculus

To striatum

From striatum

To basal forebrain

SN compacta

SN reticulata

Crus cerebri

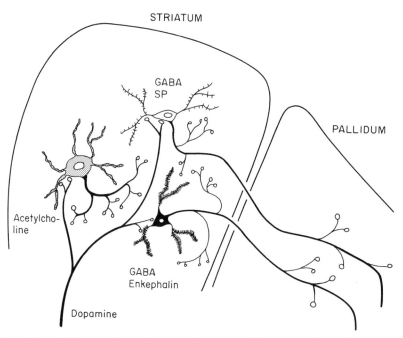

Fig. 10.11. *Three different cell types in the striatum.* Most of striatal efferent neurons are GABAergic. Note the large, cholinergic interneurons. There are other cell types in the striatum than those shown here.

ferent and efferent connections of the basal ganglia have a high degree of topographic order. Connections from functionally different parts of the cortex end differently in the striatum, and this localization goes much further than depicted in Figure 10.5. The next links from the striatum to the pallidum and the substantia nigra are also topographically arranged. For example, by the use of two fluorescent tracers in the same experiment, it has been shown in the monkey that the caudate nucleus projects primarily to the nigra, whereas the putamen is more strongly connected with the pallidum. Accordingly, few cells in the striatum send axon collaterals to both the nigra and the pallidum.

On the basis of such data, it has been suggested that there are four (or more) lines or *circuits through the basal ganglia,* in which the flow of information is kept segregated. Such circuits presumably handle different kinds of information and participate in different tasks. Thus, recent studies indicate that *the basal ganglia process different kinds of information in parallel, rather than being* *primarily concerned with integration of information from large parts of the cortex.*

Cortex–Basal Ganglia–Cortex Parallel Circuits

One circuit appears to arise in the *SMA, MI and SI,* passes through the putamen, and finally (via the pallidum and the thalamus) ends in the SMA. This circuit is probably most directly involved in control of movements. Recordings of single-cell activity in the putamen support this assumption. Another circuit arises in parts of the frontal and parietal lobes concerned with oculomotor control—that is, *area 8* immediately in front of area 6, and *area 7* (Fig. 17.3). Via particular parts of the caudate nucleus, this circuit appears to end in area 8. This area is also called the *frontal eye field* and is of particular importance for certain kinds of voluntary eye movements (see Chapter 13). Two circuits are postulated to arise in different parts of the *prefrontal cortex* and pass via the caudate nucleus, the substantia nigra (to a lesser degree the pallidum), the VA, and the mediodorsal thalamic nucleus (MD in Figs. 10.2, 17.7, and 17.8) and back to prefrontal cortical areas.

This prefrontal circuit presumably enables the basal ganglia to influence higher mental functions. Finally, one postulated circuit arises in *"limbic" parts of the cortex* (the cingulate gyrus, orbitofrontal areas of the frontal lobe, and parts of the temporal lobe cortex, which are parts of or closely connected with the limbic structures; see Chapter 16). This "limbic" circuit passes through the ventral striatum, ventral pallidum, and the MD of the thalamus and back to the cortical areas from which the circuit started.

FUNCTIONS OF THE BASAL GANGLIA

In spite of enormous research activity and rapid progress during recent years, the functions of the basal ganglia are still far from fully understood. Even the most voluminous textbooks often restrict themselves to vague statements, such as "movement control," "control of muscle tone," "assist in cognitive tasks," and "influence mood and motivation."

Taking the connections of the basal ganglia as a starting point, it is noteworthy that their major output goes to the SMA, PMA, and the prefrontal cortical areas. The properties of these areas suggest that the basal ganglia would be important in the planning phase of a movement, such as when several single-joint movements have to be put together to produce a complex movement, or when sensory stimuli or stored information has to be translated into an adequate motor response. It has been suggested, for example, that the basal ganglia participate when movements are learned by pure repetition and not by gaining insight into the nature of the task and, furthermore, that the basal ganglia enable automatic performance of well-rehearsed movements by the use of motor programs located elsewhere in the central nervous system.

It is also possible that the basal ganglia contribute to the linking of motivation and emotions to the execution of movements. Thus, recording of the activity of single cells in the striatum indicates that many respond best when a stimulus is linked with memory of an event that has a particular significance for the animal. Certain cells in the substantia nigra are, for example, active just before a rapid eye movement, but only when the movement is directed toward a target the animal cannot see and therefore has to remember where the target is.

Are the Basal Ganglia Concerned with Initiation of Movements?

In the example above, with an eye movement temporally linked with activity of neurons in the basal ganglia, a crucial question is whether the movement is triggered by the basal ganglia activity. In other words, is the disinhibition of premotor neurons brought about by basal ganglia outputs sufficient to elicit specific movements, or is the excitability of the premotor neurons merely increased so they can react with action potential to another input? The latter appears to be the case, as judged from experiments in behaving monkeys. Thus, microinjection of a GABA agonist (muscimol) in the substantia nigra did not evoke rapid eye movements but gave a strong tendency to direct the gaze toward a certain point in the environment. Thus, to elicit a specific movement, the disinhibition induced by the basal ganglia (in the thalamus or the superior colliculus) probably must coincide in time with a command signal from another source.

Judged from the symptoms occurring in humans with diseases of the basal ganglia, it seems likely that in some manner they contribute to the speed of movements, with regard to both their start and further execution. Observations of symptoms in monkeys with lesions of the globus pallidus indicate that *learned movements primarily are slower than normal, whereas the manner in which the task is performed is not significantly altered.* Therefore, neither the movement command nor the movement program appears to be located within the basal ganglia themselves.

DISEASES OF THE BASAL GANGLIA

Since we do not understand the tasks of the basal ganglia and how they are carried out, it should come as no surprise that we are unable to explain fully the symptoms occurring in diseases of the basal ganglia. Nevertheless, considerable progress has been made recently with regard to the relationships between certain symptoms and the elements responsible within the basal ganglia.

As mentioned, the most obvious symptoms in diseases of the basal ganglia are motor ones. As a rule, there is a mixture of symptoms due to *loss of neuronal activity* (compare with pareses after destruction of central motor pathways) and symptoms due to *abnormally increased neuronal activity*[5] (compare with spasticity occurring after lesions of central motor pathways). The most frequent diseases of the basal ganglia make movements difficult to initiate—this is called *akinesia*—and when started, the movements are slower and smaller than normal—this is called *bradykinesia*. Since movements are difficult to initiate, there is also a conspicuous paucity of movements, usually implied in the term akinesia. In addition, there are more or less pronounced involuntary movements called *dyskinesia*.

The most frequent disease affecting the basal ganglia is *Parkinson's disease* or *parkinsonism* (another name is *paralysis agitans*). Typically, voluntary movements are hard to initiate (akinesia) and they are slower and smaller than normal (bradykinesia). The akinesia also leads to a conspicuous lack of facial movements—the face becomes like a "mask." In addition, there is an increased muscular resting tone (rigidity) and involuntary, rhythmic, alternating movements at rest (resting tremor). Patients with Parkinson's disease have regularly been found to have a pronounced cell loss in the substantia nigra and a corresponding decrease of dopamine in the striatum.

In *Huntington's disease* (Huntington's chorea), in which there is a marked cell loss in the striatum, the most pronounced symptom is involuntary, jerky, often "dance-like" movements (chorea).

Violent, large involuntary movements of one side of the body, called *hemiballismus,* occur typically after damage to the subthalamic nucleus of the opposite side.

Parkinson's Disease

This disease of unknown etiology usually starts during the fifth or sixth decade of life. The syndrome includes, as mentioned, *akinesia, bradykinesia, tremor, and rigidity*. In addition, there are also disturbances of *postural reflexes*. Notably, the body balance during walking is disturbed, so that the patient appears to be "running after his center of gravity." The steps are typically very short, which is due to the bradykinesia (the movements are not only slower than normal but also reduced in amplitude). When being pushed from behind, the patient has difficulty stopping and continues to move forward. The normal pendulum movements of the arms during walking are absent. There is also a conspicuous loss of facial expression, as mentioned. There are disturbances of the autonomic nervous system, such as increased salivation and secretion from sebaceous glands of the skin. We do not know how the basal ganglia would influence the autonomic nervous system, and the autonomic symptoms perhaps may be caused by a more general disturbance of monoamine metabolism (not only dopaminergic cell groups are affected in Parkinson's disease).

The *tremor* is typical, with its frequency of 3–6 per second, and it is most pronounced at rest. When the patient uses the hand, the tremor disappears or is reduced in amplitude. The increased muscle tone, the *rigidity,* is different from the spasticity occurring after lesions of central motor pathways. The resistance to passive movements is equal in extensors and flexors and is independent of whether the muscle is stretched slowly or rapidly. There is no clear-cut increase in the strength of the monosynaptic stretch reflex (such as the patellar reflex), whereas the long-latency stretch reflexes are increased, and this may perhaps contribute to the difficulties with balance and locomotion. The rigidity is apparently not caused by overactivity of γ motoneurons but rather by descending influences increasing the excitability of the α motoneurons so that they fire continuously—perhaps like the situation in a nervous person who is unable to relax his muscles.

The plantar reflex is normal in patients with Parkinson's disease, indicating that there is no damage to the central motor pathways. It is an old clinical observation that the tremor and rigidity disappear if a patient with Parkinson's disease has a capsular hemiplegia, and corresponding observations are made in experimental animals. The last central link in the pathways mediating the tremor and rigidity must therefore be pathways from the cerebral cortex to the motoneurons.

The most pronounced structural change in the brain of patients with Parkinson's disease is a profound loss of pigmented (melanin-containing) neurons in the pars compacta of the substantia nigra. These are the dopamine-containing neurons. As a consequence of the loss of dopaminergic nigrostriatal fibers, the dopamine content of the striatum is reduced (symptoms first appear when the dopamine content of the striatum is reduced by 80–90%). This latter finding led to attempts to alleviate the symptoms by giving the patients dopamine, to substitute for the loss of dopaminergic neurons. For various reasons, a precursor of dopamine—L-dopa—has to be used. This is converted to dopamine in the brain. This treatment had a beneficial effect on the symptoms, particularly on the very troublesome bradykinesia. Even though L-dopa has proved to be a very helpful drug, the first hopes turned out be unrealistic. The course of the disease is not affected by the drug, and the therapeutic effect decreases as the disease progresses. There probably must be a certain number of remaining dopaminergic neurons in the nigra for L-dopa to be converted to dopamine in the striatal dopaminergic boutons. More profound changes of the striatal neurons and their ability to react to dopamine may also occur. One might perhaps think that when the brain is unable to produce enough dopamine itself, it would not be able to produce dopamine from a supplied precursor either. However, enzymes converting L-dopa to dopamine are present not only in dopaminergic neurons in the nigra but also in glial cells and in other types of neuron.

The L-dopa treatment has *side effects,* as one might expect when giving a drug that acts not only in the striatum but also in many cell groups in the brain. For example, dopamine is present in the hypothalamus, and side effects like nausea, loss of appetite, and reduced control of blood pressure may perhaps be caused by actions there. Other side effects are sleep disturbances and changes of mood. In some cases the treatment can precipitate a psychosis. Such side effects may perhaps be related to actions of dopamine on the prefrontal cortex and parts of the limbic structures (see Chapter 17: "The Frontal Lobes and Psychiatric Disease"). Long-term treatment may provoke motor symptoms that are different from those caused by the disease, such as chorealike and athetoid dyskinesias (athetosis is used of slow, "worm-like," involuntary movements of the fingers and toes).

Not all symptoms occurring in Parkinson's disease can be explained on the basis of our present knowledge. One difficulty is represented by the apparently complex and not fully understood effects of dopamine in the striatum. The highly complex organization of the striatum with regard to both connections and distribution of neuroactive substances and their receptors further complicates the matter. Furthermore, pathological changes, although most marked in the pars compacta of the substantia nigra, also occur elsewhere, such as in the pars reticulata, in the nucleus locus coeruleus, and in some of the raphe nuclei. Dopaminergic projections from the midbrain to the frontal lobe are also affected by the disease.

Assuming for the moment that dopamine has a predominantly excitatory effect on striatal projection neurons (which are inhibitory), loss of dopamine would decrease striatal firing, with subsequent increased inhibitory output from the internal pallidal segment to the thalamus. This would presumably reduce the excitation received by cells in motor cortical areas from the thalamus and might be compatible with akinesia and bradykinesia in patients with Parkinson's disease. It would not readily explain the tremor and rigidity, however.

On the other hand, assuming that the effects of dopamine are predominantly inhibitory in the striatum, loss of dopamine would presumably lead to disinhibition of thalamic neurons. This might explain tremor and rigidity (as a consequence of increased cortical excitation received from the thalamus) but hardly akinesia and bradykinesia. That tremor and rigidity are mediated by changed activity in the VL and VA of the thalamus is supported by the results of surgical interruption of the pallidothalamic fibers. This operation usually reduces the tremor and rigidity significantly, with much less effect on akinesia and bradykinesia.

Another observation supports the concept that hyperactivity of striatal neurons may be an important factor in symptom production. Thus, anticholinergic drugs have a beneficial effect on the symptoms, suggesting that there may be hyperactivity of the cholinergic interneurons of the striatum in Parkinson's disease. Acetylcholine has a slow excitatory action on striatal neurons, and, as mentioned, there is evidence that dopamine inhibits cholinergic interneurons. Thus, anticholinergic drugs may perhaps act by reducing the hyperactivity of cholinergic interneurons caused by dopamine depletion in the striatum.

The effects of dopamine in the striatum are apparently multifarious, with different actions on subpopulations of projection neurons and interneurons. As mentioned, there is some evidence that dopamine excites striatal GABAergic neurons projecting to the internal pallidal segment (and the nigra), whereas the GABAergic neurons projecting to the external pallidal segment may be inhibited.[6] Furthermore, there is some experimental evidence that loss of dopamine in the ventral striatum is responsible for the akinesia, whereas loss of dopamine in the putamen is responsible for the rigidity.

The possibility of replacing by *transplantation* the lost dopaminergic neurons in Parkinson's disease is now under intense investigation. Animal experiments—pioneered by, among others, the Swedish neurobiologist Björklund—show that transplantation can eliminate virtually all symptoms produced by lesions of the substantia nigra in adult rats. The transplanted cells must come from an embryo, and a sufficient number must be put into the striatum in the adult lesioned animal. The best results are obtained when embryonic cells in a suspension are injected rather than being implanted as a solid piece of tissue. Because the transplanted cells are embryonic, they are not rejected, and start growing apparently normal processes in their new location. The cells synthesize and liberate dopamine. The method is now under trial for use in patients with Parkinson's disease, but it is not yet clear whether the method will work in humans. One major problem is presumably to obtain a sufficient number of transplanted embryonic cells for survival. Furthermore, the huge size of the human striatum poses problems that are not encountered in the small brain of the rat.

Huntington's Disease (Huntington's Chorea)

This disease is dominantly inherited and usually starts in the fourth decade of life. It has a steadily progressing course. The disease is characterized by rapid, jerky, involuntary movements of the face, arms, and legs. In advanced stages the patient is never at rest. The dancelike quality of the movements led to the terms *chorea* and *choreatic movements* (Greek: chorea = dance). The most prominent pathological change involves the striatum, with a marked reduction in the number of GABAergic projection neurons in the nucleus caudatus and the putamen.

The mechanism whereby loss of striatal neurons produces the choreatic movements is not known. Presumably, the loss of GABAergic striatal neurons leads to increased activity of inhibitory neurons in the external pallidal segment projecting to the subthalamic nucleus, and in the internal pallidal segment and in the substantia nigra projecting to the thalamus. Since the subthalamic nucleus most likely has excitatory effects on the internal pallidal segment, reduced activity of the subthalamic nucleus would reduce inhibition of the VL/VA neurons, with increased activity as a result (disinhibition). On the other hand, the loss of inhibitory striatal input to the internal pallidal segment would increase the inhibitory influence of the VL/VA neurons. One report claims, however, that in the early stages of the disease, the cell loss in the striatum mainly concerns the neurons projecting to the external pallidal segment (cells containing GABA and enkephalin), whereas the loss of neurons projecting to the internal pallidal segment (containing GABA and substance P) occurs at a later stage. Another hypothesis focuses on the possible hyperactivity of dopaminergic nigrostriatal neurons, which are normally inhibited by GABAergic striatonigral neurons. Even though there are several problems with this hypothesis, it fits with the observation that L-dopa worsens the choreatic movements of patients with Huntington's disease.

The disease also leads to mental deterioration with dementia, which probably may be explained by cell loss occurring also in the cerebral cortex (particularly the frontal lobes).

The etiology of the disease is unknown. One hypothesis is that the cell death is caused by a toxin produced in the brain, mimicking the action of glutamate on the striatal neurons, probably involving the NMDA receptor (see Chapter 1, "Ischemic Cell Damage"). It has recently been shown that the genetic defect is located on the short arm of chromosome 4, and this makes it possible to decide whether a person is a carrier of the disease long before the symptoms occur. However, to provide individuals with such knowledge as long as there is no effective treatment poses obvious ethical questions.

NOTES

1. The claustrum and the amygdaloid nucleus were also included in the term basal ganglia by the early anatomists. The function of the claustrum is still largely unknown, even though it is known to receive its main afferents from the cerebral cortex

and to send efferents directly back to the cortex. The amygdaloid nucleus differs with regard to both connections and function from the other parts of the basal ganglia and is now usually considered a part of the so-called limbic structures (Chapter 16).

2. The ventral striatum receives afferents mainly from parts of the limbic structures, such as the hippocampal formation and the amygdaloid nucleus, and from parts of the cortex closely related to limbic structures, such as the orbitofrontal cortical areas and parts of the temporal lobe.

3. The dopamine-containing neurons in the mesencephalon that are not located within the substantia nigra are mostly confined to a region called the *ventral tegmental area*. It is located dorsomedial to the substantia nigra. Since the main efferent connections of these scattered cell groups go to the ventral striatum and to other regions included in or closely related to limbic structures, the term *mesolimbic dopaminergic system* is often used.

4. The efferent fibers from the pallidum form two bundles, the *ansa lenticularis* and the *fasciculus lenticularis*. They arise from somewhat different parts of the internal pallidal segment and fuse to form the *fasciculus thalamicus* after having traversed the internal capsule.

5. Some authors distinguish between *hyperkinetic* and *hypokinetic* disorders. The hypokinetic disorders are characterized by reduced motor activity (akinesia and bradykinesia), whereas the hyperkinetic disorders are characterized by excessive, involuntary motor activity (dyskinesia). The best-known example of hypokinetic disorders is Parkinson's disease, whereas Huntington's chorea is an example of a hyperkinetic syndrome. It should be noted, however, that the hypokinetic disorders are usually combined with rigidity and tremor, whereas the hyperkinetic disorders are often combined with muscular hypotonia.

6. Loss of dopamine would in that case lead to reduced firing of thalamic neurons via two routes: one "direct" from the striatum to the internal pallidal segment and further to the VL/VA, and another "indirect" via the external pallidal segment and the subthalamic nucleus. In the direct route, there would be reduced excitation of inhibitory striatal neurons, leading to reduced inhibition of inhibitory pallidal neurons, which in their turn would cause increased inhibition of the VL/VA. Striatal neurons projecting to the external pallidal segment would increase their activity as a consequence of dopamine depletion, which in turn would produce decreased inhibition of subthalamic neurons. Provided that subthalamic neurons excite neurons in the internal pallidal segment, the latter would receive more excitation and thus provide the VA with more inhibition. Both routes would in that case produce increased inhibition of the VL/VA.

11

The Cerebellum

That the cerebellum is important for the execution of movements has been known for a long time from clinical observations. Its fiber connections also suggest a motor function: It is mainly connected with parts of the central nervous system involved in motor control, such as the spinal cord and the motor cortex. There are certain similarities between the cerebellum and the basal ganglia; both are involved in motor control without being responsible for the initiation of movements, and both are built into "side loops" of the motor cortical areas and the central motor pathways.

Damage to the cerebellum produces characteristic symptoms primarily with respect to the execution of voluntary movements. Our normal movements are always *coordinated*—that is, the various muscles participating contract at the proper time and with the proper force. This is a prerequisite for our ability to hit a nail with a hammer, for writing even and rounded letters, for the words to follow each other with proper loudness and rhythm during speech, and so forth. After cerebellar damage such coordination is lacking, and the movements become uncertain and jerky.

The cerebellum receives information from many sources. Sensory impulses come from the skin, joints, muscles, the vestibular apparatus, and the eye. In most instances, this sensory information appears to be related to aspects of movements, such as signals from muscle and joint receptors about positions and ongoing movements. Information is also coming from other parts of the central nervous system, especially from the cerebral cortex—primarily from cortical areas treating information about movements or involved in planning or initiation of movements. The cerebellum sends information primarily to cell groups that give origin to the central motor pathways, like the motor cortical areas and the reticular formation of the brain stem. (Some cerebellar connections, however, suggest that it may also be involved in functions other than motor ones.)

It is a striking feature of cerebellar organization that the number of afferent fibers leading to the cerebellum is much larger than the number of fibers leading out—in humans, the relationship is about 40:1. This would indicate that considerable integration and processing of the information reaching the cerebellum must take place before an answer is issued. *How* this processing is done is still largely unknown, despite very detailed knowledge of the structure and properties of the neuronal elements of the cerebellum.

In Figure 11.1, the thickness of the arrows

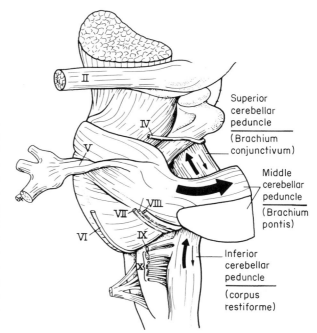

Fig. 11.1. *The cerebellar peduncles.* The brain stem seen from the left. The arrows indicate the peduncle used by the main afferent and efferent connections on entering or leaving the cerebellum. The thickness of the arrows indicates the magnitude of the various connections. Note the massive afferent pathway from the pontine nuclei entering through the middle cerebellar peduncle (the brachium pontis). The largest number of efferent fibers leave the cerebellum through the superior cerebellar peduncle (the brachium conjunctivum). From Brodal (1981).

indicates roughly the relative number of afferent and efferent fibers in the three cerebellar peduncles. The major afferent contingent enters through the middle cerebellar peduncle (the branchium pontis), whereas most of the efferent fibers leave the cerebellum through the superior cerebellar peduncle (the brachium conjunctivum).

SUBDIVISIONS, STRUCTURE, AND CONNECTIONS OF THE CEREBELLUM

The macroscopic anatomy of the cerebellum was described in Chapter 2, but some points bear repetition here. The external part of the cerebellum is a thin, highly convoluted sheet of gray matter, the *cerebellar cortex*. The folds are preponderantly arranged transversely and form *folia*. The underlying white matter contains the afferent and efferent fibers of the cerebellar cortex. In addition, masses of gray matter, the *intracerebellar nuclei,* are embedded in the white matter in the central parts of the cerebellum. These nuclei are relay stations in the efferent

connections of the cerebellar cortex (Figs. 11.10 and 11.12).

The Cerebellum Consists of Three Functionally Different Parts

The structure of the cortex is the same all over the cerebellum. Various parts of the cerebellum differ in function because of differences in fiber connections: The various subdivisions of the cerebellum receive afferents from and act on different parts of the nervous system. A subdivision of the cerebellum on the basis of functional differences corresponds closely with a subdivision on the basis of differences in where the afferent fibers come from (Fig. 11.2). Furthermore, such a subdivision corresponds also with one based on the cerebellar phylogenetic development from lower to higher animals.

The most primitive part of the cerebellum—the part occurring first during phylogeny—is the small *flocculonodular lobe* (Fig. 11.2). With reference to its phylogenetic age, it is also called the *archicerebellum.* It consists of the nodulus in the midline (a part of the vermis) connected laterally

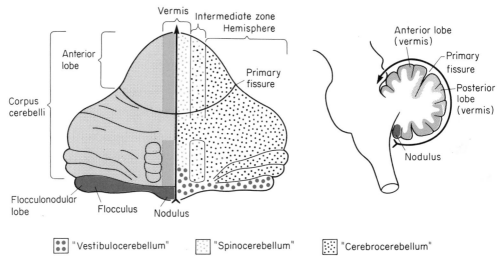

Fig. 11.2. *Main cerebellar subdivision.* To the **left,** a schematic drawing of a partly unfolded cerebellum. The **right** drawing shows how the unfolding was performed. The dots indicate roughly the cerebellar terminal regions of the main afferent contingents from the spinal cord, from the vestibular apparatus, and from the cerebral cortex via the pontine nuclei.

with a thin stalk to the flocculus. The size of this part of the cerebellum varies little among mammals. The flocculonodular lobe receives afferents primarily from the vestibular apparatus and the vestibular nuclei and is therefore also called the *vestibulocerebellum.* The rest of the cerebellum is called the *corpus cerebelli.* This comprises all of the *vermis* (except the nodulus), which forms a narrow zone on both sides of the midline, and the large lateral parts called the *cerebellar hemispheres.* The medialmost part of the hemispheres, bordering the vermis medially, is called the *intermediate zone* (Fig. 11.2). This zone cannot be distinguished from the rest of the cerebellum on a macroscopic basis but only on the basis of fiber connections. The corpus cerebelli is divided by a deep, transversely oriented fissure, the *primary fissure.* The parts of the corpus cerebelli in front of and behind the primary fissure are called the *anterior lobe* and the *posterior lobe,* respectively. The anterior and posterior parts of the vermis constitute the phylogenetically oldest parts of the corpus cerebelli and are together called the *paleocerebellum.* The midportion of the vermis and the hemispheres are younger and are therefore called the *neocerebellum.* The

anterior and posterior portions of the vermis and the adjoining parts of the intermediate zone of the corpus cerebelli receive afferents primarily from the spinal cord and are therefore also termed the *spinocerebellum.* The hemispheres receive their main input from the cerebral cortex, synaptically interrupted in the pontine nuclei, and are therefore termed the *cerebrocerebellum* or the *pontocerebellum.*

With regard to the *efferent connections* of the cerebellum, the three main subdivisions of the cerebellum *act on the parts of the central nervous system from which they receive their afferents;* that is, the vestibulocerebellum sends fibers mainly to the vestibular nuclei, the spinocerebellum influences the spinal cord, and the cerebrocerebellum acts on the cerebral cortex.

Afferent Connections from the Labyrinth and the Vestibular Nuclei

Primary vestibular afferents bring sensory impulses from the vestibular apparatus in the inner ear (the vestibular part of the labyrinth). They enter the cerebellum through the inferior cerebellar peduncle (Fig. 11.1) and end in the flocculonodular lobe and ad-

"VESTIBULOCEREBELLUM"

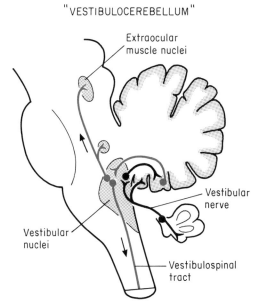

"SPINOCEREBELLUM"

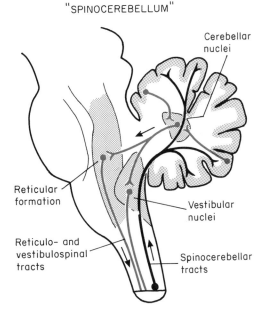

Fig. 11.3. *The main connections of the vestibulocerebellum.* Afferents are shown in black and efferents in red in a schematic drawing of a sagittal section through the brain stem. Note primary and secondary vestibulocerebellar fibers and the projection back to the vestibular nuclei. In addition to afferents from the vestibulocerebellum, the vestibular nuclei also receive cerebellar afferents from the anterior lobe vermis and from the fastigial nucleus.

joining parts of the vermis (Fig. 11.3). Most of the primary vestibular afferents do not end in the cerebellum but in the vestibular nuclei. Many neurons in the latter send axons to the cerebellum. In this manner, the cerebellum receives vestibular information also via *secondary vestibular afferents.* The vestibular input provides the cerebellum with information about the position and movements of the head. Efferents from the flocculonodular lobe end in the vestibular nuclei and can thereby influence the body equilibrium (via the vestibulospinal tracts) and eye movements (Fig. 11.3). This is treated more fully in Chapter 13.

Afferent Connections from the Spinal Cord

Several pathways bring impulses from the spinal cord to the cerebellum (Fig. 11.4).

Fig. 11.4. *The main connections of the spinocerebellum.* Note that the spinocerebellum can influence spinal motoneurons via reticulospinal and vestibulospinal pathways.

Some of these pathways go uninterrupted from the cord to the cerebellum and are called *direct spinocerebellar tracts,* whereas others are synaptically interrupted in brain stem nuclei and are therefore termed *indirect spinocerebellar tracts* (not shown in Fig. 11.4). The spinocerebellar tracts originate from neurons with their perikarya located in various lamina of the spinal cord (Fig. 2.12). They are therefore influenced by different kinds of receptors and spinal interneurons and bring different kinds of information to the cerebellum. *The spinocerebellar axons end mostly in the spinocerebellum of the same side* (as their perikarya). Some pass uncrossed; other fibers cross twice (first in the spinal cord and then back again in the brain stem). The fibers are located in the lateral funiculus as they ascend. The tracts are *somatotopically organized,* so that signals from different body parts are kept segregated. The somatotopic pattern is maintained within the cerebellum (Fig. 11.5) so that the leg is represented anteriorly within the anterior lobe, with the arm and the face represented successively more pos-

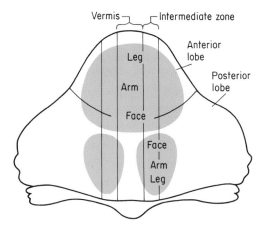

Fig. 11.5. *Somatotopic localization of the cerebellar cortex.* Based on experiments with electrical stimulation of peripheral nerves and of various subdivisions of the SI and the MI.

teriorly. In the posterior lobe the arrangement is the reverse, with the face represented anteriorly.

Functionally, the direct spinocerebellar tracts consist of two main groups. One group of tracts conveys information from *muscle spindles, tendon organs, and cutaneous low-threshold mechanoreceptors*. Physiological studies show that many of the neurons of the direct spinocerebellar tracts are activated monosynaptically by primary afferent (sensory) fibers. The tracts conduct very rapidly and appear to give precisely timed information about movements and skin stimuli (which also often are related to movements).

Another group of direct spinocerebellar tracts does not convey signals from receptors but provides information about *the level of activity among specific groups of spinal interneurons*. Such interneurons are as a rule intercalated in spinal reflex arcs and between descending motor pathways and motoneurons (that is, forming so-called premotor networks). Information about their activity is therefore presumably highly relevant for cerebellar operations.

Together, the spinocerebellar tracts provide the cerebellum with information about the activity both *before* and *after* the motoneurons—that is, about the commands issued to the motoneurons and the movements produced by the motoneuronal activity. The cerebellum can probably judge whether the command led to the desired result. When, for example, an unexpected increase of external resistance to a movement reduces the velocity compared with what was intended, the cerebellum will be informed immediately. Via its connections to the spinal cord, the cerebellum can then help to adjust the firing of the motoneurons to the new situation, so that the correct velocity is regained.

There are several *indirect spinocerebellar tracts*, but here we will only mention the one synaptically interrupted in the *inferior olive* in the medulla (Fig. 2.18). Neurons at all levels of the cord send fibers to the inferior olive of the opposite side. The spino-olivary fibers end in parts of the inferior olive that project to the spinocerebellum of the opposite side; thus, like the direct spinocerebellar tracts, the spino-olivocerebellar tract conveys information mainly from one side of the cord to the cerebellar half of the same side. This pathway, too, is precisely somatotopically organized. The kind of information conveyed by the spino-olivocerebellar tract appears to be different from that conveyed by the other spinocerebellar tracts. We will return to the inferior olive below, because this nucleus plays a unique role among cell groups sending fibers to the cerebellum.

The Dorsal, Ventral, and Some Other Spinocerebellar Tracts

Originally, two direct spinocerebellar tracts were described, differing with regard to the position of their fibers in the lateral funiculus of the cord. The fibers of one of the tracts are located dorsally and the tract was called the *dorsal spinocerebellar tract;* the fibers of the *ventral spinocerebellar tract* are located more ventrally (Fig. 11.6).

The *dorsal spinocerebellar tract* comes from a distinct cell group with fairly large cells at the base of the dorsal horn, forming the *column of Clarke* located in the spinal segments from T_1 to L_2 only. The axons of the cells in the column of Clarke ascend on the same side and enter the cerebellum through the inferior cerebellar peduncle.

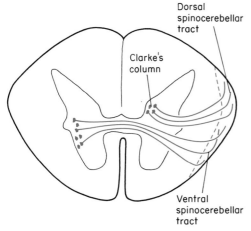

Dorsal
spinocerebellar
tract

Clarke's
column

Ventral
spinocerebellar
tract

Fig. 11.6. *The dorsal and ventral spinocerebellar tracts.* Schematic drawing of a transverse section through the thoracic cord, showing the position of the perikarya in the gray spinal matter and the tracts in the white matter. Most of the fibers of the ventral spinocerebellar tract cross twice (once in the cord and once in the brain stem), so that most spinocerebellar impulses reach the cerebellar half on the same side as the perikarya are located.

Primary afferent fibers—of which many come from muscle spindles and tendon organs—end monosynaptically on the neurons of the column of Clarke. Primary afferent fibers entering the cord through spinal nerves below the L_2 ascend in the dorsal columns before entering the lowermost part of the column of Clarke. The dorsal spinocerebellar tract conveys information only from the trunk and the lower extremities and ends in the corresponding parts of the spinocerebellum. The same kind of information from the upper extremities is mediated by another cell group, the *external cuneate nucleus,* located laterally in the medulla oblongata. Functionally, this nucleus corresponds to the column of Clarke, and primary afferents from the arms ascend in the dorsal columns to end in the nucleus. The cells of the external cuneate nucleus send their axons to the arm regions of the spinocerebellum of the same side (forming the cuneocerebellar tract).

The *ventral spinocerebellar tract* originates from cells located mainly laterally in lamina VII (Fig. 11.6)—that is, in the lamina containing the largest number of interneurons. Most of the axons cross at the segmental level in the cord to the lateral funiculus of the opposite side. However, after having reached the cerebellum through the superior cerebellar peduncle (Fig. 11.1), many of the fibers cross once more. The perikarya of the neurons giving origin to the ventral spinocerebellar neurons are found only below the midthoracic level of the cord and have a rostral counterpart conveying information from higher levels of the cord (the rostral spinocerebellar tract). These tracts convey information about the activity of the spinal interneurons, as mentioned above. Physiological experiments indicate that they primarily inform about the activity of inhibitory interneurons.

In addition to the spinocerebellar tracts mentioned so far, other cell groups in the spinal cord also send fibers to the cerebellum. Among such cell groups is the *central cervical nucleus,* located in the upper cervical segments. The fibers end in the anteriormost folia of the anterior lobe and transmit signals primarily from receptors around the cervical joints.

An additional indirect spinocerebellar pathway is relayed in the *lateral reticular nucleus,* located in the medulla just lateral to the inferior olive. This spinoreticulocerebellar pathway, too, is mainly uncrossed and appears to convey information about the activity of certain groups of spinal interneurons. Since most of the spinal interneurons are strongly influenced by descending motor pathways, the ascending tract to the lateral reticular nucleus probably informs about their activity as well. The lateral reticular nucleus also receives afferents from sources other than the spinal cord, notably the red nucleus, the vestibular nuclei, and the motor cortex. Many cells, for example, are strongly influenced by tilting of the head (stimulating vestibular receptors).

Information from sensory receptors can reach the cerebellum not only through some of the spinocerebellar tracts but also through fibers sent to the spinocerebellum from the dorsal column nuclei and the trigeminal nuclei.

Afferent Connections from the Cerebral Cortex

In humans, by far the largest number of cerebellar afferent fibers arises in the pontine nuclei (Figs. 2.19 and 11.7). The *pontocerebellar tract* ends primarily in the cerebellar hemispheres, which constitute the major part of the cerebellum in humans. The vast majority of afferents to the pontine nuclei

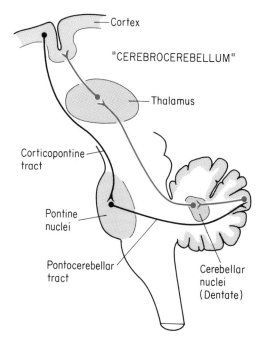

Fig. 11.7. *The main connections of the cerebro-cerebellum.* Note that the ascending connections to the cerebral cortex are synaptically interrupted in the dentate nucleus and in the thalamus. The projection to the cerebellar nuclei is GABAergic and inhibitory, whereas the thalamocortical fibers exert excitatory actions in the cortex.

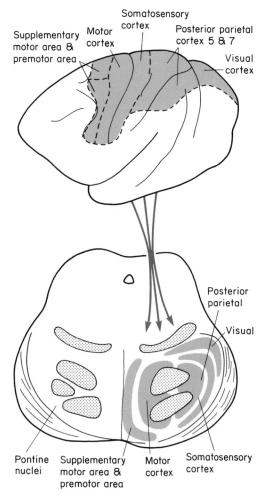

Fig. 11.8. *The corticopontine pathway.* Areas of the cerebral cortex that are strongly connected with the cerebellar hemispheres via the pontine nuclei are shown in red. Note the topographic arrangement of the corticopontine pathway in the pontine nuclei—each cortical region has its own territory.

arise in the cerebral cortex and form the *corticopontine tract* (Fig. 11.8).[1]

The main task of the pontine nuclei therefore is to process information from the cerebral cortex and forward it to the cerebellar cortex. The corticopontine tract is uncrossed, whereas most of the pontocerebellar fibers cross; thus *the cerebral cortex of one side acts mainly on the cerebellar hemisphere of the opposite side.*

The corticopontine tract runs in the *internal capsule* and then in the *crus cerebri* (Fig. 2.22), where it occupies a large part; of the approximately 19 million fibers in the crus of the human brain, the corticopontine fibers constitute the majority (the pyramidal tract, in comparison, contains only about 1 million fibers).

A large fraction of *the corticopontine fibers arise in the MI and SI.* There are, however, substantial contributions also from the

SMA and PMA and from *areas 5 and 7* of the posterior parietal cortex (Fig. 11.8). All of these areas are, in various ways, active during or before movements (see Chapter 9). Presumably, the cerebellum thus receives information about movements that are being planned and about the commands that are sent out from the motor cortex; in response it can modulate the activity of the motor cortex so that the movements are performed smoothly and accurately. The pontine nuclei also receive afferents from the *visual cor-*

tex, and physiological experiments indicate that these fibers inform primarily about moving objects in the visual field. Such connections may be of importance to the execution of visually guided movements.[2]

The pontine nuclei also receive connections from parts of the hypothalamus and limbic structures, particularly the *cingulate gyrus* and the *mammillary bodies.* The information conveyed from these regions is probably not directly related to movement, but may perhaps contribute to the well-known influence of motivation and emotions on movements.

Both the corticopontine and the pontocerebellar projections are topographically organized. This and other data indicate that there is a functional localization within the cerebellar hemispheres, so that smaller parts take care of specific tasks. In contrast to the cerebral cortex, the cerebellar cortex has no association and commissural connections—different parts of the cerebellum do not "talk" to each other. Thus, each subdivision of the cerebellar hemispheres that differs from its neighbors with regard to its afferent

connections from the cerebral cortex may probably be considered a separate functional unit. In this respect, the *cerebellum resembles the basal ganglia, which appear to be organized in several parallel circuits starting and ending in the cerebral cortex.*

The Intermediate Zone Is a Meeting Place for Impulses from the Cord and the Cerebral Cortex

The intermediate zone of the cerebellum is mainly defined on the basis of its efferent connections. It also has special features with regard to afferents, however (Fig. 11.9). Whereas the lateral parts of the hemispheres are strongly dominated by inputs from the cerebral cortex, and the vermis is dominated by spinal inputs, the intermediate zone receives connections from both the cerebral cortex and the spinal cord (Fig. 11.2). Experiments in the cat indicate that the cortical input to the intermediate zone comes primarily from the MI and SI. Single neurons in the intermediate zone can be activated from both the cerebral cortex and the spinal cord. For example, in the "arm region" (Fig. 11.5) of the anterior lobe, intermediate-zone single neurons receive converging input from the arm region of the MI and SI and from sensory receptors in the arm. Perhaps

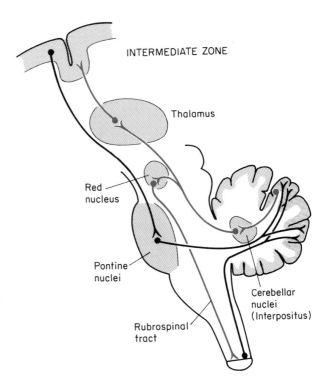

INTERMEDIATE ZONE

Thalamus

Red nucleus

Pontine nuclei

Rubrospinal tract

Cerebellar nuclei (Interpositus)

Fig. 11.9. *The main connections of the intermediate zone.* Both the spinal cord (via the red nucleus) and the cerebral cortex (via the thalamus) can be influenced by the intermediate zone.

the cerebellum in this case compares copies of the motor commands sent from the cerebral cortex with the signals from the periphery providing information about the actual movement that was produced by the command.

The Inferior Olive Also Conveys Information from the Cerebral Cortex and from the Mesencephalon

The inferior olive consists of subdivisions that receive afferents primarily from the spinal cord via several precisely organized tracts and of other, larger parts (in humans) that receive fibers mainly from various mesencephalic nuclei, such as the superior colliculus, the pretectal nuclei, the red nucleus, and several smaller nuclei. These parts of the olive send most of their fibers to the cerebellar hemispheres. There is also a modest direct projection from the cerebral cortex (especially the MI) to the inferior olive. In addition, the red nucleus and several other mesencephalic nuclei receive cortical afferents from the MI, SMA, and PMA and may therefore mediate cortical influences on the inferior olive.

The pretectal nuclei, which receive visual signals from the retina, project to a small distinct part of the inferior olive, which in its turn projects to the flocculonodular lobe (Fig. 13.28). These connections are of importance for adaptations of the vestibulo-ocular reflex (see below, "The Cerebellum and Motor Learning"). The superior colliculus, also in receipt of visual signals from the retina and the cerebral cortex, influences other parts of the cerebellum via the inferior olive and contributes to control of eye movements. The kind of information sent from the red nucleus to the cerebellum via the inferior olive is largely unknown.

As we will return to later, the kind of information conveyed to the cerebellum from the inferior olive is most likely fundamentally different from that sent from the pontine nuclei.

Structure of the Cerebellar Cortex

Before discussing the efferent connections of the cerebellum, we need to know something about the cerebellar cortex (Figs. 11.10 and 11.11). Here, the vast amount of information provided by all of the afferents is processed. To some extent, different kinds of information are integrated, and then "an-swers" are issued to various motor centers of the brain and spinal cord.

As mentioned, the cerebellar cortex has the same structure all over the cerebellum (it cannot be subdivided into cytoarchitectonic areas, differing also in this respect from the cerebral cortex). The structural arrangement of the neuronal elements is strictly geometric, so the individual elements can be distinguished fairly easily. This helps to explain why the structure and internal connections of the cerebellar cortex are much better known than that of the cerebral cortex.

The cerebellar cortex consists of *three layers*. The superficial, outermost layer is the *molecular layer*. It contains mainly dendrites and axons from cells in the deeper layers but only a few perikarya. The middle layer is dominated by the large, so-called *Purkinje cells*, arranged in a monolayer (Fig. 11.10), and is called the *Purkinje cell layer*. The deepest, lowermost layer is called the *granular layer* because it is packed with tiny *granule cells*. The Purkinje cells are the only ones that send their axons out of the cerebellar cortex and thus constitute the efferent channel. The axons of the granule cells ascend through the Purkinje cell layer into the molecular layer, in which they divide at a right angle into two branches running parallel with the surface of the cortex (Figs. 11.10 and 11.11). These branches are called *parallel fibers* and run in the direction of the long axis of the folia. The parallel fibers form numerous synapses with the Purkinje cell dendrites. The Purkinje cell dendritic tree is unusual: In the first place, it has an enormously rich branching pattern, and second, the whole dendritic tree is compressed into one plane, forming an espalier oriented perpendicular to the long axis of the folia and the parallel fibers. This arrangement ensures that each parallel fiber forms synapses with many Purkinje cells (the parallel fibers can be several millimeters long). At the same time, each Purkinje cell is contacted by an enormous number of parallel fibers. Thus, a Purkinje cell integrates the activity of a large

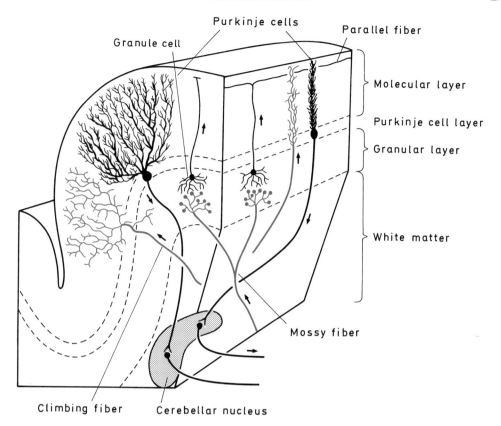

Fig. 11.10. *The structure of the cerebellar cortex.* The three layers and the main cell types are shown schematically in a piece of cerebellar folium. Note the arrangement of the Purkinje cell dendrites perpendicular to the long axis of the folium and the parallel fibers. The two main kinds of afferent fibers (mossy and climbing fibers) are also shown. The mossy fibers end on the granule cells, whereas the climbing fibers enter the molecular layer to end on the Purkinje cell dendrites.

number of granule cells. *The Purkinje cells contain GABA,* and they inhibit their target cells, as shown physiologically. The granule cells have an excitatory action on the Purkinje cells, most likely by releasing an amino acid transmitter.

Afferents to the Cerebellar Cortex Are of Two Main Kinds: Mossy and Climbing Fibers

The numerous afferent fibers to the cerebellar cortex fall in two categories, which differ in how the fibers end in the cerebellar cortex. Both kinds have an excitatory synaptic action, mediated most likely by an amino acid transmitter (glutamate or aspartate). The

climbing fibers all come from the *inferior olive,* whereas afferents from nearly all other nuclei end as *mossy fibers* (such as the vestibulocerebellar, the spinocerebellar, and the pontocerebellar fibers).[3]

The *mossy fibers* conduct signals relatively rapidly and end in the granular layer, establishing synapses with the granule cell dendrites (Figs. 11.10 and 11.11). One mossy fiber branches extensively and contacts a large number of granule cells, each of which in its turn contacts many Purkinje cells. Thus, each mossy fiber influences many Purkinje cells, but the excitatory effect on each is weak, so that *many mossy fibers must be active together to provide sufficient excitation* (via the parallel fibers) *to fire a Purkinje*

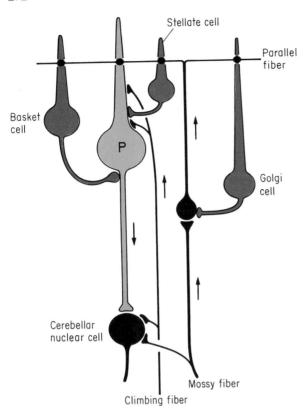

Stellate cell

Parallel
fiber

Basket
cell

P

Golgi
cell

Cerebellar
nuclear cell

Mossy fiber

Climbing fiber

Fig. 11.11. *The cerebellar cortex.* Schematic presentation of the main cell types and their synaptic arrangements. Red signifies inhibitory action; black, excitatory. Note the three kinds of inhibitory interneurons. Redrawn from Eccles, Ito, and Szentágothai (1967).

cell (as mentioned, the parallel fibers excite the Purkinje cells). A typical feature of the mossy fibers is that they transmit action potentials with a high frequency and produce Purkinje cell firing with a frequency of 50–100/sec.

The *climbing fibers* end very differently from the mossy fibers: The fibers ascend directly to the molecular layer and divide into several branches, each "climbing" along a Purkinje cell dendrite (Figs. 1.6B, 11.10, and 11.11). As they climb, they form numerous synapses with the dendrites. Each Purkinje cell receives branches from only one climbing fiber (that is, from only one cell in the inferior olive). Each olivary cell, however, innervates more than one Purkinje cell, since the number of Purkinje cells is higher than the number of olivary cells. Because each climbing fiber forms so many synapses with a Purkinje cell, the total excitatory action is strong. Thus, even a *single action potential in a climbing fiber elicits a burst of action po-*

tentials in the Purkinje cells it contacts (note the difference from the mossy fibers: Many of these have to be active simultaneously, and with a high frequency, to fire the Purkinje cells). The firing frequency of the climbing fibers is very low under natural conditions (often less than one impulse per second). Even maximal stimulation does not bring the firing frequency above 10 sec.

In conclusion, the Purkinje cells receive excitation from both mossy and climbing fiber afferent inputs, but with very different spatial and temporal characteristics of their actions.

In addition, the signal traffic within the cerebellar cortex is influenced by several kinds of *inhibitory interneurons* (Fig. 11.11). These interneurons are also excited by afferent impulses to the cortex and serve in general to increase the precision of signal traffic through the cerebellar cortex (like inhibitory interneurons in nuclei of the sensory pathways).

The Cerebellar Cortex Contains
Three Kinds of Inhibitory Interneurons

All cerebellar interneurons contain GABA (some may also contain glycine, another inhibitory neurotransmitter). One main type of interneuron is the *stellate cell,* located in the molecular layer (Fig. 11.11). It receives afferent excitatory input from the granule cells (parallel fibers), and its axons form synapses with the Purkinje cell dendrites.

Another kind of interneuron, the *basket cell,* is located close to the Purkinje cell layer. Basket cells are also contacted by parallel fibers, whereas their axons end with synapses around the initial segment of the Purkinje cell axons—a location that enables the basket cells to inhibit the Purkinje cells very efficiently. The axonal branches of the basket cells are arranged perpendicular to the long axis of the folia, so that they inhibit Purkinje cells lateral to those that are being activated by parallel fiber excitation. Activation of a group of granule cells would lead to a narrow band of excitation of the Purkinje cells along the folium, flanked by a zone of inhibition on each side. Thus it appears to be a kind of lateral inhibition, which is common in sensory systems to increase the spatial precision of sensory transmission. Correspondingly, the cerebellar cortical region activated by each mossy fiber is reduced in extension.

The third kind of inhibitory interneuron, the *Golgi cell,* is located in the granular layer. The dendrites of the Golgi cells extend upward into the molecular layer and are therefore contacted by parallel fibers (like the stellate cells and the basket cells). The axonal branches form synapses with the dendrites of the granule cells and thus reduce the excitation received by the Purkinje cells after a mossy fiber input.

Mossy and Climbing Fibers Are
Functionally Different

The great differences between the mossy and climbing fibers with regard to both structural and physiological properties strongly suggest that they convey different kinds of information and thus play different roles in cerebellar functions. Because of their ability to vary their impulse frequency over a wide range, the *mossy fibers* are presumably well suited for providing precisely graded information about movements (the muscles involved, and the direction, speed, and force of movements), localization and characteristics of skin stimuli, details concerning motor commands issued from the cerebral cortex, and so forth. Such assumptions also fit with the physiological properties of spinocerebellar fibers, known to end as mossy fibers (less is known about the corticopontocerebellar pathway in this respect).

The *climbing fibers,* because of their low range of firing frequency, are less likely to provide precisely graded information. Recording of the climbing fiber activity and the firing of the Purkinje cells in response to climbing fiber activation also suggests that the climbing fibers have a unique functional role. Thus, a single action potential in a climbing fiber is sufficient to trigger a burst of Purkinje cell action potentials (complex spikes). This would suggest an all-or-none action rather than a graded one. Several theories of cerebellar functions postulate that *the climbing fibers inform about errors in the execution of a movement* (giving an "error signal") when the movement does not correspond to what was intended). There is some experimental support for this hypothesis. Thus, some studies show that the firing frequency of climbing fibers increases in relation to a perturbation of an ongoing movement, whereas the firing frequency is unrelated to, for example, the direction and velocity of the movement. In experiments with walking cats, the firing frequency of climbing fibers leading from the forelimb increases when the foot meets an obstacle, so that the walking pattern has to be changed. In monkeys learning a new movement, there is increased climbing-fiber activity from the relevant body parts. When the movement is well rehearsed—that is, the learning phase is over—the climbing fiber firing frequency does not increase during execution of the movement (no more error signals?). A specific role of the climbing fibers during *motor learning has been postulated* on the basis of this and other kinds of experiments. The climbing fiber input is thought to alter for a long time (days, perhaps years) the responsiveness of the Purkinje cells to mossy fiber inputs. This appears to happen only when specific sets of climbing and mossy fibers simultaneously activate a Purkinje cell, leading to a change of Purkinje cell excitability, so that the following mossy fiber impulses have a different effect than previously. There is no agreement yet, however, whether the excitability of the Purkinje cells is increased or decreased by conjunctive climbing and mossy fiber activation. Furthermore, the kind of result referred to above can be interpreted in various ways, and, consequently, the special role of the climbing fibers in motor learning is not generally accepted.

Efferent Connections of the Cerebellum: The Cerebellar Nuclei

As mentioned, the three main subdivisions of the cerebellum act largely on the parts of the nervous system from which they receive afferent inputs (Figs. 11.2, 11.4, 11.7, and 11.9).

With regard to the *vestibulocerebellum*, the Purkinje cells send their axons directly to the vestibular nuclei as corticovestibular fibers (Fig. 11.3). The fibers from the vestibulocerebellum end primarily in parts of the vestibular nuclei that send ascending connections to the external ocular muscles (the medial longitudinal fasciculus, Fig. 13.17) and, to a lesser extent, in parts of the nuclei sending fibers to the spinal cord. The vestibulocerebellum can thus contribute to the control of eye movements. In addition, the vestibulocerebellum may also influence pos-

tural mechanisms via the vestibulospinal tracts.[4]

For the rest of the cerebellum, *the axons of the Purkinje cells as a rule end in the cerebellar nuclei* (corticonuclear fibers). The neurons of these nuclei forward the information to the various targets of the cerebellum. The *cerebellar nuclei* (Figs. 11.12 and 11.13) are located in the deep white matter of the cerebellum, just above the roof of the fourth ventricle. In humans, there are four nuclei on each side. Close to the midline, under the vermis, lies the *fastigial nucleus* (medial cerebellar nucleus), then follow two small nuclei, and most laterally lies the large, folded *dentate nucleus* (lateral cerebellar nucleus). The two small nuclei have specific names in humans (the globose and the emboliform nuclei) and correspond to the *anterior and posterior interposed nuclei* in animals.

The corticonuclear connections are precisely organized with a topographic pattern, so that, for example, fibers from the anterior and posterior parts of the cerebellum end in anterior and posterior parts of the nuclei, re-

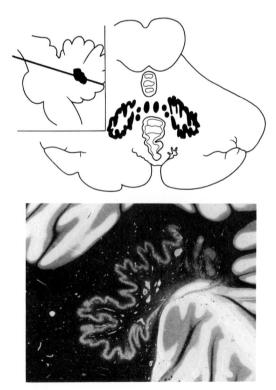

Fig. 11.12. *The cerebellar nuclei.* The photomicrograph shows a myelin-stained section placed slightly more dorsally than the drawing **above**. Therefore, only the dentate and the interposed nuclei are seen in the photomicrograph.

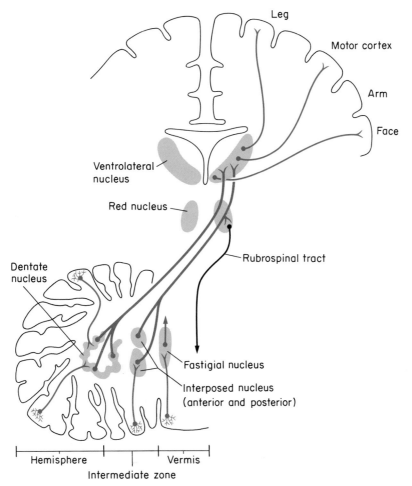

Fig. 11.13. *Ascending connections from the cerebellum.* The Purkinje cells of the hemispheres send their axons to the dentate nucleus, which in turn projects to the thalamus (the VL nucleus) of the opposite side. The last link from the VL reaches primarily the MI. The connections are somatotopically organized. The figure also shows that the Purkinje cells of the intermediate zone and the vermis project to the interposed and the fastigal nuclei, respectively.

spectively. There is a somatotopic pattern of the corticonuclear projections from parts of the cerebellum that receive somatotopically organized afferent input. Particularly marked is the longitudinal localization, with *the vermis sending fibers to the fastigial nucleus, the intermediate zone to the interposed nuclei, and the hemispheres to the dentate nucleus* (Figs. 11.13 and 11.15). Each of the nuclei sends fibers to a separate target region, as shown in a very simplified manner in Figures 11.3, 11.4, 11.7, and 11.9. On the whole, impulses from different parts of the cerebellum are kept segregated through the nuclei and further on to other parts of the brain. However, there is a marked convergence of the corticonuclear connections, since the number of Purkinje cells is much higher than the number of nuclear cells.

The Neurons of the Cerebellar Nuclei Are Spontaneously Active

The nuclear cells fire with a high frequency even in an animal sitting quietly. When neurons fire without any obvious excitatory input, they are said to be *spontaneously active*. Because all Purkinje cells are inhibitory (GABA), a continuous firing of the nuclear cells is a prerequisite for the information from the cerebellar cortex to be passed on (increased Purkinje cell activity leads to reduced nuclear cell firing). The cause of the high spontaneous activity of the nuclear cells is not entirely clear, however. They may have intrinsic properties that depolarize the membrane even in the absence of an excitatory input (pacemaker properties). In addition, the nuclear cells receive other afferents than those coming from the Purkinje cells. Thus, some of the pathways ending in the cerebellar cortex, such as the spinocerebellar and olivocerebellar projections, give off collaterals to the cerebellar nuclei. As mentioned, these pathways are excitatory. It is noteworthy, however, that the major afferent pathway to the cerebellar cortex, the pontocerebellar projection, does not appear to give off collaterals to the dentate nucleus. What maintains the high firing frequency of this largest of the cerebellar nuclei is therefore still unsettled.

The lack of pontocerebellar collaterals to the intracerebellar nuclei does not readily fit with the widely held notion that—as a fundamental basis—*all* afferent sources send collaterals to both the cerebellar cortex and the nuclei. Some theories of how the cerebellum operates are nevertheless based on the assumption of such an arrangement; the route via the cerebellar cortex is then regarded as a side loop in relation to the main transmission line through the nuclei. The cerebellar cortex is assumed to modulate the transmission through the nuclei rather than providing them with their main afferent, specific information.

Organization of Efferent Connections from the Cerebellar Nuclei

The fibers from the *dentate nucleus* leave the cerebellum through the *superior cerebellar peduncle* (Figs. 11.1 and 11.13). They cross the midline in the mesencephalon, and some fibers end in the red nucleus of the opposite side. Most fibers continue rostrally, however, to end in the *thalamus*. Here, the dentate fibers end primarily in the *ventrolateral nucleus (VL)* (some also reach the ventral anterior nucleus, VA) (Figs. 11.13 and 11.14). These nuclei also receive fibers from the basal ganglia, but they end in different parts than the cerebellar fibers (as shown schematically in Fig. 11.14), which implies that the basal ganglia and the cerebellum also influence somewhat different parts of the cortex. *Impulses from the cerebellar hemispheres*

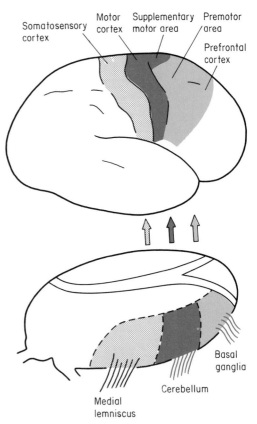

Fig. 11.14. *Thalamocortical connections.* Schematic presentation of the arrangement within the ventral thalamic nucleus of afferents from the somatosensory pathways, the cerebellum, and the basal ganglia and their further projections to the SI, MI, and the premotor cortex.

pass primarily to the MI and SMA, whereas the basal ganglia via the thalamus act mainly on the PMA and the prefrontal cortex.

Because both the ascending fibers from the cerebellum to the motor cortex and the descending fibers from the cerebral cortex to the spinal cord are crossed, *the cerebellar hemisphere exerts its influence on the body half of the same side.* Consequently, with diseases of the cerebellum, *the symptoms occur on the same side as the lesion.*

As mentioned, the efferents from the *intermediate zone* reach the *interposed nucleus.* This sends its efferents both to the contralateral thalamus (to the VL mainly, like the dentate) and the *red nucleus* (Figs. 11.9, 11.13, and 11.15). This enables the interposed nucleus to influence motorneurons

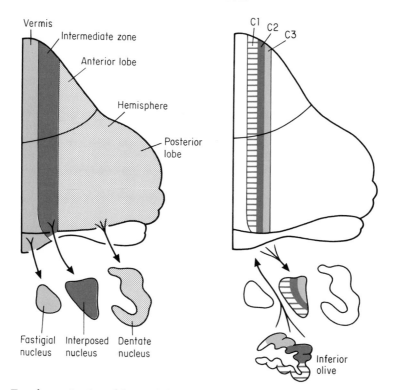

Fig. 11.15. *Zonal organization of the cerebellar cortex.* Very simplified illustration of the precise topographic pattern of cerebellar efferent and afferent connections. The cortex can be divided into longitudinal zones projecting to different parts of the cerebellar nuclei and receiving afferents from different parts of the inferior olive (**right drawing**). Note that each of the zones shown to the **left** can be further subdivided.

via both the rubrospinal tract and the pyramidal tract. Since the rubrospinal tract is crossed, the interposed nucleus (and the intermediate zone) acts on the body half of the same side.

The *fastigial nucleus* (receiving Purkinje cell axons from the vermis) sends its efferents to both the *vestibular nuclei* and the *reticular formation*. Thus, motoneurons can be influenced via the vestibulospinal and the reticulospinal tracts. On the basis of what we discussed in Chapter 9, it seems likely that *the cerebellum via the fastigial nucleus can influence posture and relatively automatic movements like locomotion.* This is supported by the results of animal experiments and by clinical observations.

Sagittal Zones and Somatotopic Organization of the Cerebellum

We have so far described that the main subdivisions of the cerebellum—such as the flocculonod- ular lobe, the vermis, and the hemispheres—differ with regard to connectivity. Furthermore, we have seen that the lateral parts of the hemispheres, the intermediate zone, and the vermis differ with regard to their efferent connections (Fig. 11.15). This *organization of the cerebellum into three longitudinal zones,* each projecting to separate parts of the cerebellar nuclei, was first described by the Norwegian neuroanatomists Jansen and Brodal in the 1940s.

But the localization within the cerebellum is far more sophisticated than what could be revealed by the fairly primitive methods 50 years ago. Each of the three longitudinal zones of Jansen and Brodal can thus be further subdivided, as shown for the intermediate zone in Figure 11.15. The numerous narrow zones differ not only with regard to their projections to the cerebellar nuclei but also from which part of the inferior olive they receive climbing fibers, as shown by the Dutch neuroanatomist Voogd. The neurons located within a particular small part of the olive send their fibers to a narrow longitudinal zone, whereas the neighboring zones receive climbing fibers from other parts of the olive (Fig. 11.15). The Purkinje cells of the zones also send their axons to different parts of the cerebellar nuclei. Apart from the parallel fibers, extending for a couple of millimeters perpendicular to the longitudinal zones, there are no association fibers interconnecting different parts of the cerebellar cortex. Thus, the cerebellar cortex and the cerebellar nuclei consist of numerous *compartments* that appear to be able to function (at least largely) independently of each other. In this respect the cerebellar cortex differs from the cerebral cortex, which is characterized by extensive association connections. The parcellation of the cortex into sagittal zones in fact goes further than shown in Figure 11.15. Physiological studies show that within the anterior lobe each zone consists of several *microzones* differing with regard to the information they receive. A microzone may perhaps represent a functional unit, taking care of a particular, well-defined aspect of a motor task.

Another aspect of cerebellar localization is that cortical cell groups representing different body parts are spatially segregated—that is, there is a *somatotopic organization*, as already mentioned (Fig. 11.5). The mossy fiber projections to the cerebellum, carrying impulses from the spinal cord and the cerebral cortex, are somatotopically organized, as are the climbing fiber projections from the inferior olive. The somatotopic localization within the cerebellar cortex was first described by the British neurophysiologist Adrian and the Americans Snider and Stowell, using electrophysiological methods. Later investigations, also with anatomic methods, have verified their findings and provided further details. Lesions restricted to, for example, the forelimb region of the anterior lobe in experimental animals produce characteristic changes of muscle that are restricted to the forelimb of the same side as the lesion.

A novel aspect of the somatotopic localization within the cerebellum was described by the American neurophysiologist Welker and collaborators, using very precise micromapping methods. Thus, the mossy fibers, formerly thought to end with a fairly diffuse somatotopic pattern, were shown to end in numerous, discrete patches in the cortex, each patch being defined by its sensory input from a specific minor part of the body. Each patch is usually less than 1 mm in diameter (in the rat and cat). Thus, the leg region within the posterior lobe consists in reality of a mosaic of patches. A salient feature is that adjacent patches can receive inputs from body parts that are widely separated. Furthermore, the same body part is usually represented in several widely separated patches. This arrangement of the mossy fibers was termed *fractured somatotopy* by Welker. How this pattern of mossy fiber inputs is coordinated with the climbing fiber inputs is not clear. As mentioned, the climbing fibers terminate in narrow sagittal strips or zones, and one such strip is often related to one body part only. In any case, the incredibly precise and complicated pattern of mossy and climbing fiber inputs to the cerebellar cortex indicates that the cerebellum is divided into numerous smaller functional units. Each unit has the same kind of neuronal machinery to treat incoming information, whereas they differ in the nature of information they receive and the part of the brain to which they send their "answers."

CEREBELLAR FUNCTIONS AND SYMPTOMS IN DISEASE

We will finally discuss the function of the cerebellum, with special reference to the motor disturbances occurring in humans after damage to the cerebellum.

Even though a multitude of symptoms have been produced in experimental animals after lesions of the cerebellum (among them, disturbances of autonomic functions) clinically, only certain motor symptoms can with certainty be referred to cerebellar lesions. This is probably explained by the fact that in humans the lesions that give clear-cut symptoms most often are large and not confined to particular functional or anatomic cerebellar subdivisions. Furthermore, they are usually combined with lesions in other parts of the central nervous system (for example, in parts of the brain stem). It is therefore often difficult to decide whether a particular symptom is caused by the cerebellar lesion. Modern imaging techniques (CT, MRI, PET; see Chapter 3), however, provide the opportunity to localize accurately even fairly small lesions in living subjects and, furthermore, to study cerebellar neuronal activity (indirectly) in healthy and diseased subjects performing specific tasks. As mentioned, derangement of motor functions dominates the clinical picture caused by cerebellar disorders. To judge from the cerebellar connections as we have discussed them above, it is clear that the cerebellum influences movements by acting on the neuronal groups that give origin to the central motor pathways (the pyramidal tract, the reticulospinal tracts, the rubrospinal tract, and the vestibulospinal tracts). These pathways, of course, control the activity of spinal and cranial nerve motoneurons. The three main subdivisions of the cerebellum (Fig. 11.2) act on different neuronal groups, and lesions restricted to each of the subdivisions give different symptoms. On this basis one usually distinguishes three cerebellar syndromes (a syndrome is a constellation of several symptoms that occur together): *the flocculonodular syndrome, the anterior lobe syndrome, and the neocerebellar syndrome.* The existence of three distinct syndromes is most clear-cut in experimental animals. In humans, the neocerebellar syndrome is most often seen, which is not surprising since the hemispheres (the neocerebellum) make up the major part of the human cerebellum.

The "Flocculonodular" and "Anterior Lobe" Syndromes

Isolated damage to the flocculonodular lobe in animals produces *disturbances of the equilibrium*—that is, unsteadiness in standing and walking. When the body is supported, movements of the extremities can be performed normally, however. Sometimes, similar symptoms occur in humans with a special kind of tumor in the posterior cranial fossa, most often arising from the nodulus (medulloblastoma).

Eye movements may also be disturbed in patients with cerebellar lesions (particularly with affection of the vestibulocerebellum). This manifests itself as *spontaneous nystagmus.*[5] It is not quite clear, however, whether such symptoms are caused by the cerebellar damage itself or by concomitant damage to the vestibular nuclei or their connections.

Damage to *the anterior lobe in experimental animals* produces primarily *a change of the muscle tone.* In decerebrate animals, the

decerebrate rigidity increases (see Chapter 9), as do the postural reflexes. This fits with the observation that electrical stimulation of the anterior lobe reduces the decerebrate rigidity (as mentioned, the Purkinje cells inhibit the cells of the cerebellar nuclei, whereas the nuclear cells have excitatory actions on reticulospinal and vestibulospinal neurons).[6] In addition, some Purkinje cells in the anterior lobe vermis send axons directly to the vestibular nuclei, and removal of this inhibitory action would also tend to increase the activity of the vestibulospinal neurons and thus the decerebrate rigidity.

In humans it is doubtful, however, whether increased muscle tone is produced by lesions including the anterior lobe. More marked is the *unsteadiness of walking* (gait ataxia) in patients with damage mainly affecting *the anterior lobe vermis and intermediate zone* (this occurs in cerebellar degeneration caused by alcohol abuse). The anterior lobe, via its efferent connections to the reticular formation and probably the red nucleus, must therefore be assumed to play a role in coordination of the half-automatic movements of walking.

The "Neocerebellar" Syndrome

The neocerebellum plays a different functional role than the phylogenetically older parts of the cerebellum: It is primarily concerned with *the coordination of the (least automatic) voluntary movements.* This stands to reason, since the cerebellar hemispheres send their main output to the MI (via the dentate nucleus and the thalamus) and thus influence the neurons of the pyramidal tract. After removal of one cerebellar hemisphere in a monkey, the voluntary movements become uncertain on the same side of the body; they become *incoordinated* or *ataxic.* The same effect can be produced by cooling the dentate nucleus (by the use of a cooling electrode) in an animal performing a well-rehearsed movement (as soon as the cooling is reversed, the movements again become normal). Movements that were performed quickly and smoothly become unsteady and jerky by the cooling. The monkey misses repeatedly when trying to grasp an object, even though it knows perfectly well where it is and what is demanded. Sometimes the hand is moved too far in relation to the object, sometimes too short. The movements tend to be *decomposed;* that is, instead of occurring simultaneously in several joints, they take place in one joint at a time, and the velocity is uneven—sometimes too high and sometimes too low. Ataxia of this kind is also the most prominent symptom in humans with damage to the cerebellar hemispheres. In clinical neurology, the various elements of ataxia have particular names, such as *dysmetria* (movement is not stopped in time), *asynergia* (decomposition of complex movements), *dysdiadochokinesia* (reduced ability to perform rapidly alternating movements of, for example, the hand), and *intentional tremor* (tremor arising when trying to perform a movement, such as grasping an object). All of these elements of ataxia are probably expressions of the same *fundamental defect in control of the force and of the exact timing of the starting and stopping of movements.* Speech is also often disturbed in cerebellar diseases. It has been called *speech ataxia,* to emphasize that it also appears to be caused by incoordination (in this case, of the respiratory muscles, the muscles of the larynx, and others), making the strength and velocity of the speech uneven.

In *acute* damage to the cerebellar hemispheres in humans, the muscle tone often appears to be reduced when tested by passive stretch (the symptom is transient). This is called *cerebellar hypotonia.* The underlying mechanism is not clear, but animal experiments indicate that it may be caused by reduced γ motoneuron activity (see also Chapter 8 for a discussion of muscle tone).

How the Cerebellum Operates Is Still Largely Unknown

Even though the study of cerebellar symptoms provides reasonable insight into the functions of the cerebellum, we are far from understanding how the cerebellum performs its tasks. The striking uniformity and strictly geometric structure of the cerebellar cortex has led to comparison with a computer, which can perform the same kinds of computations on various kinds of information. The subdivision of the cerebellum into numerous, apparently independent units may fit such a concept. Several rather different theories have been put forward to explain how the cerebellum operates. None of them has so far been universally accepted, however, and there is disagreement with regard to interpretation of some experiments said to support one theory or the other.

The Cerebellum and Motor Learning

Recent animal experiments suggest that long-lasting changes in synaptic efficacy may take place in the cerebellar cortex during motor learning. Thus, the cerebellum may not only be a machine used every time a movement is performed but may also be capable of remembering what was done and thereby adapting its influence on motoneurons in accordance with the outcome of a movement. In particular, the altered synaptic effects of the parallel fibers on the Purkinje cell dendrites have been thoroughly investigated. There is evidence that changed synaptic efficacy is produced by the simultaneous firing of mosssy and climbing fibers acting on the same Purkinje cell. The climbing fiber influence—although in itself excitatory—probably renders the Purkinje cells less excitable for a long time (at least hours). Thus, the next time a certain mossy fiber input arrives, the Purkinje cell response is reduced (that is, it fires fewer action potentials).

One example of such synaptic changes is the adaptability of the vestibulo-ocular reflex, as shown by the Japanese neurophysiologist Ito. The *vestibulo-ocular reflex* (VOR) ensures that when the head moves in one direction, the eyes move in the opposite direction with exactly the same speed. This makes it possible to keep the gaze fixed on a stationary object even though the head moves. The strength of the reflex response to a certain head movement (that is, the sensitivity of the reflex) needs to be adjusted when, for example, the head grows and alters its proportions. Via relay stations (Fig. 13.28), signals from the retina provide information about retinal slip (the image is not kept stationary on the retina but moves). Most likely, climbing fibers ending in the flocculus provide such signals and thus tell the cerebellum that the velocity of the eye movement is incorrect. Information about head movements from the vestibular apparatus is provided by mossy fibers, also ending in the flocculus. The sensitivity of the vestibulo-ocular reflex can be altered experimentally in a short time, as shown by making experimental animals wear prismatic glasses that displace the image on the retina. The most drastic experiment is when the movement of the surroundings appears to be the opposite of the real movement, leading to a complete reversal of the reflex response. Destruction of the cerebellar flocculus prevents adaptation of the reflex. It is disputed, however, whether the change in synaptic efficacy—that is, the learning—underlying the adaptability of the vestibulo-ocular reflex is caused by changes in the cerebellum or elsewhere.

Certain conditioned responses are examples of possible cerebellar participation during motor learning. Especially the so-called nictitating membrane reflex (a part of the blink reflex) in rabbits has been investigated. When a jet of air hits the eye, the nictitating membrane moves together with the eyelid. This is an unconditioned reflex, in which the trigeminal nerve is the afferent link, the reflex center is in the brain stem involving the sensory trigeminal nucleus, the reticular formation, and the facial nucleus, and the efferent link is the facial nerve to the muscles around the eye. If the jet of air is regularly preceded by a tone (conditioning stimulus), the rabbit will eventually react with a nictitating membrane movement even when the tone is presented alone. The impulse pathway for the conditioned response is much more complicated than that for the unconditioned reflex (for example, the auditory pathways and parts of the cerebral cortex are involved). What is interesting in this connection, however, is that after destruction of certain parts of the cerebellum, the reflex can no longer be conditioned (that is, only the unconditioned response occurs, and the animal can no longer be trained to react to the tone only). Damage to the cerebellum after having made the response conditioned abolishes the conditioned (but not the unconditioned) response. It is sufficient to remove a small part of the cerebellar "face area" of the intermediate zone to get these effects (this is a further example of the cerebellar functional localization). Other conditioned responses appear to be dependent on the integrity of the cerebel-

lum, but they have been less rigorously studied than the nictitating reflex. As with the vestibulo-ocular reflex, however, it is not quite settled whether the learning of the conditioned response—that is, the memory traces coupling the conditioning stimulus to the response—is located in the cerebellum or elsewhere. If learning takes place in the cerebellum in such rather primitive motor responses, it is tempting to assume that corresponding changes occur in the cerebellar hemispheres when humans learn complex voluntary movements (such as learning to play a musical instrument).

Perhaps the cerebellum may participate also in other kinds of learning. Thus, measurements of regional cerebral oxidative metabolism with positron emission tomography in humans indicate that the posterior parts of the cerebellar hemispheres increase their neuronal activity when learning a tactile recognition task (more than during just tactile recognition of an object).

NOTES

1. Other precerebellar nuclei—that is, brain stem nuclei that send their efferents to the cerebellum—also receive afferents from the cerebral cortex. This concerns the *reticular tegmental nucleus,* located just dorsal to the pontine nuclei, and the *lateral reticular nucleus.* In quantitative terms, however, these pathways play minor roles compared with the corticopontocerebellar one.

2. There are modest connections to the pontine nuclei from the *frontal eye field, area 8,* and from *parts of the auditory cortex.* There are, however, few if any pontine fibers from prefrontal areas and major parts of the temporal lobe.

3. In addition to the climbing fibers and mossy fibers—demonstrated with the Golgi method a long time ago—a third kind of cerebellar afferent has been demonstrated with the histofluorescence method (that is, fibers containing catecholamines). Such fibers come from the raphe nuclei and from the nucleus locus coeruleus and contain serotonin and norepinephrine, respectively. They appear to end rather diffusely in both the granular and molecular layers. Fibers coming from the hypothalamus also end in this manner.

4. The vestibular nuclei also receive direct projections from Purkinje cells of the vermis of the anterior and the posterior lobes. These fibers end primarily in the lateral vestibular nucleus (nucleus of

Deiters), which projects to the spinal cord. Therefore, the vermal projection to the vestibular nuclei appears to influence primarily postural mechanisms. To make this even more complicated, the vestibular nuclei (mainly the nucleus of Deiters) also receive indirect cerebellar afferents from the anterior and posterior lobe vermis. These are relayed in the medial cerebellar nucleus (the fastigial nucleus).

5. *Nystagmus* is movements in which the eyes move slowly in one direction (as when following a moving object with the gaze), and rapidly back. When nystagmus occurs in a person at rest with no kind of stimulation, it is called spontaneous. Nystagmus is discussed further in Chapter 13.

6. Electrical stimulation with electrodes surgically implanted at the cerebellar surface has been used in patients with neurological disorders such as epilepsy and cerebral palsy. The theoretical basis is the inhibitory action of the Purkinje cells with subsequent reduction of abnormally increased neuronal excitability and muscle tone. Even though some report favorable results with such stimulation, there is no agreement as to whether the effect is due to the cerebellar stimulation or some other factor.

IV

The Brain Stem and the Cranial Nerves

The definition of the term *brain stem* varies. We use it here to refer to the medulla oblongata, the pons, the mesencephalon, and in addition the diencephalon. Often the term is applied only to the macroscopically distinct part, however, which consists of the medulla, pons, and mesencephalon. Which definition is used is of no great importance, since the brain stem is a topographically and embryologically defined unit; it does not represent a uniform functional "system." Neuronal groups within the brain stem take part in virtually all the tasks of the central nervous system.

Functionally, the brain stem may be said to have two levels of organization. On the one hand, most of the cranial nerves and their nuclei represent "the spinal cord of the head." On the other hand, many cell groups in the brain stem represent a superior level of control over the spinal cord and the cranial nerve nuclei. This section deals with both aspects. Chapter 12 deals with the reticular formation, which represents the superior level of control. Chapter 13 describes most of the cranial nerves and their nuclei.

12

Reticular Formation

The reticular formation attends primarily to tasks involving the nervous system and the organism as a whole. This fits with the fact that it is phylogenetically old and is present even in lower vertebrates. Structurally and functionally, the reticular formation has close relations with many other parts of the central nervous system and is therefore mentioned in all the system chapters. In this chapter we cannot avoid some reference to matters that are systematically treated in later chapters (particularly in Chapter 13 on the cranial nerves, and in Chapters 14 and 15 on the autonomic nervous system).

The reticular formation extends from the lower end of the medulla to the upper end of the mesencephalon, where it gradually fuses with certain thalamic cell groups.[1] At all levels it occupies the central parts (Figs. 2.17, 2.21, 12.1, 12.4, 12.7, and 12.10) and fills the territories not used by cranial nerve nuclei and other distinct nuclei (such as the dorsal column nuclei, the pontine nuclei, and the colliculi) and by the large fiber tracts (such as the medial lemniscus and the pyramidal tract).

Two cell groups that have close topographic and other relations with the reticular formation (and which are often considered a part of the reticular formation) have

attracted much interest recently. These are the *raphe nuclei* (Figs. 12.1 and 12.5) and a small cell group called the *nucleus locus coeruleus* (Fig. 12.6). A characteristic feature of these nuclei is that their axons have extremely widespread ramifications, reaching many parts of the brain and the spinal cord. Another special feature is that they send fibers directly to the cerebral cortex—that is, without synaptic interruption in the thalamus, as is typical of most cortical afferent pathways from lower levels.

STRUCTURE AND CONNECTIONS OF THE RETICULAR FORMATION

Structure and Subdivisions

The reticular formation received its name from the early anatomists because of its networklike appearance in microscopic sections (Figs. 12.2 and 12.4). It is built of cells of various forms and sizes that appear to be rather randomly mixed. Between the cells, there is a wickerwork of fibers passing in many directions. These fibers are partly axons and dendrites of the neurons of the reticular formation, partly afferent axons from other parts of the central nervous system. The reticular neurons have typically

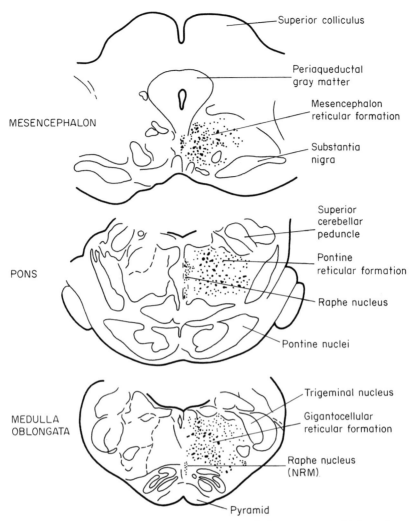

Fig. 12.1. *The reticular formation.* Transverse sections through various levels of the brain stem (cat) showing the position of the reticular formation. The size of the black dots indicates the size of the neurons, which varies considerably among subdivisions of the reticular formation. Based on Brodal (1957).

very long and straight dendrites, so that they cover a large volume of neuropil (Fig. 12.4). This distinguishes the reticular neurons from those found in specific nuclei of the brain stem, such as the cranial nerve nuclei (see the nucleus labeled XII in Fig. 12.4).

A more detailed analysis of the reticular formation makes clear, however, that it consists of several subdivisions, among which the cells differ in shape, size, and arrangement even though the borders between such subdivisions are not sharp (Fig. 12.1). It is especially important that such cytoarchitec-

tonically defined subdivisions also differ with regard to fiber connections and content of neurotransmitters. Not surprisingly, therefore, they differ functionally as well. In the pons and the medulla, approximately the medial two-thirds of the reticular formation consists of many large cells, in part so-called giant cells (Figs. 12.1 and 12.2). The lateral one-third contains almost exclusively small cells. Tract-tracing methods have shown that the medial part sends out many long, ascending and descending fibers, whereas the lateral small-celled part receives

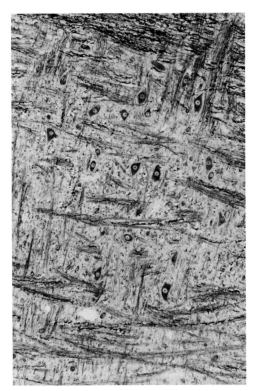

Fig. 12.2. *The reticular formation.* Photomicrograph of section of the medulla, stained to show fibers (myelin) and cell bodies. Note how the perikarya—some of them very large—are distributed diffusely without clear nuclear borders, and with small fiber bundles coursing in various directions. The section is from the so-called gigantocellular subdivision of the reticular formation (see Fig. 12.1). Magnification, ×300.

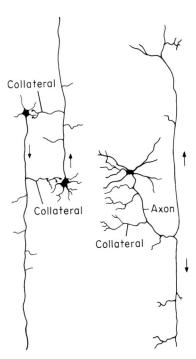

Fig. 12.3. *Neurons in the medial part of the reticular formation with long ascending and descending axons.* To the **right** is an example of a neuron with a bifurcating axon, with one ascending and one descending branch. Both branches give off collaterals as they course through the reticular formation. To the **left** are shown two neurons with ascending and descending axons, respectively. In this way, neurons with ascending axons can influence the activity of neurons with descending axons.

most of the afferents coming to the reticular formation. In general, therefore, we may say that *the lateral part is receiving, whereas the medial part is efferent and conveys the influence of the reticular formation to higher parts, such as the thalamus, and lower parts, such as the spinal cord.*

Studies with the Golgi method (and recently with intracellular tracers) give evidence of how complexly the reticular formation is organized. The long ascending and descending efferent fibers give off numerous collaterals on their way through the brain stem (Fig. 12.3). As can be seen in Figure 12.4, the collaterals run primarily in the transverse plane. Most dendrites of reticular

cells have the same preferential orientation, so the reticular formation may be described as consisting of numerous transversely oriented disks (Fig. 12.4). The numerous collaterals of the axons from the cells in the medial parts ensure that signals from each reticular cell may reach many functionally diverse cell groups (such as other parts of the reticular formation, cranial nerve nuclei, the dorsal column nuclei, the colliculi, the spinal cord, certain thalamic nuclei, and the hypothalamus).

The Raphe Nuclei

The raphe nuclei (raphe = seam) together form a narrow, sagittally oriented plate of neurons in the midline of the medulla, pons, and mesenceph-

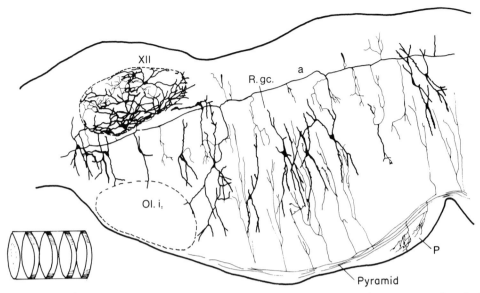

Fig. 12.4. *Orientaion of dendrites in the reticular formation.* Sagittal section through the medulla (rat). Note the long, straight dendrites, which are typical of the neurons of the reticular formation, in contrast to the neurons of a cranial nerve nucleus (XII) and other specific brain stem nuclei. A long axon (a) with numerous collaterals extending ventrally in the transverse plane is also shown. Collaterals of the pyramidal tract fibers (Pyr.) also enter the reticular formation. P = pontine nuclei; R.gc. = the gigantocellular nucleus of the reticular formation; Ol.i. = the inferior olivary nucleus. From Scheibel and Scheibel (1958).

alon (Figs. 12.1 and 12.5). In many ways, these nuclei have similarities with the reticular formation proper and are often considered part of it. On the basis of cytoarchitectonic and connectional differences, several raphe nuclei have been identified (Fig. 12.5) even though their borders are far from sharp. Together, the raphe nuclei receive afferents from many sources, such as the cerebral cortex, the hypothalamus, and the reticular formation. The efferent connections are special because *each axon ramifies extensively and reaches large parts of the central nervous system* with little topographic arrangement. Some topography is nevertheless present since the caudal raphe nuclei send their efferents to the spinal cord, whereas the rostral nuclei send fibers upstream to the cerebral cortex, among other places (Fig. 12.5).

Their *direct projections to the cerebral cortex* place the raphe nuclei among other nuclei with this same characteristic: dopaminergic cell groups in the mesencephalon, the nucleus locus coeruleus and adjoining scattered cell groups, and the basal nucleus. Another characteristic feature of the raphe nuclei is that most of the neurons contain *serotonin*. The actions of serotonin appear to be multifarious, depending on the kinds of receptor that are present postsynaptically. Most neurons in addition contain one or more *neuropeptides*, which presumably contribute to the synaptic effects of efferent fibers from the raphe nuclei.

The functions of the raphe nuclei are only incompletely known. In Chapter 4, we discussed the inhibitory actions of raphespinal fibers on the *central transmission of signals from nociceptors.* Later in this chapter we will briefly discuss the nuclei's relation to *sleep.* Lesions of the raphe nuclei have also been reported to evoke various kinds of behavioral changes, such as aggression and increased motor activity (to destroy the raphe nuclei in isolation however, is, virtually impossible).

A final peculiarity of the raphe nuclei is that they send fibers ending in close relation to the ependymal cells (which cover the interior aspect of the brain ventricles). The function of these fibers is unknown but may perhaps be related to regulation of transport processes through the ependyma.

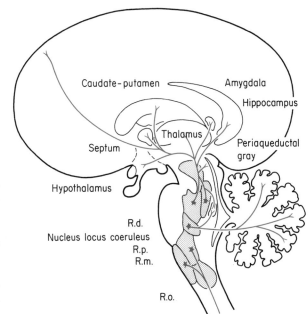

Fig. 12.5. *The raphe nuclei.* Schematic midsagittal section through the brain, showing the various subdivisions of the raphe nuclei and some main connections. The most rostral nuclei send their fibers rostrally to the thalamus, cortex, and other cell groups, whereas the caudal nuclei project to the spinal cord. R.m. = the nucleus raphe magnus (NRM); R.o. = the nucleus raphe obscurus; R.p. = the pontine raphe nucleus; R.d. = the dorsal raphe nucleus.

The Nucleus Locus Coeruleus

This nucleus consists of a small group of strongly pigmented cells located under the floor of the fourth ventricle (Fig. 12.6). It appears to be present in all mammalian species. After it was shown in the 1960s that the cells contain *norepinephrine,* the nucleus attracted considerable interest. The nucleus locus coeruleus has clear borders except ventrally, where it merges gradually with the adjoining reticular formation—which also contains many noradrenergic neurons. This is one reason why the nucleus locus coeruleus is often considered a part of the reticular formation.

The *efferent* fibers from the nucleus locus coeruleus are highly branched and reach virtually all parts of the central nervous system. It sends direct fibers to the cerebral cortex, the hypothalamus, the hippocampus, and other limbic structures. Direct fibers also reach the spinal cord and large parts of the brain stem.

The *afferent* connections of the nucleus are incompletely known but most likely come from many cell groups. Fibers terminating in the nucleus locus coeruleus have been traced from the hypothalamus, the amygdaloid nucleus, the raphe nuclei, and the substantia nigra.

The nucleus appears to be related to certain phases of *sleep* (see below). The highly branched

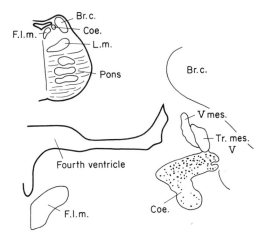

Fig. 12.6. *The nucleus locus coeruleus.* Its position just below the floor of the fourth ventricle is shown in a transverse section of the pons. This nucleus and other noradrenergic cell groups in the vicinity have neurons with highly branched axons ending rather diffusely in most parts of the central nervous system. Coe. = the nucleus locus coeruleus; Br.c. = the superior cerebellar peduncle (the brachium conjunctivum); F.l.m. = the medial longitudinal fascicle; L.m. = the medial lemniscus; V.mes. = the mesencephalic trigeminal nucleus; Tr.mes. = mesencephalic tract of the trigeminal nerve.

and widespread organization of its fibers and the lack of topographic organization suggest other, *nonspecific effects on large parts of the brain* as well. In Chapter 9, we mentioned possible *facilitatory effects on spinal motoneurons.* The nucleus is probably also instrumental in *the activating system of the brain stem* discussed later in this chapter.

The Efferent Connections of the Reticular Formation

The reticular formation sends fibers to (and thereby acts on) four main regions: the *thalamus,* the *spinal cord, brain stem nuclei,* and the *cerebellum.* The influence on brain stem nuclei, such as the cranial nerve nuclei, is mediated in large part by collaterals of the long ascending and descending fibers destined for the thalamus and the cord. The reticular cell groups sending fibers to the thalamus overlap with cell groups sending fibers to the cord. The overlap is only partial, however, so that areas can be distinguished which send either ascending or descending efferent fibers (Fig. 12.9).

The *descending reticular fibers* to the cord run in the ventral part of the lateral funiculus and in the ventral funiculus (Fig. 12.7). Such *reticulospinal fibers* end primarily on interneurons, which in turn can influence motoneurons. The *ventral reticulospinal tract*[2] was discussed in Chapter 9 in relation to motor control. This is in reality not *one* tract but several that differ with regard both to anatomic organization and functional properties. The ventral reticulospinal tracts are both crossed and uncrossed and mediate both inhibitory and excitatory effects on spinal motoneurons. The reticulospinal neurons are further characterized by their axonal branching pattern, with collaterals given off at several levels of the spinal cord. Thus, muscles in different parts of the body can be influenced by each neuron. As discussed in Chapter 9, the *ventral reticulospinal tracts are of particular importance for postural mechanisms, for the orientation of the head and body toward external stimuli, and for voluntary movements of proximal body parts.*

The *ascending fibers* from the reticular formation end in the *intralaminar thalamic nuclei* (Figs. 2.23, 4.19, and 12.8) unlike the specific sensory tracts ending in the lateral thalamic nucleus. Some fibers also end in the *hypothalamus.* We will discuss the functional significance of the ascending reticular connections later in this chapter; suffice it here to say that they are of particular importance for the general level of activity of the cerebral cortex, which in turn is related to consciousness and attention.

Figure 17.9 shows that the cell groups giving off ascending axons are located somewhat more caudally than those emitting descending axons. By means of the numerous collaterals of both the ascending and descending fibers in the reticular formation (Figs. 12.3 and 12.4), the two kinds of cell groups can influence each other. Furthermore, there are also many interneurons connecting different parts of the reticular formation. Thus a close cooperation is possible between the parts of the reticular formation acting on the cerebral cortex and those acting on the spinal cord.

Connections from the Reticular Formation to the Cerebellum

Three distinct cell groups within the reticular formation send most of their efferent fibers to the cerebellum. They are therefore regarded as being among the *precerebellar nuclei.* This first of these is the *reticulotegmental nucleus* (nucleus reticularis tegmenti pontis), situated immediately dorsal to the pontine nuclei. It receives afferent connections from the pretectal nuclei and the superior colliculus among other cell groups, and sends fibers in particular to regions of the cerebellum known to participate in the control of eye movements. The second cell group, the *lateral reticular nucleus,* lies in the medulla, lateral to the inferior olive. It receives its main afferent input from the spinal cord and is therefore a link in one of the indirect spinocerebellar pathways (see Chapter 11). It also receives vestibular inputs (from the vestibular nuclei), however, and may therefore serve to integrate information about the activity in motor-related spinal interneurons with information about the position of the body (head). The smallest of the precerebellar reticular nuclei is the *paramedian reticular nucleus,* lo-

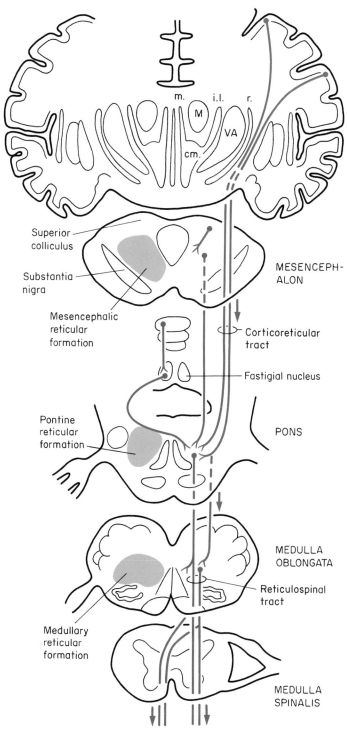

Labels in figure:
m. i.l. r.
M
VA
cm.

Superior colliculus

Substantia nigra

Mesencephalic reticular formation

MESENCEPH-ALON

Corticoreticular tract

Fastigial nucleus

Pontine reticular formation

PONS

MEDULLA OBLONGATA

Reticulospinal tract

Medullary reticular formation

MEDULLA SPINALIS

Fig. 12.7. *The descending connections of the reticular formation and afferents from higher levels.* Note that descending fibers from the cerebral cortex end on reticulospinal neurons. Most of the long connections are both crossed and uncrossed, although this is not shown in the figure. Numerous shorter fibers interconnecting subdivisions of the reticular formation are not shown.

291

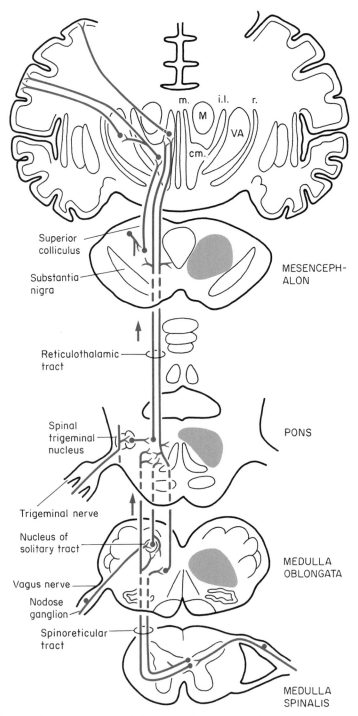

Fig. 12.8. *The ascending connections of the reticular formation and afferents from lower levels.* The afferents from lower levels arise in the cord (spinoreticular neurons) and in the cranial nerve nuclei. The ascending fibers from the reticular formation end in the intralaminar thalamic nuclei. In addition, there are direct connections to the cerebral cortex from the raphe nuclei and the nucleus locus coeruleus, not shown in this figure (Figs. 12.5 and 12.6).

cated medially in the medulla. It receives afferents from the spinal cord and some other sources. Its functional role is not known.

The Afferent Connections of the Reticular Formation

Various cell groups send fibers to the reticular formation (Figs. 12.7 and 12.8). *Spinoreticular fibers* were discussed in Chapter 4. They ascend in the ventral part of the lateral funiculus together with the spinothalamic tract,[3] but diverge in the lower medulla. Among other destinations, the fibers end in the parts of the reticular formation giving off long ascending axons to the thalamus. This provides a spinoreticulothalamic pathway that is anatomically and functionally different from the major sensory pathways discussed in Chapter 4. Some of the spinoreticular fibers end in areas where neurons send axons back to the spinal cord, thus establishing feedback loops between the reticular formation and the cord.

Corticoreticular fibers arise mainly in the cortical areas that give origin to the pyramidal tract. They end preponderantly in the regions of the reticular formation sending axons to the spinal cord. Therefore, a corticoreticulospinal pathway exists. It is known to be of importance for the control of voluntary and automatic movements, as discussed in Chapter 9.

The *superior colliculus* sends fibers to parts of the reticular formation. These connections make it possible for visual signals to influence the reticular formation, since the superior colliculus receives visual information directly from the retina and from the visual cortex.

In addition to spinal neurons that send their axons only to the reticular formation, many *secondary sensory neurons send collaterals to the reticular formation*. This concerns many of the fibers of the spinothalamic tract, which, presumably, mediate *nociceptive and thermoceptive signals* to the reticular formation. The same kind of information from the face is provided by collaterals of ascending axons from the sensory (spinal) trigeminal nucleus. *Visceral sensory* impulses reach the reticular formation by collaterals of ascending fibers from the nucleus of the solitary tract (which receives afferents from the vagus nerve, for example). *Auditory* signals reach the reticular formation by collaterals of ascending fibers in the auditory pathways. *Vestibular* signals come from the vestibular nuclei. Finally, the reticular formation receives afferents from the *cerebellum* (primarily the fastigial nucleus, Fig. 11.4). This is an important pathway for the cerebellar influence on α and γ motoneurons.

The Reticular Formation Integrates Various Kinds of Information

The above description of afferents indicates that *signals from virtually all kinds of receptors can influence neurons of the reticular formation*. This is also shown by physiological experiments. Electrodes placed in the reticular formation can record potentials evoked by stimulation of receptors for light, sound, smell, and taste. Furthermore, stimulation of peripheral nerves carrying signals from cutaneous receptors and proprioceptors and of visceral nerves evokes activity. Whenever a receptor is stimulated, the signals reach not only the cortical areas of importance for the perception of the stimulus but also the reticular formation. Finally, stimulation of the cerebral cortex, the hypothalamus, and limbic structures can produce changes in the activity of the reticular formation. Thus, under normal conditions, there are always signals coming into the reticular formation, keeping it in a state of tonic activity. The extent of the tonic activity depends on how strongly the reticular formation is "bombarded" by receptors and by other parts of the brain.

Anatomic and physiological data indicate that large parts of the reticular formation are characterized by *integration* of various kinds of information. The efferent signals from the reticular formation do not provide specific information about features such as stimulus modality. The very long dendrites and numerous interneurons with widely branching axons form a structural basis for integration. Such findings, together with physiological data showing that electrical stimulation of the reticular formation typically produces widespread and unspecific effects, led to the assumption that the reticular formation functions as a unity (without regional specialization). More recent investigations with more refined methods have shown, however, that the reticular formation is heterogeneous both anatomically and functionally, even though the borders between different subregions are not sharp.

FUNCTIONS OF THE RETICULAR FORMATION

It follows from the above discussion of its efferent connections that the reticular formation can act on virtually all other parts of the central nervous system. We have previously considered its effects on the spinal cord (Chapters 4 and 9), and we will add more below on this point. In addition, we will discuss the effects on the cerebral cortex, which are of particular importance. Parts of the reticular formation that are involved in the control of eye movements are discussed in Chapter 13, whereas the parts involved in the control of autonomic functions are described briefly in Chapter 15.

The Activating System

It is striking that the efferent connections of the reticular formation can *activate* both lower and higher levels of the central nervous system. Electrical stimulation alters several functions mediated by the spinal cord, such as muscle tone, respiration, and blood pressure. Also, the general activity of the cerebral cortex—which is closely related to the level of consciousness—can be altered by stimulation of the reticular formation. *The activating system of the brain stem* was therefore introduced as another name for

the reticular formation. Stimulation of the reticular formation, however, can also produce inhibitory effects on several processes.

As mentioned above, we believe that there is a tonic activity of the reticular formation maintained by a constant inflow of impulses from various sources. The level of tonic activity is reflected by the level of consciousness, among other things. The activity of the reticular formation is in fact essential for the conscious awareness of specific sensory stimuli and for adequate behavioral responses to them. When our attention is caught by a novel stimulus, this is mediated by the reticular formation. At the same time, the reticular formation produces the motor responses that ensure automatic orientation of the head and the body toward the source of the stimulus. The motor apparatus is mobilized, together with alterations of respiration and circulation.

Actions on Skeletal Muscles

Animal experiments during the 1940s led to the identification of two regions within the reticular formation that influence *the tone of the skeletal muscles.* Stimulation of a region in the medulla that sends particularly strong connections to the spinal cord (Figs. 12.9 and 12.10) could inhibit stretch reflexes and also movements induced by stimulation of the motor cortex. This region was therefore called the *inhibitory region.* A region with opposite effects, the *facilitatory region,* was found rostral to the inhibitory one. It extends rostrally into the mesencephalon and is located somewhat more laterally than the inhibitory region.[4] The actions in the cord concern not only α but also γ motoneurons, so that the reticular formation can control the sensitivity of the muscle spindles. The activity of the γ motoneurons is increased by stimulation of the facilitatory region and inhibited by the inhibitory region. The muscle tone can therefore be up- and down-regulated by changes in the balance between the influences from the two regions. Since the cerebral cortex, the cerebellum, the basal ganglia, and other regions

Fig. 12.9. *Position of efferent reticular cell groups.* Drawing of sagittal section through the brain stem (cat). To the **left,** the areas with neurons sending axons to higher levels (the thalamus) are indicated with dots, whereas areas sending fibers to the spinal cord are shown in the **right** drawing. Note that the cell groups sending descending fibers are located somewhat more rostrally than the regions sending ascending fibers, providing opportunity for mutual influences by collaterals (as shown in Fig. 12.3). NVII, VI, X, XII = cranial nerve nuclei; P. = pontine nuclei; Tr. = trapezoid body; N. cun. = cuneate nucleus; N. rub. = red nucleus; Or. inf. = inferior olive.

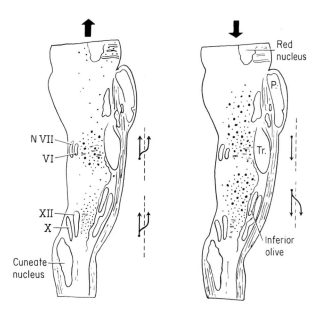

send fibers to the reticular formation, it is not unexpected that muscle tone can be influenced from these parts as well. It should be recalled, however, that other cell groups than the reticular formation also have direct access to the motoneurons, notably the vestibular nuclei with their strong facilitatory effects on the tone of muscles maintaining the upright position (the concept of muscle tone is discussed in Chapter 8).

In addition to the rather diffuse effects on muscle tone obtained by electrical stimulation of the reticular formation, its role in the control of certain kinds of voluntary and reflex movements was discussed in Chapter 9. There is, however, no principal difference between the influence of motoneurons in eliciting a movement and in maintaining a (static) posture. On the basis of the present state of knowledge of the organization of the reticular formation, the emphasis is more on its control of fairly specific motor tasks than on its diffuse effects on the muscle system as a whole. Certain subregions have, for example, a particular role in control of the *rhythmic locomotor movements* (Chapter 9), whereas other regions are devoted to the control of *eye movements* (Chapter 13), and some are concerned primarily with *orienting movements of the head and the body* in response to optic and vestibular stimuli. In such cases, parts of the reticular formation—often consisting of fairly extensive networks—collect the relevant information about, for example, the position of the head

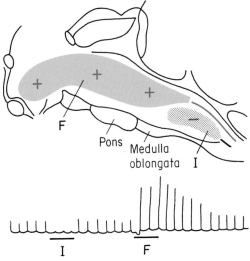

Fig. 12.10. *Facilitatory (F) and inhibitory (I) regions of the reticular formation.* Schematic sagittal section through the brain stem (cat). The diagram **below** shows the amplitude of the patellar reflex (measured with EMG). In the period marked I, the inhibitory region was stimulated electrically, and the reflex response is almost abolished. In the F period, the facilitatory region was stimulated, and the patellar reflex response is markedly enhanced. From Kaada (1950).

and body, and ensure through their output signals the coordinated activity of all the muscles that are necessary to produce a proper response. Such reticular cell groups are often called *premotor centers*. Common to premotor centers is their control of the activity of large groups of muscles.

Effects on Respiration and Circulation

The early investigations with stimulation of the reticular formation indicated that inspiratory movements are evoked from a region that coincides roughly with the inhibitory region (Fig. 12.10). Expiratory movements were produced by stimulation within the facilitatory region in the medulla. Later studies with microelectrodes have shown, however, that neurons with respiratory movement-related activity are found in several regions of the reticular formation, and not only in the medulla. Furthermore, a clear-cut separation of an inspiratory and an expiratory region appears not to be tenable.

Several kinds of information reaching reticular neurons are relevant for the *control of respiration*, such as signals from receptors within the lung tissue and from receptors in the walls of the large arteries, which monitor the blood concentration of oxygen and carbon dioxide.

The reticular formation also receives all information necessary to *control blood pressure, the distribution of the blood volume among the organs, the stroke volume, and the heart rate* (see Chapter 14). To some extent, a distinction can be made between inhibitory and facilitatory regions for circulatory control, too. A "pressor" region producing increased blood pressure on stimulation and a "depressor" region with the opposite effect were originally identified in the medulla. Conditions have turned out to be more complex, however. As with respiratory control, rather extensive parts of the reticular formation participate in the coordination of the proper adjustments of the work of the heart and the diameter of the vessels. The effects are mediated chiefly by

reticulospinal fibers that act on preganglionic sympathetic neurons and by reticular efferents to the dorsal motor nucleus of the vagus.

Effects of the Reticular Formation on the Cerebral Cortex

The ascending effect of the reticular formation was brought into focus by a paper published by the neurophysiologists Moruzzi (Italian) and Magoun (American) in 1949. Suddenly, new perspectives were opened on important aspects of brain functioning, especially consciousness, sleep, and wakefulness. On the basis of their animal experiments, Moruzzi and Magoun formulated a new concept: *the ascending activating system of the brain stem.*

Electrical stimulation of the reticular formation in anesthetized animals produces certain changes of the electrical activity in the cortex, as recorded by *electroencephalography (EEG)*. This method samples the collective activity of neurons in large parts of the cerebral cortex. Depending on how coordinated, or *synchronized,* the neuronal activity is, different kinds of waves are seen in the encephalogram. Under anesthesia (without stimulation), relatively slow waves dominate (Fig. 12.11). On stimulation of the reticular formation, the slow waves of the EEG are replaced by waves with a faster and more irregular rate and with a lower amplitude. We say that the EEG changes from *synchronization* to *desynchronization*. Together with desynchronization or *activation* of the EEG occur signs of increased attention and alertness—that is, an *arousal* is produced. Such an arousal can be produced also in unanesthetized animals with implanted electrodes. For example, a cat lying still with no obvious interest in its surroundings becomes suddenly alert and attentive when the reticular formation is stimulated with a high-frequency train of impulses. Various kinds of experiments confirmed the hypothesis of Moruzzi and Magoun that *the reticular formation is necessary for the mainte-*

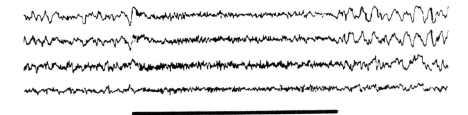

1 sec.

Fig. 12.11. *EEG recordings from the classic studies of Moruzzi and Magoun of the activating system of the brain stem.* The four tracings are recorded over different parts of the cerebral cortex of a cat. The thick line shows the period of electrical stimulation of the reticular formation. The stimulation produces desynchronization of the EEG (activation), which returns to a synchronized pattern when the stimulation stops.

nance of normal wakeful consciousness. The reticular formation determines the level of wakefulness, with its many variations from tense alertness to drowsiness and sleep. Marked reduction of the activity of the reticular formation is associated with unconsciousness, as shown experimentally in animals with selective lesions. In humans with prolonged periods of unconsciousness after head injuries, there is often damage of the mesencephalic reticular formation. The lesion can be surprisingly small and yet produce deep unconsciousness.

As mentioned above, the reticular formation can have either activating or inhibiting effects on functions mediated by the spinal cord, depending on which region is stimulated (Fig. 12.10). Similar findings were made with regard to the ascending effects on the cerebral cortex, even though we so far have discussed only the activating effects. It appears that inhibition—that is, synchronization of the EEG—is evoked most easily from the caudal parts, whereas activation or desynchronization is evoked from the rostral parts (corresponding to the effects on skeletal muscles).

Electroencephalography

Direct recording from the surface of the cerebral cortex of animals shows that the patterns of electrical waves differ among parts of the hemispheres. In humans, too, direct recordings from the exposed cortex can be done during brain surgery (electrocorticography). The electrical waves are conducted through the skull and the soft tissues of the scalp and can therefore be recorded with electrodes placed on the skin of the head. With this method, *electroencephalography*, the electrical signals are dispersed and attenuated on their way through the skull and soft tissues, so that the origin of the signals within the hemisphere can only be roughly determined. Nevertheless, the method has been of great importance both for research and diagnostically since its introduction around 1930.

The electroencephalogram or EEG varies considerably with age; most marked are the changes during the first couple of years. There are also individual variations. Furthermore, the EEG pattern changes during sleep and during general anesthesia. Hyperventilation, which leads to a reduced carbon dioxide concentration in the blood, changes the excitability of cortical neurons, and this is reflected in the EEG. Finally, several drugs affect the EEG.

When analyzing the EEG, one can discern various wave forms and patterns. The α *waves* are relatively slow, with a frequency of 8–12/sec (Fig. 12.12). They occur typically in an awake person who is relaxed and resting with her eyes closed. When the person opens her eyes or starts to think about a mental task (Fig. 12.12), the EEG immediately changes to a pattern with more irregular waves with a higher frequency and lower amplitude. These are called β *waves*. The change of wave pattern from α to β waves is called *desynchronization* or *activation* of the EEG. During sleep, other wave forms and patterns occur that are typical of specific stages of sleep. Various neurological diseases can be diag-

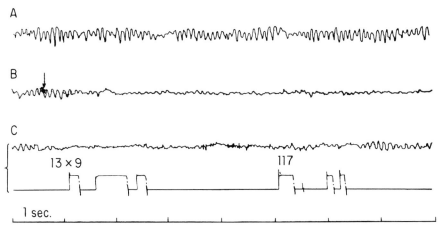

Fig. 12.12. *EEG (electroencephalography).* Three traces are shown, all of them recorded over the occipital lobes. **A.** The person is in a relaxed state, with his eyes closed. There are α waves typical of synchronization. **B.** At the arrow, the person opens his eyes and the α waves are replaced by faster, irregular waves with smaller amplitude, called β waves. The EEG is desynchronized. **C.** Desynchronization produced by solving a mental task. The person is asked to make a calculation (13×9). After the calculation is completed (117), the slower waves return.

nosed because they are associated with characteristic changes of the EEG. To some extent, the EEG can also help to localize the disease process. EEG is particularly important in the diagnosis of epilepsy.

It is not fully understood how the various wave forms in the normal EEG arise, but it is clear that they depend in large measure on different activity states in thalamocortical neurons. Thalamocortical neurons (functioning as relay cells for transmission of sensory and other signals to the cortex) have unique membrane properties owing to the presence of a special kind of Ca^{2+} channel that opens only when the cell is hyperpolarized to a certain level. Thalamocortical neurons generate action potential in two different patterns or modes: They may fire in bursts (that is, they fire 2–8 action potentials with a high frequency followed by a pause), or they fire single spikes with a varying overall frequency. The bursting pattern is associated with synchronization of the EEG (in states of drowsiness and so-called slow-wave sleep), whereas the single-spike firing occurs together with desynchronization (during attentiveness and during rapid-eye-movement sleep). It appears that these different functional states of the thalamocortical (relay) neurons determine whether they transmit signals to the cortex; only in the single-spike mode do the cells transmit to the cortex the information they receive from, for example, peripheral receptors.

Impulse Pathways for the Activation of the Cerebral Cortex

What are the pathways used by the reticular formation to influence consciousness, attention, and sleep? All of the major specific sensory pathways (the spinothalamic tract, the medial lemniscus, and the visual and auditory pathways) can be interrupted without affecting consciousness or the activation of the EEG produced by stimulation of the reticular formation. On the other hand, when these sensory pathways are left intact but the ascending connections of the reticular formation are interrupted by a cut in the mesencephalon, the animal becomes unconscious. Electrical stimulation of the reticular formation can no longer activate the EEG, even though stimulation of peripheral receptors evokes potentials in the cortical sensory regions. Thus, the sensory signals reach the cortex, but they are restricted to the sensory regions, and, most importantly, they are unable to arouse the animal.

Pathways other than the major sensory ones must therefore be responsible when the reticular formation activates the EEG over major parts of the cerebral hemisphere and produces behavioral changes indicating increased attention. Connections from the reticular formation to the intralaminar thalamic nuclei are likely candidates. Thus, electrical stimulation of these nuclei can produce activation of the EEG similar to that seen after stimulation of the reticular formation itself. The intralaminar thalamic nuclei send widespread efferents to the cerebral cortex. Therefore, a reticulothalamocortical pathway probably is important for the actions of the reticular formation on the cerebral cortex. Many, but not all, of the reticulothalamic fibers to the intralaminar nuclei are cholinergic. In addition to this indirect reticulothalamocortical pathway, there are direct projections to the cerebral cortex from monoaminergic cell groups in the brain stem—usually considered parts of the reticular formation—such as the raphe nuclei and the nucleus locus coeruleus. These projections are also related to attentional mechanisms and the states of sleep and wakefulness, as indicated by physiological and pharmacological studies.

The Reticular Formation and the Control of Sensory Information

In Chapter 4, we discussed how the central transmission of sensory signals can be controlled from higher levels of the central nervous system. Descending connections to the spinal cord from the raphe nuclei and various (other) parts of the reticular formation have been shown to suppress the central conduction of signals from nociceptors. Furthermore, the central transmission of visual, auditory, and other sensory impulses is subjected to control by the reticular formation. Thus, even though it is not alone in this capacity, the reticular formation plays an important role in the elimination of sensory signals that are considered irrelevant, so that our attention can be focused on the relevant signals.

Together with other mechanisms, inhibition from the reticular formation can ensure that, for example, we do not notice that someone is talking to us while we are absorbed in a book. This role is closely related to the one played by the reticular formation in attention and consciousness. Thus, the reticular formation is perhaps more concerned with the focusing of our attention on certain stimuli or internal events—that is, restricting our awareness—than with a global control of consciousness.[5]

Sleep

Sleep consists of several phases that can be distinguished on the basis of differences in the EEG. The transition from alertness to drowsiness changes the EEG in the direction of synchronization. When a subject is falling into a deep, quiet sleep, the α waves disappear altogether and are replaced by irregular slow waves with greater amplitude. After an initial light *phase I,* the sleep becomes gradually deeper, until *phase IV.* To waken a person in sleep phase IV requires relatively strong stimuli, whereas only weak stimuli are necessary in phase I. *Phase V* is special because the EEG is desynchronized, and there are conjugated movements of the eyes, much like a person looking at moving objects. Because of these *rapid eye movements* (REM), this phase is also called *REM sleep* or *paradoxical sleep.* Muscle tone is generally reduced, with occasional muscular twitches, and there are changes of blood pressure and heart rate. Dreaming occurs—at least mainly—during REM sleep. The various phases of sleep follow each other with the same order throughout the night. Usually, the first REM phase occurs after about 1½ hours of sleep and lasts for about 10 minutes. Thereafter the REM phases return at intervals of 1 to 2 hours. When waking up (or being wakened) just after a REM phase, a person remembers the content of the dream vividly.

The neural basis of sleep and its various phases is still not fully clarified and has turned out to be very complex. Several brain regions and neurotransmitters are of importance. Lesions of the *hypothalamus,* for example, can lead to increased or reduced amounts of sleep, but it is clear that the neuronal groups directly involved in sleep control are located in the brain stem, especially in the pons. Initially, after the discovery of the activating system, it was assumed that sleep was simply the result of reduced activity of the activating system—that is, a purely passive process. Further studies showed, however, that sleep could be induced by electrical stimulation of the lower parts of the reticular formation and that lesions of the same region prevented sleep (insomnia). The *raphe nuclei* (especially the dorsal raphe nucleus) are of importance for sleep, perhaps especially for the REM phase. Typically, raphe neurons reduce their activity at the start of a REM phase ("REM-off neurons"). Since many of the raphe neurons are *serotoninergic*, it seems reasonable that this transmitter is involved in REM sleep. Attempts to test this hypothesis have given conflicting results, however. The *nucleus locus coeruleus*—with mainly *noradrenergic* neurons—also appears to play a role in sleep mechanisms, although its exact role is debated. Relatively specific cooling of the nucleus (which is a reversible way of making the neurons inactive) induces REM sleep, in agreement with the presence of many "REM-off neurons" in this nucleus. Destruction of descending fibers from the nucleus locus coeruleus (and from some other cell groups in the vicinity) abolishes the inhibition of motor activity that is characteristic of the REM phase. After such lesions, animals still have REM sleep, but behave as if they were acting out their dreams with orienting movements, more complex exploratory behavior, and attack or flight. Neurons that increase their activity in relation to REM sleep ("REM-on neurons") are found in the dorsolateral part of the pons (laterodorsal tegmental nucleus, the pedunculopontine tegmental nucleus, and the parabrachial nucleus). Many of these neurons are *cholinergic*. It now appears that REM sleep is characterized by increased activity of cholinergic neurons, and reduced activity of monoaminergic neurons in the dorsolateral pons. The effects produced by the activity of the cholinergic REM-on neurons is most likely mediated largely via connections to several other parts of the reticular formation. Several neuropeptides (substance P, somatostatin, VIP) are colocalized with the classical transmitters in REM-related neurons.

The monoaminergic REM-off neurons and the cholinergic REM-on neurons are largely intermingled in the dorsolateral part of the pons, which may explain why lesion experiments have yielded conflicting results.

Narcolepsy, which is a genetically linked disease with sudden, irresistible attacks of REM sleep (or components of REM sleep), may be related to an increased concentration of muscarinic receptors within the brain stem. Furthermore, there is evidence that monoamine metabolism is deficient. Both drugs that block muscarinic receptors and drugs that increase synaptic concentration of monoamines (such as amphetamine and tricyclic antidepressants) are reported to reduce the narcoleptic attacks.

The Reticular Formation and the Relationship between Mental and Bodily Processes

Variations in the activity of the reticular formation are reflected in virtually all aspects of the nervous processes and also in the activity of the endocrine organs controlled by the hypothalamus. Knowledge of such interactions may help to explain how mental and bodily processes are so intimately correlated and often change in parallel. There is much evidence to suggest that the activity of the reticular formation is influenced by our mental state. The thought of a forthcoming, unpleasant event or the memory of an embarrassing or agonizing situation may suddenly make a drowsy person alert and tense (increased muscle tone), produce sweating, increase the heart rate, and so forth. Every doctor who routinely tests reflexes knows that apprehension and anxiousness is accompanied by increased reflex responses and increased muscular tone. An exaggerated patellar reflex at the start of a consultation becomes "normal" as the patient relaxes. Another everyday example is the difficulty in falling asleep when one is preoccupied with distressing thoughts.

All of the above effects are expressions of increased activity of the reticular formation produced by the influence of psychic processes—presumably closely linked with neuronal activity in the cerebral cortex, limbic structures, and the hypothalamus. Thus, stimulation of certain cortical areas can increase the activity of reticular neurons, and this is followed by desynchronization of the EEG. Nonanesthetized animals at the same time become attentive. These effects are mediated by direct and indirect connections from the cortex to the brain stem. There are also connections from the hypothalamus and limbic structures (such as the amygdaloid nucleus) to the reticular formation, which may be of particular importance because emotionally colored psychic phenomena are most effective in causing activation.

That insomnia is related to increased activity in the reticular formation is suggested by the fact that most drugs used against insomnia reduce the activity of reticular neurons. General anesthesia abolishes the transmission through central parts of the reticular formation (resulting in lack of activation of the EEG and unconsciousness), whereas the transmission in the specific sensory pathways is less affected.

It is also well known that bodily processes can influence our mental state. For example, a treatment that leads to muscle relaxation usually also reduces mental tension. Again, the effects are probably mediated by a reduction of the activity of the reticular formation. At the same time there are alterations of respiration, blood pressure, heart rate, and other autonomic functions, such as sweat secretion, peristaltic movements of the bowel, and secretion of gastric juice. Most likely, some of the autonomic expressions of anxiety may by themselves serve to maintain and increase the anxiety.

NOTES

1. Some authors include certain thalamic cell groups—especially the intralaminar nuclei—in the term "the reticular formation of the brain stem."

2. Reticulospinal fibers are located also in the dorsal part of the lateral funiculus (dorsal reticulospinal tract). Many of these fibers are monoaminergic and come from, among other places, the raphe nuclei and adjoining parts of the reticular formation, as discussed in Chapter 4. These dorsal pathways appear to be primarily concerned with control of sensory transmission from the dorsal roots to motoneurons (segmental reflex arcs) and to second-order sensory neurons, which are links in the ascending sensory pathways.

3. The medial lemniscus does not give off collaterals to the reticular formation. Information from low-threshold mechanoreceptors must therefore reach the reticular formation via spinoreticular neurons.

4. The distinction between inhibitory and facilitatory regions is less sharp than originally believed. In several places, single neurons with inhibitory or facilitatory actions on muscles are intermingled.

5. The term consciousness is used here without attempting to define it precisely. Indeed, no satisfactory definition appears to have been put forward. Such attempts soon end in a discussion of how nervous impulses can be translated into a mental experience. Even though the term consciousness is an abstraction—it cannot be imagined without a content, that is, consciousness *of* something—it is of clinical value to distinguish between levels of consciousness (from attention to coma, as the extremes).

13

Cranial Nerves

We usually count 12 cranial nerves, even though neither the first (the olfactory nerve) nor the second (the optic nerve) are true nerves. These two and, in addition, the cochlear nerve were dealt with in Chapters 5, 6, and 7. A brief survey of the anatomy of the cranial nerves was given in Chapter 2 (Figs. 2.15 and 2.16).

GENERAL ORGANIZATION OF THE CRANIAL NERVES

Before dealing with specifics for each of the cranial nerves (Fig. 13.1), we will discuss some features that are common to them all. Like the spinal nerves that connect the spinal cord with the body, the cranial nerves connect the brain stem with the peripheral organs. Several structural features are shared by the spinal cord and the brain stem, and thus also by the spinal and cranial nerves. Nevertheless, the brain stem is less regularly built and more complex in its organization than the spinal cord, and the cranial nerves are not as schematic in their composition as the spinal nerves. Most of the cranial nerves, for example, lack a distinct ventral (motor) root and a dorsal (sensory) root. Some of the cranial nerves are purely sensory, others are

purely motor, and others are mixed. Like the spinal nerves, several of the cranial nerves contain autonomic (preganglionic) fibers supplying smooth muscles and glands. Finally, some also contain afferent fibers from visceral organs.

The Cranial Nerves Can Contain Four Different Kinds of Nerve Fibers

The cranial nerves can contain the following kinds of fibers:

1. *Somatic efferent* fibers innervating skeletal (striated) muscles;
2. *Visceral efferent* fibers supplying smooth muscles and glands and belonging to the *parasympathetic* part of the autonomic nervous system;
3. *Somatic afferent* fibers with sensory impulses from the skin and mucous membranes of the face, from muscles and joints, and from the vestibular apparatus;
4. *Visceral afferent* fibers with sensory impulses from the visceral organs.

The *efferent fibers* of the cranial nerves have their perikarya in brain stem nuclei corresponding to the columns of spinal motoneurons (Fig. 8.2) and the intermediolateral cell column of the cord (Fig. 14.2). We use the

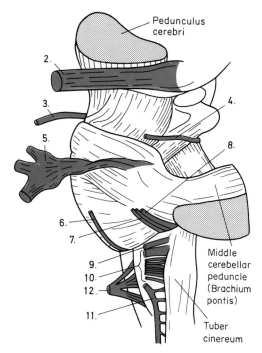

Pedunculus
cerebri

2.

3.

5.

4.

8.

6.

7.

9.

10.

12.

11.

Middle
cerebellar
peduncle
(Brachium
pontis)

Tuber
cinereum

Fig. 13.1. *The brain stem and the cranial nerves.* Seen from the left side. See also Figures 2.15 and 2.16.

terms *somatic efferent* and *visceral efferent cranial nerve nuclei* of these cell groups (Figs. 13.2 and 13.3). The *afferent fibers* have their perikarya in ganglia close to the brain stem, corresponding to the spinal ganglia. The central process of the ganglion cells enters the brain stem and ends on neurons in nuclei corresponding to the spinal dorsal horn and the dorsal column nuclei (Fig. 13.4). We use the terms *somatic afferent* and *visceral afferent cranial nerve nuclei* for such groups. From such afferent (sensory) nuclei, signals are conducted centrally to the thalamus and the cortex, and via brain stem interneurons to the somatic and visceral efferent (motor) cranial nerve nuclei (as links of brain stem reflex arcs).

The Cranial Nerve Nuclei Are Formed Like Longitudinal Columns

In early embryonic life, all neurons giving origin to a particular kind of fiber lie together in one longitudinal column in the brain stem. During further development, however, these columns break up into smaller groups, and some of these groups move away from the original column. Nevertheless, the tendency for cranial nerve nuclei of the same category to form columns can be recognized also in the adult brain (Fig. 13.2). The demonstration of this regular pattern has been of value in understanding the functions of the cranial nerves. Furthermore, knowledge of this pattern aids us in learning about the cranial nerves and their nuclei.

The Position of the Cranial Nerve Nuclei

It is helpful at the outset to remember the following general rule (evident from Figs. 13.2 and 13.3): *The efferent (motor) nerve nuclei lie medially in the brain stem, whereas the afferent (sensory) nuclei are located laterally.*

The *somatic efferent nuclei* are in early embryonic life all arranged in a column close to the midline, but later some move away in a ventrolateral direction (Fig. 13.3). Those remaining in the medialmost column are termed *general somatic efferent* and comprise (from caudal to rostral) *the nucleus of the accessory nerve (11), the nucleus of the hypoglossal nerve (12), the nucleus of the abducent nerve (6), and the nucleus of the oculomotor nerve (3).* (In the following we will for practical reasons use abbreviated names, such as the accessory nucleus and the hypoglossal nucleus.) All of these nuclei innervate *myotome muscles*—that is, muscles that are developed from the segmentally arranged somites of early embryonic life. The somatic efferent nuclei that have moved away from the medial column all innervate *branchial muscles*—that is, striated muscles developed from the branchial arches (facial and masticatory muscles, and muscles of the pharynx and larynx). We call these nuclei *special somatic efferent.* This group comprises the *nucleus ambiguus (9, 10), the facial nucleus (7), and the motor trigeminal nucleus (5).*

The *visceral efferent* (parasympathetic)

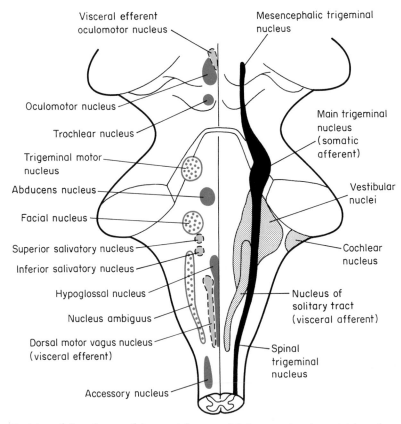

Visceral efferent
oculomotor nucleus

Mesencephalic trigeminal
nucleus

Oculomotor nucleus

Trochlear nucleus

Trigeminal motor
nucleus

Abducens nucleus

Facial nucleus

Superior salivatory nucleus

Inferior salivatory nucleus

Hypoglossal nucleus

Nucleus ambiguus

Dorsal motor vagus nucleus
(visceral efferent)

Accessory nucleus

Main trigeminal
nucleus
(somatic
afferent)

Vestibular
nuclei

Cochlear
nucleus

Nucleus of
solitary tract
(visceral afferent)

Spinal
trigeminal
nucleus

Fig. 13.2. *Position of the columns of the cranial nerve nuclei.* Schematic drawing of the brain stem seen from the dorsal aspect. The somatic efferent nuclei innervating myotome muscles are shown in dark red. The special somatic efferent nuclei innervating branchial arch muscles are marked with red dots. The visceral efferent nuclei are shown in red. In the right half, the sensory nuclei are shown.

column of cranial nerve nuclei is located immediately lateral to the somatic efferent column (Fig. 13.3) and comprises the *dorsal motor nucleus of the vagus* (10), the small *inferior and superior salivatory nuclei* (9, 7), and the *parasympathetic oculomotor nucleus of Edinger-Westphal* (3). The *visceral afferent* fibers all end in one long nucleus, the *nucleus of the solitary tract,* which is located lateral to the visceral afferent column (Fig. 13.3).

Most laterally we find the *somatic afferent* nuclei. This group comprises the *sensory trigeminal nucleus* (5), the *vestibular nuclei* (8), and the *cochlear nuclei* (8). The sensory trigeminal nucleus consists of three functionally different parts (the spinal, the principal, and the mesencephalic nuclei). Together the three parts form one continuous column, however, which extends from the upper cervical segments of the cord into the mesencephalon (Fig. 13.2).

The fibers of the vestibulocochlear nerve are often classified as *special somatic afferent* because they originate from special sense organs; the trigeminal fibers are then termed *general somatic afferent.*

Figures 13.2 and 13.3, and the above account, show that fibers of one kind all come from one of the columns of nuclei only, even though the fibers peripherally may follow several of the cranial nerves. Thus, all (general) somatic afferent fibers end in the sensory trigeminal nucleus, whereas the fibers

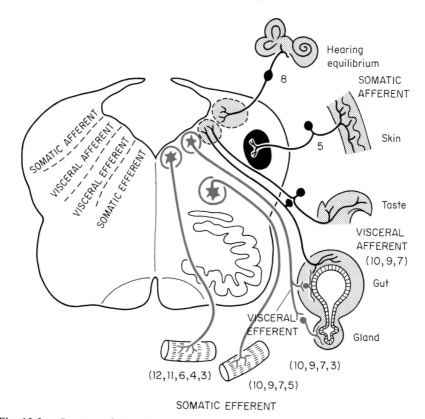

Fig. 13.3. *Position of the columns of the cranial nerve nuclei.* Schematic cross section of the medulla.

peripherally follow not only the trigeminal nerve but also the glossopharyngeal and the vagus nerves.

The Development of the Cranial Nerve Nuclei

The positions and arrangement of the cranial nerve nuclei can be understood on the basis of some knowledge of the development of the nervous system. In the part of the neural tube that later becomes the spinal cord, there is first on each side of the central canal a distinct dorsal part, the *alar plate,* and a ventral part, the *basal plate* (Fig. 13.5A). The efferent (motor) nuclei of the cord develop from the basal plate, whereas the afferent (sensory) nuclei, which receive afferents from the spinal ganglia, develop from the alar plate. In the brain stem part of the neural tube, the central canal widens to form the fourth ventricle, and the alar plate is then bent laterally (Fig. 13.5B). Thus, the alar plate comes to lie laterally rather than dorsally, and the basal plate medially rather than ventrally. The border between them is marked by the *sulcus limitans.* By further differentiation, the pattern arises that was described above for the cranial nerve nuclei—for example, by division of the somatic efferent column, with one part remaining close to the floor of the fourth ventricle and one part moving ventrolaterally (Fig. 13.5C).

Some of the columns of cranial nerve nuclei extend through only a limited part of the brain stem. For example, the visceral afferent nucleus (the nucleus of the solitary tract) is present only in the medulla oblongata (Fig. 13.2). This is probably caused by regression of certain components of the cranial nerves during evolution of the species, resulting in regression also of the corresponding parts of the nuclear column.

The Cranial Nerves and Their Nuclei Are Links in Reflex Arcs: Brain Stem Reflexes

Like the spinal nerves that are links in spinal reflex arcs, the cranial nerves constitute af-

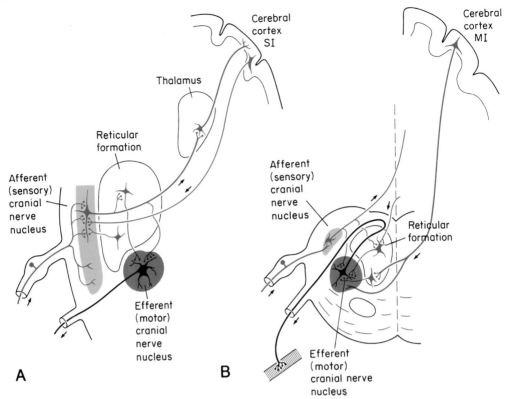

Fig. 13.4. *Main features of the organization of the cranial nerve nuclei.* **A.** Sensory nucleus (for example, the trigeminal nucleus). The efferent fibers of the nucleus ascend to the thalamus of the opposite side, and from there the next neuron projects to the cerebral cortex. The fibers destined for the thalamus give off collaterals on their course through the reticular formation and the motor cranial nerve nuclei. Thus, a reflex arc with reflex center in the brain stem is established. The sensory nucleus is influenced by descending fibers from the cerebral cortex. **B.** Motor nucleus (for example, the facial nucleus) sending its efferent fibers out of the brain stem to striated muscles. The neurons of the nucleus are influenced by the cerebral cortex, by the reticular formation, and by collaterals of the ascending fibers from the sensory nuclei.

ferent and efferent links of reflex arcs with reflex centers in the brain stem (Fig. 13.4). Often, such reflex centers are fairly complex, comprising neurons at several levels of the brain stem (for some, even at the cortical level). Thus, the afferent fibers may enter the brain stem at one level, whereas the efferent fibers leave at another. One example is the corneal reflex (touching of the cornea elicits an eye wink), in which the afferent fibers of the trigeminal nerve, entering at the midpontine level, descend in the brain stem and form synapses in the lower medulla (the spinal trigeminal nucleus). From the medulla, the impulses are conveyed by interneurons to the facial nucleus on both sides, located in the lower pons. The reflex center is in this case rather extensive, and as a consequence lesions at various levels of the brain stem may produce a weakened or abolished corneal reflex. However, depending on the location of the lesion, the change of the corneal reflex will be accompanied by various other symptoms, which helps in determining the exact site of the lesion.

Some brain stem reflexes are simple, such as the monosynaptic stretch reflex that can be elicited of the masticatory muscles.

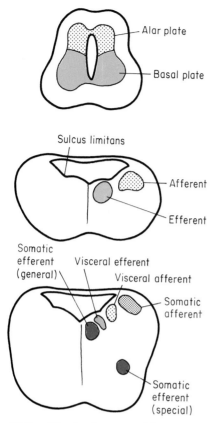

Alar plate

Basal plate

Sulcus limitans

Afferent

Efferent

Somatic
efferent   Visceral efferent
(general)
                Visceral afferent

Somatic
afferent

Somatic
efferent
(special)

Fig. 13.5. *The development of the cranial nerve nuclei.*

cranial nerve nuclei are influenced by the *pyramidal tract*—that is, by fibers forming the *corticobulbar tract* (Fig. 13.4). An important difference between the corticospinal and corticobulbar fibers is that several of the cranial nerve nuclei receive both crossed and uncrossed fibers. Unilateral damage to the descending fibers (for example, in the internal capsule) produces clear-cut pareses only in some of the muscle groups innervated by the cranial nerves.[1]

Examination of the cranial nerves is of great importance in clinical neurology because it can provide exact information about the site of a disease process. A prerequisite, however, is that the examiner has reasonably precise knowledge of where the cranial nerves exit from the brain stem (Figs. 2.16 and 13.1) and the position of their nuclei both rostrocaudally and mediolaterally (Figs. 13.2 and 13.3). Furthermore, the functions of the various nerves must be known in sufficient detail as a basis for the necessary tests.

Figures 2.17–2.19, 2.21, and 13.6 show the location of the cranial nerve nuclei in cross sections of the brain stem.

The Cranial Nerve Nuclei Are Connected with Central Sensory and Motor Tracts

As mentioned, the cranial nerves and their nuclei are organized in accordance with the same general rules as the spinal nerves (with some exceptions). This means that the cranial nerves are the first links in sensory pathways corresponding to the *dorsal column–medial lemniscus system* and the *spinothalamic pathway* (Fig. 13.4). Furthermore, like the nuclei involved in the sensory pathways conducting from the spinal cord, those of the brain stem are subjected to descending control of the sensory transmission. This concerns influences from parts of the reticular formation and from the cerebral cortex.

Several of the somatic efferent (motor)

THE HYPOGLOSSAL NERVE

The twelfth cranial nerve, the hypoglossal nerve (Fig. 13.1), is the motor nerve of the tongue. It is composed of only *somatic efferent fibers*. The fibers come from the hypoglossal nucleus, which forms a slender, longitudinal column close to the midline in the medulla (Figs. 13.1 and 13.6). The nucleus produces an elongated elevation in the floor of the fourth ventricle (the hypoglossal trigone) (Fig. 2.20). The root fibers of the nerve pass ventrally and leave the medulla just lateral to the pyramid (Figs. 2.17, 13.1, and 13.6). Several small fiber bundles join to form the nerve, which leaves the skull through the *hypoglossal canal* in the occipital bone. The nerve then forms an arc as it courses downward and forward in the upper neck—external to the carotid artery—to the root of

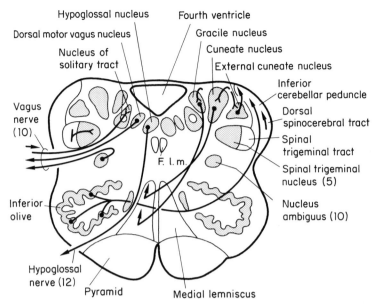

Fig. 13.6. *Position of cranial nerve nuclei,* some other nuclei, and the main tracts in the medulla.

the tongue. The fibers innervate the striated muscle cells of the tongue.

The muscles of the tongue are used *voluntarily* during speech and eating. At such times the neurons of the hypoglossal nucleus are influenced by fibers of the pyramidal tract coming from the face region of the motor cortex of the opposite hemisphere. The descending fibers cross in the medulla just above the nucleus. A central motor lesion above the nucleus (for example, in the internal capsule) can produce pareses of the opposite half of the tongue, together with the more obvious pareses of the extremities. No clear-cut atrophy of the tongue occurs in cases of central motor lesions.

Reflex movements of the tongue occur in swallowing (and vomiting). The hypoglossal motoneurons are then activated from brain stem reflex centers, located in the reticular formation. Various kinds of stimuli can activate the reflex center for swallowing, notably touch and pressure receptors at the back of the tongue.

A *unilateral lesion of the hypoglossal nerve or nucleus* produces paralysis of the tongue on the same side. Since this is a peripheral paresis, a pronounced atrophy of the tongue muscles ensues. This is witnessed by a wrin-

kled surface of the tongue because the mucous membrane becomes too big for the reduced volume (Fig. 13.7). When the tongue is stretched out, it deviates to the paretic side, because of paresis of the genioglossus muscle. This muscle passes backward and laterally into the tongue from its origin at the inside of the mandible; its normal action when acting unilaterally is to draw the tongue forward and to the opposite side.

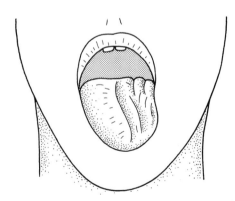

Fig. 13.7. *Peripheral paralysis of the hypoglossal nerve on the left side.* The tongue deviates to the side of the lesion when the patient tries to stretch it out. Atrophy of the intrinsic muscles of the tongue makes the surface wrinkled.

The Ansa Cervicalis

Some of the motor fibers from the first cervical spinal segment join the hypoglossal nerve and follow it for some distance before leaving it and descending in the neck. The descending fibers join other motor fibers from the second and third cervical segments and thereafter form a (fairly obvious) arc external to the internal jugular vein, called the *ansa cervicalis* (*ansa* means handle). The fibers of the ansa cervicalis innervate the infrahyoid muscles and have no relation to the hypoglossal nucleus or the muscles of the tongue. Damage to the hypoglossal nucleus or the proximal part of the nerve (before the fibers from C_1 join it) therefore produces no pareses of the infrahyoid muscles.

THE ACCESSORY NERVE

The eleventh cranial nerve, the accessory nerve, brings *somatic efferent fibers* to two muscles in the neck, the sternocleidomastoid and the trapezius. The accessory nucleus is located in a column in the upper part of the cervical cord (Fig. 13.2) and contains neurons that are of the ordinary motoneuron type. The root fibers leave the cord and ascend to enter the posterior fossa through the foramen magnum. The nerve then leaves the skull through the jugular foramen together with the vagus and the glossopharyngeal nerves. Outside the skull, the nerve passes internal to the sternocleidomastoid muscle and superficially through the upper part of the lateral triangle of the neck before continuing under the upper part of the trapezius muscle.

The accessory nerve is joined for a short distance intracranially by some fibers from the nucleus ambiguus. These fibers leave the nerve just outside the jugular foramen and follow the vagus nerve in their further course. They should therefore be considered a part of the vagus with a somewhat aberrant course rather than a part of the accessory nerve.

In *central motor lesions* (of the corticobulbar component of the pyramidal tract), pareses of the contralateral sternocleidomastoid and the trapezius are usually observed.

Because of its superficial position, the nerve may be damaged in the lateral triangle, producing a *peripheral paresis*. In such a case only the trapezius is paretic, since the fibers innervating the sternocleidomastoid leave the nerve higher up. Furthermore, the upper part of the trapezius muscle is usually most seriously affected, the lower part being supplied also from the cervical plexus. Paresis of the trapezius muscle makes it difficult to elevate the arm, because the trapezius is necessary for the rotation of the shoulder blade around its anteroposterior axis.

THE VAGUS NERVE

The vagus nerve is the tenth cranial nerve and is characterized by containing *fibers of all four kinds described above.*[2] Correspondingly, it is connected with four different nuclei in the medulla. The root fibers emerge in a row at the lateral aspect of the medulla (Figs. 13.1 and 13.6) and join to form one nerve, which leaves the skull through the *jugular foramen.*

In the jugular foramen and immediately below, the nerve has two swellings, the *jugular* and the *nodose ganglia* (Fig. 13.8), which contain the pseudounipolar perikarya of the sensory vagus fibers.

As implied by the name (Latin: vagus = wandering), the vagus nerve sends branches to widespread regions of the body. After leaving the skull, the nerve passes as a fairly thick cord downward in the neck together with the common carotid artery, further through the thorax, and into the abdomen through the diaphragm. It gives off branches in the neck, in the thorax, and in the abdomen.

Visceral Efferent (Parasympathetic) Vagus Fibers

The visceral efferent neurons belong to the parasympathetic part of the autonomic nervous system. The perikarya are found in the *dorsal motor nucleus of the vagus* (Figs. 2.18, 13.2, and 13.6). The fibers do not pass di-

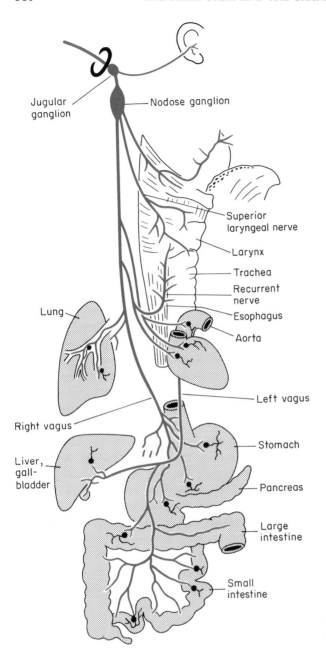

Jugular ganglion

Nodose ganglion

Superior laryngeal nerve

Larynx

Trachea

Recurrent nerve

Esophagus

Aorta

Lung

Left vagus

Right vagus

Stomach

Liver, gall-bladder

Pancreas

Large intestine

Small intestine

Fig. 13.8. *The course and distribution of the vagus nerve.*

rectly to the organs, but end on a second set of neurons in *parasympathetic ganglia* close to or in the wall of the organs (Fig. 13.8)— as is the case for all parasympathetic nerves (Fig. 14.1). The neurons leading from the central nervous system to the ganglia are called *preganglionic,* and those leading from the ganglion to the organ are called *postganglionic.*

In the neck, the vagus gives off visceral ef-

ferent fibers to the *heart* (Fig. 13.8). The perikarya of the postganglionic neurons are located in the wall of the heart and around the great vessels in the vicinity of the heart, and the postganglionic fibers end among the muscle cells of the heart, especially those of the sinus node, which determines the heart rate.

Other branches from the vagus supply the *esophagus* and the *trachea* and, further down in the thorax, the *bronchi* of the lung. The postganglionic fibers innervate smooth muscles and glands in these structures.

In the *abdomen*, the vagus sends fibers to the *stomach*, the *small intestine*, and the *first half of the large intestine*. The vagus also supplies the *liver*, the *gallbladder*, and the *pancreas* with parasympathetic fibers. To reach the various organs, the fibers follow the arteries and form plexuses around them together with sympathetic fibers.

Impulses in the vagus nerve *reduce the heart rate, constrict the bronchi, and increase bronchial secretion*, whereas the *peristaltic movements and secretion are increased in the stomach and intestine*. The *secretion of the pancreas is also increased*.

Visceral Afferent Vagus Fibers

All branches of the vagus with visceral efferent fibers also contain afferent (sensory) fibers. These neurons have their pseudounipolar perikarya in the large *nodose ganglion* (Fig. 13.8). When the fibers enter the brain stem, they form a small bundle that passes caudally: the solitary tract (this is not a true tract, however, but the central course of a nerve). The fibers establish synapses in the *nucleus of the solitary tract* (Figs. 2.18, 13.2, and 13.6). The efferent fibers from this nucleus pass to the reticular formation and other cranial nerve nuclei in the vicinity and to higher levels such as the thalamus and the hypothalamus (Fig. 13.21).

All of the sensory fibers from the *larynx* and some from the *pharynx* follow the vagus.[3] The sensory fibers from the larynx follow the superior laryngeal nerve (from the part above the vocal cords) and the recurrent laryngeal nerve (from the lower part of the larynx).

Visceral Reflexes

The visceral afferent impulses in the vagus nerve do not reach consciousness, apart from perhaps feelings of hunger or satiety and more vague sensations. The visceral afferents are, however, links in *reflex arcs* that control *secretion and peristaltic movements*

of the gastrointestinal tract (and vomiting). Such reflexes also mediate alterations of airway secretion and of the airway resistance by changing the tone of the bronchial smooth muscles. The reflex centers of all these reflexes are located in the medulla, and the efferent links are visceral efferent fibers coming from the dorsal motor nucleus of the vagus.

Visceral afferents from *baroreceptors* in the wall of the large vessels provide information about the blood pressure in the aorta. Increased blood pressure gives rise to increased firing frequency of the afferent fibers. This in turn produces increased firing of visceral efferent vagus fibers, which reduces the heart rate. The reflex center must involve connections from the nucleus of the solitary tract to the dorsal motor nucleus of the vagus (these two nuclei are close neighbors, as can be seen in Fig. 13.2).

The dorsal motor nucleus of the vagus can be influenced also by impulses other than those coming from the viscera. For example, the sight, the smell, or even the thought of food can produce increased secretion of gastric juice. These are examples of conditioned responses, whereas the stimulation of taste receptors produces an unconditioned (true reflex) response.

Somatic Efferent Vagus Fibers

The somatic efferent vagus fibers come from the *nucleus ambiguus* (Figs. 13.2 and 13.6), which belongs to the special somatic efferent nuclei. The fibers supply all striated muscles of the *larynx* and parts of the muscles of the *pharynx*. The fibers to the pharynx take off from the vagus as several small branches, whereas most of the fibers to the larynx are collected in the *recurrent laryngeal nerve*. This nerve takes off from the main vagus trunk at the level of the aortic arch on the left side and the subclavian artery on the right. It then arches behind the vessels and ascends in the furrow between the trachea and the esophagus, to reach the larynx. One of the laryngeal muscles located on the outside, the cricothyroid muscle, receives motor fibers in the superior laryngeal nerve (which

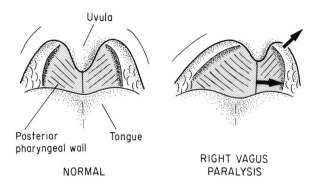

Fig. 13.9. *Paralysis of the right vagus nerve.* The uvula and the posterior pharyngeal wall are pulled toward the normal side when the patient says "aah." Redrawn from Mumenthaler (1979).

is a predominantly sensory nerve, as mentioned above). The vagus also innervates one of the muscles of the soft palate (the levator veli palatini muscle).

A *lesion of the vagus nerve* above the exit of the motor branches to the pharynx and the soft palate produces deviation of the uvula and the posterior pharyngeal wall to the normal side (as can be seen, for example, when a patient is asked to say "aah") (Fig. 13.9). Pareses of the soft palate and the pharynx cause fluid and food to enter the nasal cavity when swallowing (owing to inadequate closure of the nasopharynx). Furthermore, the voice becomes hoarse because the vocal cords cannot be properly adducted. Such a symptom will obviously also occur after a lesion of the recurrent laryngeal nerve anywhere along its course. In case of a unilateral lesion, the voice hoarseness will gradually disappear, because the muscles of the normal side adapt to the changed conditions.

The neurons of the nucleus ambiguus are influenced by, among other sources, the pyramidal tract during speech. They can also be activated reflexly, however, by irritating stimuli of the respiratory tract (cough reflex).

Somatic Afferent Vagus Fibers

This is the smallest contingent of fibers in the vagus nerve. They have their perikarya in the small *jugular ganglion*. They come from a small region of the skin of the external ear (the auricular ramus) and terminate in the trigeminal sensory nucleus.

THE GLOSSOPHARYNGEAL NERVE

The ninth cranial nerve, the glossopharyngeal, resembles the vagus but is smaller and innervates a more restricted region. The root fibers leave the medulla immediately rostral to the vagus fibers (Fig. 13.1). The root fibers fuse to form one trunk that leaves the cranial cavity through the jugular foramen (together with the vagus and the accessory nerves). The nerve follows an arched course (ventrally) lateral to the pharynx, which it penetrates to reach the base of the tongue. Close to the jugular foramen, the nerve contains two small sensory ganglia with pseudounipolar ganglion cells (the superior and petrous ganglia).

Of the peripheral branches, some innervate *the muscles and the mucous membrane of the pharynx* (together with the vagus, which appears to be the most important quantitatively); other sensory fibers reach *the posterior part of the tongue, to innervate taste buds, and the mucous membrane* (and also the mucous membrane of the soft palate and the tonsillar region).

The glossopharyngeal nerve also contains *visceral efferent* (parasympathetic) fibers to the *parotid gland* (and to the salivary glands in the posterior part of the tongue).

The Sinus Nerve and Baroreceptors

A special contingent of visceral afferent fibers in the glossopharyngeal nerve come from the wall of the *carotid sinus* (the thin-walled, dilated part of the internal carotid artery). The fibers conduct impulses from mechanoreceptors recording the tension of the arterial wall; that is, the receptors monitor the blood pressure and are therefore called *baroreceptors.* The afferent fibers end in the nucleus of the solitary tract, and from there the impulses are conveyed to the dorsal motor nucleus of the vagus. Increased impulse frequency of the cardiac vagus fibers reduces the heart rate, and the blood pressure thereby is reduced. When the blood pressure falls, there will be reduced firing of the cardiac vagus fibers, with increased heart rate and blood pressure. This is one of several mechanisms to ensure that the blood pressure is maintained within certain limits and that the cerebral blood flow is sufficient at all times.

The Nuclei of the Glossopharyngeal Nerve

The somatic efferent fibers to the striated pharynx muscles come from the *nucleus ambiguus,* whereas the visceral efferent fibers have their perikarya in the small *inferior salivatory nucleus* (Fig. 13.2). The impulses from this nucleus follow a somewhat complicated course to reach the parotid gland (as is the case for several of the parasympathetic fiber components of the cranial nerves). The preganglionic parasympathetic (visceral efferent) fibers from the inferior salivatory nucleus end in a small *otic ganglion* just outside the cranial cavity. The axons from the ganglion cells (postganglionic) join one of the trigeminal branches—the *auriculotemporal nerve,* which passes close to the ganglion—to the gland.

The *visceral afferent* fibers carrying impulses from the *taste buds* in the posterior third of the tongue end in the nucleus of the solitary tract. From there, the impulses are sent to the thalamus and further on to the cerebral cortex. The sensory fibers from the posterior part of the tongue, the tonsils, the soft palate, and the pharynx end in the sensory trigeminal nucleus.

THE VESTIBULOCOCHLEAR NERVE: THE SENSE OF EQUILIBRIUM

The eighth cranial nerve, although consisting of only one trunk, is in reality two functionally different nerves, the *cochlear nerve*

(dealt with in Chapter 6) and the *vestibular nerve,* which we will describe here. The nerves fuse after leaving the labyrinth (the cochlea and the vestibular apparatus) and follow the internal acoustic meatus. At the lower end of the pons, in the *cerebellopontine angle* (Fig. 13.1), the nerve enters the brain stem. Most of the fibers in the vestibular nerve end in the *vestibular nuclei.* The perikarya of the primary (afferent) vestibular fibers are located at the bottom of the internal meatus, forming the *vestibular ganglion.*[4] The main structural features of the labyrinth were described in Chapter 6 (Figs. 6.1 and 6.2) and will not be repeated here.

The Vestibular Apparatus

The vestibular apparatus, together with the cochlea, constitute the labyrinth. Unlike the cochlea, however, it does not depend on the external ear and the tympanic cavity to function. Like the cochlear duct with the organ of Corti (Figs. 6.3 and 6.7), the membranous labyrinth containing the vestibular receptors is embedded in the temporal bone and surrounded by a space containing perilymph (Fig. 13.10). The membranous labyrinth is filled with endolymph.

The vestibular part of the labyrinth consists of two small vesicles, the *utricle* and the *saccule,* and three circular tubes connected to the utricle, the *semicircular ducts* (Fig. 13.11). Each of the semicircular ducts has a swelling, the *ampulla,* in the end close to the utriculus. The ducts are oriented in three planes perpendicular to each other. In the erect position and with the head in a neutral position, the *lateral semicircular duct* lies approximately in the horizontal plane, whereas the posterior and the anterior ducts are oriented vertically (Fig. 13.11).

Sensory epithelium with *hair cells* (Fig. 13.13) is found at five places in the vestibular labyrinth. The hair cells are similar to those in the cochlea. In each of the ampullae of the semicircular ducts, there is a transversely oriented elevation, the *ampullar crista* (Fig. 13.12). Hair cells with long cilia are present between the epithelial cells forming the

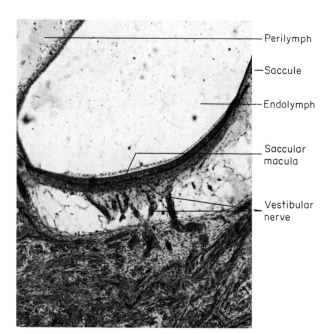

Perilymph

Saccule

Endolymph

Saccular
macula

Vestibular
nerve

Fig. 13.10. *The sacculus.* Photomicrograph through the region of the saccular macula. Compare Figure 13.12.

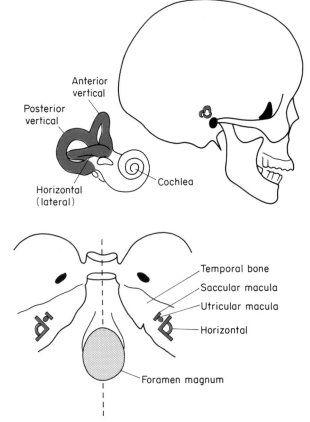

Anterior
vertical

Posterior
vertical

Horizontal
(lateral)

Cochlea

Temporal bone

Saccular macula

Utricular macula

Horizontal

Foramen magnum

Fig. 13.11. *The position of the skull of the vestibular apparatus.* Note the orientation of the semicircular ducts in relation to the conventional planes of the body. The **lower** figure shows the base of the skull seen from above with the vestibular apparatus projected to the surface of the pyramid of the temporal bone.

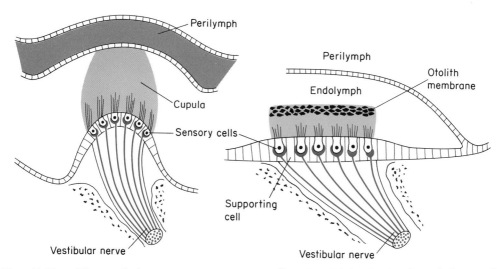

Fig. 13.12. *The vestibular receptor regions.* Schematic. **Left:** Longitudinal section through the ampulla of a semicircular duct with the am- pullar crista. **Right:** Section through the saccular macula. Compare Figure 13.10.

crista. The cilia project into a jellylike mass, the *cupula.* In the utricle and the saccule there are small patches of hair cells like those in the ampullae, the *utricular and saccular maculae* (Figs. 13.10 and 13.12). The macular hair cells are also covered by a jellylike mass, which is special because of its content of small "stones," the *otoliths* (Figs. 13.12 and 13.14). The otoliths are crystals of calcium salts. The utricular macula lies in approximately the same plane as the lateral semicircular duct (that is, horizontally in the neutral position), whereas the saccular macula is oriented almost vertically (Fig. 13.11).

The Adequate Stimulus for the Semicircular Ducts Is Rotation of the Head

Flow of the fluid (the endolymph) inside the semicircular ducts displaces the cupula, thereby bending the cilia. This activates or inhibits the sensory cells, depending on the direction of bending. *Flow of the endolymph in the semicircular ducts is produced by rotational movements of the head.* This is explained by the inertia of the fluid: When the head starts to rotate, the fluid "lags behind." When the rotation stops, the fluid continues to flow for a moment (like the water in a bowl that is rotated rapidly for a couple of turns). If the head rotation continues at even velocity, the fluid and the head will after a short time move with the same speed and in the same direction, which means that the cilia are not bent. Thus, it is clear that not every rotational movement is recorded by the receptors of the semicircular ducts: *Alteration of the velocity of the rotational movement—that is, positive or negative angular acceleration—is the adequate stimulus for the semicircular duct receptors.* Thus these receptors have *dynamic sensitivity* (see Chapter 4). Linear acceleration does not affect (or affects only slightly) the semicircular ducts. By linear displacement of the head (a translatory movement) without concomitant rotation, there is no stimulation of the semicircular duct receptors. An example of linear acceleration is a car that starts or brakes on a flat, straight road. If the road goes up and down and is curved, rotational accelerations of the car (and the heads of its passengers) are superimposed on the linear ones.

The orientation of the semicircular ducts ensures that rotation of the head in any conceivable plane produces change of activity of the receptors in one or more of the ducts. The pattern of activity produced by all the

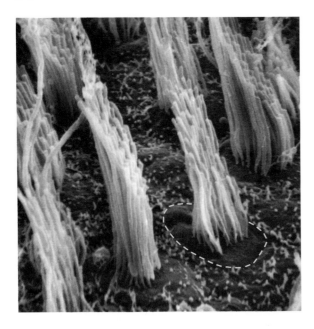

Fig. 13.13. *Sensory (hair) cells of the utricular macula.* Scanning electron micrograph. The apical surface of one sensory cell is indicated. Magnification, × 10,000. Compare Figures 13.12 and 13.15. Courtesy of Prof. H. Lindeman.

receptors is used by the brain to monitor the rotational movements of the head at all times. The semicircular ducts of both sides must function normally to supply the brain with the necessary information. A pair of ducts (for example, the right and left lateral ones) gives complementary signals to a given rotation—that is, increased impulse frequency from the one and reduced from the other.

Sacculus and Utriculus Signal the Position of the Head and Linear Acceleration

The small otoliths have higher specific weight than the endolymph and the substance in which they are embedded and are therefore more strongly influenced by gravitational forces. Taking as an example the utricular macula, which in the neutral head position is oriented horizontally, a change of head position tilts the macula, and the otoliths "pull" the cilia in that direction. Different angles of tilt produce different patterns of activity of the macular hair cells. Owing to their different orientations in space, *the utricular and saccular hair cells together provide information about all possible head positions.*[5] Its ability to provide information about the position of the head at any one time (in the absence of movement) shows that the vestibular apparatus has *static sensitivity.* This property depends on the presence of receptors that adapt slowly or not at all (as discussed in Chapter 4), so that the receptors give a constant signal as long as a certain position is maintained. The static sensitivity of the vestibular apparatus depends, as we have seen, on the force of gravity and disappears in a state of weightlessness (such as in space travel).

Since the static sensitivity is a property of the utricle and the saccule, these parts of the vestibular apparatus are called the *static labyrinth.* We will see, however, that this part of the labyrinth also has dynamic properties.

The *dynamic sensitivity* of the utricle and the saccule is seen when their activity is recorded during *linear acceleration.* The response increases (that is, the firing frequency of the afferent fibers) with increasing acceleration. This is again explained by the inertia of the otoliths. On linear displacement of the head with changing velocity, as in a car that is accelerating, the otoliths "lag" behind and thereby bend the cilia backward (in relation to the direction of the movement).

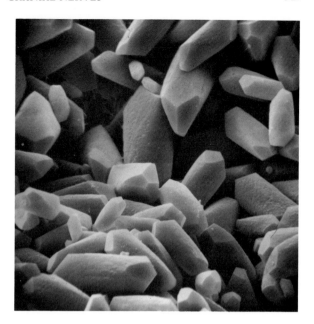

Fig. 13.14. *Otoliths from the utricular macula* (cat). Scanning electron micrograph. Magnification, ×2100. Courtesy of Prof. H. Lindeman.

The opposite happens when the car slows down; the otoliths continue to move for a moment and bend the cilia forward (compare with the forces acting on a loose object in a car when the car speeds up or slows down).

More about the Vestibular Receptor Cells

Electron microscopic studies have shown that there are two kinds of vestibular receptor cells, which are found both in the cristae of the semicircular ducts and in the maculae of the saccule and utricle (Fig. 13.15). One kind, the *type 1* cell, is bottle-shaped, whereas the *type 2* cell is slender. The sensory fibers (the peripheral process of the vestibular ganglion cells) end differently on the two cell types (Fig. 13.15A). On the apical end of the cells there are numerous (50–110) stereocilia and one longer and thicker kinocilium. The stereocilia are unusually long microvilli and contain actin filaments like other microvilli. The kinocilium contains microtubuli (like cilia of the respiratory epithelial cells), indicating that the kinocilium is capable of active movements. The stereocilia are arranged regularly in accordance with their height (Figs. 13.13 and 13.15). This structural *polarization* of the receptor cells corresponds with the functional polarization mentioned above. Thus, bending of the stereocilia *toward* the kinocilium increases the firing frequency of the sensory fibers in contact with the cell, whereas bending in the opposite direction reduces the firing frequency. This is because the receptor cell is *depolarized* or *hyperpolarized* by bending of the cilia. The transmission of the signal from the receptor to the afferent nerve fiber is chemical, but the substance involved is not known. The alteration of the membrane potential of the receptor cell is believed to be caused by mechanical deformation of various parts of the so-called basal plate to which the cilia are anchored. The deformation changes the permeability of cation channels. Even a displacement of 0.2 μm at the tip of a cilium—corresponding to a displacement in the apical membrane of only 10 nm—elicits a robust response from the receptor!

Displacement of the cilia perpendicular to the direction of the polarization produces no response, whereas oblique displacements give a reduced response compared with a stimulus that is properly aligned with the polarization. This means that a given firing frequency of an afferent fiber is ambiguous—it can, for example, be caused by a weak stimulus in the direction of the polarization or a stronger obliquely oriented one. This may be the reason why the hair cells in the maculae are arranged differently with regard to the orientation of the polarization axes, so that all the cells together cover 360° (Fig. 13.15C). This ensures that the information received by the brain about head position in space is unambiguous. This requires, of course, that the brain be

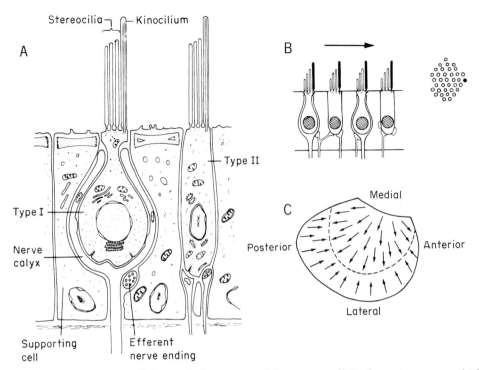

Fig. 13.15. *Sensory cells of the vestibular apparatus.* **A** and **B**. Note the polarization of the cilia. **C**. The utricular macula seen from above. The arrows indicate the direction of polarization of the sensory cells in the various parts, which altogether cover all directions of deflection of the sensory hairs. From Brodal (1981).

able to compare the magnitude of the signals from various parts of the maculae to reach a conclusion.

The Primary Afferent Vestibular Fibers and the Vestibular Nuclei

The primary afferent fibers end in various parts of the vestibular nuclei. The collection of large and small vestibular nuclei is collectively called the *vestibular complex*. It covers a large area in the floor of the fourth ventricle and consists of four large nuclei and several small cell groups. (Not all cell groups within the vestibular complex receive primary vestibular fibers, however, and are therefore not vestibular, strictly speaking.) Figure 13.16 shows the location of the four major nuclei: the *superior*, the *lateral* (or nucleus of Deiters), the *medial*, and the *descending* (or inferior).

Most of the afferent fibers from the *semi-circular ducts* end in the superior nucleus and the rostral part of the medial nucleus, whereas the fibers from the *utricular macula* end primarily in the lateral nucleus. In agreement with the distribution of primary afferents, neurons in the superior nucleus are found to respond best to rotational head movements (angular acceleration), whereas the cells in the lateral nucleus are particularly sensitive to static head position.

The Vestibular Nuclei Receive Afferents from Regions Other Than the Labyrinth

The physiological properties of neurons in the vestibular nuclei are not copies of those of the primary afferent fibers. This is explained by convergence on the cells of various kinds of afferents (such as fibers from the semicircular ducts and the utricle) and by interconnections between the nuclei (for example, commissural fibers linking the two sides). Furthermore, the vestibular complex receives afferents from other parts of the central nervous system, especially the *spinal cord*, the *re-*

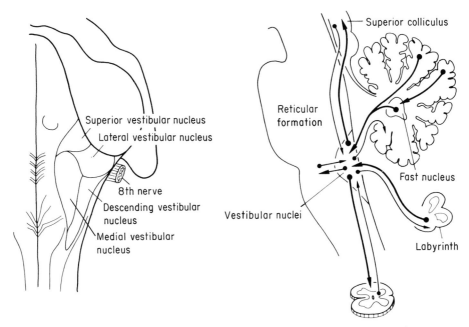

Fig. 13.16. *The vestibular nuclei.* To the **left,** the location of the nuclei is shown in a dorsal view of the brain stem. To the **right,** the main afferent and efferent connections are shown. Note reciprocal connections with the spinal cord, the cerebellum, the reticular formation, and the nuclei of the extraocular muscles and other visually related nuclei of the mesencephalon.

ticular formation, certain mesencephalic nuclei, and the *cerebellum.* Afferents from the mesencephalon arise, for example, in the superior colliculus, and the cerebellar fibers come from both the flocculonodular lobe and the anterior lobe.

Efferent Connections of the Vestibular Nuclei

Schematically, the vestibular nuclei (and therefore also the vestibular receptors) act on three main regions (Fig. 13.16): (1) the *spinal cord,* and especially the motoneurons, as discussed in Chapter 9; (2) the *cranial nerve nuclei of the extraocular muscles;* and (3) the *cerebellum.*

Information from the vestibular apparatus is used primarily to influence muscles that contribute to the equilibrium and to eye movements that ensure that the retinal image is kept stationary when the head moves.

Most of the *fibers to the spinal cord* come from the lateral vestibular nucleus and form the *(lateral) vestibulospinal tract.* The fibers descend in the ventral funiculus on the same side as the nuclei from which they come. In the ventral horn they end—in part monosynaptically—on α and γ motoneurons (Fig. 13.17). The tract is somatotopically organized, so that various body parts can be selectively controlled. The vestibulospinal tract has strong effects on muscles contributing to equilibrium and posture (see Chapter 9). As mentioned, the lateral nucleus receives afferents from the utricular macula; these provide information about the static position of the head in space and thereby indirectly about the position of the body. Change of body position also changes its center of gravity, with a resulting need to adjust muscle tone to maintain equilibrium.

A smaller *(medial) vestibulospinal tract* arises in the medial nucleus. It also descends in the ventral funiculus and acts on motoneurons. The fibers do not reach below the upper thoracic segments, however, and are thought to be of importance primarily for

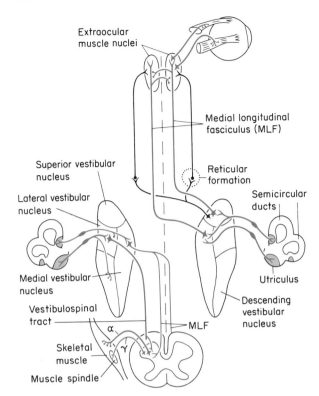

Extraocular
muscle nuclei

Medial longitudinal
fasciculus (MLF)

Superior vestibular
nucleus

Reticular
formation

Lateral vestibular
nucleus

Semicircular
ducts

Medial vestibular
nucleus

Utriculus

Vestibulospinal
tract

Descending
vestibular
nucleus

MLF

α

Skeletal
muscle

γ

Muscle spindle

Fig. 13.17. *The connections of the vestibular nuclei* with the spinal cord and the nuclei of the extraocular muscles.

head movements elicited by the vestibular receptors.

Fibers to the *nuclei of the extraocular muscles* arise mainly in the superior and medial nuclei, which receive many primary afferent fibers from the semicircular ducts (Fig. 13.17). The fibers leave the nuclei medially and join to form a distinct fiber bundle, the *medial longitudinal fasciculus,* located close to the midline below the floor of the fourth ventricle (Figs. 2.19, 13.17, and 13.29). Some of the fibers cross to the other side as they ascend, to end in the *abducent,* the *trochlear,* and the *oculomotor nuclei.* The connections are precisely organized so that the vestibular nuclei can select the combinations of muscles to be influenced. In addition to the direct connections in the medial longitudinal fasciculus, there are indirect pathways from the vestibular nuclei to the eye muscle nuclei via the reticular formation (Fig. 13.17). We will return to this below when discussing vestibular reflexes.

Vestibular fibers to the *cerebellum* were described in Chapter 11. They end primarily in the vestibulocerebellum and arise in the medial and descending nuclei (in restricted parts of these nuclei that do not appear to receive primary vestibular afferents). Fibers from the vestibulocerebellum to the vestibular nuclei can adjust the sensitivity (the gain) of the vestibulo-ocular reflex, as will be discussed below (see also Fig. 13.28).

Connections to the *thalamus* from the vestibular nuclei have been demonstrated anatomically, and there is physiological evidence that impulses from the vestibular apparatus can reach the cerebral cortex. The impulses reach a limited area close to the *face area of SI* (Fig. 4.20). It is not clear what such impulses contribute to consciously perceived sensations. They may, perhaps, mediate the signals producing a feeling of dizziness (vertigo) during certain kinds of vestibular stimulation. Furthermore, whereas the maintenance of body balance is caused by reflex control of muscle tone, the conscious awareness of how the body is oriented in space presumably depends on signals from the utricular and saccular maculae transmitted to the cerebral cortex.

Impulses from the utricle and the saccule are indeed necessary for the *proper orientation of the body in space* when visual information is prevented, as can be shown in animals whose otoliths have been removed and in persons with loss of vestibular function. Whereas such persons manage well as long as they can see, they have serious problems in maintaining the body's equilibrium in the dark.

Vestibular Reflexes

The anatomic basis and the physiological mechanisms underlying reflexes elicited from the vestibular apparatus have been intensively investigated recently. This interest is in part caused by the special problems encountered in space journeys. As with other parts of the brain being comprehensively investigated, conditions turn out to be more complex than initially thought. We will discuss only a few salient points.

Tonic and *phasic labyrinthine reflexes,* mediated by the vestibulospinal tracts, were described in Chapter 9. Here we will primarily address reflex actions on movements of the eye, *vestibulo-ocular reflexes.* This topic is also discussed toward the end of this chapter, when dealing with the cranial nerves supplying the extraocular muscles.

In general, *tonic* vestibular reflex effects are produced by impulses from the utricle and the saccule, whereas *phasic* reflex responses are caused by signals from the semicircular ducts when the stimulus is rotation of the head (angular acceleration) and from the utricle or saccule when the stimulus is linear acceleration.

There are several vestibulo-ocular reflexes, mediated by reflex arcs of various complexities. The simplest one consists of *three neurons* (Fig. 13.28):

1. Primary afferent fibers from the cristae of the semicircular ducts;

2. Neurons in the vestibular nuclei that send their axons to the nuclei of the extraocular muscles (passing in the medial longitudinal fasciculus); and

3. Motoneurons in these nuclei, which send their axons to the extraocular muscles.

There are, furthermore, other impulse pathways with additional synapses, interrupted in the reticular formation and some other brain stem nuclei. The vestibulo-ocular reflexes ensure, as mentioned, that *the image is kept stationary on the retina when the head moves (rotates).* A movement of the head in any direction is accompanied by a compensatory movement of the eyes in the opposite direction and with exactly the same velocity as the head movement. Rotation of the head produces movement of the endolymph inside the semicircular ducts. Taking a rotation in the horizontal plane (turning the head from one side to the other) as an example, mainly the lateral semicircular duct records the movement and elicits a compensatory eye movement in the horizontal plane.

When the head movement is relatively small, the eyes move with exactly the same velocity as and in the opposite direction of the head, and the image is kept in the same position on the retina all the time. This kind of movement, in which the eyes track an object accurately, is called the *smooth pursuit movement.* When the head movement becomes larger, so that it becomes impossible to keep the image stationary even with maximal excursion of the eyes, a fast *saccadic movement* occurs in the same direction as the head movement. Then the gaze is fixed again on the object and another smooth-pursuit phase follows (as long as the head continues to move in the same direction). Such an alternation between smooth-pursuit and saccadic eye movements is called *nystagmus.* In this case, the nystagmus was produced by stimulation of the semicircular ducts (rotation of the head) and is therefore called *vestibular nystagmus.* Nystagmus can, however, also be elicited by movement of the surroundings when the head is stationary, as we will discuss below.

As mentioned, the vestibular nuclei receive afferents from sources other than the labyrinth, such as nuclei in the mesencephalon, the reticular formation, and the cerebellum. Some of these sources mediate visual information that can modify the vestibular reflex responses. This convergence of various inputs seems logical. Thus, to achieve optimal control of the eye movements, *the responsible neural cell groups must receive and integrate vestibular information about movements of the head, visual signals about movements of the image on the retina, and proprioceptive signals about movements of the eyes relative to the head.*

The Cerebellum Can Adjust the Vestibuloocular Reflex to Changing External Conditions

The *magnitude* of the reflex response (not the response itself) to a certain rotational stimulus depends on signals to the vestibular nuclei from the cerebellum (Fig. 13.28). The Purkinje cells of the vestibulocerebellum receive primary vestibular fibers (ending as mossy fibers) that provide information about direction and velocity of the head movement. In addition, the same Purkinje cells receive information, via the inferior olive and climbing fibers, about whether the image is stationary or "slips" on the retina. A retinal slip indicates that the velocity of the compensatory head movement is too high or too low. The cerebellum is then capable of adjusting the excitability of the neurons in the vestibular nuclei— that is, in the reflex center of the vestibulo-ocular reflex. We also say that the cerebellum can change the *gain* of the reflex. Such adaptive change of gain of the reflex is presumably needed continuously during growth and also in situations of muscular fatigue. How much the gain can be altered is shown by experiments in which animals wear optic prisms that deflect the light so that it appears to come from another direction than it really does.

Nystagmus and Falling Tendency Can Be Caused by Vestibular Stimulation

When an upright person rotates fairly rapidly a few times around his axis and then stops, the eyes can be seen to move rapidly one way (saccade) and slowly the other (slow pursuit) for some seconds afterwards. Obviously, the rotation has induced nystagmus. By using special instruments, it can be seen that there is nystagmus also at the start of the rotation, but in the opposite direction of that occurring after the rotation has stopped. When the person rotates to the right, the saccade movement is to the right and the slow pursuit movement is to the left—as if the person fixes her gaze on a stationary point and then moves the eyes rapidly when this point is slipping out of the visual field. The eyes then move to a new fixation point, and the same sequence of events is repeated. When the rotation of the body continues for some time, the nystagmus disappears and the person gets dizzy (compare with ballet dancers who deliberately ensure that the head does *not* move with even velocity during pirouettes; this way they have sufficient time for fixation so that the brain gets information to determine the orientation of the body in space).

The nystagmus is caused by stimulation of the receptors in the semicircular ducts. As mentioned, at the start of the movement the inertia of the endolymph makes it lag behind, thereby bending the cilia of the receptor cells, whereas the endolymph continues to flow for a moment after the rotation has stopped. The person who had just stopped rotating feels as if he were still rotating, but now in the opposite direction. The direction of the nystagmus corresponds to the illusion of such a rotation—that is, with the saccade phase to the left after a rotation to the right.

After stopping the rotation, the person is also unsteady and tends to fall to one side, especially if he is asked to keep his eyes closed. Furthermore, the arm deviates to the right if the person is asked to point straight ahead (with his eyes closed). This is called *postrotational past pointing.* After the rotation stops, the illusion of the opposite movement (that is, the person feels he is turning to the left) causes the past pointing to the right: The person feels that the room is moving to the right.

The postrotational effects on postural muscles are mediated via the vestibulospinal tracts (Fig. 13.17) and show that the receptors of the semicircular ducts also influence the spinal cord and the postural muscles, and not only the cranial nerve nuclei and the extraocular muscles.

Nystagmus, falling tendency, and past pointing can also be produced by irrigation of the external auditory meatus with hot or cold water.

The change of temperature makes the endo-lymph flow in the semicircular ducts and thus produces stimulation of the receptors. Such a *caloric test* is used clinically to examine the function of the vestibular labyrinth and the conduction of impulses to the brain stem.

Various diseases affecting the vestibular receptors or the impulse pathways to the motoneurons of the extraocular muscles (the vestibular nerve, the vestibular nuclei, and the medial longitudinal fasciculus) can produce nystagmus in the absence of vestibular or visual stimulation. This is called *spontaneous nystagmus*. In certain cases, the nystagmus may be present only in certain positions of the head (positional nystagmus).

THE FACIAL AND INTERMEDIATE NERVES

The seventh cranial nerve belongs to the second branchial arch and innervates structures developed from this. The facial nerve is the motor nerve of the facial (mimetic) muscles, supplying them with *special somatic efferent* fibers. The small *intermediate nerve* follows the facial nerve and is usually considered to belong to it. Thus, parts of the intermediate nerve can be said to represent a sensory root of the facial nerve with its *visceral afferent* fibers. The intermediate nerve also contains *visceral efferent* (parasympathetic) fibers, however.

The facial nerve (together with the intermediate nerve) leaves the brain stem laterally at the lower border of the pons, just ventral to the eighth nerve (Figs. 2.16 and 13.1). It then follows the eighth nerve to the bottom of the internal auditory meatus. The *facial nerve proper* (with the special somatic efferent fibers) then arches first posterolaterally and thereafter downward in a canal in the temporal bone. It leaves the skull through the *stylomastoid foramen* immediately medial and anterior to the mastoid process. The nerve then passes forward through the parotid gland and divides into several branches, spreading out like a fan to all the facial muscles.

The fibers of the *intermediate nerve* leave the facial nerve in the bottom of the internal meatus and in the facial canal. The *visceral efferent* (parasympathetic preganglionic) fibers bring secretory impulses to the *lacrimal gland* and two of the large *salivary glands* (the submandibular and the sublingual glands). See Figure 14.9 for details of the complicated route followed by the parasympathetic fibers. We also return to the intermediate nerve in some detail below. The *visceral afferent* fibers of the intermediate nerve innervate *taste buds in the anterior two-thirds of the tongue.*

The Facial Nerve

The motor fibers of the facial nerve have their perikarya in the *facial nucleus,* located in the lower pons. It belongs to the column of special somatic efferent nuclei (Figs. 13.2 and 13.3). The nucleus consists of several subdivisions, each supplying small groups of muscles. The root fibers of the facial nerve have a peculiar course before they leave the brain stem (Fig. 13.18). First, the fibers pass medially and lie dorsal to the abducent nucleus, forming the genu of the facial nerve, before they bend in the lateral and ventral direction. The facial fibers pass just beneath

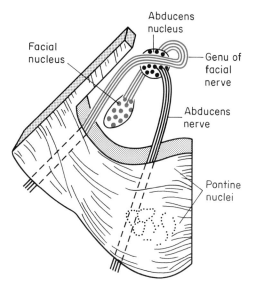

Fig. 13.18. *The course of the facial nerve and its relation to the abducent nucleus.* Schematic cross section through the lower pons.

the floor of the fourth ventricle and form a small elevation, the facial colliculus (Fig. 2.20). Owing to the course of the nerve, symptoms of a peripheral facial paresis may occur in lesions located considerably more medial and dorsal than the nucleus itself. Figure 13.18 shows that damage to the abducent nucleus (affecting the lateral rectus muscle of the eye) is also likely to be accompanied by signs of pareses of the facial muscles of the same side.

Central and Peripheral Facial Pareses

Impulses from the facial nucleus evoke contractions of the mimetic muscles and are therefore responsible for our facial expressions. These muscles are used also in conjunction with speech, eating, blinking, and so forth. Impulses for voluntary movements of the facial muscles are conveyed through the pyramidal tract (corticobulbar fibers). The fibers arise from the face region of the MI in the precentral gyrus.

The part of the facial nucleus supplying the muscles in the forehead and around the eyes receive both uncrossed and crossed pyramidal tract fibers, whereas the muscles in the lower part of the face receive purely crossed fibers. A lesion of the pyramidal tract (for example, in the internal capsule) therefore produces clear-cut pareses only in the lower part of the face on the opposite side of the lesion. Most obvious is the sagging corner of the mouth. The patient can still wrinkle the forehead and close the eyes voluntarily. A *peripheral lesion* (of the facial nucleus or the nerve), however, produces pareses of *all* the facial muscles on the same side as the lesion (Fig. 13.19). For example, the eye cannot be closed, with consequent danger of drying and ulceration of the cornea (and permanent loss of vision).

Peripheral lesions of the facial nerve may be caused by hemorrhage, infarctions, or tumors in the pons, by infections of the middle ear (to which the nerve passes in close proximity), or damage to the branches in the face. Most often, however, the cause of peripheral facial paresis is unknown. In such

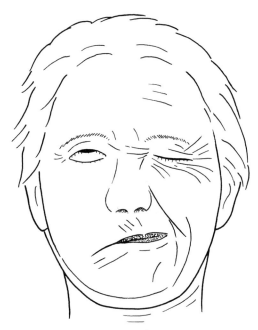

Fig. 13.19. *Peripheral facial paralysis* (right side). The patient is asked to close her eyes and to retract the corners of the mouth. Based on Monrad-Krohn (1954).

cases the muscle power usually returns after some time.

The Mimetic Muscles

The facial or mimetic muscles originate from the facial skeleton and insert with elastic tendons in the dermis. There is a large number of small muscles, with the majority located around the mouth and the eyes. Of particular practical value are the muscles responsible for blinking and closure of the eye (the orbicularis oculi muscle) and the muscles around the mouth (the orbicularis oris and several other muscles), which move the lips. The buccinator muscle prevents the cheeks from being pressed out when the intraoral pressure is increased and, perhaps more important, prevents the cheeks from being sucked in between the teeth.

Facial Expressions of Emotion Do Not Depend on the Integrity of the Pyramidal Tract

Whereas impulses mediated by the pyramidal tract activate the motoneurons of the facial nucleus in voluntary movements (such as speech and eating), other descending pathways are responsible for facial expressions of emotions, such as sorrow and pleasure. As most of us know from personal experience, a genuine smile cannot be produced on command but arises independent of any conscious will. In contrast, our facial expressions often reveal emotions we would rather have concealed. A voluntary effort is required to suppress our spontaneous facial expressions, which most likely are controlled by descending connections from the hypothalamus and possibly the basal ganglia. Thus, lesions of the pyramidal tract do not abolish spontaneous facial expressions. The patient smiles and laughs when told a good joke but is unable to present a polite social smile. In contrast, in central pareses (such as capsular hemiplegia) emotional facial expressions are often exaggerated, and the patient cannot suppress a smile or prevent crying. Diseases of the basal ganglia, such as Parkinson's disease, present the opposite picture: The emotional, spontaneous expressions are lacking, whereas a voluntary, social smile is possible.

The Facial Nerve Is the Efferent Link of the Corneal Reflex

The facial nucleus is also a link in some important reflex arcs. One is the *corneal* or *blink reflex*. It is elicited by touch or irritation of the cornea, and the sensory impulses are conducted centrally in the trigeminal nerve to the spinal trigeminal nucleus (Fig. 13.2). From there the impulses are transferred via interneurons in the reticular formation to the facial nucleus of both sides, and a contraction of the muscles of the eyelid is produced. The corneal reflex can be weakened or abolished by a lesion anywhere along the course of the afferent and efferent links or in the rather extensive reflex center.

Another reflex mediated by the facial nerve is the *stapedius reflex,* in which the response is contraction of the tiny stapedius muscle in the middle ear. The stimulus is an intense sound conducted centrally in the cochlear (acoustic) nerve to the cochlear nu-

clei. Most likely, interneurons in the reticular formation transfer the signals to the facial nucleus. The stapedius muscle pulls the stapes a little out of the oval window (Fig. 6.7) and thereby dampens the transmission of sound waves to the cochlear duct. Accordingly, peripheral facial paresis can produce hypersensitivity to sounds (hyperacusis).

The Intermediate Nerve

Where the facial nerve bends posteriorly in the temporal bone, there is a small ganglion (the geniculate ganglion) containing the perikarya of the sensory fibers of the intermediate nerve. Here a branch of the intermediate nerve, the *greater petrosal nerve,* leaves the main trunk of the facial nerve. It leaves the skull behind the orbit and contains visceral efferent (parasympathetic) fibers. These preganglionic fibers end in the small parasympathetic *pterygopalatine ganglion* located behind the orbit. From there postganglionic fibers follow trigeminal branches to the *lacrimal gland* and *glands in the nasal cavity* (Fig. 14.9). The rest of the intermediate nerve fibers leave the facial nerve as it passes downward posterior to the middle ear. This branch is called the *chorda tympani* because it passes through the middle ear (tympanic cavity) on its way forward to join the lingual nerve (a trigeminal branch) outside the skull. The chorda tympani contains *visceral afferent* fibers from taste buds in the anterior two-thirds of the tongue. These fibers have their perikarya in the geniculate ganglion. In addition, the chorda tympani carries *visceral efferent* (parasympathetic) fibers that end in the small *submandibular ganglion.* From this ganglion, postganglionic parasympathetic fibers pass to the *submandibular* and the *sublingual (salivary) glands.*

Secretion of Tears and Saliva

The preganglionic parasympathetic fibers of the intermediate nerve—acting on the lacrimal, the submandibular, and sublingual glands—have their perikarya in the small *superior salivatory nucleus.* This nucleus belongs to the column of visceral efferent nuclei (Fig. 13.2). As mentioned, preganglionic parasympathetic fibers acting on the parotid gland have their perikarya in the *inferior salivatory nucleus* and follow the glossopharyngeal nerve.

The secretion of saliva is brought about primarily by stimulation of the taste receptors but also by impulses from higher levels of the brain (such as the thought of tasty food; it is especially effective to imagine that one is eating a lemon).

The secretion of tears, even more than the salivary secretion, is an example of how visceral functions can be influenced from higher levels of the brain. The continuous secretion of tears is of course primarily a physiological protection of the eyes and is increased in response to any irritation of the cornea or the conjunctiva; nevertheless, the most profuse tear production occurs when we express strong emotions by crying. The impulses to the superior salivatory nucleus producing the flow of tears when crying are not mediated by the pyramidal tract or other efferent cortical fibers descending in the internal capsule—in correspondence with the fact that tears cannot be produced voluntarily nor can the secretion of tears be suppressed. Most likely, fibers from the hypothalamus are responsible for the activation of the visceral efferent neurons during crying. But the hypothalamus is under the influence of higher levels, such as parts of the cerebral cortex and the limbic structures. Thus, it is the conscious experience of the emotions (such as sorrow or pity) that starts the train of neural events leading to tear secretion.

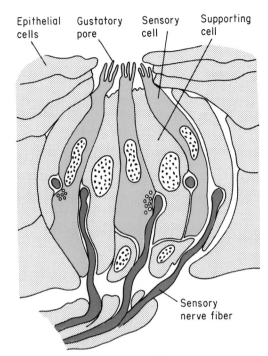

Fig. 13.20.   *Taste bud.* Semischematic drawing based on electron micrographs.

THE SENSE OF TASTE

The sense of taste is not among the most important of the special senses in humans, and much of what we usually call taste experience is in reality brought about by stimulation of olfactory receptors (compare the reduced sense of taste during a common cold). In addition, signals from oral thermoreceptors and mechanoreceptors contribute.

The Taste Receptors

The true taste impulses come from chemoreceptors in the *taste buds* located primarily in the epithelium of the tongue (Fig. 13.20). The taste buds are concentrated along the lateral margins of the tongue and the root of the tongue and are found in small elevations of the mucous membrane called *papillae.* The largest (vallate) papilla lies along a transverse line posteriorly on the tongue (Fig. 13.21).

The *taste buds* are composed of around 100 elongated sensory cells and supporting cells (Fig. 13.20). The sensory cells have long microvilli at their apical surface, protruding into a small opening in the epithelium, the *taste pore.* Here the membrane of the sensory cell comes in contact with substances that are dissolved in the saliva. Around the basal ends of the sensory cells are found terminal endings of sensory (afferent) axons. The sensory cells of the taste buds are constantly renewed; each cell lives probably only about 10 days.

We usually distinguish only four *elementary taste qualities:* salt, sour, sweet, and bitter. Each of these are most easily perceived (have the lowest threshold for identification) in a particular region of the tongue (sweet at the tip of the tongue, then salty, sour, and bitter more posteriorly in that order). Such differences are only relative, however. Recordings of the activity of single afferent fi-

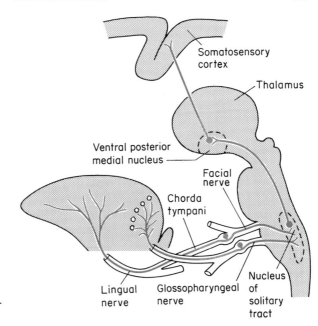

Somatosensory
cortex

Thalamus

Ventral posterior
medial nucleus

Facial
nerve

Chorda
tympani

Lingual
nerve

Glossopharyngeal
nerve

Nucleus
of
solitary
tract

Fig. 13.21. *Pathways for taste impulses.*

bers from taste buds indicate that each sensory unit reacts to several of the four elementary qualities, but with the lowest threshold to only one.

Flavors Act on Ion Channels in the Apical Membranes of the Sensory Cells

Depolarization of the sensory cells is the immediate cause of action potentials in the afferent fibers. The transmission from the sensory cells to the afferent nerve fibers is chemical but the substance responsible is unknown. Studies of isolated sensory cells show that for some of the taste qualities there are no specific membrane receptors; the taste stimulus acts directly on ordinary ion channels in the apical membrane. The specificity of the sensory cell depends on the fact that the cell is exposed to the stimulus only at the apical membrane. The cells of the taste bud are interconnected with special cell contacts (zonula occludens) sealing the lateral membranes off from the taste pore. Thus, fluid in the mouth cannot penetrate between the cells.

Sour substances appear to act primarily by virtue of their concentration of hydrogen ions, which act by closing K^+ channels in the apical membrane. This depolarizes the cell. Hydrogen ions, however, act on various kinds of channels, such as channels for Na^+ and Ca^{2+}. One might therefore think that closure of such channels would counteract the effect on K^+ channels.

Specificity is achieved because the concentration of K^+ channels is particularly high at the apical membrane, whereas the other kinds of channels are evenly distributed. Sour substances will therefore close many K^+ channels but only a few other channels. *Salty substances* act primarily on passive Na^+ channels in the apical membrane. When the concentration of Na^+ increases in the fluid in contact with the apical membrane, Na^+ ions enter the cell and thereby depolarize it.

Sweet and *bitter* substances do not act directly on membrane ion channels but on specific receptors in the apical membrane. Ion channels are influenced via intracellular second messengers, with subsequent depolarization of the sensory cell.

Pathways for Taste Impulses

The intermediate nerve (accompanying the facial nerve) contains the taste fibers from the anterior two-thirds of the tongue, whereas the fibers from the posterior third follow the glossopharyngeal nerve (Fig. 13.21).[6] All taste fibers end in the rostral part of the *nucleus of the solitary tract*. The neurons in the nucleus send their axons to the *visceral efferent nuclei of the salivary glands* and to the *dorsal motor nucleus of the vagus*. Such connections mediate reflex secretion of saliva and gastric juice (and other digestive fluids). Some of the cells in the nucleus of the solitary tract send their axons to the *hypothalamus.* This enables taste impulses to influence the higher autonomic centers.

Fibers from the nucleus of the solitary tract also end in the *thalamus,* enabling taste impulses to reach the cerebral cortex. The synaptic interruption in the thalamus is in the VPM nucleus (Figs. 4.19 and 13.21), which serves as a relay for impulses from the face in general. Taste impulses are transmitted to the face region of the SI (Fig. 4.20).

Our conscious experience of taste is not caused only by stimulation of taste receptors, as mentioned above. Furthermore, numerous taste cells with different specificities are presumably always stimulated while eating or drinking. The synthesis in the cerebral cortex of all these varied impulses forms the basis of our subjective experience of taste.

THE TRIGEMINAL NERVE

The fifth cranial nerve is first and foremost the sensory nerve of the face, with mainly *somatic afferent* fibers. In addition, it contains a small portion with *special somatic efferent* fibers to the masticatory muscles. The trigeminal nerve is the nerve of the first branchial arch and innervates structures that are developed from this arch.

The nerve leaves the brain stem laterally on the pons (Figs. 2.16 and 13.1) with a small (medial) motor root and a large (lateral) sensory root. Shortly after leaving the pons, the nerve expands to form the large *semilunar ganglion,* which contains the perikarya of the pseudounipolar (sensory) ganglion cells (Fig. 13.22). Three large branches continue anteriorly from the ganglion: the ophthalmic, the maxillar, and the mandibular nerves (Figs. 13.22 and 13.25).

The *ophthalmic nerve* enters the orbit and supplies the eye bulb (including the cornea), the upper eyelid, the back of the nose, and the skin of the forehead with sensory fibers (Fig. 13.23). It also sends fibers to the mucous membranes of the anterior part of the nasal cavity. The *maxillary nerve* runs forward in a sulcus in the bottom of the orbit and sends fibers to the lower eyelid, the skin above the mouth, the upper teeth and the gingiva, and,

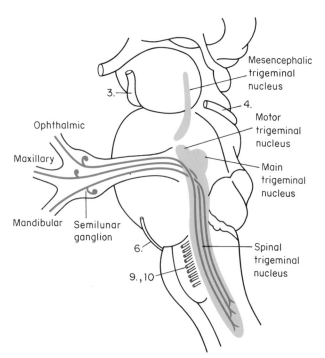

Fig. 13.22.   *The positions of the trigeminal nuclei.*

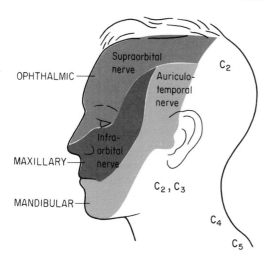

Fig. 13.23. *Distribution in the facial skin of the three main trigeminal branches.* The location of some further branches is indicated. The segmental origins of sensory fibers to the rest of the head and the neck are also indicated.

the face. As with other spinal nerves, fibers leading from different kinds of receptors are intermingled in the nerve but have become arranged by receptor type when entering the central nervous system. Then the fibers are distributed to three subdivisions of the long sensory trigeminal nucleus (Figs. 2.17–19, 13.2, and 13.22). Fibers from *proprioceptors* (muscle spindles, joint receptors) end in the *mesencephalic nucleus*, fibers from *low-threshold mechanoreceptors* end in the *main* or *principal nucleus*, whereas impulses from *nociceptors* end in the *spinal trigeminal nucleus.*[7]

More about the Subdivisions of the Sensory Trigeminal Nucleus

The *thinnest fibers* of the trigeminal nerve (Aδ and C fibers), conducting primarily from nociceptors and thermoreceptors, bend caudally after entering the pons (Fig. 13.22). They continue as a small bundle, the *spinal tract of the trigeminal nerve,* located just beneath the medullary surface. It is joined by somatic afferent fibers, which have followed the glossopharyngeal and the vagus nerves peripherally. Just like the solitary tract, the spinal tract, strictly speaking, is not a tract, since it consists of the central process of the pseudounipolar ganglion cells. The spinal tract continues down into the upper cervical segments and corresponds to the bundle of Lissauer in the cord (Fig. 2.10). The fibers enter the *spinal trigeminal nucleus* (or nucleus of the spinal trigeminal tract), which corresponds largely to the dorsalmost laminae of the cord. For example, a layer very similar to the substantia gelatinosa is present. The spinal trigeminal nucleus can be further subdivided in a rostrocaudal sequence. The caudal part or subnucleus appears to be especially involved in pain mechanisms and corresponds most closely with the dorsal laminae of the cord. It also receives dorsal root fibers from the upper cervical segments. This may perhaps explain why a certain condition with paroxysms of facial pain of unknown origin (trigeminal neuralgia) may sometimes irradiate outside the area innervated by the trigeminal nerve (see the explanation of referred pain in Chapter 4). The spinal tract of the trigeminal nerve is sometimes surgically transected to alleviate severe, chronic facial pain (medullary trigeminal tractotomy). This abolishes pain and temperature sensitivity in the face on the same side.

finally, the hard palate and the posterior (major) part of the nasal cavity. The *mandibular nerve* innervates the lower teeth and gingiva, the tongue, and the skin of the lower jaw and upward, well into the temporal region (Fig. 13.23). The branch of the mandibular nerve supplying the tongue with somatic sensory afferent fibers is called the *lingual nerve.* This nerve receives visceral afferent (taste) fibers from the chorda tympani, destined for the anterior two-thirds of the tongue.

The motor fibers of the trigeminal nerve follow the mandibular nerve but leave this in several smaller twigs to the masticatory muscles (and some other muscles with relation to the lower jaw and the soft palate).

The Sensory Trigeminal Nucleus

With regard to function and fiber composition, the sensory part of the trigeminal nerve corresponds to the spinal dorsal roots. The trigeminal nerve, therefore, belongs to the somatosensory system and conducts impulses from *low-threshold mechanoreceptors, thermoreceptors,* and *nociceptors* in the face and in the mucous membranes of

Thick myelinated fibers (Aα and β) in the trigeminal nerve from the *skin* end mostly in *the main (principal) sensory trigeminal nucleus* (Fig. 13.22) with a precise somatotopic pattern. This part of the trigeminal nucleus corresponds functionally to the dorsal column nuclei.

The *mesencephalic trigeminal nucleus* stretches as a slender column from the upper part of the pons and into the mesencephalon. This is a very unusual nucleus, since its neurons look like pseudounipolar ganglion cells and indeed send one process peripherally into the trigeminal nerve. Afferent fibers from the *muscle spindles* of the masticatory muscles follow the mandibular nerve, whereas those from the extraocular muscles follow the ophthalmic and perhaps the oculomotor nerve. Impulses from mechanoreceptors in the root sheaths of the teeth end in the mesencephalic nucleus.

The trigeminal nucleus, especially the spinal subdivision, has numerous connections with the *reticular formation*. This is partly by means of reflex arcs involving the trigeminal nerve as the afferent link but also as links in ascending pathways to the thalamus with signals from nociceptors.

Central Transmission of Signals from the Trigeminal Nucleus

Functionally, the spinal trigeminal nucleus (especially its caudal part) corresponds to the dorsalmost laminae of the cord, whereas the main sensory nucleus corresponds to the dorsal column nuclei. These similarities are evident also in the central pathways. The secondary sensory fibers from the cells in the spinal nucleus join the spinothalamic tract and end in the thalamus. Fibers from the main nucleus join the medial lemniscus. The somatotopic pattern within the thalamic terminal region is such that the fibers from the trigeminal nucleus—carrying impulses from the face—end most medially, in the *ventral posteromedial nucleus (VPM)* (Fig. 4.19). The ascending fibers from the trigeminal nucleus cross to the opposite side before they join the large sensory tracts.[8] From the thalamus, the signals are transmitted to the *face region of the SI* in the postcentral gyrus (Figs. 4.20 and 4.21).

Reflexes Involving the Trigeminal Nerve

Like the spinal dorsal root fibers, the trigeminal nerve constitutes the afferent link of several reflex arcs. We have described the *corneal reflex* (the blink reflex) above, in conjunction with the facial nerve that constitutes the efferent link of this reflex. Other reflexes are the *sneeze reflex,* elicited from the mucous membrane of the nasal cavity, and the *sucking reflex,* elicited in the newborn from mechanoreceptors of the lips. A stretch reflex can be produced by a brief tap downward on the chin, stretching the masticatory muscles (among them, the masseter muscle). This *masseter reflex* is monosynaptic and involves the mesencephalic trigeminal nucleus. The peripheral processes of the neurons of this nucleus innervate the muscle spindles, and the central processes reach the motor trigeminal nucleus in the pons. This reflex, with its reflex center in the mesencephalon and pons, is one of those routinely tested in clinical neurology.

The Motor Trigeminal Nucleus

The *special somatic efferent* fibers in the trigeminal nerve come from the motor trigeminal nucleus, located in the pons at the level of the main sensory nucleus (Figs. 2.19 and 13.22). All of the motor fibers follow the mandibular nerve. A *peripheral paresis* of the motor fibers of the trigeminal nerve (or the nucleus) leads to atrophy of the masticatory muscles and reduced force of biting on the side of the lesion. A unilateral paresis of the masticatory muscles is most easily detected by asking the patient to open his mouth widely; the lower jaw then deviates toward the side of the paretic muscles. This is caused by paresis of the lateral pterygoid muscle, which normally pulls the mandible forward in conjunction with opening of the mouth.

Voluntary movements of the jaws during speech and chewing depend on the pyramidal tract (corticobulbar fibers). The fibers from the MI to the motor trigeminal nucleus are often both crossed and uncrossed (bilateral), but in some persons they appear to be purely crossed. Only in the latter case will there be clear-cut signs of pareses of the masticatory muscles after a lesion of the internal capsule (capsular hemiplegia). There may also be other signs of a central paresis, such as an increased masseter reflex on the paretic side.

Reflex movements of the masticatory muscles occur during swallowing, sucking, and vomiting. The afferent fibers of such reflexes are partly sensory trigeminal fibers from the oral cavity and partly sensory fibers passing in the vagus and the glossopharyngeal nerves.

THE ABDUCENT, TROCHLEAR, AND OCULOMOTOR NERVES

These three cranial nerves (the sixth, fourth, and third) supply the extraocular muscles with *somatic efferent* fibers. In addition, the oculomotor nerve contains *visceral efferent (parasympathetic)* fibers to the smooth, intrinsic eye muscles. Simplified, we may say that by moving the eye in the orbit, the extraocular muscles ensure that the images we look at fall on the central part of the retina (the macula), whereas the intrinsic muscles control the amount of light that reaches the retina and adjust the curvature of the lens so that the retinal image is always in focus. Most of these tasks are performed reflexly, and usually eye position, light access, and lens curvature are all controlled simultaneously.

Before describing the nerves to the eye muscles and their nuclei, we will discuss a few salient features of eye movements in general. The central connections of the eye muscle nuclei are best treated collectively in a discussion of central control of eye movements.

Horizontal, Vertical, and Rotatory Movements of the Eye

The eye is a sphere, lying in the orbit, surrounded by fat. The eye can rotate freely in any direction around its center, whereas translatory movements are prevented. To describe the rotatory movements of a sphere, we define three axes, all passing through the center, oriented perpendicular to each other. For convenience, we describe the movements as taking place in three planes: a frontal, sagittal, and a transverse or horizontal plane. A movement in the horizontal plane takes place around a vertical axis, and the anterior part of the eye—and therefore the gaze—moves from side to side. Such *horizontal eye movements* are performed when we look to one side; when looking to the left, the left eye rotates laterally and the right eye rotates medially. A movement in the sagittal plane takes place around a transverse axis, and the anterior part of the eye moves up and down. Such movements, directing the gaze up and down, are called *vertical eye movements*. Movements in the frontal plane take place around a sagittal axis, and the eye rotates without any horizontal or vertical movement. For practical reasons only, such movements around a sagittal axis are called *rotatory eye movements* (even though, strictly speaking, all eye movements are rotations around the center of the eyeball).

The *six extraocular (extrinsic) muscles* ensure that the optical axes of the eyes (Fig. 5.3) can be directed precisely toward any point in the visual field. The scheme in Figure 13.26 shows the main movements produced by each of the extraocular muscles when acting alone. It can be seen that most of the muscles produce vertical, horizontal, and rotatory movements. We can nevertheless simplify matters by stating that *two muscles produce predominantly horizontal movements* (the medial and lateral rectus muscles), *two produce predominantly vertical movements* (the superior and inferior rectus muscles), whereas *two muscles produce mainly rotatory movements* (the superior and inferior oblique muscles).

The Extraocular Muscles

The small extraocular muscles (Figs. 13.24 and 13.25) all attach to the sclera and originate from the wall of the orbit (a brief account of the structure of the eye bulb is given in Chapter 5).

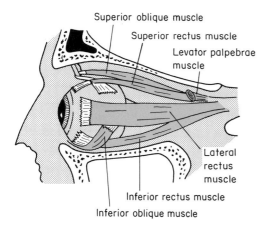

Superior oblique muscle

Superior rectus muscle

Levator palpebrae muscle

Lateral rectus muscle

Inferior rectus muscle

Inferior oblique muscle

Fig. 13.24. *The extraocular muscles* seen from the lateral aspect. The lateral wall of the orbit is removed. Note that the straight muscles insert in front of the equatorial plane of the eye, whereas the oblique muscles insert behind.

We analyze the actions of the extraocular muscles in relation to the above-defined three axes through the center of the eyeball. We then need to know the direction of the force exerted by the muscles in relation to

the axis. We must furthermore know whether the muscle insertion in the sclera is anterior or posterior to the *equatorial plane of the eye,* a frontal plane dividing the eye in an anterior and a posterior half.

There are *four straight* and *two oblique* extraocular muscles (Figs. 13.24 and 13.25). The straight ones (the rectus muscles) come from the posterior end of the orbit and run forward to insert in front of the equatorial plane. This means that the *lateral rectus* muscle pulls the eye (the cornea) laterally, whereas the *medial rectus* muscle pulls it medially. These two muscles thus produce *pure horizontal movements.* Correspondingly, the *superior rectus* muscle pulls the eye (the cornea) upward, whereas the *inferior rectus* muscle pulls it downward. These two therefore produce *vertical movements.* Because the superior and inferior rectus muscles run anteriorly in a lateral direction, however, they do not produce purely vertical movements but also some horizontal movement (in the medial direction). Thus, when the su-

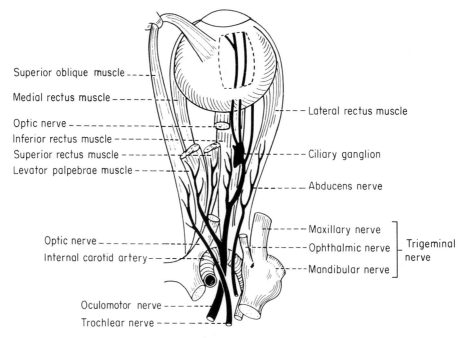

Superior oblique muscle

Medial rectus muscle

Optic nerve

Inferior rectus muscle

Superior rectus muscle

Levator palpebrae muscle

Lateral rectus muscle

Ciliary ganglion

Abducens nerve

Maxillary nerve

Ophthalmic nerve

Mandibular nerve

Trigeminal nerve

Optic nerve

Internal carotid artery

Oculomotor nerve

Trochlear nerve

Fig. 13.25. *The right orbita seen from above.* Note the three cranial nerves innervating the muscles of the eye. Some of the extraocular muscles and the optic nerve have been cut. The external layers of the eye bulb have been partly re-

moved to expose the postganglionic fibers from the ciliary ganglion on their way to the intrinsic eye muscles. Note also the position of the trigeminal ganglion and the internal carotid artery. From Brodal (1981).

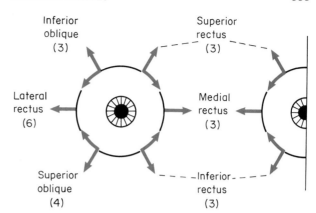

Inferior
oblique
(3)

Superior
rectus
(3)

Lateral
rectus
(6)

Medial
rectus
(3)

Superior
oblique
(4)

Inferior
rectus
(3)

Fig. 13.26. *The actions of the extra-ocular muscles.* The arrows indicate the direction of the action (but not the force). Note that all muscles except the medial and lateral recti rotate the eye, in addition to their other actions.

perior rectus muscle acts alone, it produces an upward movement combined with a (smaller) medial—that is, an oblique movement (Fig. 13.26). In addition, the muscle produces a small medial rotation of the eye (around the sagittal axis).

The *superior oblique muscle* has a rather complicated course (Figs. 13-24 and 13.25). It originates posteriorly in the orbit and runs forward medially. Just behind the anterior margin of the orbit, it bends sharply around a small hook of connective tissue and continues in a posterolateral direction to insert posterior to the equatorial plane. The muscle has actions around all three axes: It rotates the eye so that the upper part moves medially and directs the gaze downward and laterally. The *inferior oblique* muscle originates from the bottom of the orbit in its anteromedial part and runs, like the superior oblique, posterolaterally to insert behind the equator. It directs the gaze laterally and upward and rotates the eye with its upper part laterally. The main action of the oblique muscles is to rotate the eyes (in the opposite direction around the sagittal axis).

The Eye Muscles Are Built for Precise Control

The structure of the extraocular muscles reflects their use in extremely delicate and precisely controlled movements. The muscle fibers are very thin compared with ordinary skeletal muscle fibers, and the motor units are among the smallest in the body (only 5–10 muscle fibers per motoneuron). Consequently, the nerves to the extra-

ocular muscles contain many nerve fibers: The abducent nerve in humans (supplying only one muscle) contains around 6000 axons. The extraocular muscles are composed of a mixture of fibers with fast and with slow twitch contractions. The muscles are required both to hold a certain tension for a long time (static position holding) and to produce extremely fast movements. The maximal speed of contraction is, accordingly, high compared with other skeletal muscle fibers. Furthermore, the maximal firing frequency of the motoneurons innervating the extraocular muscles is unusually high and occurs during saccadic movements. EMG recordings in awake human subjects with their eyes open show that there is some activity in virtually all of the extraocular muscles. The tension produced by each muscle varies, of course, with the position of the eyes.

There is a high density of *muscle spindles* in the extraocular muscles. Apart from the general rule that muscles subject to precise control have a high density of muscle spindles, their functional role in the extraocular muscles is not clear. Thus, signals from extraocular muscle spindles are apparently not consciously perceived—that is, they do not contribute to the awareness of eye position and movements (in this respect differing from muscle spindles elsewhere, as discussed in Chapter 4). Nor do signals from extraocular muscle spindles evoke stretch reflexes. In general, it seems highly likely that muscle spindle signals, providing information about the length and the change of length of the extraocular muscles, are integrated with signals providing information about movements of the head from the labyrinth and with signals from the retina. The latter signals can, for example, supply information about whether the image is stationary or is slipping on the retina. Experiments with transection of the ophthalmic nerve (assumed to contain most of the muscle spindle afferents from the extraocular muscles) produce pronounced instability of the eyes and slow pendular movements in darkness.

The Eye Movements Are Conjugated

Virtually all natural eye movements are combinations of the various movement directions described above. By combining proper amounts of vertical and horizontal movements, any oblique movement can be produced. Furthermore, all natural eye movements are *conjugated*—that is, the two eyes move together to ensure that the image always falls on *corresponding points* of the two retinae (Fig. 5.3). Double vision (diplopia) results if the eye movements do not occur in conjugation. This is a typical symptom of pareses of the extraocular muscles (caused, most frequently, by lesions of one of the nerves to the muscles). Other typical symptoms are strabismus (squint), vertigo (dizziness), and an altered position of the head (the latter to avoid diplopia).

Almost all eye movements require a complicated cooperation of numerous muscles, with activation of synergists and inhibition of antagonists. When, for example, we look to the left, the left lateral rectus is activated and the left medial rectus is inhibited, whereas the right medial rectus is activated and the right lateral rectus is inhibited. This is the simplest possible example, with a purely horizontal movement. In most other situations the cooperation between various muscles becomes much more complicated and requires an extensive, sophisticated neural network for control. We return to this below.

The Abducent Nerve

The abducent nerve leaves the brain stem close to the midline at the junction of the medulla and the pons (Figs. 2.16 and 13.1). Figure 13.18 shows the location of the abducent nucleus and its relation to the facial nerve. The abducent nerve runs forward intracranially and passes through the cavernous sinus before entering the orbit through the superior orbital fissure (Fig. 13.25). It supplies only one muscle, the *lateral rectus*. The muscle pulls the eye so the cornea faces laterally (abducts the eye) (Fig. 13.26). Even though other muscles can abduct the eye somewhat (the superior and the inferior oblique muscles), the lateral rectus is necessary for more than a slight lateral movement. A person with a unilateral lesion of the abducent nerve usually keeps the head turned somewhat to the side of the lesion to compensate for the loss of lateral motion of the eye.

The Trochlear Nerve

This is the only one of the cranial nerves to leave the brain stem on the dorsal side (just below the inferior colliculus) (Figs. 2.20 and 13.1).[9] The trochlear nucleus is situated a little ventrally to the aqueduct in the mesencephalon (Figs. 2.20 and 13.29). Like the abducent nerve, the trochlear traverses the cavernous sinus and enters the orbit through the superior orbital fissure. It innervates the *superior oblique muscle* (Figs. 13.25 and 13.26), which directs the gaze downward and laterally.

The Oculomotor Nerve

The nerve emerges from the ventral aspect of the mesencephalon, in the interpeduncular fossa (Figs. 2.16 and 2.21). This is the largest of the three nerves supplying the extraocular muscles and, as mentioned, contains somatic efferent and visceral efferent fibers. The *somatic efferent fibers* come from the large *oculomotor nucleus* (or nucleus of the oculomotor nerve) situated close to the midline in the mesencephalon, ventral to the aqueduct (Figs. 2.21 and 13.29). The medial longitudinal fasciculus, with ascending fibers from the vestibular nuclei, lies close to the oculomotor nucleus (and to the abducent and trochlear nuclei as well). The *visceral efferent* (parasympathetic) fibers come from the small *nucleus of Edinger-Westphal* located in the vicinity of the oculomotor nucleus. Often the term *oculomotor complex* is used of the somatic efferent and visceral efferent nuclei together.

The oculomotor nerve passes forward to the orbit through the cavernous sinus together with the other nerves to the eye (entering through the superior orbital fissure). The somatic efferent and parasympathetic fibers part in the orbit (Fig. 13.25). The somatic efferent fibers innervate the following extraocular muscles: the *superior and inferior rectus,* the *medial rectus,* and the *inferior oblique.* These muscles can move the eye medially, upward, and downward and rotate it around the sagittal axis (Fig. 13.26). In addition, the oculomotor nerve supplies the *levator palpebrae superioris* muscle, which serves to lift the upper eyelid.

The *visceral efferent* (preganglionic parasympathetic) oculomotor fibers end in the small *ciliary ganglion* situated behind the eye (Fig. 13.25). Here the fibers establish synapses with the postganglionic neurons, which send their axons anteriorly in the wall of the eye to innervate the *intrinsic (smooth) muscles of the eye:* the *sphincter pupillae* and the *ciliary muscle* (Fig. 5.2). Contraction of the ciliary muscle increases the lens curvature when looking at near objects (accommodation, see Chapter 5). The sphincter pupillae constricts the pupil to reduce the amount of light reaching the retina.

A *lesion of the oculomotor nerve* produces, among other symptoms, an abnormal position of the eye, which is directed laterally (due to the unopposed pull of the lateral rectus) and downward (due to the superior oblique muscle). As in lesions of the abducent or the trochlear nerves, the patient will have double vision. In addition, the upper eyelid droops (ptosis) because of paralysis of the levator palpebrae. The interruption of the parasympathetic fibers makes the pupil larger (due to loss of action of the sphincter pupillae), and the light reflex is absent (in an incomplete lesion of the nerve, the pupil may be slightly larger and the reaction to light more sluggish than on the normal side). The ability to accommodate the lens is abol-ished, making it impossible to see near objects sharply. The intracranial course of the oculomotor nerve makes it especially vulnerable in cases of temporal herniation caused by increased intracranial pressure (see Chapter 2). Thus, examination of the size of the pupils, and their reaction to light, is of great practical value in patients who are unconscious after head trauma.

The Light Reflex and the Accommodation Reflex

The oculomotor nerve is the efferent link of both of these reflexes, even though they are quite different in other respects. The *light reflex* is relatively simple, with its reflex center in the brain stem (Fig. 13.27A). An increase in the amount of light reaching the retina elicits a contraction of the sphincter pupillae muscle. Both pupils constrict even when the light hits only one eye. The afferent link consists of fibers of the optic nerve that leave the optic tract before it reaches the lateral geniculate body. The fibers end in the *pretectal nuclei* on both sides (Fig. 13.27A). From these nuclei, the impulses are conveyed to the Edinger-Westphal nuclei on both sides, and via the ciliary ganglion the impulses reach the sphincter pupillae. The bilaterality of the connections explains why a unilateral stimulus produces a bilateral response.

Interruption of the oculomotor nerve abolishes the light reflex in the eye on the side of the lesion, but the reflex is present in the other eye. In case of interruption of the afferent link on one side (damage to the retina or the optic nerve), the light reflex is absent in both eyes when light is shone into the eye on the lesioned side but is present in both sides when the other eye is illuminated. Thus, examination of the light reflex can provide valuable information with regard to the site of a lesion.

The *accommodation reflex* is a cortical reflex: The reflex arc passes via the cerebral cortex. The afferent link is fibers passing in the optic nerve from the retina, and the efferent link consists of parasympathetic fibers

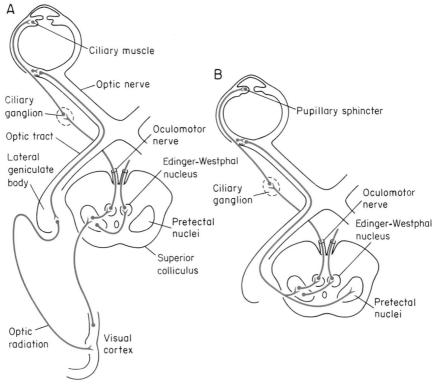

Fig. 13.27. *Visual reflexes.* The reflex arcs for (**A**) the accommodation reflex and (**B**) the light reflex.

in the oculomotor nerve to the ciliary ganglion (Fig. 13.27). From there the postganglionic fibers pass to the ciliary muscle. Details concerning the reflex center are not known, however. The accommodation reflex is elicited only when we fix the gaze on an object that is moving toward us. Together with the accommodation, a pupillary constriction occurs as the object comes closer.

CONTROL OF EYE MOVEMENTS

All ocular movements are produced by impulses to the extraocular muscles from the nuclei of the sixth, fourth, and third cranial nerves. The activity of the motoneurons in these three nuclei must be precisely coordinated and is indeed controlled by a highly complex set of interconnected neuronal groups. Studies of such "preoculomotor"

nuclei and networks have provided a wealth of interesting data. Best known are the networks involved in control of the saccadic (fast) eye movements, whereas the anatomic basis of the control of smooth-pursuit movements is less well understood.

Before going into some main features of the nuclei of the extraocular muscles' connections, we will discuss briefly the kinds of eye movement we are dealing with. This topic has been discussed to some extent also in connection with the vestibular nerve.

Classification of Eye Movements

In general, the control system for eye movements must ensure that the gaze can be moved quickly from one point of fixation to another—that is, by *saccadic movements,* or *saccades*—but also that the gaze can be kept stationary on an object even when the object or the head moves: by *slow-pursuit move-*

ments. Rhythmic alternation between saccades and pursuit movements is called *nystagmus* (see also "Vestibular Reflexes" above). The eye movements may be *voluntary,* as when we follow a moving object with the eyes, or *reflex,* when the head moves (the vestibulo-ocular reflex) or the surroundings move (optokinetic reflex). Nystagmus can be produced by vestibular stimulation or optokinetically.

More about Classification of Ocular Movements

A schematic classification of eye movements is given below. Several of the points have been discussed previously in this chapter, but a collective treatment and more details are given here.

1. *Saccades* are conjugated movements that change the optical axis of the eyes from one point of fixation to another with maximal speed. Saccades can (at least in a certain sense) be *voluntary,* as when we look at a stationary landscape and fix the gaze at one point for a moment, and then move on (with a saccade) to another point of fixation. Saccades can also be *reflex,* as with vestibular or optokinetic nystagmus. When awake, we perform saccades all the time, often several per second.

2. *Smooth-pursuit* movements are performed when we follow a moving object to keep the image stationary on the central part of the retina. As a rule, we use pursuit movements both of the eyes and of the head when looking at a moving object. One might think that the movements of the head would elicit conjugated eye movements in the opposite direction of the head (the vestibulo-ocular reflex). Since this does not occur, the vestibulo-ocular reflex must be suppressed during such smooth-pursuit movements.

3. *Optokinetic reflex* movements are saccadic or smooth-pursuit movements intended to stabilize the retinal image when the whole visual field moves relative to the head.

4. *Vestibulo-ocular reflex* movements are smooth-pursuit movements and saccades elicited by movements of the head (Fig. 13.28).

5. *Vergence* movements change the visual axes of the eyes in relation to each other when the point of fixation moves away from or toward the eyes. This is necessary to keep the image on corresponding points of the retina. Vergence movements are a prerequisite for fusion

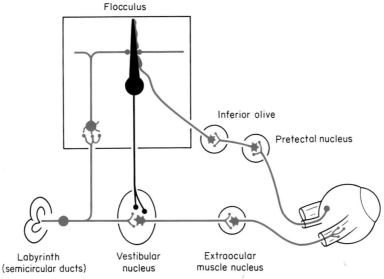

Fig. 13.28. *Main structural elements of the vestibulo-ocular reflex.* Only excitatory connections are shown (even though there are inhibitory neurons in the vestibular nuclei that influence the motoneurons of the antagonists). The reflex arc consists of three neurons from the semicircular duct to the extraocular muscles. The cerebellar flocculus receives signals from the labyrinth and from the retina, and the output of the Purkinje cells can adjust the sensitivity of the vestibular neurons, if necessary, to avoid retinal slip. Based on Ito (1984).

of the two images and for stereoscopic vision. Convergence of the optic axes, which takes place when an object is approaching the eyes, depends primarily on the activity of the medial rectus muscles, with some contribution also from the superior and inferior recti (Fig. 13.26). Convergence movements are accompanied by accommodation and pupillary constriction.

Each of the above movement types is controlled at least partly by different central neural structures, finally focusing on the motoneurons of the eye muscle nuclei.

Afferent Connections to the Nuclei of the Eye Muscle Nerves

We have previously mentioned connections from the *vestibular nuclei,* which, via the *medial longitudinal fasciculus,* reach all the cranial nerve nuclei of the eye muscles (Fig. 13.17). These connections are both crossed and uncrossed. Some of the vestibular neurons sending their axons into the medial longitudinal fasciculus are excitatory; other neurons are inhibitory (GABA). The connections are precisely organized, enabling the activation of specific synergists and the inhibition of their antagonists (with regard to the intended eye movement). Other efferent fibers from the vestibular nuclei end in cell groups situated in the vicinity of the eye muscle nuclei, which send their axons to the latter. The *perihypoglossal nuclei* are examples of such preoculomotor cell groups. These nuclei (the most prominent one is the prepositus nucleus) are situated around the hypoglossal nucleus in the medulla. In addition to afferents from the vestibular nuclei, the perihypoglossal nuclei receive afferents from other structures involved in eye movement control, such as parts of the reticular formation and the cerebellum.

The direct and indirect impulse pathways from the vestibular nuclei to the eye muscle nuclei mediate the vestibulo-ocular reflexes (Fig. 13.28) and are probably also involved in optokinetic reflexes. In the latter case, signals from the retina reaching the vestibular nuclei (synaptically interrupted in several

nuclei) must be involved, rather than signals from the labyrinth.

Proprioceptive impulses from muscle spindles of the extraocular muscles reach the eye muscle nuclei from the mesencephalic trigeminal nucleus.

Optic impulses do not pass directly from the retina to the eye muscle nuclei but are mediated by several brain stem nuclei, which also receive impulses other than visual information. This concerns the *superior colliculus* and the *pretectal nuclei* (situated rostral and ventral to the superior colliculus; Fig. 13.27). These nuclei receive afferents from the retina and from parts of the cerebral cortex involved in control of eye movements (the frontal eye field, the posterior parietal cortex, and parts of the extrastriatal visual areas; Fig. 13.31).

There are no direct connections from the *cerebral cortex* to the eye muscle nuclei. Activation of the extraocular muscles from the cortex in conjunction with voluntary eye movements is mediated via other brain stem cell groups, primarily specific regions of the reticular formation in the vicinity of the eye muscle nuclei (Fig. 13.30).

Many of the signals from the various sources mentioned above are integrated by cell groups in the reticular formation, situated close to the eye muscle nuclei. From these *premotor* cell groups, the final commands are issued to the motoneurons. The premotor groups receive, for example, signals from the cerebral cortex, the vestibular nuclei, and the superior colliculus. One *center for horizontal eye movements* has been identified close to the abducent nucleus in the pons, and another *center for vertical eye movements* close to the oculomotor nucleus in the mesencephalon (Fig. 13.29).

More about Brain Stem Centers for Control of Eye Movements

By combining anatomic data on the fiber connections with physiological results (obtained by single-cell recordings, electrical stimulation, and lesions), we have identified brain stem cell groups of particular importance for eye movements. A *center for horizontal eye movements* has been

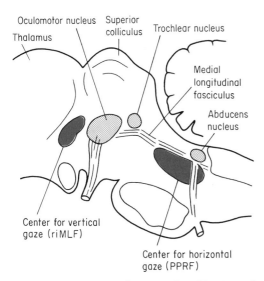

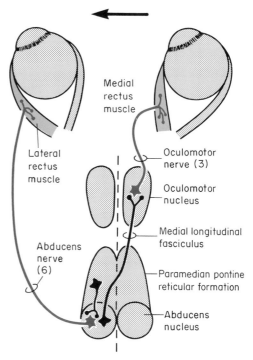

Fig. 13.29. *Centers for vertical and horizontal eye movements.* Sagittal section through the monkey brain stem. Redrawn from Büttner-Ennever (1988).

Fig. 13.30. *Control of horizontal conjugate eye movements.* Highly simplified scheme to show some of the connections responsible. Only excitatory connections are included. The figure also shows how interruption of the medial longitudinal fascicle produces a paralysis of the gaze in the medial direction (internuclear ophthalmoplegia).

identified in the paramedian pontine reticular formation. This center, called the *PPRF*, is situated close to, and sends fibers to, the abducent nucleus. It also sends fibers to the parts of the oculomotor nucleus containing the motoneurons of the medial rectus muscle. Together with the lateral rectus (innervated by the abducent nucleus), the medial rectus participates in horizontal movements. In addition, there are so-called internuclear neurons in the abducent nucleus that send axons to the medial rectus motoneurons of the opposite side (Fig. 13.30). This premotor network ensures simultaneous activation of the lateral rectus on one side and the medial rectus on the other, and inhibition of the antagonists.

A lesion in the region of the PPRF reduces horizontal conjugate movements to the side of the lesion. Especially marked is the reduction in saccadic movements. A unilateral *lesion of the medial longitudinal fasciculus* between the abducent and the oculomotor nucleus produces so-called *internuclear ophthalmoplegia* with abolished ability to adduct the eye on the same side (the medial rectus muscle). This may be understood on the basis of the diagram in Figure 13.30. However, vergence movements are possible even though the medial rectus is responsible also in that case. Thus, pathways other than the medial longitudinal fasciculus are responsible for the activation of the medial rectus muscle during vergence movements.

As mentioned, the PPRF receives impulses directly and indirectly from the vestibular nuclei, the superior colliculus, and the frontal eye field. It appears to function as the last premotor station for the initiation of conjugate horizontal saccadic movements. In agreement with this, there are neurons in the PPRF that are active immediately before and during a saccade to the same side, whereas they are inactive during slow-pursuit movements and fixation. These so-called *excitatory burst neurons* are believed to establish excitatory connections with the motoneurons responsible for the saccade. There are also *inhibitory burst neurons,* located close to the PPRF, with a pattern of activity similar to the excitatory burst neurons. They inhibit monosynaptically the motoneurons in the abducent nucleus of the opposite side. The activity of both kinds of burst neurons appears to be controlled by a third kind of neuron in the PPRF, which is tonically active. Such *omnipause neurons* probably inhibit the burst neurons tonically, except in relation to saccades. Thus, the omnipause neurons are silent immediately before and during saccades, regardless of the direction and amplitude of the movement. Recent studies indicate that the omnipause neurons receive direct connections from both the superior colliculus and the frontal eye field (they must presumably also receive impulses from the vestibular nuclei, since saccades can be elicited by vestibular signals as well).

A *center for vertical and rotatory eye movements* has been identified in the reticular formation close to the oculomotor nucleus. This region includes a nucleus called the *riMLF* (the rostral interstitial nucleus of the medial longitudinal fasciculus) and probably also another small cell group (the interstitial nucleus of Cajal). This region receives, most likely, afferents from the vestibular nuclei, the pretectum (and thereby indirectly from the superior colliculus), and frontal eye field. Physiological studies indicate that there are monosynaptic connections from the region of the riMLF to the trochlear nucleus and motoneuron groups within the oculomotor nucleus that produce vertical eye movements.

The PPRF and the region of the riMLF are interconnected, indicating that they do not operate independently of each other. The fact that many natural eye movements are neither purely horizontal not purely vertical but combinations of both strongly suggests that the centers for horizontal and vertical movements must coordinate their activity.

Cortical Centers for Control of Eye Movements

The *frontal eye field* (area 8 of Brodmann, Figs. 13.31 and 17.3) is located immediately frontal to the premotor area. It is of particular importance for *voluntary saccades* (regions in the parieto-occipital region also contribute to control of saccades). Electrical stimulation of the frontal eye field elicits conjugated eye movements to the opposite side. The effect is mediated by fibers descending in the internal capsule to brain stem premotor cell groups, such as the superior colliculus, the pretectal nuclei, and the PPRF, which in their turn activate motoneurons in the eye muscle nuclei. A unilateral lesion of the frontal eye field makes the patient unable to move the gaze voluntarily to the side opposite the lesion (for example, when asked by the examiner to

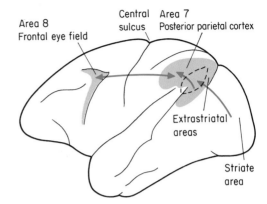

Fig. 13.31. *Cortical areas involved in control of eye movements* (monkey). The arrows show some association connections of these areas. The dashed line indicates that some of the area is hidden in a sulcus.

move the gaze). The ability to move the gaze laterally is not completely lost, however. Thus, smooth-pursuit movements occur when an object is brought into the visual field and then moved slowly laterally—that is, the patient is able to follow the object with her gaze.

With regard to *cortical control of smooth-pursuit movements,* a region in the occipitotemporal region seems to be of particular importance. This notion is based on, among other things, observations of the activity of single cells in relation to eye movements. The subcortical cell groups intercalated between these cortical regions and the eye muscle nuclei are, however, not identified with certainty. The ability to *fix the gaze* is a prerequisite for slow-pursuit movements. A *fixation center* is assumed to be localized within the cortical region responsible for the initiation of slow-pursuit movements.

The term *fixation reflex* implies that the tendency to fix the gaze on an object is not really voluntary, at least not in the strict sense of that word (even though fixation is dependent on the person being conscious). *Optokinetic nystagmus* is an expression of the fixation tendency or reflex. When a screen with alternating black and white vertical stripes is moved horizontally in front of a person, nystagmus occurs. The gaze is fixed automatically on one of the stripes and follows it until it leaves the visual field. Then the eyes move rapidly back to the starting position and the gaze is fixed again on another stripe. This sequence repeats itself as long as the screen moves.

NOTES

1. The accessory, the hypoglossal, and the part of the facial nucleus supplying the lower part of the face—and often also the motor trigeminal nucleus—receive only crossed fibers, as judged from clinical observations (Monrad-Krohn).

2. Embryologically, the vagus nerve belongs to the fourth, fifth, and sixth branchial arches, and this explains the peculiar course of some of its branches.

3. On an embryological basis, all sensory fibers from the pharynx (and the posterior part of the tongue) should be classified as visceral afferent. There is evidence, however, that such fibers end in the somatic afferent trigeminal nucleus and not in the visceral afferent nucleus. Functionally, they may therefore be considered somatic afferent rather than visceral afferent.

4. There are also *efferent cholinergic fibers* in the vestibular nerve, ending in contact with the vestibular receptors. Their actions are not known in man. In lower mammals, they have been shown to have an inhibitory action, whereas the action in monkeys appears to be excitatory. The efferent fibers come from a small cell group in the lower pons close to the vestibular nuclei.

5. The utricle records especially head positions that vary around a sagittal axis (that is, a lateral tilt), whereas the saccule probably records positions mainly around a transverse axis (that is, flexion–extension in the cervical joints).

6. There are also some taste buds on the soft palate, which are innervated by the intermediate nerve. The few taste buds present on the most posterior part of the tongue and on the upper side of the epiglottis are innervated by the vagus nerve.

7. The separation of fibers of different kinds is not quite as sharp as this account may indicate, however. Thus, many trigeminal fibers divide after entering the brain stem into an ascending and a descending branch (just like the sensory fibers entering the cord). In this manner, single ganglion cells may end in more than one nuclear subdivision.

8. A lesion affecting lateral parts of the medulla is likely to interrupt the spinothalamic tract and the spinal trigeminal nucleus. This will cause reduced or abolished pain and temperature sensation in the opposite body half but on the same side of the face (Fig. 4.14).

9. Another peculiarity of the trochlear nerve is that it crosses the midline before leaving the brain stem, so that the left trochlear nucleus innervates the right superior oblique muscle and vice versa. Some of the fibers of the oculomotor nerve also cross before leaving the brain stem.

V

The Autonomic Nervous System

The *autonomic nervous system* (or visceral system) is not a term that can be defined precisely, either anatomically or functionally. The old belief that the somatic and the autonomic parts of the nervous system are completely independent is not tenable. The more we have learned about the structure and function of the nervous system, the clearer it has become that simplistic divisions like this are rather arbitrary. The somatic and visceral processes are so intimately interrelated that any subdivision becomes by necessity artificial. For practical reasons, it is nevertheless helpful to use the term autonomic nervous system and to define it very broadly as *the neuronal groups and fiber connections that control the activity of visceral organs, vessels, and glands* (also the vessels and glands that are not parts of visceral organs). Visceral organs contain smooth-muscle cells and glands. We can therefore also define the autonomic system as *the parts of the nervous system that control the activity of smooth muscles and glands,* regardless of their location in the body (in contrast to the somatic or cerebrospinal system, which controls striated skeletal muscles). Mostly, we are not aware of the processes going on in the organs controlled by the autonomic nervous system, and their activities are not subject to voluntary, conscious control. The autonomic nervous system cooperates with the endocrine system, as we will see in this section.

The autonomic system can be subdivided in different ways. As with the somatic system, we distinguish *peripheral* and *central* parts. Whereas the peripheral parts of the autonomic and somatic systems can be separated fairly well, the division becomes much less clear within the central nervous system. The peripheral parts of the autonomic system are described in Chapter 14, whereas the central parts, notably the hypothalamus, are treated in Chapter 15.

The autonomic system can also be divided into a *sympathetic* and a *parasympathetic* part, differing anatomically and functionally (again, the separation is most obvious in the peripheral nervous system). The actions of the two parts of the autonomic system are mainly antagonistic: Where the sympathetic system activates, the parasympathetic reduces the activity, and vice versa.

14

Peripheral Autonomic Nervous System

Although the nerves to visceral organs contain both efferent (motor) and afferent (sensory) fibers, the structural and functional differences between the autonomic and the somatic systems concern primarily the efferent side. Therefore, this chapter deals mainly with the visceral efferent neurons, briefly describing special features of visceral afferent neurons and visceral sensibility.

In general, the actions of the sympathetic system suggest that it is of special importance in situations of stress, requiring mobilization of bodily resources. The parasympathetic system, on the other hand, contributes primarily to processes of maintenance, such as digestion and reproductive behavior. The actions of the two systems, however, are much more varied than this, and such generalized statements should be taken only as useful rules of thumb.

GENERAL ORGANIZATION OF THE AUTONOMIC SYSTEM

Two Succeeding Neurons Constitute the Efferent Pathway

Despite their different actions, the sympathetic and the parasympathetic systems have certain features of peripheral organization

in common. These should be known before going into the differences between them.

In contrast to the somatic efferent fibers (leading from motoneurons to skeletal muscles), the visceral efferent fibers do not pass nonstop to the organs. The transmission of signals is interrupted by *autonomic ganglia* (Fig. 14.1). The multipolar cells in the ganglia send their axons to the effectors (smooth-muscle cells and glands) in visceral organs. The neurons conducting impulses to the ganglia are called *preganglionic,* whereas the ganglion cells and their axons are called *postganglionic.* The *perikarya of the preganglionic neurons* are located in the spinal cord and the brain stem. The preganglionic neurons, both the sympathetic and the parasympathetic ones, use *acetylcholine* as neurotransmitter.

Another typical feature of the autonomic nervous system is that the postganglionic fibers as a rule form extensive *plexuses* around the organs they innervate.

Postganglionic Fibers Do Not Establish Typical Synapses

The thin, unmyelinated postganglionic fibers do not form typical synapses with the effector cells, in contrast to the somatic ef-

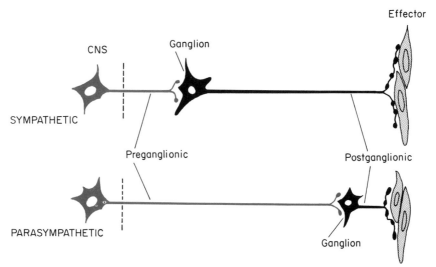

Fig. 14.1. *Basic organization of the peripheral part of the autonomic system.* Two consecutive neurons conduct the impulses from the central nervous system to the effectors. Note the differ-ence in length between the pre- and postgangli-onic fibers in the sympathetic and the parasym-pathetic systems. Effectors may be glandular cells and not only smooth-muscle cells, as shown here.

ferent fibers innervating skeletal muscle cells (Fig. 8.4). When the postganglionic fibers reach the vicinity of the effector cells, they branch extensively, and there are small swellings—*varicosities*—along the branches (Fig. 14.1). In each varicosity there are vesi-cles with neurotransmitter. The varicosities do not form synapses but can be located fairly close to the effector cells. Often the distance between the varicosities and the ef-fectors is so great that the transmitter, after being released, must diffuse over fairly long distances to reach its target. This means that the neurotransmitter acts on several effector cells within a certain distance. When the dif-fusion distance is great, the transmitter acts slowly—that is, with a fairly long latency and a prolonged action (compared with the fast action at the neuromuscular junction). Often, only a few of the smooth-muscle cells in the wall of a hollow organ—such as a ves-sel—are close enough to the varicosities to be directly influenced by the transmitter. In such cases, the action potential elicited in some smooth-muscle cells is propagated from cell to cell via gap junctions between them (which couple the cells electrically). In

general, therefore, *the actions of the auto-nomic nervous system are more diffusely dis-tributed, both spatially and temporally, than is the case in the somatic system.* The prop-erties of the smooth-muscle cells contribute to increase this difference, because their ac-tion potentials last much longer than those of skeletal muscles. Furthermore, smooth-muscle cells (for example, in the wall of the gastrointestinal tract) can be made to con-tract by stimuli other than nervous ones, such as by stretching and by the actions of hormones. The autonomic system therefore *contributes* to the regulation of the contrac-tion of smooth-muscle cells in the gastroin-testinal tract and in the walls of the vessels, but it is not alone in this capacity (again in contrast to the control of skeletal muscle cells by the motoneurons).

There are, nevertheless, *great differences between different organs with regard to the precision of their autonomic innervation.* Some visceral organs require much faster and more accurate control than others. The smooth muscles of the eye (the ciliary muscle and the sphincter pupillae, regulating the curvature of the lens and the diameter of the pupil) must be subject to very precise control. The same holds for the muscles of the ductus deferens, in which the propulsive contractions must be fast and well coordinated. Such demands are not made of the smooth muscles of the gastrointestinal tract and the vessels. Corresponding to different functional requirements, the pattern of autonomic innervation varies in different organs. The intrinsic eye muscles, for example, receive a large number of nerve fibers so that all muscle cells come in close contact with varicosities of nerve fibers. This arrangement is called *multiunit,* because it is similar to the conditions in the somatic system with many precisely controlled motor units. In places with few nerve fibers to supply a large number of smooth-muscle cells, so that only a few cells are close to nerve varicosities, we use the term *single-unit* arrangement. Thus, numerous muscle cells behave as a unit when one or a few are activated.

Differences between the Sympathetic and the Parasympathetic Systems

The two systems differ in several respects. The *preganglionic neurons* are situated in different parts of the central nervous system: The *sympathetic* ones are found in the T_1–L_2 spinal segments, whereas the *parasympathetic* preganglionic neurons lie in the brain stem and the $(S_2)S_3$–S_4 spinal segments (Figs. 14.5 and 14.9). Furthermore, the *ganglia* are located differently: *Sympathetic* ones lie close to the central nervous system, whereas the *parasympathetic* ganglia are located close to the target organs. Thus, the sympathetic preganglionic fibers are short, and the parasympathetic ones are long (Fig. 14.1).

Another difference between the two systems is the *neurotransmitters* utilized by the postganglionic fibers: The sympathetic fibers release *norepinephrine,* whereas the parasympathetic fibers release *acetylcholine* from their varicosities.

Finally, the distribution of postganglionic fibers is different. Thus, virtually *all parts of the body receive sympathetic fibers, whereas the parasympathetic fibers are mostly restricted to the true visceral organs.* The body wall and the extremities (skin, muscles, joints) do not receive parasympathetic fibers.

The Parasympathetic Innervation Is Usually More Precise Than the Sympathetic

As a general rule (with notable exceptions), the sympathetic system is more diffusely organized than the parasympathetic. This is shown, for example, in the relation between the number of preganglionic and postganglionic fibers. In the parasympathetic ciliary ganglion (Figs. 13.25 and 13.27), two postganglionic fibers leave the ganglion for each preganglionic fiber reaching it— that is, a 2:1 relationship (in the cat). For the sympathetic superior cervical ganglion (Fig. 14.5), the relationship is 30:1 in the cat and 60–190:1 in humans (this ganglion contains more than 1 million neurons in man). Furthermore, the parasympathetic innervation is in several places arranged with *multiunits*—that is, small "motor units" and the possibility of precise control. This concerns, for example, the innervation of the intrinsic eye muscles. The sympathetic innervation is often (but not always) arranged with *single units*—that is, a large number of smooth muscle cells are activated from one postganglionic fiber and behave as a functional unit.

Another difference concerns the topographic arrangement of the preganglionic neurons. Whereas the sympathetic neurons show only a fairly rough topography within the intermediolateral column in relation to the location of the target (Fig. 14.5; Table 14.1), the parasympathetic neurons are as a rule collected in distinct nuclei (Fig. 14.9) or subdivisions of a nucleus (like the dorsal motor nucleus of the vagus), each related to one target organ.

The difference in innervation precision between the sympathetic and the parasympathetic systems mentioned above have several exceptions, however. One example is the ductus deferens, in which the rhythmic contractions are elicited by sympathetic fibers. A multiunit arrangement is required to ensure the necessary precision and speed of the contractile wave moving the sperm during ejaculation. On the other hand, the parasympathetic innervation of the gastrointestinal tract, eliciting contractile activity, is rather diffuse (single-unit arrangement).

Table 14.1. *The Principal Features of the Autonomic Innervation of Some Organs*

Organ	The Sympathetic System			The Parasympathetic System		
	Preganglionic neuron	Postganglionic neuron	Action	Preganglionic neuron	Postganglionic neuron	Action
Eye	Th_{1-2}	Superior cervical ganglion	Pupillary dilatation	Edinger-Westphal nucleus	Ciliary ganglion	Pupillary constriction accommodation
Lacrimal gland	Th_{1-2}	Superior cervical ganglion	?	Superior salivatory nucleus	Pterygopalatine ganglion	Secretion of tears
Submandibular & sublingual glands	Th_{1-2}	Superior cervical ganglion	Vasoconstriction	Superior salivatory nucleus	Submandibular ganglion	Secretion of saliva, vasodilation
Parotid gland	Th_{1-2}	Superior cervical ganglion	Vasoconstriction	Inferior salivatory nucleus	Otic ganglion	Secretion of saliva, vasodilation
Heart	$Th_{1-4(5)}$	Superior, middle, inferior cervical & upper thoracic ganglia	Increased heart rate and stroke volume, dilation of coronary arteries	Dorsal motor nucleus, vagus nerve	Cardiac plexus	Reduced heart rate (bradycardia)
Bronchi, lungs	$Th_{2-7(2-4?)}$	Inferior cervical & upper thoracic ganglia	Vasodilation, bronchial dilation	Dorsal motor nucleus, vagus nerve	Pulmonary plexus	Bronchial constriction and secretion
Stomach	Th_{6-10} Greater splanchnic nerve	Celiac ganglion	Inhibition of peristaltic movement & secretion, vasoconstriction	Pulmonary plexus	Myenteric & submucosal plexus (ganglia)	Peristaltic movement & secretion
Pancreas	Th_{6-10} Greater splanchnic nerve	Celiac ganglion	Vasoconstriction	Pulmonary plexus	Periarterial plexus	Secretion
Small intestine ascending & transverse large intestine	Th_{6-10} Greater splanchnic nerve	Celiac, superior & inferior mesenteric ganglia	Inhibition of peristaltic movement & secretion	Pulmonary plexus	Myenteric & submucosal plexus (ganglia)	Peristaltic movement & secretion
Descending large intestine, sigmoid, rectum	$Th_{11}-L_2$	Inferior mesentery hypogastric & pelvic plexus (ganglia)	Inhibition of peristaltic movement & secretion	S_{3-4}	Myenteric & submucosal plexus (ganglia)	Peristaltic movement & secretion
Ureter, bladder	$Th_{11}-L_2$	Hypogastr. & pelvic plexus (ganglia)	Relaxation of detrusor muscle & contraction of internal sphincter	S_{3-4}	Pelvic plexus (ganglion)	Contraction of detrusor & inhibition of internal sphincter
Head, neck (skin & skeletal muscles)	Th_{1-4}	Superior & middle cervical ganglia				
Upper extremity	Th_{3-6}	Stellate & upper thoracic ganglia	Sweat secretion, vasoconstriction, pilo-erection			No parasympathetic innervation
Lower extremity	$Th_{10}-L_2$	Lower lumbar & upper sacral ganglia				

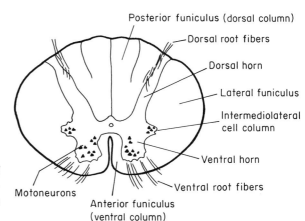

Fig. 14.2. *The intermediolateral cell column* contains the perikarya of the preganglionic sympathetic neurons. Cross section of the thoracic cord.

PERIPHERAL PARTS OF THE SYMPATHETIC SYSTEM

Preganglionic Fibers and the Sympathetic Trunk

The peripheral parts of the sympathetic system consist of neurons conveying impulses to visceral organs, and sensory fibers leading in the opposite direction. The efferent, *preganglionic sympathetic fibers* belong to neurons with perikarya in the *intermediolateral column* in the spinal cord (Fig. 14.2). The fibers leave the cord (like other efferent fibers) through the ventral roots, but because the intermediolateral column is present only in the T_1–L_2 segments (Fig. 14.5), only the ventral roots of these segments contain preganglionic sympathetic fibers (the sympathetic system is also called the *thoracolumbar* system). The sympathetic fibers follow the somatic ones only for a short distance, however. Just after the ventral and the dorsal roots fuse, the sympathetic preganglionic fibers leave the spinal nerve to end in a sympathetic ganglion (Fig. 14.3). In early embryonic life, one ganglion is produced on each side for every spinal segment, but during further development some ganglia fuse, so the final number is smaller than the number of segments. This reduction is most marked in the cervical region.

The ganglia are located just outside the intervertebral foramen, laterally on the vertebral column (Fig. 14.4). The row of such *paravertebral ganglia* extends from the base of the skull to the coccygeal bone in the pelvis minor. Since the ganglia are interconnected by fiber bundles, a continuous string called the *sympathetic trunk* is formed (Figs. 14.4 and 14.5). The ganglia form small

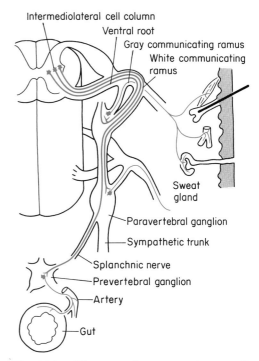

Fig. 14.3. *The sympathetic system.* Postganglionic neurons are located in the ganglia of the sympathetic trunk and in the prevertebral ganglia. Sympathetic fibers to the trunk and the extremities follow the spinal nerves, whereas fibers to the visceral organs form separate nerves and follow the main vessels to the organs.

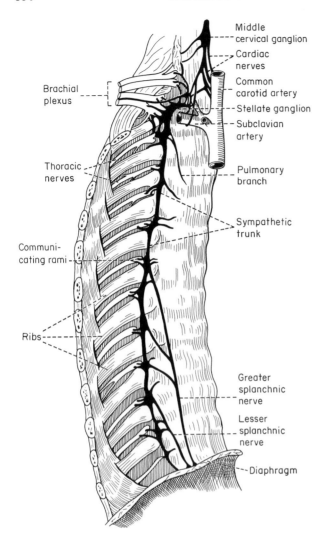

Middle
cervical ganglion

Cardiac
nerves

Common
carotid artery

Stellate ganglion

Subclavian
artery

Pulmonary
branch

Brachial
plexus

Thoracic
nerves

Sympathetic
trunk

Communi-
cating rami

Ribs

Greater
splanchnic
nerve

Lesser
splanchnic
nerve

Diaphragm

Fig. 14.4. *The sympathetic trunk.* A part of the thoracic vertebral column and the ribs seen from the right. Note the communicating rami and the splanchnic nerves. Redrawn from Spalteholz (1929).

swellings along the trunk. There is usually one ganglion for each pair of spinal nerves, except in the cervical region, where there are only three: the *superior, middle,* and *inferior cervical ganglia.* The middle ganglion can be missing, and the inferior cervical ganglion is usually fused with the uppermost thoracic ganglion to the large *stellate ganglion* (Fig. 14.4). In the lumbar and sacral parts of the sympathetic trunks, some cross-connections are present.

The preganglionic sympathetic fibers leave the spinal nerve as a small bundle called the *white communicating ramus,* which connects the nerve with the sympathetic trunk (Figs. 14.3 and 14.4). Since

many of the preganglionic fibers are myelinated, this communicating ramus is whitish. Because of the restricted extension of the intermediolateral column, *only the thoracic and the upper two lumbar spinal nerves give off white communicating rami.*

When reaching the ganglia of the sympathetic trunk, some preganglionic fibers establish synapses with postganglionic neurons in that ganglion, whereas others continue uninterrupted through the ganglion (Fig. 14.3). In the upper part of the trunk, the fibers continue rostrally, in the lower part caudally, to establish synapses with ganglion cells in ganglia at levels above and below the intermediolateral column

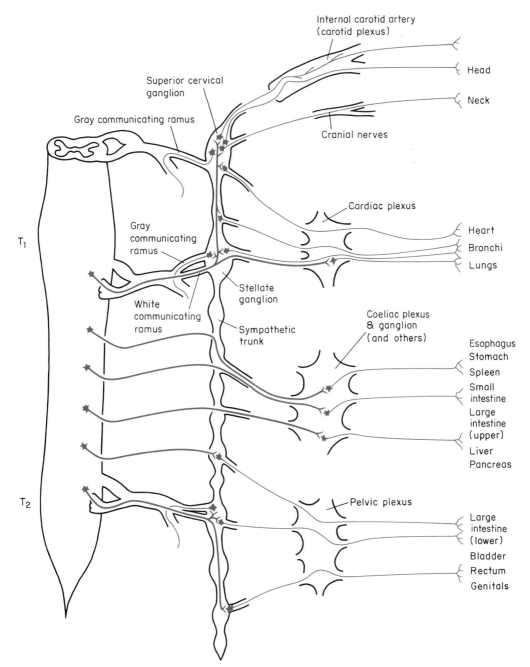

Fig. 14.5.   *The sympathetic system,* highly schematized.

(Figs. 14.5, 14.7, and 14.8). This arrangement ensures that *preganglionic fibers reach all the ganglia of the sympathetic trunk (the paravertebral ganglia).*

Some of the preganglionic fibers pass directly through the ganglia and form separate nerves destined for *prevertebral sym-pathetic ganglia* (Figs. 14.3–14.5). We will return to this point later in this chapter.

Autonomic Ganglia

The autonomic ganglia contain *multipolar neurons* of various sizes (Fig. 14.6) with long, branching dendrites. The axons are mostly unmyelin-

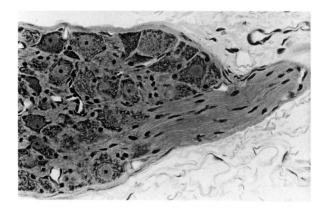

Fig. 14.6. *Autonomic ganglion.* Microphotograph of thionine-stained section. To the right, a nerve is seen to enter the ganglion with preganglionic fibers.

ated and very thin. The perikarya of the ganglion cells are embedded in a meshwork of fibers consisting of afferent fibers, ganglion cell dendrites, and axons of the ganglion cells. At least some of the ganglia receive *sensory fibers* from visceral organs. There are also *interneurons* in the autonomic ganglia. Such features, and other data, indicate that the ganglia are not just simple synaptic interruptions of purely motor (efferent) pathways but can serve as *reflex centers* for some visceral reflexes.

Postganglionic Sympathetic Fibers

The postganglionic fibers from the ganglia of the sympathetic trunk take different routes. From all of the ganglia, some fibers pass back to the spinal nerve as the thin *gray communicating ramus* (Figs. 14.3 and 14.4). This ramus is more grayish than the white ramus because most of the postganglionic fibers are unmyelinated.[1] *All of the spinal nerves are supplied with postganglionic fibers through the communicating rami* (Fig. 14.5). The postganglionic fibers follow the spinal nerves out into all their branches.

Other postganglionic fibers leave the trunk and *pass to larger arteries in the vicinity* and follow them peripherally (such as the subclavian artery to the arm, the common iliac artery with branches to pelvic organs and the lower extremity) (Figs. 14.7 and 14.8). Some of these fibers innervate the smooth-muscle cells of the artery. Many of the postganglionic sympathetic fibers that follow the spinal nerves leave them periph-

erally to innervate small vessels. Other fibers from the spinal nerves innervate sweat glands and smooth muscles attached to hair follicles (Fig. 14.3).

Sympathetic Innervation of the Head and Extremities

The head, neck, and upper extremity are supplied with preganglionic sympathetic fibers from the upper thoracic segments. The fibers enter the sympathetic trunk through the communicating rami. Some establish synaptic contacts with postganglionic neurons in the upper thoracic ganglia, whereas other fibers pass through these ganglia to end in the cervical ganglia (Figs. 14.5 and 14.7). From these ganglia, postganglionic fibers enter the spinal nerves to the neck (C_1–C_4) and the upper extremity (C_5–T_1).

The *head* receives postganglionic fibers from the superior cervical ganglion. From the ganglion, the fibers follow arteries and cranial nerves to the skin, the eye, the lacrimal gland, and the salivary glands.

With regard to the *lower extremities,* the arrangement corresponds to that described for the upper extremity, with postganglionic fibers following partly the spinal nerves and partly the large arteries (Fig. 14.8).

Sympathetic Innervation of the Viscera

As mentioned above, the postganglionic sympathetic fibers to the extremities and the body wall follow to a great extent the spinal nerves. The visceral organs of the thorax and the abdomen do not receive branches from the spinal nerves, however. Therefore, the sympathetic fibers destined for these organs have to form separate nerves.

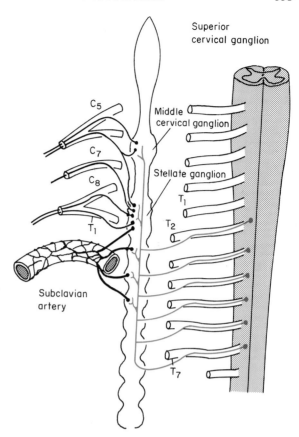

Fig. 14.7. *Sympathetic innervation of the upper extremity.* The preganglionic fibers come from the upper thoracic segments of the cord and synapse in the ganglia of the sympathetic trunk up to the middle cervical ganglion. The postganglionic fibers follow partly the spinal nerves and partly the subclavian artery to the arm. Redrawn from Haymaker and Woodhall (1945).

Such *splanchnic nerves* are fairly thin twigs that leave the sympathetic trunk at various levels.

The sympathetic fibers to the *heart* follow the superior, middle, and inferior cardiac nerves leaving the corresponding cervical ganglia. The perikaryon of the postganglionic neuron is located in the cervical ganglia (Fig. 14.5). In addition, some smaller branches to the heart take off from the upper thoracic sympathetic ganglia.

Most sympathetic fibers to the *abdominal viscera* form *the greater and lesser splanchnic nerves* (Fig. 14.4). These nerves consist mainly of preganglionic fibers from spinal segments T_6–T_{11}, which pass uninterrupted through the ganglia of the sympathetic trunk (Figs. 14.3 and 14.5). The nerves penetrate the diaphragm and end in ganglia located on the ventral side of the abdominal aorta in the upper abdomen. These are called *prevertebral ganglia,* to distinguish them from the paravertebral ganglia of the sympathetic trunk. The largest among the prevertebral ganglia is the *celiac ganglion,* located where the celiac artery emerges from the aorta. Smaller prevertebral

ganglia are found where the superior and inferior mesenteric arteries emerge. The postganglionic fibers follow the arteries to the various organs.

The greater and lesser splanchnic nerves and the corresponding prevertebral ganglia supply the visceral organs in *the upper and middle part of the abdomen,* such as the stomach, pancreas, gallbladder, small intestine, and the large intestine to the descending part. The *adrenal medulla,* which also receives preganglionic fibers from the splanchnic nerves, is special. The medullary endocrine cells (chromaffin cells)—which are transformed postganglionic neurons—release epinephrine (and small amounts of norepinephrine) into the bloodstream on sympathetic stimulation.

The visceral organs of the *lower abdomen* receive their sympathetic innervation from the intermediolateral column in the lower thoracic and upper two lumbar segments. These fibers also leave the sympathetic trunk as separate nerves (lumbar splanchnic nerves) to reach prevertebral

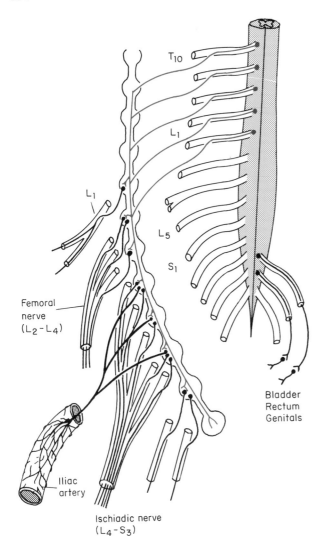

Fig. 14.8.   *Sympathetic innervation of the lower extremity.* In the **right** side of the figure, pre- and postganglionic parasympathetic fibers from the sacral cord are also shown. Redrawn from Haymaker and Woodhall (1945).

ganglia. The postganglionic fibers follow the arteries to the organs (Fig. 14.5).

The prevertebral ganglia are embedded in a meshwork of fibers, forming *prevertebral plexuses*, with names corresponding to those of the ganglia (Fig. 14.5).

PERIPHERAL PARTS OF THE PARASYMPATHETIC SYSTEM

As mentioned, the preganglionic parasympathetic (visceral efferent) neurons have their perikarya in the brain stem and in the sacral cord. The cells are morphologically similar to the sympathetic preganglionic neurons of the intermediolateral column.

The Cranial Nerves Contain Preganglionic Parasympathetic Fibers

The preganglionic fibers of the *cranial part* of the parasympathetic system follow the *oculomotor*, the *facial (intermediate)*, the *glossopharyngeal*, and the *vagus nerves*. The fibers come from the visceral efferent column of cranial nerve nuclei (Figs. 13.2 and 13.3). The preganglionic fibers of the cranial nerves supplying structures in the head end in several parasympathetic ganglia, located outside the skull close to large cranial nerve trunks (Fig. 14.9). These are the *ciliary*, the *pterygopalatine*, the *otic*, and the *submandibular ganglia*. From these ganglia, the

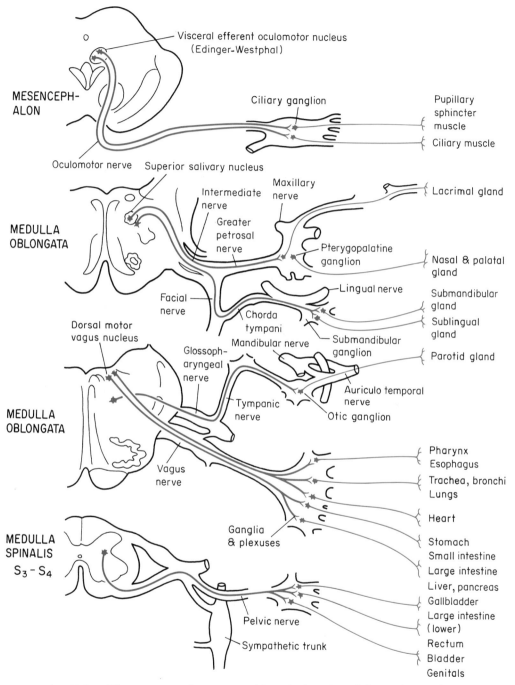

Fig. 14.9. *The parasympathetic system.* Note the location of the perikarya of the preganglionic neurons in the brain stem and in the sacral cord.

MESENCEPH-ALON

Visceral efferent oculomotor nucleus (Edinger-Westphal)

Ciliary ganglion

Pupillary sphincter muscle

Ciliary muscle

Oculomotor nerve

Superior salivary nucleus

MEDULLA OBLONGATA

Intermediate nerve

Maxillary nerve

Lacrimal gland

Greater petrosal nerve

Pterygopalatine ganglion

Nasal & palatal gland

Facial nerve

Lingual nerve

Submandibular gland

Chorda tympani

Sublingual gland

Dorsal motor vagus nucleus

Mandibular nerve

Submandibular ganglion

Parotid gland

Glossoph-aryngeal nerve

Auriculo temporal nerve

MEDULLA OBLONGATA

Tympanic nerve

Otic ganglion

Vagus nerve

Pharynx
Esophagus

Trachea, bronchi
Lungs

Heart

Ganglia & plexuses

Stomach
Small intestine
Large intestine

MEDULLA SPINALIS
$S_3 - S_4$

Liver, pancreas
Gallbladder

Large intestine (lower)

Pelvic nerve

Rectum

Sympathetic trunk

Bladder

Genitals

postganglionic fibers pass to the effector organs (the intrinsic muscles of the eye, the lacrimal gland, and the salivary glands). The preganglionic fibers of the *vagus nerve* do not end in well-defined ganglia but in more diffusely distributed collections of postganglionic neurons in the walls of (or just out-side) the organs. These postganglionic neurons have short axons running in the wall of the organ and innervate smooth-muscle cells and glands. As mentioned in Chapter 13, the vagus nerve sends parasympathetic fibers to the heart, the lungs, the gastrointestinal tract down to the descending colon, the gall-bladder, the liver, and the pancreas (Fig. 13.8).

The Enteric Nervous System

The postganglionic parasympathetic fibers of the gastrointestinal tract are embedded in two plexuses in the wall. Postganglionic sympathetic fibers also contribute to these plexuses. Largest is the *myenteric plexus*—located between the circular and the longitudinal external smooth-muscle layers, whereas the smaller *submucous plexus* is situated below the mucous membrane.

It has become clear that these plexuses and ganglia represent a part of the peripheral nervous system that is to some extent independent, as expressed by the name *enteric nervous system.* Thus, the neurons in the myenteric and submucous ganglia are able to function even after the sympathetic and parasympathetic nerves to the gastrointestinal have been cut. The number of neurons in the enteric system is large, and only a few of these are under direct control from the central nervous system (by means of parasympathetic preganglionic fibers). Numerous neurotransmitters, in particular many neuropeptides, have been demonstrated in the enteric ganglion cells. Only a few of them contain acetylcholine, the classic transmitter of postganglionic parasympathetic neurons.

Some of the enteric neurons are most likely *sensory* and send their central process to prevertebral ganglia. Thus, local reflex arcs not involving the central nervous system are established.

The enteric nervous sytem plays a decisive role for the *peristaltic movements of the bowel,* moving the content toward the anus.

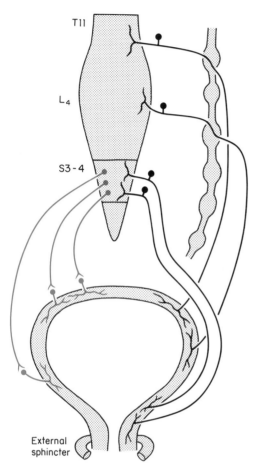

Fig. 14.10. *Innervation of the bladder.* To the left is the parasympathetic innervation of the smooth muscles responsible for emptying the bladder. The preganglionic neurons are located in the spinal segments S_3–S_4, whereas the postganglionic perikarya are found just outside or in the wall of the bladder. To the right is the course of the sensory fibers from the bladder. From the lower part, the sensory fibers follow the efferent parasympathetic fibers, whereas the sensory fibers from the upper part (the fundus) follow the sympathetic fibers (via the sympathetic trunk). The striated, external sphincter muscle is innervated by motoneurons in the sacral segments S_3–S_4 (not shown).

The Sacral Part of the Parasympathetic System Supplies the Genitals, Bladder, and Rectum

The perikarya of the preganglionic neurons in the sacral cord are located in the $(S_2)S_3$–S_4 segments, with a position corresponding to the intermediolateral column of the sympathetic system (Figs. 14.9 and 14.10). The parasympathetic preganglionic fibers leave the cord through the ventral roots and follow the spinal nerves for a short distance. Then they leave the spinal nerves as separate, small *pelvic nerves*. In contrast to the sympathetic preganglionic fibers, the parasympathetic ones do not pass to the sympathetic trunk but join postganglionic sympathetic fibers in the *pelvic plexus,* located immediately lateral to the rectum, the bladder, the prostate gland (in the male), and the cervix (in the female). Many of the postganglionic parasympathetic neurons are located in the pelvic plexus.

Postganglionic parasympathetic fibers innervate all the organs of the pelvis and, in addition, the corpora cavernosa (erectile tissue) of the penis and the clitoris. The descending and sigmoid colon and the rectum are innervated from the sacral parasympathetic division. Of particular practical importance is the parasympathetic innervation of the rectum and the bladder, which is responsible for emptying these organs.

Peripheral Autonomic Plexuses

When an organ is innervated by both sympathetic and parasympathetic fibers, these two components intermingle and form autonomic plexuses just outside or in the wall of the organs. For example, the *cardiac plexus* on the outside of the heart contains both kinds of fibers and, in addition, the perikarya of the postganglionic parasympathetic neurons. Especially well-developed plexuses are found around the large vessels in the upper abdomen, where vagus fibers intermingle with sympathetic fibers from (mainly) the splanchnic nerves. The plexuses get their names from the arteries they surround and follow peripherally: the *celiac plexus,* the *superior* and *inferior mesenteric plexus,* and the *renal plexus.* Together with these plexuses are collections of sympathetic ganglion cells. Thus, there are ganglia with the same prefix as the plexuses (the celiac ganglion, and so forth).

Plexuses formed mainly by sympathetic fibers stretch from the lower part of the abdominal aorta into the pelvis minor as the *hypogastric plexus*. In the pelvis, the hypogastric plexus mixes with parasympathetic fibers from the pelvic nerves and forms the pelvic plexus around pelvic organs, as mentioned above.

FUNCTIONAL ASPECTS OF THE AUTONOMIC NERVOUS SYSTEM

When the autonomic system is considered as a whole, certain main functional features are clear. The *parasympathetic system* controls primarily processes that are necessary for the maintenance of the organism over the long term. The parasympathetic system thus activates the digestive processes, ensures that waste products are expelled by contraction of the bladder and rectum, protects the eye against strong light, ensures focused vision, reduces the activity of the heart, reduces the diameter of the airways, and increases bronchial secretion. The *sympathetic system* as a whole is more concerned with mobilizing the resources of the body when an extra effort is required. In situations of fear and anger, there are usually signs indicating increased sympathetic activity, such as increased blood pressure, increased heart rate, and dilatation of the pupils. At the same time, stored energy is mobilized by epinephrine secreted into the bloodstream from the adrenal medulla (increased blood level of glucose and fatty acids). Epinephrine also activates the heart and dilates the bronchi (relaxation of smooth-muscle cells). The activity of the gastrointestinal tract is inhibited. In general, such responses are adequate in flight-or-fight situations.

Actions of Sympathetic Fibers on the Circulatory and Respiratory Organs

The postganglionic sympathetic fibers innervate *vessels in all parts of the body*. Because the vascular smooth-muscle cells are arranged circularly, contraction reduces the diameter and increases the vascular resistance. Such *vasoconstriction* is most marked in the smallest arteries, the *arterioles,* which are especially concerned with the regulation of blood flow to the organs. Action potentials in the sympathetic fibers ending in the vessel walls produce vasoconstriction and, thus, reduced blood flow. By varying the impulse frequency of the sympathetic nerves, they can vary the diameter of the vessels.[2]

When there are no impulses in the sympathetic fibers innervating the vessel (and no other substances act to produce contraction), the arterioles are maximally widened by the internal blood pressure. This is called *vasodilation.*

In many situations the task of the sympathetic system is to ensure that there is a sufficient blood flow through "high-priority" organs, primarily the brain and the heart. When the blood flow through these organs diminishes, sympathetic neurons to vessels in other parts of the body increase their firing rate. Thus, the blood flow through skeletal muscles and the visceral organs is reduced. Sudden vasodilation in large parts of the body leads to a fall in blood pressure and fainting, because the cerebral blood flow is reduced.

Sympathetic innervation of the *large veins* is also of importance for the maintenance of adequate blood pressure. Constriction of such capacity vessels distributes more of the blood volume to the arterial side— that is, the effective blood volume increases. This mechanism is of importance in case of reduced blood volume (on bleeding or dehydration).

Impulses in sympathetic fibers to arterioles in *skeletal muscles* produce vasoconstriction. Epinephrine—released from the adrenal medulla on sympathetic stimulation—may, however, inhibit the vascular smooth-muscle cells and thereby produce vasodilation.

The *heart* receives sympathetic fibers partly through separate nerves from the cervical sympathetic ganglia (Figs. 14.4 and 14.5) and partly through direct branches from the upper thoracic ganglia. Sympathetic impulses produce increased heart rate (by action on the pacemaker cells in the sinus node), increased stroke volume, and dilation of the coronary arteries.

In general, the sympathetic innervation of the circulatory system ensures that the cardiac output can be increased, that the blood pressure can be maintained, and that the blood flow is directed to the organs needing it the most.

The vessels of the *lungs* receive sympathetic fibers producing vasodilatation. It is doubtful whether postganglionic sympathetic fibers act on the bronchial smooth musculature in humans[3] (even though such innervation is present in several animal species). Epinephrine, however, has a powerful inhibitory effect on the bronchial musculature; that is, it produces bronchial dilation. Thus the sympathetic system, by its stimulation of the adrenal medulla, acts indirectly on the resistance of the airways.

Cardiac Muscle Cells and Impulse Conduction in the Heart

The heart is built of a special kind of striated muscle cell but does not receive somatic nerve fibers. The cardiac muscle cells differ from skeletal muscle cells by, for example, being electrically coupled by gap junctions (nexus). Thus the action potential spreads from cell to cell. In this respect, the cardiac muscles resemble smooth musculature. Another difference is that the cardiac muscles do not require nerve impulses to produce action potentials. The heart muscle cells have pacemaker properties—the cells depolarize spontaneously and produce regular action potentials. The speed of depolarization and thus the frequency of spontaneous action potentials vary considerably, however, among muscle cells in different parts of the heart. The highest frequency is found among the cells in a small bundle of specialized muscle cells, the *sinus node,* located in the upper part of the right atrium. Normally the impulse that triggers contraction of the whole heart starts in the sinus node. From there it spreads outward to the rest of the atria and further on to the ventricles through a bundle of specialized muscle cells. Cardiac muscle cells with a lower spontaneous firing frequency than the cells of the sinus node are activated by spread of the impulse from the sinus node before the spontaneous depolarization has reached the threshold for an action potential.

The sympathetic and parasympathetic fibers to the heart end partly in the sinus node, whereby the heart rate can be regulated either up or down. At rest, the heart is under a certain dominance of the parasympathetic system (the vagus nerve), which "restrains" the cardiac activity. Actions on the stroke volume by the autonomic system are mediated by fibers ending near the muscle cells of the ventricles.

Effects of Sympathetic Fibers in Other Organs

The *sweat glands* of the skin are innervated by sympathetic fibers, producing sweat secretion. Sweat secretion normally occurs together with dilatation of cutaneous vessels when there is a need for increased loss of heat. Sweat secretion may, however, also occur in extreme situations with a large drop in blood pressure or with strong pain. In such situations, the skin vessels are maximally constricted and the skin is, consequently, pale and cold (cold sweat). A special feature of the innervation of sweat glands is that the neurotransmitter released from the postganglionic fibers is *acetylcholine* (and not norepinephrine).

Impulses in sympathetic fibers also activate the small smooth muscles attached to the hair roots, which make the hairs stand up. This is called *piloerection*. At the same time, the muscles compress the sebaceous glands, so that they empty their product into the hair follicle. In humans, the sympathetic control of hair position is of minor importance, whereas in animals it is of great significance for control of body temperature.

In the *abdominal viscera,* impulses in sympathetic fibers produce vasoconstriction and reduced contractile activity of the smooth muscles of the walls of hollow organs (that is, reducing the amplitude and frequency of the peristaltic movements). At the same time, the secretion of the glands of the digestive tract is reduced. In sum, these effects result in a marked reduction of the digestive processes. The sympathetic system also inhibits the emptying of the rectum, both by inhibition of the smooth muscles of the wall and by activating the smooth muscles of the internal anal sphincter. In addition, the smooth muscles of the *bladder* wall are inhibited.

The sympathetic innervation of the *genital organs* concerns vessels and the smooth musculature. The innervation of the *ductus deferens* is of particular importance because impulses in sympathetic fibers are responsible for the rhythmic contractions during ejaculation. The *uterus* receives sympathetic fibers, even though their functional role is not clear. Even after complete denervation the uterus may function normally in pregnancy and in parturition.

The sympathetic fibers to the *eye* have their perikarya in the superior cervical ganglion. They produce dilation of the pupil by activating the *dilatator pupillae muscle* and by causing contraction of the radially oriented vessels of the iris (the latter effect is probably most important for pupillary dilation). A small smooth muscle attached to the upper eyelid, the *tarsal muscle,* is also innervated by sympathetic fibers. The tonic activity of this muscle helps to keep the eyelid up while we are awake.

Irritation of Peripheral Nerves Can Produce Changes in the Skin

The effects of sympathetic fibers to the skin—that is, sweat secretion, vasoconstriction, and piloerection—can be reproduced by electrical stimulation of the ventral roots or the peripheral branches of the spinal nerves. Under abnormal conditions, the sympathetic fibers can be irritated by infections or by compression or traction of the nerves. In such cases there is abnormal sweat secretion from areas of the skin that are pale and cold. Destruction of the sympathetic fibers (by, for example, prolonged compression) leads to abolished sweat secretion and vasodilation, resulting in areas of the skin that are abnormally warm and red and at the same time dry. Observations of such local changes of the skin can be helpful in the diagnosis of diseases affecting the peripheral nerves.

Interruption of the Sympathetic Innervation of the Head

Sympathetic denervation of the head is usually caused by lesions of the sympathetic trunk in the neck. Because all preganglionic fibers enter the trunk below the inferior cervical ganglion (Fig. 14.5), a lesion anywhere above the level of the thoracic outlet can interrupt the sympathetic innervation of the head. It may be caused, for example, by a tumor in the apex of the lung, in the thyroid gland, or in any of the numerous lymph nodes in the neck. The ensuing symptoms can be understood on the basis of what has been described above about the effects of sympathetic fibers on the skin and the eye. In the case of a uni-lateral lesion, the *facial skin* on the side of the lesion becomes redder (warmer) and drier than that on the other side (caused by vasodilatation and lack of sweat secretion). The *pupil* is smaller (miosis) on the side of the lesion (paralysis of the sphincter pupillae), and the eyelid usually droops a little (ptosis) owing to paralysis of the tarsal muscle. This constellation of symptoms (red and dry skin, miosis, and ptosis) affecting half of the face is called *Horner's syndrome*.

Vasomotor Reflexes

Normally, the sympathetic neurons are activated reflexly, and many of them are links in arcs for so-called vasomotor reflexes—that is, reflexes in which the response is a change of vascular diameter (and thus resistance). The superior aim of the control of *blood pressure* is to ensure that the brain (and the heart) always has a sufficient blood flow. *Baroreceptors* in the large arteries in the neck and the aortal arch record the slightest fall in blood pressure and produce an automatic increase of the impulse frequency of sympathetic fibers. This is most marked for the sympathetic fibers to *skeletal muscles* but if necessary, fibers to the heart are also activated. In this manner, vasoconstriction of the skeletal muscle arterioles is produced. This increases the vascular resistance and the blood pressure is elevated, with the end result that the blood flow to the brain is increased to an adequate level.

Such vasomotor reflexes have been studied with the *microneurographic technique* (see Chapter 4), enabling the recording of the activity of small groups of postganglionic sympathetic fibers in humans. This makes it possible to study the relationship between the sympathetic impulse frequency and, for example, blood pressure.

The activity of the postganglionic sympathetic fibers to the *skin* appears not to be clearly related to the blood pressure, in contrast to the activity of fibers supplying vessels in skeletal muscles. On the other hand, skin sympathetic fiber activity is closely correlated with the ambient temperature; the sympathetic innervation of the skin serves first and foremost the *control of body temperature*. Increased activity of fibers innervating the sweat glands occurs together with reduced activity of fibers to the small vessels. This produces vasodilation and sweat secretion with increased loss of heat.

The activity of sympathetic fibers to the skin is, however, also strongly influenced by *emotions*—as witnessed by blushing when "having made a fool of oneself" and paleness when frightened. In case of very strong emotions or extreme physical stress (shock, intense visceral pain), simultaneous sympathetic activation of vascular smooth muscles and sweat glands can occur (cold sweat).

The above shows that various categories of sympathetic fibers can be controlled independently. There is not a uniform "sympathetic tonus" for all parts of the sympathetic system. High activity in some parts must coexist with low activity in others if the sympathetic system is to fulfill its tasks in controlling blood pressure and body temperature, in reproduction, and so forth.

There are striking differences between various persons with regard to the level of activity of sympathetic fibers under identical circumstances, as shown with the microneurographic technique. Postganglionic fibers to skeletal muscles—which constitute a large fraction of all postganglionic fibers in peripheral nerves—have been studied in particular. As mentioned, the activity of these fibers changes in close correlation with changes of the central blood pressure. Comparison of persons with normal blood pressure shows that the resting activity of sympathetic fibers varies by a factor of ten from person to person. Thus, each person appears to have his own characteristic pattern, which is unchanged over a long time. From this "baseline" value, the impulse frequency is up- or down-regulated in response to alterations in blood pressure caused by, for example, the change of body position from sitting to standing. No clear correlation has been found in the level of activity between sympathetic fibers to muscles and elevated blood pressure (hypertension).

The Effects of Parasympathetic Fibers

As mentioned, the sympathetic and the parasympathetic systems have mostly antagonistic effects (on the organs innervated by both).

The parasympathetic postganglionic fibers produce *glandular secretion* (for example, from the lacrimal gland, salivary glands, and glands of the respiratory and gastrointestinal tracts). Parasympathetic fibers are furthermore responsible for increased strength and frequency of *peristaltic contractions in the gastrointestinal tract and the bladder*. The *heart rate is lowered,* and the pupil is reduced in diameter. Parasympathetic fibers are also responsible for the *accommodation of the lens* (see Chapter 5).

Most of the vessels of the body do not receive parasympathetic innervation. Exceptions are vessels of glands and of the *external genitals,* in which parasympathetic impulses cause vasodilation (that is, they inhibit the smooth-muscle cells). Increased activity of the parasympathetic fibers to the penis (and the clitoris) produces erection.

NEUROTRANSMITTERS IN THE AUTONOMIC NERVOUS SYSTEM

The impulse transmission between neurons of the autonomic system is mediated by neurotransmitters, as elsewhere in the nervous system. The preganglionic fibers end with typical synapses on the dendrites of the postganglionic neurons. As mentioned, all (or the vast majority of) *preganglionic neurons use acetylcholine;* that is, they are cholinergic. Many (perhaps all) preganglionic neurons contain in addition *neuropeptides* (enkephalin, somatostatin, neurotensin, and others), as demonstrated with immunocytochemical techniques. The functional significance of these neuropeptides, which coexist with acetylcholine in preganglionic neurons, is so far not clear, but the two substances are most likely released together. The released acetylcholine binds to *nicotinic receptors* in the membrane of the postganglionic neurons (in the autonomic ganglia).

Most *postganglionic parasympathetic neurons* release *acetylcholine.* In the peripheral organs, acetylcholine binds to *muscarinic receptors* in the membrane of cardiac, smooth-muscle, and glandular cells.

Most *postganglionic sympathetic neurons* release *norepinephrine* and are noradrenergic. The effects on the effector cells are mediated by two kinds of receptors, the α- and the *β-adrenergic receptors,* which are differently distributed and have different effects on the postsynaptic cells. In the heart, norepinephrine produces increased heart rate by its binding to β receptors. By binding to α receptors, norepinephrine produces con-

traction of smooth-muscle cells in most blood vessels, in the ductus deferens, and in the dilatator pupillae muscle of the eye. Binding to β-receptors elicits relaxation of smooth-muscle cells in the wall of the bladder, the uterus, and the airways.

Subgroups of Adrenergic Receptors

Each of the two main kinds—α- and β-adrenergic receptors—has several subtypes with different distributions and actions. When norepinephrine binds to the α_1-receptor, this produces opening of Ca^{2+} channels, which leads to depolarization, and in turn elicits contraction or secretion. The action of the α_1-receptor is not directly on the Ca^{2+} channel but indirectly via intracellular second messengers (diacylglycerol and activation of protein kinase C). The α_2-receptor is mostly localized presynaptically and modulates the transmitter release. The β_1-receptor is mostly localized postsynaptically in the heart, on adipose cells, and in the central nervous system. It acts via cAMP as a second messenger. The β_2-receptor has a different distribution than the β_1-receptor, being primarily found in smooth-muscle cells of the respiratory tract. Binding of epinephrine (or drugs with similar action) to β_2-receptors causes relaxation of the smooth-muscle cells, notably in the walls of the bronchi. This produces dilation of the bronchi and reduces airway resistance.

Noncholinergic and Nonadrenergic Transmission in the Autonomic System

In addition to the classical neurotransmitters acetylcholine and norepinephrine, several other neuroactive substances have been demonstrated in the autonomic nervous system. The majority of pre- and postganglionic neurons probably contain neuropeptides in addition to acetylcholine or norepinephrine. Furthermore, some autonomic neurons contain neither acetylcholine nor norepinephrine. Such *noncholinergic and nonadrenergic* autonomic fibers are found in the respiratory tract, the gastrointestinal tract, the bladder, and the external genitals. Some of these release *adenosine triphosphate (ATP)* as neurotransmitter; others contain neuropeptides such as *somatostatin, substance P, VIP,* and *cholecystokinin (CCK).* Recent evidence also indicates that *nitric oxide* (NO) may act as an inhibitory transmitter in some autonomic nerves to pelvic organs.

The coexistence of norepinephrine and other transmitters was first suggested by the observation that blocking the receptors for norepinephrine did not prevent all effects of sympathetic nerve stimulation. In the ductus deferens—which receives a very dense sympathetic innervation—stimulation of the nerves produces first a fast contraction caused by release of ATP and subsequently a slow contraction produced by norepinephrine. In the salivary glands, the parasympathetic postganglionic fibers release both acetylcholine and VIP. The acetylcholine produces secretion from the glandular cells, whereas the VIP produces vasodilatation. Another example concerns the arteries of the penis, which dilate to cause erection. This vasodilatation is caused by parasympathetic postganglionic fibers that release VIP (and not acetylcholine). A final example of exceptions to the general rules about neurotransmitters and the autonomic system concerns the sweat glands. As mentioned, these are innervated by sympathetic fibers that use acetylcholine instead of norepinephrine.

Epinephrine, which is released from the chromaffin cells of the adrenal medulla by sympathetic stimulation, has largely the same effects as norepinephrine. Thus, epinephrine binds to α- and β-adrenergic receptors of the heart, vessels, and the respiratory tract. In addition, epinephrine stimulates the release of free fatty acids from adipose tissue and the breakdown of glycogen to glucose. These metabolic effects are mediated by β-receptors in fat and liver cells.

Presynaptic Receptors Modulate the Transmitter Release from Postganglionic Nerve Terminals

Neurotransmitters released from the postganglionic neurons bind not only to postsynaptic receptors in the membrane of smooth-muscle and glandular cells but also to *presynaptic receptors* in the membrane of the varicosities along the fibers. Thus, for example, norepinephrine that is released from sympathetic fibers can bind presynaptically and inhibit further release of norepinephrine or bind to parasympathetic cholinergic terminals in the vicinity. In the heart, sympathetic fibers inhibit the release of acetylcholine in this manner. The sympathetic inhibiting effect on the peristaltic contractions of the gastrointestinal tract is mediated, at least partly, by binding of norepinephrine to α-receptors on the parasympathetic, cholinergic terminals—that is, the release of acetylcholine is inhibited.

Sensitization

When the postganglionic autonomic fibers to an organ are interrupted, the sensitivity of the organ to the transmitter (which is no longer released) is increased. Epinephrine and norepinephrine in the bloodstream, for example, have a more powerful action after an organ has lost its sympathetic innervation, and the same holds for adrenergic drugs. This phenomenon, called *sensitization,* is not restricted to the autonomic system, however. It occurs, presumably, after denervation of any neuron. For example, skeletal muscle cells have increased sensitivity to acetylcholine after having lost their nerve supply. The underlying mechanism is probably increased postsynaptic density of receptors, as though the neuron attempts to maintain normal synaptic activity.

Drugs with Actions on the Autonomic Nervous System

Several drugs influence the synaptic transmission in the autonomic nervous system. *Atropine* blocks the action of acetylcholine (released from postganglionic parasympathetic fibers) on muscarinic receptors. Other drugs have similar *anticholinergic* effects, often as a side effect. This is the case for several psychopharmaceuticals. The peripheral actions of the parasympathetic system are inhibited, causing symptoms such as dilated pupils (mydriasis) and reduced accommodation of the lens (causing difficulties in seeing close objects clearly). The heart rate increases, and the secretory activity is reduced in several glands. Atropine, for example, is used to reduce secretion of glands in the respiratory tract during surgical anesthesia. The reduced salivary secretion causes dryness of the mouth, a very bothersome side effect of anticholinergic drugs. The peristaltic contractions of the bowel are reduced, causing obstipation. The bladder contractility is reduced, with danger of incomplete emptying (especially in cases of prostatic enlargement causing increased urethral resistance, the danger of urinary retention should be kept in mind). Because the sweat glands receive a cholinergic innervation, their secretion may also be reduced (most antiperspirants contain substances with an anticholinergic action).

Pilocarpine is an example of a drug with a *parasympathicomimetic* action: that is, a cholinergic drug. Administration of pilocarpine causes increased salivation, tear flow, reduced heart rate, and increased secretion from and peristaltic movements of the gastrointestinal tract. The pupil is small (miotic), causing reduced vision in dim light.

Many drugs activate adrenergic receptors—

that is, they have *sympathicomimetic* effects. Some act on both α- and β-receptors, others act preferentially on one or the other receptor type (or on subtypes). *Isoprenaline* (isoproterenol) acts selectively on β-receptors. It thus produces increased heart rate and bronchial dilatation. *Metaraminol* acts preferentially on α-receptors and causes peripheral vasoconstriction and, thereby, increased blood pressure.

Drugs that *block α-receptors* (such as phentolamine) produce peripheral vasodilatation and fall in blood pressure, whereas drugs that block β-receptors mainly cause reduced heart rate and stroke volume and bronchial constriction. The development of more selective *β-blockers,* acting selectively on β_1-receptors present in the heart, has made it possible to treat hypertension without unwanted bronchial constriction (β_2-receptors are found primarily in the lungs). On the other hand, the development of adrenergic drugs acting selectively on β_2-receptors (and not on β_1-receptors) has made it possible to treat patients with bronchial obstruction (as asthmatics) without such side effects as increased cardiac activity and hypertension.

The impulse *transmission in the autonomic ganglia* can also be influenced by drugs. As mentioned, acetylcholine is the main transmitter in both sympathetic and parasympathetic ganglia. The nicotinic receptors in the ganglia are nevertheless somewhat different from those present at the neuromuscular junction. This makes it possible to influence one of these targets without affecting the other.

All neurotransmitters present in the peripheral parts of the autonomic system are also found in the central nervous system, together with adrenergic and cholinergic receptors (see Chapter 1). Thus, drugs designed to act on peripheral parts of the autonomic nervous system may produce side effects through actions on central neurons—that is, in case they pass the blood–brain barrier.

SENSORY INNERVATION OF VISCERAL ORGANS

Together with the visceral efferent (sympathetic and parasympathetic) fibers in the nerves to the internal organs, there are afferent fibers conveying sensory information from the viscera to the central nervous system (Fig. 14.11). Sensory fibers follow the sympathetic splanchnic nerves leaving the

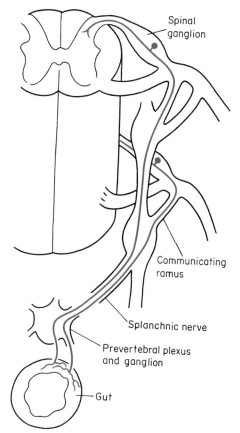

Fig. 14.11. *Sensory fibers of sympathetic nerves to the visceral organs.* Note that the fibers pass through the prevertebral plexuses and ganglia before entering the spinal nerves via the communicating rami.

sympathetic trunk at various levels (Fig. 14.5), the parasympathetic cranial nerves (the oculomotor, the intermediate, the glossopharyngeal, and the vagus nerves; Fig. 14.9), and, finally, the parasympathetic pelvic nerves leaving the sacral spinal nerves to innervate pelvic organs (Figs. 14.9 and 14.10).

The visceral afferent neurons are structurally indistinguishable from the somatic afferent ones—that is, they have their pseudounipolar perikarya in ganglia of the spinal and cranial nerves (Fig. 14.11). The peripheral process follows the sympathetic or parasympathetic nerves to the organs, whereas the central process enters the dorsal horn or the brain stem sensory nuclei (the nucleus of the solitary tract). The vast majority of the visceral afferent fibers are thin (Aδ and C fibers).

With some exceptions, such as taste and fairly diffuse sensations of hunger, fullness, and so forth, the sensory signals from the viscera are not consciously perceived. Under abnormal conditions, sensory signals from the viscera can, of course, produce the sensations of intense pain and nausea. The normal function of the sensory innervation of the internal organs is probably related to their mediation of *visceral reflexes*, such as coughing, vomiting, swallowing, circulatory and respiratory reflexes, emptying of the rectum and bladder, and so forth. Many of these reflexes have their reflex centers in the reticular formation.

As a general rule, *fibers conducting impulses from visceral nociceptors (producing sensations of pain) follow sympathetic nerves*, whereas *the parasympathetic nerves contain fibers conducting from other kinds of receptors*. Thus, there is no evidence of fibers leading from nociceptors in the vagus nerve. The above conclusions are based primarily on the clinical results of cutting various nerves in attempts to alleviate visceral pain.

Visceral Receptors

Morphologically, most of the visceral receptors are free nerve endings (Fig. 4.1).[4] They respond to various kinds of stimuli, even though they are structurally identical. A large group consists of *mechanoreceptors* recording the tension of the tissue in which they are located. Such receptors are found, for example, in the heart, lungs, and in the walls of hollow abdominal organs. They provide information about the degree of filling of hollow organs and can elicit reflex contractions aimed at emptying the organ or moving the content. Some stretch receptors may give rise to sensations of pain by responding to strong dilatation of a hollow organ and to forceful contractions of the smooth musculature. Most visceral nociceptors are, however, believed to be sensitive to substances in the tissue produced by inflammation or ischemia (chemoreceptors).

Other chemoreceptors, strategically placed in the vascular system (at the aortic arch and at the bifurcation of the common carotid artery), react to the carbon dioxide and oxygen concentration in the blood.

Central Pathways and Visceral Reflexes

The sensory impulses from the visceral organs pass through the dorsal roots and end in the *dorsalmost parts of the dorsal horn* (Fig. 4.10). The sensory fibers following the cranial nerves end in the *nucleus of the solitary tract* in the medulla (Fig. 13.2). From these receiving cell groups in the cord and in the brain stem, the signals are transmitted to motor nuclei (especially those consisting of preganglionic autonomic neurons), to the reticular formation, and to the hypothalamus and the thalamus. Visceral afferent signals arriving through the dorsal roots are transmitted centrally, at least for the most part, through the *spinothalamic tract* (Fig. 4.14). Details are not known, however, with regard to the central transmission of visceral afferent impulses.

Many of the *visceral reflexes* elicited by signals from visceral receptors and receptors in the walls of vessels have their reflex centers in the spinal cord. The more complex reflexes, however, requiring coordination of activity in several parts of the body, have reflex centers in the brain stem or in the hypothalamus. We will return to this in Chapter 15.

Vasomotor reflexes were discussed earlier in this chapter. Other important visceral reflexes are produced by stimulation of receptors in the *lungs* and the *airways,* such as coughing and respiratory adjustments.

The *emptying reflexes of the rectum and the bladder* are elicited by stimulation of stretch receptors in their walls and have reflex centers partly in spinal segments (S_2)S_3–S_4 and partly in the brain stem. These visceral reflexes are unusual because they can be suppressed voluntarily. The *vomiting reflex* can be elicited by irritation of the mucosa of the stomach but also in various other ways. In the case of irritation of the stomach, the sensory signals are probably conducted centrally in the vagus nerve. The reflex center is located in the brain stem, and the efferent links include several cell groups; the dorsal motor nucleus of the vagus elicits contraction of the musculature of the stomach, whereas descending connections from the reticular formation activate motoneurons supplying the abdominal muscles, the diaphragm, and the sphincter muscles of the pelvic floor.

Reflexes Elicited from Receptors of the Lungs

Signals from stretch receptors in the bronchial walls contribute to *inhibition of inspiratory movements* when the lungs have been inflated to a certain extent (the Hering-Breuer reflex). Receptors producing *coughing* are probably free endings between the epithelial cells of the airways, in part located very close to the epithelial surface (irritation receptors). Such free nerve endings contain substance P (as do many other sensory neurons).

A special kind of receptor—the *J- or juxtapulmonary receptor*—is located close to the lung alveoles. It responds to increased pulmonary capillary pressure. Increased pressure in the left atrium (which receives the blood from the lungs) immediately leads to increased pulmonary capillary pressure, with the danger of developing lung edema. Thus, it seems reasonable that the capillary pressure must be monitored closely. Stimulation of the J-receptors produces increased heart rate but may also cause bronchial constriction (this is known to occur in patients with heart failure and increased pulmonary capillary pressure). It is furthermore believed that signals from the J-receptors can reach consciousness and cause a feeling of dyspnea.

Visceral Pain

As mentioned, visceral afferent signals do not usually reach consciousness. Under abnormal conditions, one may experience sensations from the visceral organs and vessels. Pain is of special interest in this connection. Most fibers carrying signals from visceral nociceptors follow the sympathetic nerves of the organs.[5] Fibers conveying signals from nociceptors in the walls of the arteries of the extremities follow the peripheral (spinal) nerves, just like the efferent sympathetic fibers.

Surgery of visceral organs (for example, of the abdomen) can be performed without the patient feeling pain as long as the abdominal wall is anesthetized. Pain is felt only when the mesenteries or the peritoneum is pulled. Cutting with a sharp knife, for example, is not painful. That the abdominal viscera are not insensitive, however, is witnessed by the intense pain accompanying certain diseases, such as stones blocking the ureter or the gall ducts, or intestinal obstruction. In other diseases, pain can be completely lacking for a long period, such as in many cases of cancer of the lungs, the kidneys, or the gastrointestinal tract. The adequate stimuli for visceral nociceptors are obviously different from those of somatic nociceptors in the skin. This is perhaps not surprising since the visceral organs are not normally exposed to harmful stimuli that the organism has to respond to with a certain behavior.

As mentioned, visceral pain can be provoked by *stretching* the tissues. When the wall of a hollow organ is distended above an obstruction, forceful contractions of the smooth musculature are produced in an attempt to overcome the obstruction. Such spasmic contractions usually occur with regular intervals, explaining the typical bouts of pain experienced when, for example, a stone is stuck in the ureter.

Another cause of visceral pain is *ischemia*, which can occur when an artery is thrombosed. The commonest example is the pain felt when a coronary artery is narrowed (angina pectoris) or occluded (heart infarction).

Pain is also felt when *irritating substances* come in contact with the peritoneum, as in cases of perforation of a gastric ulcer or an inflamed gallbladder. The spread of bile, gastric content, or blood to the peritoneal cavity causes extreme pain and shock.

The arteries are also sensitive to painful stimuli. An arterial puncture (for example, to draw a blood sample) is painful. Furthermore, spasmic contractions or strong dilatation of arteries is also painful.

Special Features of Visceral Sensation: Referred Pain

Visceral pain differs in many respects from pain originating in somatic structures. Often the pain is not felt where the organ is located but in some other place, often in the body wall or the extremities. The pain is referred to another site than where it originates, and this phenomenon is called *referred pain*. This pain (for example, in the left arm in the case of angina, and under the right scapula in the case of a gallstone) can be localized fairly precisely by the patient. At the site of the diseased organ, however, there is usually only a diffuse pain, difficult both to localize and to describe. Another example of referred pain is the pain felt in the shoulder region in cases of irritation of the diaphragm.

The explanation of this phenomenon was discussed in Chapter 4. It is most likely caused by the convergence on spinothalamic neurons in the cord of signals from somatic structures (especially the skin) and viscera innervated from the same spinal segments. The signals coming from the visceral organs are interpreted as arising in the skin and not in the visceral organ, presumably because impulses from the visceral organs are never consciously perceived under normal circumstances (for example, nociceptors of the heart are not normally stimulated). The pain arising in the heart is usually referred to the ulnar aspect of the left arm or the upper part of the chest because these regions of the skin and the heart both receive sensory innervation from the upper thoracic segments of the cord. The gallbladder and the skin in the region of the lower end of the scapula are both innervated from the eighth thoracic segment. The shoulder pain on irritation of the diaphragm is explained by the common innervation from the fourth and fifth cervical segments.

The phenomenon of *cutaneous hyperesthesia* in cases of visceral diseases was also explained in Chapter 4.

Pain Can Be Relieved by Sympathectomy

Knowledge of the special features of visceral pain and of the segmental innervation of visceral organs is of importance for surgical interventions of the autonomic nervous system. Such operations are performed occasionally, especially on the sympathetic system, to interrupt the pathways for pain impulses and sometimes to increase the blood flow of the extremities (to interrupt vasoconstrictor fibers). Thus, interruption of the lumbar sympathetic trunk interrupts the sympathetic outflow to the lower extremities (Fig. 14.8).

There is also good evidence that abnormal activity of sympathetic efferent neurons can contribute to a certain kind of painful condition that occurs especially after trauma to the extremities (*causalgia, reflex dystrophy*). The pain in such cases has an intense, burning character and can be provoked by trivial, normally innocuous stimuli (such as light touch). Often the pain is accompanied by signs of abnormal efferent sympathetic activity, such as pale, cold skin. If the condition lasts, the skin becomes thin and glossy with loss of hairs. There may also be atrophy of muscles and osteoporosis of the skeleton. The cause of the pain is unknown, but interruption of the sympathetic outflow to the painful extremity can often reduce or completely remove the pain—for example, by blocking the stellate ganglion in case of pain in the arm (Fig. 14.7). In the latter case there has been no interference with the sensory innervation of the arm, since this passes in the spinal nerves.

The Axonal Reflex

It has been known for a long time that electrical stimulation of dorsal roots can produce vasodilatation in the dermatome of the root concerned. Originally, this was interpreted as evidence of the existence of efferent fibers in the dorsal root, but this has not been verified by modern methods. The phenomenon is undoubtedly caused by impulses conducted in the peripheral direction by the sensory fibers. Such impulses, conducted in the direction opposite the normal direction, are called *antidromic*. The action potentials are of course exactly the same as those conducted in the normal direction (orthodromically). Antidromic impulses in C fibers appear to release *substance P* from the peripheral branches. Substance P probably causes the release of *histamine* (presumably from mast cells). Histamine causes vasodilatation, especially of the capillaries, and at the same time the capillaries become leaky. Thus, a local edema is produced.

Various phenomena can probably be explained by this phenomenon. When the skin is stroked with a fairly sharp object, it reddens (vasodilatation) after a few seconds on both sides of the stripe. This can be explained as follows: The stroking of the skin stimulates C fiber nociceptors, and action potentials are conducted to the central nervous system (and we experience a sharp pain). At the same time, however, the action potential is also conducted peripherally in the branches of the C fiber not innervating the stimulated skin stripe. These branches end in the skin outside the stripe, where they liberate substance P and cause vasodilatation. The process is called a reflex, and since it only utilizes the peripheral process of a pseudounipolar ganglion cell, it is called an *axon reflex*. The reflex cannot be elicited in an area of the skin that has been deprived of its sensory innervation.

Under normal conditions, the antidromic impulses in sensory fibers hardly play any role. They may, however, help to explain certain pathological phenomena. An example from the airways can be mentioned. In disposed individuals, irritating gases can produce a marked edema of the mucous membranes. The edema is apparently caused by histamine release, which in turn is caused by substance P released by an axon reflex from sensory fibers innervating the mucous membrane (partly coming close to the surface of the epithelium).

NOTES

1. White and gray rami are often fused into one, so that even at the levels T_1–L_2 there may be only one communicating ramus on each side. This contains, as will be understood, both the pre- and postganglionic fibers. In the case of two rami, the color difference between them is not very marked.

2. The degree of vasoconstriction is influenced not only by the nervous system but also by circulating hormones, in particular epinephrine. Furthermore, substances produced by the local metabolism in the tissue influence the degree of contraction of the vascular smooth-muscle cells.

3. Studies in humans with histofluorescence techniques, which visualize catecholaminergic nerve fibers in tissue sections, have shown the presence of such fibers around the vessels but not around the bronchi.

4. There are some encapsulated nerve endings in the visceral organs. Thus, Pacinian corpuscles are present in the pancreas, the mesenteries, and the vessel walls. Their functional role at these sites is unknown.

5. An exception to this rule is the transmission of signals from nociceptors in the neck of the bladder, the prostate, the cervix uteri, and the rectum. "Pain fibers" from these organs follow the parasympathetic pelvic nerves to the sacral spinal nerves (Fig. 14.10). Signals from nociceptors in the fundus of the uterus and of the bladder, however, follow the sympathetic nerves of the hypogastric plexus ending in segments T_{11}–L_2.

15

Central Autonomic System: Hypothalamus

Sympathetic and parasympathetic parts cannot be clearly separated in the higher centers that control autonomic functions. Thus, the cell groups at higher levels are centers for *coordination of reflex responses* involving various autonomic processes that require cooperation of sympathetic and parasympathetic neuronal groups at the lower levels. This chapter will be concerned mainly with the hypothalamus, which is the most important higher center for control of autonomic (visceral) functions. The control exerted by the hypothalamus is mediated by the peripheral parts of the autonomic system and by the endocrine system. In addition, the hypothalamus serves to coordinate endocrine, autonomic, and somatic motor responses to behavior that is appropriate for the immediate needs of the body, such as feeding, drinking, and reproduction. The role of the hypothalamus in the interactions between bodily and mental processes will also be discussed briefly.

the control of autonomic processes, as mentioned in Chapter 12. Electrical stimulation and lesions of restricted parts of the reticular formation of the pons and medulla produce changes in blood pressure, cardiac activity, respiration, sweat secretion, gastrointestinal activity, and other processes. Such higher-level centers exert control of the lower autonomic reflex centers of the spinal cord and coordinate their activities. They ensure, for example, that the segmental vasomotor reflexes operate together to serve the needs of the whole organism, and not only its individual parts. A perfect coordination cannot be performed by the brain stem autonomic centers, however. This is witnessed by the poor control of autonomic functions such as blood pressure and body temperature in decerebrate animals (see Chapter 9). Optimal atuonomic control requires that the brain stem and spinal centers be supplied with afferent fibers from higher centers, especially in the hypothalamus.

AUTONOMIC CENTERS IN THE BRAIN STEM

Physiological experiments have localized several regions of the *brain stem* involved in

STRUCTURE AND CONNECTIONS OF THE HYPOTHALAMUS

The hypothalamus is the principal higher center for control of autonomic processes.

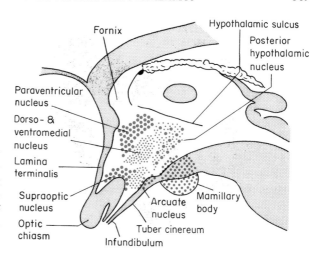

Fig. 15.1. *The hypothalamus.* Median section through the third ventricle. Some of the major hypothalamic nuclei are shown with red dots. The size of the dots indicates the relative size of the neurons of the various nuclei. Redrawn after Le Gros Clark et al. (1936).

This small part of the brain, weighing only 4–5 g in humans, is a mosaic of minor nuclei that can be distinguished on the basis of their cytoarchitectonics, connections, cytochemistry, and physiological properties. Only the main features will be discussed here.

In the wall of the third ventricle, below the hypothalamic sulcus, some identifiable nuclei are embedded in a more diffuse mass of neurons (Fig. 2.24); together these constitute the hypothalamus. The borders between the hypothalamic nuclei and the neighboring regions are not sharply demarcated. This explains why the borders have been drawn differently by different authors. Figure 15.1 shows the classic subdivisions of the British neuroanatomist Le Gros Clark. It is now common to distinguish a *medial part of the hypothalamus,* containing several fairly distinct nuclei, and a *lateral hypothalamic area* (or nucleus) with a diffuse structure. The latter is traversed by numerous fibers running mainly longitudinally. Collectively they are usually termed the *medial forebrain bundle,* though this is not a single tract anatomically or functionally and has no sharp borders. Some of the fibers of the medial forebrain bundle are long and come from monoaminergic cell groups in the brain stem. Other fibers arise in cell groups related to olfactory functions. Many fibers are short, presumably connecting parts of the hypothalamus with each other. Within the *medial part,* one can distinguish *anterior, middle (tuberal),* and *posterior (mammillary) nuclear groups.* Particularly well-defined are two anterior large nuclei, the *paraventricular nucleus* and the *supraoptic nucleus.* The first is located close to the wall of the third ventricle, the latter just above the optic chiasm (Fig. 15.1). In the middle or tuberal nuclear group we find the *ventromedial,* the *dorsomedial,* and the *arcuate (infundibular)* nuclei. The latter nucleus is located in the bottom of the third ventricle, below the ventromedial nucleus. In the posterior part of the hypothalamus we find the *posterior nucleus* close to the ventricular wall, whereas the characteristic *mammillary nucleus* (consisting of several subnuclei) is located in the bottom of the ventricle. The term *mammillary body* is used of the macroscopically visible part of the mammillary nuclei (Figs. 2.14, 2.24, and 15.1). In general, there is a high degree of cooperation among the hypothalamic nuclei, mediated by short intrahypothalamic fibers. Notably, there are numerous reciprocal connections between the medial nuclei and the lateral area (nucleus) of the hypothalamus.

The Connections and Functions of the Hypothalamic Nuclei Have Been Hard to Clarify

Determining the exact connections and functional roles of the various nuclei has proved more difficult in the hypothalamus than in most other parts of the brain. This is partly because the nuclei are so small and are located in a part of the brain that is difficult to reach with experimental manipulations and partly because most of the afferent and efferent fibers are unmyelinated and mixed with fibers destined for other parts of the brain. In particular, lesions or stimulations of the lateral hypothalamic area are bound to affect the medial forebrain bundle and thereby fibers destined for other regions than the hypothalamus. The hypothalamic nuclei furthermore have a rich network of mutual connections, so that, for example, a lesion of one nucleus will interfere with the functioning of several others as well. Modern methods utilizing toxic agents that destroy the cell bodies without affecting fibers of passage have helped to settle some controversies, however.

The Hypothalamus Contains Many Neurotransmitters

Numerous *neurotransmitter candidates* are present in the hypothalamus, as demonstrated with immunocytochemical and biochemical methods. Acetylcholine, norepinephrine, dopamine, serotonin, histamine, and many neuropeptides are found with a differential distribution among the hypothalamic nuclei. Norepinephrine is among the neurotransmitters found in highest concentration (some of the norepinephrine is related to terminals of fibers from the nucleus locus coeruleus). Some of the neuropeptides are involved in the hypothalamic control of the pituitary gland or released to the bloodstream in the pituitary. The functional role of the various neurotransmitters in the hypothalamus is still incompletely known (as is, indeed, why so many different neurotransmitters are needed in the brain).

Hypothalamic Neurons Are Influenced by Hormones

In addition to receptors for the endogenous neurotransmitters, many hypothalamic cells also contain *receptors for various hormones*, such as for the steroid sex hormones, the thyroid hormones, and for hormones released from the anterior pituitary. The sex and thyroid hormones pass the blood–brain barrier easily. The steroid sex hormones bind to intracellular receptors, and thereby influence the activity of hypothalamic cells (and cells in other parts of the brain, particularly in certain limbic structures). Some hormones that do not pass the blood–brain barrier easily can nevertheless act on the hypothalamus and certain other brain regions. This is possible because certain regions of the brain close to the ventricles lack a blood–brain barrier, and the neurons in such regions send axons to other parts of the brain. One example is the *subfornical organ,* located below the fornix close to the wall of the third ventricle. The hormone *angiotensin II,* the production of which is increased by a reduction of the blood volume, binds to specific receptors in the subfornical organ. The latter sends axons to the supraoptic and paraventricular hypothalamic nuclei (which produce the antidiuretic hormone). This exemplifies that hormones acting on the hypothalamus (directly or indirectly) provide feedback information of importance for the hypothalamic control of the pituitary gland. Other hormonal actions on the brain will be briefly discussed later in this chapter.

Afferent Connections

Figure 15.2 shows diagrammatically the main afferent connections of the hypothalamus. It is immediately clear that many—perhaps most—parts of the brain are able to influence the hypothalamus! (The mammillary nucleus is in several aspects different from the other hypothalamic nuclei and will be treated separately below.)

The many groups of afferents end in at least partially different parts of the hypothalamus. The *retina* supplies the hypothalamus with visual information (probably fairly unspecific information concerning the total amount of light rather than patterned vision). Olfactory information reaches the hypothalamus indirectly from regions receiving fibers from the olfactory bulb, such as the *amygdala* and the *olfactory cortex* (Fig. 7.1), which send fibers to parts of the hypothalamus (Fig. 15.2). Physiological studies show that *auditory* information can reach the hypothalamus, and the same holds

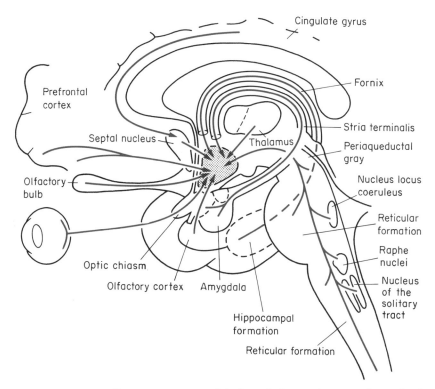

Fig. 15.2. *Main afferent connections of the hypothalamus.* Arrows indicate the direction of impulse conduction.

for signals from *cutaneous* receptors. Anatomically, direct fibers have been traced from the *spinal cord* to the hypothalamus, but most information from the cord reaches the hypothalamus indirectly via the reticular formation. In that case, the sensory information is presumably highly integrated—that is, not providing specific information about stimuli features. The hypothalamus, like many other parts of the brain, receives afferents from the *nucleus locus coeruleus* and the *raphe nuclei.* These afferents probably provide rather diffuse modulatory effects on the general level of excitability of large groups of neurons. Of special interest are hypothalamic afferents from the *nucleus of the solitary tract* (the visceral afferent cranial nerve nucleus). Such fibers can convey information about, for example, taste stimuli and the condition in the gastrointestinal tract.

The hypothalamus is also under the influence of *higher levels of the brain.* The *fornix* carries fibers from the *hippocampal formation* (Figs. 16.1 and 16.2), and many of these end in the hypothalamus. The *cerebral cortex* can influence the hypothalamus, especially via the dorsomedial thalamic nucleus, but there are also some direct fibers from the *prefrontal cortex.* The *cingulate gyrus* can act on the hypothalamus via the septal nuclei.

This brief overview of hypothalamic afferents should make it clear that the *hypothalamus can be influenced by means of most kinds of receptors and also by higher levels of the brain, such as the cerebral cortex and the limbic structures.* In addition, several hormones can bind specifically to hypothalamic neurons and thus influence their activity. Studies of the internal organization of the hypothalamus and physiological experiments indicate that considerable integration of the incoming information takes place be-

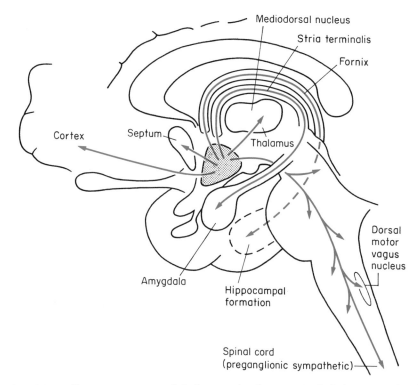

Fig. 15.3. *Main efferent connections of the hypothalamus.* The connections to the pituitary gland are not included, nor are the efferent connections of the mammillary nucleus.

fore the hypothalamus sends out its command to the endocrine and the autonomic system, as well as to somatic motor centers and higher levels of the brain.

Efferent Connections

The efferent connections of the hypothalamus are widespread, just like the afferent connections (Fig. 15.3). In addition to its characteristic projection to the pituitary, the *hypothalamus sends fibers to most of the cell groups from which it receives afferents,* such as the *amygdala,* the *septal nuclei,* nuclei of the *reticular formation,* some of the *cranial nerve nuclei,* and the *spinal cord.* The hypothalamus can also influence the *cerebral cortex.*

Hypothalamic *influences on autonomic processes* such as blood pressure, heart rate, temperature regulation, and digestion are mediated by direct and indirect *descending connections to the preganglionic sympa-thetic and parasympathetic neurons.* Many hypothalamic neurons send axons to para-sympathetic cell groups of the brain stem (such as the dorsal motor nucleus of the vagus) and to the sympathetic neurons of the intermediolateral column of the cord. In addition, effects on these cell groups are mediated via the reticular formation, which receives many afferents from the hypothalamus.

Hypothalamic *effects on the cerebral cortex* occur mainly via the thalamus (this concerns especially the mamillary nucleus). The mediodorsal thalamic nucleus may receive direct hypothalamic afferents, and, in addition, several of the nuclei mentioned above that receive fibers from the hypothalamus project to the mediodorsal nucleus (the amygdala and the septal nuclei). Direct connections from the hypothalamus to the basal parts of the prefrontal cortex have also been demonstrated (some of these direct hypothalamic fibers are GABAergic, others are histaminergic). Thus, there are probably several routes by which the hypothalamus can act on the prefrontal cerebral cortex.

The Mammillary Nucleus

Situated most posteriorly in the hypothalamus, the mammillary nucleus differs in several respects from the other nuclei. It consists of several subnuclei and forms the characteristically shaped mammillary bodies (one on each side) at the ventral aspect of the diencephalon (Figs. 2.14 and 2.24). The subnuclei differ to some extent with regard to connections, although we will disregard such differences here.

Among the *efferent* mammillary connections (Fig. 15.4), the *mammillothalamic tract* is most conspicuous. The fibers, forming a thick bundle, run anteriorly and upward in the wall of the third ventricle to end in the *anterior thalamic nucleus* (Fig. 2.25). This nucleus projects to the *cingulate gyrus* (Fig. 17.7). Thus, a major target of the mammillary nucleus is the cerebral cortex. Another large efferent fiber tract descends in the brain stem as the *mammillotegmental tract*. These fibers end primarily in certain nuclei of the mesencephalic and pontine *reticular formation*.

Most of the *afferent* fibers to the mammillary nucleus originate in the *hippocampal formation* and pass in the *fornix* (Figs. 2.24, 15.4, and 16.2). In humans, the fornix contains more than 1 million axons. In addition, the mammillary nucleus receives afferents from the septal nuclei and some brain stem nuclei.

The mammillary nucleus appears to be an important *link in the signal transmission from structures in the temporal lobe to the cingulate gyrus*. These connections, and thus the mammillary nucleus, may be related to *spatial memory* and orientation in space (see Chapter 16).

FUNCTIONAL ASPECTS

Hypothalamic "Centers"

The above account of its connections suggests that the hypothalamus functions as a coordinator of information of many different kinds, particularly pertaining to homeostasis and "bodily maintenance." The hypothalamus contains cell groups that serve as control centers for several autonomic functions, such as blood pressure, body temperature, water balance, metabolism, digestion, and reproduction. Furthermore, the rhythmic variations of several bodily processes are governed by the hypothalamus. For each of the mentioned broad functional categories, the *hypothalamus serves to coordinate endocrine, autonomic, and somatic motor responses into appropriate behavior.*

Even though the hypothalamus contains some well-defined nuclei, it is not possible to localize any of the functional centers mentioned above to one specific nucleus. The centers must be imagined as rather extensive networks of mutually interconnected hypothalamic cell groups. This agrees with the observation that many of the autonomic processes influenced by the hypothalamus are not controlled independently. Some factors, such as the diameter of the vessels, are of importance in several different processes, such as temperature regulation and control of blood pressure. Complex behavior, such as that necessary for feeding and drinking, depends on the integrity of both medial and lateral hypothalamic areas, even though subregions play different roles.

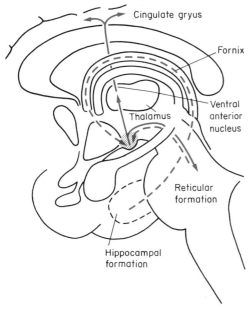

Fig. 15.4.   *Main connections of the mammillary nucleus.*

Control of Body Temperature

When the blood flowing through the anterior part of the hypothalamus is warmed, an experimental animal shows signs of increased heat loss. Cats, for example, pant and sweat through the paws. If these parts of the hypothalamus are destroyed (on both sides), the animal no longer reacts to a rise in ambient temperature. The body temperature therefore rises. When, on the other hand, the posterior parts of the hypothalamus are destroyed, the animal no longer reacts with shivering and vasoconstriction to a fall in ambient temperature. Therefore, the body temperature drops (the vasoconstriction reduces heat loss, and the shivering increases heat production). Such observations are interpreted as follows: The anterior part of the hypothalamus contains a "center" for ensuring that the body temperature does not rise above normal levels, whereas the posterior parts contain a "center" for heat conservation. In humans, abnormal rise in the body temperature, hyperthermia, can be produced by diseases affecting the hypothalamus or by an inadvertent lesion during surgery. Occasionally, hyperthermia occurs during general anesthesia.

Digestion and Feeding

Various metabolic processes are controlled by the hypothalamus. For example, lesions of certain parts can produce abnormal fat deposition, both in experimental animals and in humans. The gastrointestinal tract is influenced by the hypothalamus. Lesions can produce ulcers of the mucous membranes and bleeding in the stomach and the small intestine. Stimulation of the hypothalamus can elicit increased secretion of gastric juice and strengthening of peristaltic movements. Even though the intestinal changes are not identical after hypothalamic lesions in experimental animals and in humans with gastric and duodenal ulcers, it seems likely that the hypothalamus may be involved in the development of the latter.

Not only the digestive processes but also *feeding behavior* is controlled from the hypothalamus. Early stimulation and lesion experiments indicated that the lateral hypothalamic area can induce increased eating (or behavior directed at acquiring food), whereas the medial parts (especially the ventromedial nucleus) reduce eating (induce satiety). Further studies have shown that, although essentially correct, this scheme is too simple. The inputs to the hypothalamic "feeding" centers are multifarious, as witnessed by data from animal experiments, and by everyday experiences of the numerous factors that influence human feeding behavior. It is nevertheless remarkable how most people maintain their body weight over many years, although even the smallest daily surplus of food would cause a steady weight gain. The hypothalamic centers governing food intake are thought to operate in accordance with a *set-point* theory. Feedback loops ensure that the food intake oscillates around the set point. Overeating is automatically followed by reduced consumption. Of course, psychological factors—or occasionally, hypothalamic disease—may disturb this finely tuned control mechanism.

The Hypothalamus and Sleep

Lesions of the hypothalamus in experimental animals and in humans are often accompanied by sleep disturbances, sometimes as an abnormal amount of sleep and sometimes as insomnia or disturbed sleep rhythm. Experimental evidence has led to the assumption that a "sleep center" exists in the anterior part of the hypothalamus and a "waking center" in the posterior part. Conditions are probably much less schematic, however. Our knowledge of the role of the reticular formation in sleep mechanisms (see Chapter 12) has altered the interpretation of the experiments mentioned above. Thus, the "waking center" in the posterior hypothalamus coincides with regions known to produce an activating effect on the cortex and may not be a part of the hypothalamus. Stimulation of this region produces changes in the EEG and in behavior that are characteristic for the awake state.

The Hypothalamus and Biological Rhythms

The hypothalamus plays a role as a pacemaker for several functions showing a cyclic variation. Light stimuli from the retina (varying with length of the light/dark cycle) (Fig. 15.2) appear to be of particular importance for the set of such *circadian rhythms*. The pacemaker capacity appears to be inborn, however. Thus, in rats, rhythmic activity occurs in some hypothalamic cell groups in late embryonic life.

The retinohypothalamic fibers end in the *suprachiasmatic nucleus*. Lesions of this nucleus disturb (but do not necessarily abolish) the cyclic variations of body temperature, blood level of steroid hormones from the adrenal cortex, and sexual functions. The suprachiasmatic nucleus has connections with several other parts of the hypothalamus, which enable it to influence the various functions mentioned above (and other functions as well).

THE HYPOTHALAMUS AND THE ENDOCRINE SYSTEM

The effects of the hypothalamus on organs innervated by the autonomic nervous system can be explained by direct and indirect connections to the preganglionic sympathetic and parasympathetic neurons of the brain stem and the spinal cord. Diseases or lesions affecting the hypothalamus can, however, disturb *functions controlled by the endocrine system,* too, such as sexual functions, growth, and metabolism. Of the endocrine organs, only the adrenal medulla receives an important autonomic innervation. The effects of the hypothalamus on the endocrine organs are explained by the hypothalamic control of the superior endocrine organ, the pituitary. This control concerns both the anterior and posterior parts of the pituitary (Fig. 15.5). Two different pathways are used for the hypothalamo-pituitary interactions. The posterior pituitary is reached by a direct neural tract (often re-

ferred to as the supraopticohypophysial tract), whereas the anterior pituitary is reached by the so-called tuberoinfundibular tract and a special portal vascular system (Fig. 15.5C). We will return to this below.

The *pituitary gland* (the hypophysis) consists of an *anterior lobe,* the *adenohypophysis,* that is developed from the epithelium of the primitive foregut and is built up of clusters of epithelial cells with a rich supply of wide capillaries (sinusoids). The *posterior lobe* of the pituitary, the *neurohypophysis,* is developed from the neural tube and consists of nerve terminals of fibers from the hypothalamus and a special kind of glial cell, the *pituicytes.*

The Anterior Pituitary Produces Several Hormones

The following hormones are produced and secreted by the epithelial cells of the adenohypophysis:

1. *Growth hormone* (GH) or somatotrophic hormone, which stimulates body growth, particularly growth of long bones;
2. *Thyroid-stimulating hormone* (TSH);

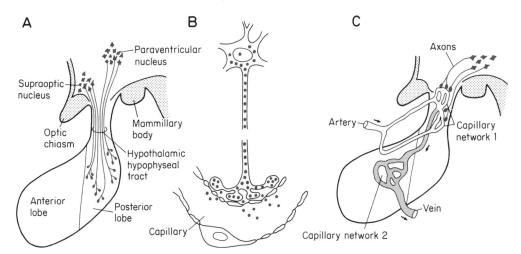

Fig. 15.5. *The relationship between the hypothalamus and the pituitary gland.* **A.** Connections from the hypothalamus to the posterior lobe. **B.** Axonal transport of peptide hormones (neuropeptides) from the hypothalamus to the pitu-

itary. **C.** The portal vessels of the pituitary stalk ensure that releasing hormones (factors) are transported from the median eminence in the upper part of the stalk to the epithelial cells of the anterior lobe.

3. *Adrenocorticotrophic hormone* (ACTH), which stimulates the production of steroid hormones, such as cortisol, in the adrenal cortex;[1]

4. Two *gonadotrophic hormones*—one follicle-stimulating hormone (FSH) that promotes the growth of the oocyte and its surrounding follicle cells and one luteinizing hormone (LH) that is necessary for the ovulation and formation of the corpus luteum from the follicle cells; and

5. *Prolactin* (or lactogenic hormone), which stimulates growth of the mammary gland during pregnancy and maintains the milk secretion during the nursing period.

Various observations indicate that as a rule each hormone is produced by a specific cell type. The cells are named for the hormone they produce, and are called somatotrophs (GH), thyrotrophs (TSH), mammotrophs (prolactin), and so forth. In routine histological sections, however, only three kinds of epithelial cells can be recognized in the anterior pituitary: acidophils, basophils, and chromophobes. The acidophils produce GH and prolactin, whereas the basophils probably produce the rest. It follows that the basophils and the acidophils both are heterogeneous groups, as indeed has been shown with immunocytochemical techniques with antibodies raised against the various hormones.

The Relation between the Hypothalamus and the Posterior Pituitary

Two peptide hormones are released to the bloodstream in the posterior pituitary: *vasopressin* or *antidiuretic hormone* (ADH) and *oxytocin*. Both hormones are synthesized in the hypothalamus and are brought to the pituitary by axonal transport. The thin, unmyelinated axons reaching the posterior lobe (in man, about 100,000) come from two hypothalamic nuclei in the anterior part of the hypothalamus: the *supraoptic nucleus* and the *paraventricular nucleus* (Figs. 15.1 and 15.5A). These two nuclei are quite similar. Most of the cells are large, with the nucleus located peripherally in the perikaryon and with large vesicles in their cytoplasm. These vesicles contain precursor molecules of the final hormones. Both nuclei are richly vascularized. Even though both ADH and oxytocin are produced in both cell groups, ADH is produced predominantly in the supraoptic nucleus and oxytocin mainly in the paraventricular nucleus. The vesicles can also be demonstrated within the axons. The axons end with large boutons in close contact with the fenestrated capillaries of the posterior lobe (Fig. 15.5B). Action potentials reaching the boutons constitute the signal for release of the hormone (just as for the release of neurotransmitter in ordinary nerve cells). The cells of the supraoptic and the paraventricular nucleus are called *neurosecretory* because they have all the characteristic features of neurons but at the same time release their product to the bloodstream.

The antidiuretic hormone was extracted from the posterior lobe quite early, before the neural connection between the hypothalamus and the posterior lobe had been ascertained. The hormone acts by increasing the water reabsorption in the kidneys—that is, it reduces the urine secretion (the hormone also elicits contraction of vascular smooth-muscle cells, which explains why it is also called vasopressin). It was known that destruction of the posterior lobe leads to a condition called *diabetes insipidus*, which is characterized by daily urine volume of 10–15 liters. Later it was discovered that the disease could be produced also by cutting the pituitary stalk. This was the beginning of a full understanding of the nature of the relationship between the hypothalamus and the pituitary.

The production of ADH varies in accordance with the osmalarity of the blood. Most likely, the cells of the supraoptic nucleus (and in some other nuclei) function as *osmoreceptors*.[2] When the osmotic pressure of the blood increases because of extraordinary loss or reduced intake of fluid (for example, by heavy sweating, diarrhea, or vomiting), the cells of the supraoptic nucleus are excited and increase the frequency of their action potentials, thus releasing more ADH into the bloodstream. This results in reduced urine volume (the urine becomes more concentrated). At the same time the synthesis of the hormone is increased. Even a salty meal is enough to stimulate the osmoreceptors. The hypothalamus is thus a control center for the body's "housekeeping" of water.

Oxytocin elicits contraction of the smooth-muscle cells in the wall of the uterus and thus plays a role during delivery. It also produces contraction of the smooth-muscle cells (myoepithelial cells) of the mammary gland, thereby assisting in emptying the breast. When the infant suckles, sensory impulses travel from the nipple (through the spinal nerves) to the cord and further to the hypothalamus, where the neurons of the paraventricular nucleus are influenced. Increased firing frequency leads to increased secretion of oxytocin to the bloodstream, and the hormone reaches the mammary gland in seconds. This is called the *milk ejection reflex*. It is special in that only the afferent link is neural, the efferent link being humoral. Although oxytocin is present in males, its function is so far unknown.

The Influence of the Hypothalamus on the Anterior Pituitary: The Hypophyseal Portal System

It has long been known that diseases affecting the hypothalamus can be accompanied by altered growth, metabolism, and sexual functions—processes that are controlled by hormones produced in the anterior pituitary (adenohypophysis). There are, however, no axonal connections from the hypothalamus to the anterior lobe. Thus, mechanisms other than those concerning the posterior lobe must be responsible for the influence of the hypothalamus on the anterior lobe. The discovery of a *special vascular arrangement in the infundibulum* (stalk) of the pituitary— the *hypophyseal portal system*—was a breakthrough in this respect (Fig. 15.5C). Most of the arteries reaching the anterior pituitary do not branch into capillaries among the epithelial cells but continue upward in the stalk (some arteries enter this directly). In the upper part of the stalk, they form wide capillaries (sinusoids) that finally collect into large veins. These *hypophyseal portal veins* course back to the anterior lobe, where they form a new set of sinusoids among the epithelial cells. From these sinusoids the blood is collected in veins that leave the pituitary. *The blood in the sinusoids of the anterior lobe has first been through a capillary net in the stalk of the pituitary.* Thus, substances can be transported from the stalk to the anterior lobe. Numerous thin axons from the hypothalamus end in the uppermost part of the hypophyseal stalk. This region is called the *median eminence*. The fibers were formerly believed to come only from the tuberal region of the hypothalamus, and especially from the *arcuate nucleus* (Fig. 15.1), as the name *tuberoinfundibular tract* implies. Hypothalamic nuclei outside the tuberal region also contribute to the tract, however. The fibers of the tuberoinfundibular tract end in contact with the capillaries in the median eminence. These fibers transport peptides from their parent cell bodies (axonal transport) and release them into the hypophyseal portal system. From the capillaries in the median eminence, the peptides are brought by the blood to the second capillary network among the epithelial cells of the anterior lobe. Most of the peptides transported by the portal system cause hormonal secretion from the epithelial cells of the anterior lobe and are therefore called *releasing factors or hormones*. One releasing hormone appears to act on one kind of anterior lobe cell only and thus produces secretion of only one hormone. Some peptides transported in the tuberoinfundibular tract have an inhibitory effect on the secretion of anterior lobe hormones and are called *inhibitory factors or hormones*.

Several of the peptides involved in the control of the pituitary are found also in neurons in other parts of the brain, where they are released at conventional synapses. Examples are somatostatin (inhibits the release of GH), thyrotrophin-releasing hormone (TRH), and corticotrophin-releasing hormone (CRH).

THE HYPOTHALAMUS AND MENTAL FUNCTIONS

The relationship between the hypothalamus and the pituitary discussed above helps explain why diseases affecting the hypothalamus can produce alterations of hormonal secretion from the pituitary itself, the thyroid, the adrenal cortex, and the gonads. But it also helps in explaining the relationship between mental and bodily processes. Thus, the hypothalamus receives afferents from many parts of the brain, among them the cerebral cortex and the limbic structures, which are closely related to what we term mental or psychic functions. Furthermore, the hypothalamus has access to bodily processes through its connections with the peripheral parts of the autonomic nervous system. In short, our mental state can produce alterations of endocrine organs and of autonomically innervated organs by acting on the hypothalamus.

Psychosomatic Interrelations

Mental processes, by acting on the hypothalamus, may produce brief reactions from visceral organs or prolonged alterations of the hormonal balance, which in turn result in somatic disease. Such bodily symptoms produced by mental processes are examples of what is called *psychosomatic interrelations*. Women may lose their menstruation for some time after psychic stress (loss of a close person, dissatisfaction, depression, and so forth). The mechanism is apparently reduced secretion of gonadotrophic hormones from the pituitary. When subjected to bodily stress (such as infections, trauma, intoxications, and major surgery), the organism responds by, among other things, increasing the secretion of corticosteroids. The same response can also be produced by mental stress by causing increased secretion of releasing hormones from the hypothalamus, which in turn increases the secretion of ACTH from the anterior pituitary. In experimental animals, this hormonal response to mental stress is prevented by transection

of the stalk of the pituitary. Functions controlled by the posterior pituitary (such as urinary volume) can be influenced by our mental state. A particularly striking example is that of a woman breast-feeding her baby, who can cause the milk to trickle from the nipples just by thinking of the child. The inner image of the child in some way influences the hypothalamus, with an increase of oxytocin secretion as the result. This reaches the mammary glands and makes the smooth muscles contract (milk ejection reflex).

The influence of the nervous system on the *immune system* has attracted much interest recently. Even though the mechanisms are not fully understood, there is now much evidence to suggest that the hypothalamus can influence the properties of cells such as natural killer cells and lymphocytes. Thus, it seems likely that mental processes can alter the bodily resistance in a broad sense (for example, against infections and cancer, and perhaps many other diseases). This is, in fact, in accordance with clinical experience.

Bodily Processes May Influence Psychic Ones

Such interactions are especially clear with regard to the hormonal effects on the brain. For example, increased production of thyroid hormones changes the mental state toward excitement, increased initiative, and lively associations, whereas reduced production leads to apathy, fatigue, and increased need of sleep. The changes of mood often associated with the menstrual cycle in women (premenstrual syndrome) are probably caused, at least in part, by effects of female sex hormones on the brain. Thus, a high density of receptors for sex hormones has been demonstrated in various parts of the brain. This concerns in particular certain hypothalamic cell groups, but also neurons in other parts such as the cerebral cortex can bind sex hormones. It seems likely, therefore, that the excitability of many neuronal groups can be influenced by circulating hormones (steroid hormones pass the blood–brain barrier easily). In cats, heat behavior may be produced by implantation of female sex hormones in the posterior part of the hypothalamus. Many other experiments give further evidence that animal behavior can be considerably influenced by circulating hormones, presumably by their actions on the brain. The male sex hormone testosterone can produce male sexual identification and behavior when given to monkeys at an early stage of their development, regardless of the sex of the monkey. Thus, a female monkey may later behave like a male if given a small amount of testosterone for a period shortly after birth.

The Hypothalamus and Emotions

The hypothalamus is among the parts of the brain most directly involved in the expression of emotions or *emotional reactions* (in an experimental context, emotional reactions can be defined as behavior in response to stimuli producing sensations with an emotional coloring). This agrees well with the fact that the hypothalamus functions as a superior center for control of autonomic processes. Emotions are expressed, as we know from everyday experience, to a large extent through changes of the functions of autonomically innervated organs, such as palpitations, dryness of the mouth, fainting, blushing, paling, alterations of the digestive tract, sweating, frequent micturition, and so forth.

So-called *sham rage* can be provoked in cats and dogs in which the whole cerebral cortex, the basal ganglia, and large parts of the thalamus have been removed. Since only the hypothalamus is connected with the brain stem in such animals, their expression of rage must depend on the hypothalamus. Such animals react much like normal animals to painful stimuli, with biting, scratching, snarling, and increased ventilation. Since the whole cortex is removed, it is unlikely that true emotions are experienced, however. It seems reasonable to conclude that the hypothalamus contains cell groups that coordinate and put into action the behavior expressing the rage. The rage of such "hypothalamic" animals is, in contrast to normal animals, not directed toward anything in particular; they seem to lack the ability to know the nature and the location of the stimulus provoking the pain (as one

might expect in an animal lacking the cerebral cortex and most of the thalamus). Furthermore, the expression of the rage dies out very quickly after the stimulus is over, whereas the reactions continue for a while in normal animals (as in humans). This observation also suggests that other parts of the brain normally act on the hypothalamus when emotional reactions are produced, as we will discuss in Chapter 16.

The above account indicates that to regard the hypothalamus as the locus of the emotions would be an impermissible oversimplification. Rather, the *hypothalamus is a superior center for the integration and coordination of emotional reactions*. This conclusion is supported by some observations in humans. During brain surgery with local anesthesia, pressure on or traction of the hypothalamic region can elicit reactions of panic, crying, laughter, or profuse talking. The patients sometimes, however, report a change of mood, such as depression or euphoria. It thus appears that the activity of the hypothalamus is not *only* of significance for emotional reactions but also in some way for the emotions themselves (perhaps mediated by connections back to the limbic structures and the cerebral cortex from the hypothalamus).

Emotions and Emotional Reactions

When discussing the relations between the hypothalamus and emotions, one must distinguish the emotions themselves from the emotional *reactions*—that is, the behavior expressing our emotions. We can experience the feelings or emotions only subjectively. Of course, we may learn that certain external stimuli or situations usually produce certain emotions in other people, but such correlations can only be tentative because so many psychological individual variations play a role. We cannot obtain information from animals about their emotions. The emotional reactions, however, can be directly observed and are often more reliable in animals than in humans. Factors such as upbringing, social conventions, and rational considerations determine to a large extent the emotional reactions in humans. That emotions in animals can only be inferred indirectly from their behavior explains why it is not quite clear how many basic emotions animals have. Commonly, however, only three basic emotions are identified (in cats, dogs, and monkeys): rage, fear, and pleasure (love). Even though the emotions of animals certainly are less schematic than this, there is no doubt that the emotions of humans have much more variation and nuances. This should be kept in mind when drawing conclusions with regard to emotions and psychosomatic interactions in humans on the basis of animal experiments.

NOTES

1. The hormone ACTH is synthesized from a large precursor protein called *pro-opiomelanocortin* or pro-ACTH/endorphin. This precursor molecule is cleaved into other peptides, notably *β-lipotropin* (β-LPH) with a yet-unsettled function, and *β-endorphin,* which is a potent opioid peptide with inhibitory actions on pain transmission. The functional role of the β-endorphin secreted from the pituitary is not clear, however. β-Endorphin is also found in a hypothalamic nucleus (the arcuate nucleus) with projections to brain stem nuclei of importance for pain transmission (see Chapter 4).

2. The ADH secretion is also influenced by other factors, although in primates these appear to be much less potent than changes of osmolarity. For example, reduced blood volume leads concentration of angiotensin II in the bloodstream, which in turn affects the supraoptic and paraventricular nuclei via the subfornical organ. Ethanol reduces the secretion of ADH, thereby increasing urine production.

VI

The Cerebral
Cortex and
Limbic Structures

This part of the book deals with the cerebral cortex and parts of the fore-brain closely associated with the cortex with regard to both development and connections. The cerebral cortex can be divided in two parts (without definite delimitations) on the basis of phylogenetic development: *the neo-cortex*, which is the most recent part and comprises most of the cortex in higher mammals, and *the allocortex*, which is the oldest part. The nomen-clature used for the oldest part of the cortex varies, but usually the term *allocortex* is used for the parts of the cortical mantle with a simple, often only three-layered structure instead of the six layers that are typical of the neocortex. In reptiles the allocortex constitutes what little cortex there is. In humans the neocortex has completely outgrown the allocortex, which forms only a ring of varying thickness at the medial aspect of the hemi-spheres, encircling the corpus callosum and the brain stem (Fig. 16.1). In addition to the fact that the structure of the allocortex is simpler than that of the neocortex, there are other differences as well. The neocortex devel-ops in parallel with the thalamus and receives most of its subcortical affer-ents from the thalamus, whereas the allocortex receives afferents from sev-eral other subcortical nuclei. Together, these nuclei and the allocortex are commonly said to comprise the so-called *limbic system*. There are wide variations among authors, however, with regard to which cell groups are included in this term.

As a first rough indication of functional differences, one may say that conscious thoughts and actions depend primarily on the neocortex, whereas the allocortex and the other parts of the limbic system are more concerned with emotions, motivation, and affective behavior. As we will discuss in the following chapter, however, there are no sharp distinctions in such functional respects between the neocortex and the limbic structures. Nor do the cell groups comprising the limbic system represent a functionally homogeneous "system."

It should finally be emphasized that higher mental functions—usually associated with the cerebral cortex—can only exceptionally be linked to specific nuclei or cortical areas. The most complex tasks of the nervous system are carried out by networks distributed between neurons in many parts of the cortex and in subcortical nuclei.

16

Limbic Structures

Coordination of autonomic functions is a major task of the hypothalamus, as discussed in Chapter 15. We have also described how the hypothalamus influences processes such as metabolism, growth, and reproduction. Hypothalamic influences on bodily functions are mediated in part via peripheral regions of the autonomic nervous system and in part through the endocrine system. The afferent connections of the hypothalamus show that it can be influenced not only by the peripheral organs and tissues it controls but also by higher levels of the nervous system, primarily the *frontal lobe, cingulate gyrus, hippocampal formation, septal nuclei,* and the *amygdaloid nucleus.* It is therefore understandable that stimulation of most of these regions can produce effects like those from stimulation of the hypothalamus.

THE "LIMBIC SYSTEM"

Several of the cell groups mentioned above (that is, the cingulate gyrus, the hippocampal formation, the septal nuclei, the amygdaloid nucleus, and sometimes also the mammillary nucleus and anterior thalamic nucleus[1]) are commonly embraced under the term "limbic system" (gyrus limbicus is another name for the cingulate gyrus). Sometimes terms like "the emotional brain" have been used to describe these regions. The cell groups comprising the limbic system coincide in part with what was formerly called the *rhinencephalin,* although this term, strictly speaking, comprises only the parts of the brain receiving olfactory fibers. The value of such collective terms is questionable. Even though some of the effects of stimulation or ablation of several of the cell groups in the limbic system are similar, there are also clear-cut differences. Furthermore, the fact that many of the nuclei are interconnected does not imply that they constitute a system with a unified function. Studies with modern methods have served to strengthen this view by showing differences between the individual nuclei with regard to connections, neurotransmitters, properties of single cells, and effects of selective lesions. In fact, *it is not possible to define "the limbic system" with a reasonable degree of precision.* Thus, we will not treat the structures included under this term as a unit but rather will discuss each separately. We also prefer to use the neutral term *limbic structures* (Fig. 16.1) because it does not give a misleading impression of functional unity.

383

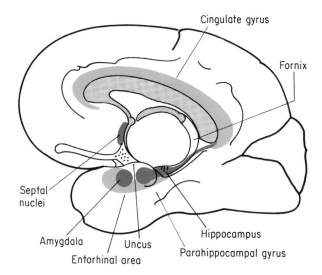

Fig. 16.1.   *The limbic structures.* The right hemisphere seen from the medial aspect. The regions and cell groups indicated in red are usually included in the term "limbic system."

The Circuit of Papez

In 1937, Papez described what he considered a closed circuit of connections starting and ending in the hippocampus. From the hippocampus, the flow of signals was postulated to pass to the mammillary nucleus, from this nucleus to the anterior thalamic nucleus, from there to the cingulate gyrus, and then finally back to the hippocampus. This circuit of interconnected cell groups was hypothesized to form the anatomic basis of emotional reactions and expressions. These suggestions formed the basis for the concept of "the limbic system," which was introduced in the early 1950s. Even though the connectional scheme of Papez is basically correct, it has been modified on several important points. For example, the afferent fibers of the mammillary nucleus (passing in the fornix) do not come from the hippocampus itself but from adjacent regions in the parahippocampal gyrus (subiculum) (Figs. 16.2 and 16.3). Each of the cell groups of the circuit has other—and sometimes more important—connections than with each other. A unified functional role of the circuit in the expression of emotions has not been corroborated by later research.

THE CEREBRAL CORTEX AND "LIMBIC FUNCTIONS": THE CINGULATE GYRUS

Experimental and clinical data show that *autonomic functions* can be influenced by the cerebral cortex. From the cingulate

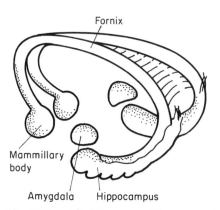

Fig. 16.2.   *The hippocampal formation, fornix, mammillary nucleus, and the amygdala.* On the

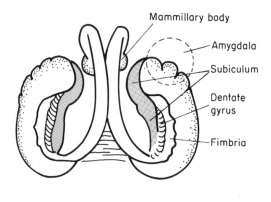

left, they are seen obliquely from behind; on the **right,** from above.

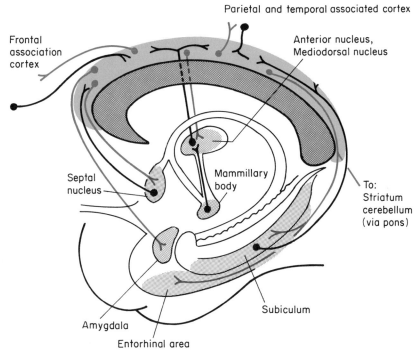

Fig. 16.3. *Main connections of the cingulate gyrus.* The cingulate gyrus has connections with cortical association areas and with limbic structures and may act as a mediator between them.

gyrus in particular (Figs. 16.1 and 16.3), electrical stimulation elicits a combination of autonomic (visceral) and somatic effects.[2] Autonomic effects include, for example, alterations of *respiration and circulation* (reduced rate of breathing, heart rate, and blood pressure), of the *digestive tract* (altered peristaltic movements and secretory activity), and *pupillary dilatation*. Somatic effects are mainly expressed as changes of *muscle tone* and of ongoing *movements* (most often inhibition).

Behavioral changes can be elicited by stimulation of the anterior part of the cingulate gyrus in particular. Most attention has been paid to *aggressive reactions*. Bilateral removal of the cingulate gyrus in monkeys makes them tamer. They may also become socially indifferent—that is, they appear to have lost interest in other members of their group and do not try to make contact.

Surgical lesions of parts of the cingulate gyrus, *cingulotomy,* has been performed in some patients with intense, chronic pain that could not be alleviated by conventional means. Some of these patients were reported to experience their pain as less intense and disabling after the operation. Cingulotomy has also been reported to have beneficial effects when performed on some patients with chronic and severe depression. Several ethical objections have been raised to *psychosurgery* of this kind. Furthermore, the outcome for the individual person appears to be difficult to predict; the effect may in some cases be the opposite of that desired.

Alterations of functions controlled by the autonomic system can be produced by stimulation of parts of the cortex other than the cingulate gyrus. Stimulation of the underside (the orbital surface) of the *frontal lobes* and of the *pole of the temporal lobe* produces effects similar to those obtained from the cingulate gyrus. This may perhaps be explained by the known connections between the frontal and temporal lobes and the connections between these parts and the cingulate gyrus (Figs. 16.3 and 17.13).

Stimulation of neocortical regions does not *only* produce effects on autonomic functions; somatic functions are altered as well.

Thus, no part of the cortex appears to serve autonomic functions only. On the other hand, alterations of autonomic functions can occur after stimulation of cortical regions one might believe to be purely somatic, such as the motor and the premotor cortical areas. Thus, stimulation of the motor cortex produces vasomotor changes (that is, changes of the blood vessel diameter and, therefore, of blood flow) of the opposite body half. On damage to these cortical areas, as seen in patients with a cerebral stroke, vasomotor changes often occur in the paralyzed parts of the body. Even alterations of the heart rate and blood pressure and of the digestive tract can occur. As a final example of combined somatic and autonomic effects, stimulation of the frontal eye field (Fig. 13.31) produces pupillary dilatation in addition to the more obvious conjugated eye movements.

Pathways for Neocortical Influence on Autonomically Innervated Organs

How the neocortex influences the autonomic nervous system (and the endocrine organs) is not entirely clear. There are few direct connections from the cortex to the hypothalamus (even though cortical connections to the reticular formation of the brain stem can explain some effects). The cingulate gyrus receives afferents from association areas of the parietal, frontal, and temporal lobes (Fig. 16.3), but it has no direct efferent connections to the hypothalamus. Indirect pathways are available, however. Thus, the cingulate gyrus projects to the hippocampal formation, to the septal nuclei, and to the amygdaloid nucleus, all of which have different connections to various parts of the hypothalamus. Furthermore, neocortical areas in the frontal and temporal lobes (Fig. 16.4) project to the amygdaloid nucleus and can therefore influence the hypothalamus indirectly.

Fairly large areas of the cerebral cortex can thus influence the hypothalamus and brain stem autonomic centers. To simplify, *neocortical effects on autonomic functions* *appear to be mediated primarily by neocortical efferents to such limbic structures as the hippocampal formation, the amygdaloid nucleus, and the septal nuclei, which mediate the effects on hypothalamic nuclei* (and to some extent directly on brain stem autonomic centers).

THE AMYGDALOID NUCLEUS

The amygdaloid nucleus (or *amygdala* for short) is located in the temporal lobe, underneath the uncus (Figs. 16.1, 16.2, and 16.4). In humans, the amygdala is a complex of subnuclei, each with a distinctive internal structure, neurotransmitters, and connections. We can distinguish between a small *corticomedial* (including a central nucleus) and a large *basolateral* nuclear group. The basolateral group increases in size from lower to higher mammals and is particularly well developed in humans. The corticomedial nuclear group lies close to the olfactory cortex (Fig. 7.2). To simplify, we may say that the *corticomedial nuclei are connected primarily with the olfactory bulb, the hypothalamus, and the visceral nuclei of the brain stem, whereas the basolateral nuclei are connected with the thalamus and parts of the cerebral cortex.* In addition, the basolateral nuclei send fibers to the *striatum* (especially the ventral striatum, see Chapter 10). This would suggest that the corticomedial part of the amygdala is concerned primarily with autonomic functions, whereas the basolateral parts are more involved in conscious processes related to the frontal and temporal lobes.

Connections of the Amygdaloid Nucleus

The *corticomedial* nuclei receive *afferents* from the *olfactory bulb*, the *hypothalamus*, and the *septal nuclei*. The *basolateral* nuclei receive fibers from the *thalamus*, the neocortex of the *frontal lobe* (prefrontal cortex), parts of the *temporal lobe*, and from the *cingulate gyrus* (Fig. 16.4).

The *efferent* connections of the amygdala are mostly reciprocal to the afferent ones. One major efferent pathway goes to the *hypothalamus*. Most of these fibers are collected in the macro-

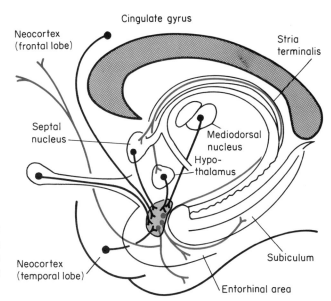

Fig. 16.4. *Main connections of the amygdaloid nucleus.* Note the close connections with the hypothalamus and with association areas in the temporal and frontal lobes.

scopically visible *stria terminalis,* which arches over the thalamus (Figs. 15.3 and 16.4). The fibers end primarily in the ventromedial hypothalamic nucleus (compare with the efferents from the hippocampal formation, which run in the fornix and end in the mammillary nucleus). Other efferents pass to the *thalamus* [especially to the mediodorsal nucleus (MD)], enabling impulses from the amygdala to reach the *prefrontal cortex* (Fig. 17.7). Parts of the allocortex are reached by fibers from the amygdala, especially the *hippocampal formation* (the entorhinal area and the subiculum) and the *septal nuclei.* As mentioned above, there are also efferents from the amygdala to the *striatum.* Finally, there are connections from the amygdala to various brain stem nuclei, such as the *periaqueductal gray,* parts of the *reticular formation,* and *parasympathetic cranial nerve nuclei.*

Since the amygdaloid complex consists of several subnuclei that differ with regard to connections and neurotransmitters, the amygdala cannot be regarded as a functional unit. Depending on their localization within the amygdaloid complex, lesions must be expected to produce different symptoms.

Behavioral Effects Are Pronounced on Stimulation of the Amygdaloid Nucleus

Many behavioral changes have been produced by electrical stimulation of the amygdala in animals with implanted electrodes.

(In such experiments the electrodes have been inserted and fixed to the skull under general anesthesia. Afterward the electrodes cause the animal no pain or obvious discomfort.) Stimulation produces a varied pattern of somatic and autonomic responses, which appear to be parts of more complex behavioral reactions.

As would be expected from the anatomic data discussed above, stimulation of medial and lateral parts of the amygdaloid complex gives different responses. *Stimulation of the corticomedial nuclear group* produces smacking, salivation, and licking and chewing movements. Emptying of the rectum and the bladder may occur, together with inhibition of voluntary movements.

Stimulation of the *basolateral nuclear group* often produces arousal and signs of increased *attention:* The animal lifts its head, its pupils are dilated, and it looks around (especially toward the side opposite of the stimulating electrode). The attention of the animal appears to be directed toward something in the surroundings. As might be expected, together with these behavioral changes occurs *activation of the EEG.* Strong stimulation can produce more dramatic effects, such as signs of strong *fear or rage.* The animal (for example, a cat) might try to escape and show other signs of fear, or it may snarl and growl and perhaps attack the examiner. Most likely, fear and rage are elicited from slightly different parts of the amygdala.

In *humans,* the amygdala has been stimulated in conjunction with brain surgery of the temporal lobe under local anesthesia. A wide spectrum of autonomic and emotional reactions have been produced in such cases, but most pronounced is a feeling of anxiety. Memorylike hallucinations and *déjà vu* experiences have also been reported. Similar effects—that is, fear and various kinds of hallucinations—have been produced by stimulation of cortical areas of the temporal lobe, which are believed to send fibers to the amygdala. A feeling of fear can occur just before an epileptic fit that starts in these regions of the temporal lobe.

The amygdala may be of importance for certain kinds of learning and memory. Experiments with monkeys after a lesion restricted as far as possible to the amygdala indicate that they have difficulties in learning the association between objects and their meanings. They can recognize objects but cannot relate them to other kinds of information, such as whether the object was associated with a reward or something unpleasant.

The Amygdaloid Nucleus, Sexuality, and Psychosurgery

Bilateral destruction of the amygdala in animals produces increased tameness with reduced aggressive and defensive reactions as the most marked symptom. Another reported behavioral change is hypersexuality. This may, however, be related to damage to allocortical areas in the vicinity of the amygdala rather than to the amygdala itself. Nevertheless, it is conspicuous that the amygdala is among the brain regions with the highest density of receptors for sex hormones. It therefore seems likely that the activity of neurons in parts of the amygdala is influenced by the level of sex hormones in the blood (the sex hormones are lipid-soluble and pass the blood–brain barrier easily).

Stereotactic destruction of the amygdala has been performed on some especially violent criminals to reduce their aggression. Bilateral destruction of the amygdala has even been performed in an attempt to cure hyperactive children. The ventromedial hypothalamic nucleus, receiving many fibers from the amygdala, has also been stereotactically lesioned in a small number of sex criminals. The ethical objections to all these psychosurgical interventions were so strong, however, that they were tried only for a short period. Furthermore, the results appear to be so unpredictable that psychosurgery of this kind would be difficult to defend even if there were no other objections.

THE SEPTAL NUCLEI

Even though the septal nuclei are small, they have attracted much interest because of their relation to autonomic functions and behavioral reactions. In humans, the septal nuclei lie just anterior to the anterior commissure[3] (Figs. 2.27 and 16.1).

The major connections of the septal nuclei are with the hippocampus (Fig. 16.7), and the development of the septal nuclei in different animals varies in accordance with the development of the hippocampus. Both the *septohippocampal* and the *hippocamposeptal fibers* follow the *fornix* (which also carries a large number of fibers from the hippocampal formation to the hypothalamus). In addition, the septal nuclei have reciprocal connections with the *hypothalamus* (Figs. 15.2 and 15.3) and with the *cingulate gyrus* (Fig. 16.3). Furthermore, the septal nuclei send efferents to the thalamus and the amygdala.

Changes of several behavioral reactions have been observed after lesions of the septal nuclei in animals, for example, altered sexual and foraging behavior. Aggressive behavior appears to be reduced (as stimulation of the septal nuclei can produce aggression). The effects are similar to those produced by lesions of the amygdala and the anterior parts of the cingulate gyrus. Symptoms specific to the septal nuclei, constituting the so-called septal syndrome, have not been convincingly demonstrated.

THE HIPPOCAMPAL FORMATION

The last among the limbic structures we will discuss are the *hippocampus* and nearby regions in the temporal lobe, the *dentate gyrus* and the *subiculum* (the latter located in the parahippocampal gyrus) (Figs. 16.1, 16.2, and 16.5). Collectively, these structures form the *hippocampal formation*. The term *hippocampal region* includes in addition the *entorhinal area* in the parahippocampal gyrus. Whereas the interest formerly was directed mainly to the hippocampus itself, recent studies of, for example, fiber connections have made us consider the function of the hippocampus in conjunction with the other structures of the hippocampal region.

The *hippocampus* (Figs. 2.28, 2.32, 16.2) forms an elongated bulge medially in the temporal horn of the lateral ventricle, produced by invagination of the ventricular wall by the hippocampal fissure (Fig. 16.5). Along the medial aspect of the hippocampus, the *dentate gyrus* forms a narrow, notched band (Figs. 2.32, 16.2, and 16.5).

The hippocampus and the dentate gyrus belong to the allocortex and have a simplified laminar pattern compared with the neocortex. Nevertheless, they are far from simply built, with several different cell types and precisely organized, highly complex patterns of connections. Only some salient features will be described here.

Most of the neurons of the dentate gyrus are small so-called *granule cells*, whereas the only well-defined hippocampal cell layer consists of large *pyramidal cells* (Figs. 16.5 and 16.6). Above and below the pyramidal cell layer are layers containing the pyramidal cell dendrites and incoming axons. There are also various kinds of interneurons, notably the GABAergic *basket cells*, which inhibit the pyramidal cells. The hippocampus can be divided into three longitudinal zones, named *CA1* to *CA3* (Fig. 16.5). The granule cell axons contact the pyramidal cell dendrites, and the pyramidal cells send axons out of the hippocampus.

The main *hippocampal afferents* come from two sources (Fig. 16.7): The largest

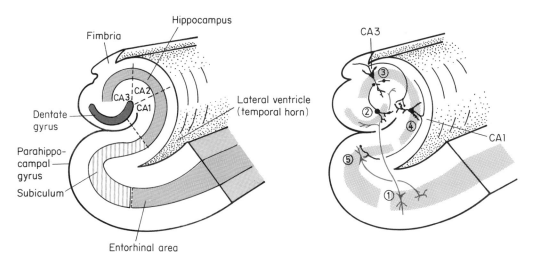

Fig. 16.5. *The hippocampus.* Schematized drawing of a frontal section through medial parts of the temporal lobe. Compare Figures 2.28 and 16.6, which show corresponding sections. The section is oriented approximately perpendicular to the long axis of the lower, thickened part of the hippocampus (cf. Figs. 2.32 and 16.2). The **right** drawing shows one (of several) impulse pathways through the hippocampus. 1 = Pyramidal cell in the entorhinal area; 2 = granule cell in the dentate gyrus; 3 = pyramidal cell in the CA3; 4 = pyramidal cell in the CA1; 5 = pyramidal cell in the subiculum projecting to the entorhinal area.

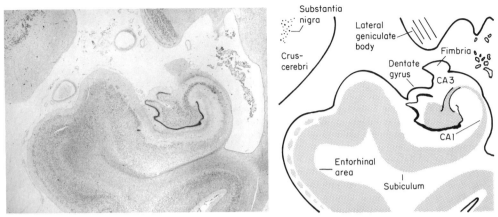

Fig. 16.6. *The hippocampal region.* Photomicrograph of thionine-stained frontal section through the human temporal lobe. The temporal horn of the lateral ventricle with some of the cho-roid plexus is seen above to the right of the hippocampus. The mesencephalon with the crus and the substantia nigra is seen to the left. The section corresponds to the drawing in Figure 2.28.

number of fibers arise in the *entorhinal area* of the parahippocampal gyrus, whereas a smaller contingent comes from the *septal nuclei*. The hippocampal *efferents* end primarily in the *subiculum*, the *entorhinal area*, and the *septal nuclei*. Thus, the hippocampus acts to a large extent on the regions from which it receives information. Indirectly, however, the hippocampus can act on other regions, too. Thus, via the subiculum and the entorhinal area, the hippocampus can influence the *mammillary nucleus* and other parts of the *hypothalamus*[4] and, not least, various parts of the *neocortex* (among them the cingulate gyrus) (Fig. 16.3).

A large number of *commissural fibers*

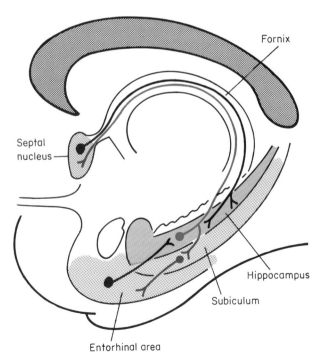

Fig. 16.7. *Some main connections of the hippocampus.*

connect the hippocampus of the two sides, indicating a close cooperation between them.

Septohippocampal Fibers and Fibers from the Brain Stem Have Modulatory Effects

Even though the number of septohippocampal fibers is modest, the pathway is probably of great functional significance. The septohippocampal neurons release *acetylcholine,* which has a long-lasting depolarizing effect on the hippocampal neurons—that is, the pathway has a *modulatory* action (see Chapter 1). Electrical stimulation of the septal nuclei does not drive the hippocampal pyramidal cells to produce action potentials but increases their excitability for seconds or even longer. Thus, this pathway appears not to provide the hippocampus with specific information but rather to control the firing rate of hippocampal cells in response to specific information from the entorhinal area (and thus from many parts of the cortex).

Other hippocampal afferents come from the *raphe nuclei* (serotonin) and the *nucleus locus coeruleus* (norepinephrine). These inputs, too, appear to have *modulatory* effects on the hippocampal cells. Thus, there is evidence that the long-term increase in synaptic effects that can be produced in the hippocampus by certain kinds of afferent stimulation (LTP; see below) are reduced after pharmacological removal of monoamines from the hippocampus.

Impulse Routes through the Hippocampus

Even though the internal architecture of the hippocampus is rather complicated, with several neuronal types with complex interconnections, a relatively simple main transmission route from input to output appears to exist, as first shown by the Norwegian neurophysiologist Andersen (Fig. 16.5). This pathway starts in the entorhinal area and has three synaptic interruptions. Neurons in the entorhinal area send their axons, forming the so-called *perforant path,* to the hippocampus, where many end in the dentate gyrus. The axons of the granule cells of the dentate gyrus, called *mossy fibers,* end primarily on the apical dendrites of the pyramidal cells of CA3 (Fig. 16.5). The CA3 pyramidal cells send so-called *Schaffer collaterals* to the apical dendrite of the CA1 pyramidal cells. From CA1 a significant part of the impulse traffic is directed to the subiculum, and from there to the entorhinal area—thus closing the circuit passing from the entorhinal area

through the hippocampus and back to the entorhinal area. All links in this pathway are excitatory. It has attracted special interest that the synapses in this pathway are modifiable or plastic: The strength of the EPSP produced by a fiber can be enhanced for a long time by specific kinds of stimulation (we will return to this below). It should be emphasized, however, that entorhinal efferents do not end exclusively on the granule cells of the dentate gyrus but also directly on pyramidal cells. Thus, there may exist several parallel pathways through the hippocampus and not only the one depicted in Figure 16.5.

On the basis of primarily physiological data, it was postulated that the hippocampus is organized in thin *lamellae* oriented perpendicular to the long axis of the hippocampus, each lamella presumably representing a functional unit (Fig. 16.5 shows the circuitry in the plane of a lamella). This cannot be the whole story, however. Anatomic investigations performed in monkeys and in lower mammals show that the efferent fibers from a narrow transverse zone of the entorhinal area extend for a considerable distance longitudinally in the hippocampus. Thus, each entorhinal efferent neuron can presumably contact neurons in many hippocampal lamellae. Furthermore, the collaterals of the hippocampal pyramidal neurons extend not only in the plane of the lamellae (as shown in Fig. 16.5) but also longitudinally. In fact, it is still not clear what should be regarded as a functional unit within the hippocampus and the degree of functional localization present.

The Medial Forebrain Bundle

Many fibers interconnecting the various limbic structures are located in a diffusely delimited, parasagittal fiber mass in the basal part of the hemisphere. This ill-defined structure is called the *medial forebrain bundle* and was referred to in Chapter 15. It extends from the region of the anterior commissure anteriorly and posteriorly into the mesencephalon. Most of the fibers are short, interconnecting nuclei located close to each other, such as the septal nuclei, various hypothalamic nuclei, and the periaqueductal gray of the mesencephalon (Fig. 15.3). Fibers from the monoaminergic cell groups of the brain stem pass through the medial forebrain bundle on their way to forebrain structures, such as the cortex (including the hippocampal formation). Functionally, the medial forebrain bundle is heterogeneous, and lesions of it cannot be expected to reveal the function of any particular cell group or fiber tract.

The Entorhinal Area Receives Afferents from Many Neocortical Association Areas

To understand the nature of the information processed by the hippocampus, we must know the afferent connections of the entorhinal area. Thus, the entorhinal area is the major source of hippocampal afferents (Fig. 16.7). Recent studies with retrograde transport of HRP (and other techniques) have shown that most association areas of the neocortex are likely to influence the entorhinal area, either directly or indirectly, by means of fibers to other areas in the parahippocampal gyrus, which in turn project to the entorhinal area. Common to all of the areas sending fibers to the entorhinal area seems to be that they receive information from various kinds of cortical primary sensory areas—that is, various kinds of sensory information converge and are presumably integrated in such *polysensory association areas*. Thus, the signals delivered to the hippocampus from the entorhinal area presumably convey, among other things, highly processed sensory information.

The entorhinal area should not be regarded as a functional unit. Several subdivisions have been identified on the basis of cytoarchitecture and connections. Each subdivision must therefore be expected to deliver a specific kind of information to the hippocampus.

Possible Functions of the Hippocampal Formation

Two aspects of the connections of the hippocampal formation are, presumably, crucial for the understanding of its functional roles: First, the extensive, two-way connections with various cortical association areas and, second, the direct and indirect connections with other limbic structures such as the cingulate gyrus and the septal nuclei (and

with the hypothalamus). As for neocortical connections, the hippocampus obviously processes large amounts of information. The parallel increase in the size of the hippocampus and the neocortex during evolution furthermore indicate that its main functions are related to the neocortex. There is now much evidence that the hippocampal formation plays an important role for certain kinds of *learning and memory*.

There Is More Than One Kind of Learning and Memory

Learning in a wide sense is a prerequisite for memory—something new must be stored that can later be recalled. The learning of skills (that is, how to perform, for example, a movement) is most likely quite different from the learning of factual knowledge, episodes, concepts, and so forth. The last kind of learning enables us to recall consciously the stored information, often in the form of pictures that may be described verbally—that is, a memory of *what*. With skills such as playing an instrument or doing arithmetic, the stored information is available only during the performance—that is, a memory of *how*.

Clinical observations and animal experiments indicate that these two broad categories of learning and memory use largely different parts of the brain.[5] For example, as discussed in Chapter 11, the cerebellum appears to be of importance for motor learning, whereas the hippocampal formation is crucial for other kinds. Observations of patients with dementia seem to favor the view that (at least partly) different neural structures are responsible for the learning of "how" and "what." Thus, whereas the ability to learn and remember new words, faces, places, events, and so forth is severely reduced in such patients, the ability to learn skills is better preserved. Also, observations of patients with memory deficits after lesions of the temporal lobe (without dementia) indicate that they learn and remember new movements better than new faces, words, places, and so forth.

The Hippocampus and Memory

The belief that the hippocampus is of importance for memory goes back to the end of the past century and was based on careful examination of patients with loss of memory as a result of brain damage. The degree and type of memory deficits were correlated with the site of the brain lesion, as determined histologically after the death of the patient. Patients with severe *amnesia* (loss of memory) that is not accompanied by intellectual reduction (dementia) typically have lesions affecting the medial parts of the temporal lobe (and often also the medial parts of the thalamus). Such lesions include the hippocampal formation as the most constant finding. In such cases the amnesia is mainly *anterograde*—that is, the memory is lost for events taking place *after* the time of the brain damage. In case of *retrograde* amnesia, the patient is unable to recall events that took place *before* the damage. Retrograde amnesia virtually never occurs without anterograde amnesia. It should be stressed, however, that such lesions affect primarily *long-term memory,* whereas *short-term memory* may be virtually unimpaired (that is, the ability to remember, for example, numbers or words for up to a minute).

Observations of numerous patients with brain lesions indicate that the hippocampus is particularly important for the memory of events, objects, words, and so forth. The interpretation of such clinical data is difficult, however, because there are very few cases published in which the lesion can be said with confidence to affect *only* the hippocampus. One such case was described recently, however (see below, "Can Destruction of CA1 Alone Produce Anterograde Amnesia?"), and it supports the notion that the hippocampus has a special role in certain kinds of memory.

The evidence in favor of a crucial role of the hippocampus in learning and memory stems to a large extent from animal experiments. These comprise studies with selective lesions and rigorous postoperative testing and studies of the properties of single hip-

pocampal cells. The interpretation of such data, however, is controversial. The transfer of data from lower mammals and even primates to humans is furthermore especially difficult with regard to higher mental functions. Studies of monkeys indicate that the hippocampus is of importance for the process of learning or *forming of the memory traces* (but not necessarily for the long-term storage of the information). As mentioned, this impairment does not concern all forms of learning and later recall. Lesions of the hippocampal formation in monkeys lead to difficulties with the recall of events, objects, and so forth, in agreement with the clinical data.

The monkeys with lesions of the hippocampal formation appear to have special difficulties with remembering *where* an object was located—the association between objects and space. This is of interest in relation to properties of single hippocampal cells, as described by O'Keefe and co-workers. Thus, the firing of single hippocampal cells changes with the position of the animal in relation to its surroundings. The firing pattern changes, for example, with the location of the animal in different corners of the cage. On the basis of such experiments, it was proposed that the hippocampal neurons together form a *cognitive map* of our surroundings.

A Famous Case of Amnesia

Patients with bilateral damage to medial aspects of the temporal lobe have pronounced anterograde (and often less severe retrograde) amnesia, as described above. The most famous case of this kind was described by Scoville and Milner. In 1953, this patient, called H.M. in the voluminous literature that deals with the results of tests to which he has been subjected, underwent surgery to remove bilaterally the medial aspects of his temporal lobes (the purpose was to cure his severe epilepsy). His lesion comprises most likely the hippocampal formation, additional parts of the parahippocampal gyrus, the uncus, and the amygdala. The epileptic fits became less frequent, but unfortunately he acquired a severe, permanent anterograde amnesia. Initially, he also had considerable retrograde amnesia that gradually improved to concern only 1 year before the operation. He remembered well the address of the place he lived before the operation, but he never learned the new address when moving afterward. He was furthermore unable to recall people he had met for the first time after the operation, even though he might have met them regularly for years. He could easily recall songs he had learned before the operation but not those he heard for the first time afterward. He never learned where the lawn mower was kept in his new house. Shortly after eating dinner, he could start on a new one without remembering that he had just eaten. Nevertheless, his intelligence, as measured with various tests, was unaltered compared with before the operation, and his capacity for abstract reasoning was normal. Interestingly, his ability to learn new movements was much better than that for learning new faces, words, and so forth.

The memory deficits described above all concern events that took place some time previously—that is, *long-term memory*. His *short-term memory* was not correspondingly impaired, however. For example, he could recognize a word among nine presented to him 40 seconds earlier.

Once H.M. described his life as follows: "Every day is alone, regardless of the pleasures I have had or the sorrows I have had." Without long-term memory, we lose the continuity between the events of the present and the past.

Can Destruction of CA1 Alone Produce Anterograde Amnesia?

An interesting case was recently described by Zola-Morgan and co-workers, which supports the importance of the hippocampus proper for learning and memory. The patient, called R.B., had an episode of brain ischemia during cardiac surgery. Afterward, he had moderate anterograde amnesia that lasted until his death some years later. He was not appreciably reduced intellectually. Even though his amnesia was much less severe than that of H.M., he had grave problems remembering the events of the day before. During his visits to his doctor, he would repeat the same story at short intervals. Histological examination of the brain after his death showed that the most pronounced alterations were in the hippocampus and, interestingly, restricted to CA1 on both sides. Within the CA1 there was an almost total loss of pyramidal cells (Fig. 16.5). That the CA1 field of the hippocampus is partic-

ularly vulnerable (to ischemia) was suggested in the past century on the basis of observations of patients with epilepsy. The mechanism in such cases may be excessive release of glutamate that activates NMDA receptors (see Chapter 1, "Ischemic Cell Damage"). This results in an uncontrolled influx of calcium, with subsequent cell damage.

As a possible explanation of the marked symptoms of R. B. caused by a seemingly minor damage to the hippocampus, Zola-Morgan and co-workers suggest that destruction of the CA1 field (in its entire length) effectively interrupts signal transmission through the hippocampus and thus isolates it from the rest of the brain (see Fig. 16.5).

Long-Lasting Changes of Synaptic Efficacy in the Hippocampus: LTP

The various links of the impulse pathway through the hippocampus are excitatory and use *glutamate* as neurotransmitter. There are several kinds of glutamate receptor in the hippocampus, among them *NMDA receptors*, which appear to be involved in the production of long-term changes of synaptic efficacy of afferents ending on the pyramidal cells (see Chapter 1, "Excitatory Amino Acid Transmitters"). This phenomenon is called *long-term potentiation* (LTP) and was first observed (long before the NMDA receptor was found) in the hippocampus by the Norwegian neurophysiologist Lømo and co-workers. LTP is produced whenever the pyramidal cells are subjected to excitatory inputs—for example, from the Schaffer collaterals—while they are in a depolarized state (caused by another excitatory input). Thus, simultaneous synaptic activation of the cell from two sources can make it "remember," in the sense that the next time the cell is activated by the same fibers, the postsynaptic effects are stronger than earlier. Binding of glutamate to the NMDA receptor opens a Ca^{2+} channel, but only when the membrane is in a depolarized state. The influx of Ca^{2+} acts as a signal to a long-lasting enhancement of the synaptic efficacy (or, in other words, LTP).

The mechanism for LTP, apart from being related to the NMDA receptor and calcium influx, is not yet fully understood. For example, it is not settled whether the increased synaptic effect of a single action potential in an afferent terminal is caused by increased transmitter release (that is, a presynaptic mechanism) or whether the changes occur postsynaptically. Electron microscopic studies indicate that LTP may be associated with sprouting of boutons; more transmitter is released because new boutons are formed. In any case, the LTP phenomenon has attracted great interest and intense investigation because of evidence that the hippocampus is of special importance for learning and memory. The hippocampus is now a fertile ground for attempts to close the gap between knowledge about the cellular mechanisms and behavior in higher mammals.

Not Only Medial Parts of the Temporal Lobe Are of Importance for Memory

One of the old arguments in favor of the hippocampus as important for memory was based on observations of patients with so-called Korsakoff's psychosis (usually a result of chronic alcoholism). This condition is characterized by severe amnesia and cell loss in the mammillary nucleus (and certain other places). Because it was believed that most of the afferents to the mammillary body passing in the fornix arose in the hippocampus, this was taken as evidence of the role of the hippocampus in memory. As mentioned, however, the fornix fibers do not arise in the hippocampus but in the subiculum. Furthermore, cell loss in Korsakoff's psychosis is marked also in parts of the brain other than the mammillary nucleus, notably in the *medial parts of the thalamus* (especially in the region of MD; Fig. 17.7). As mentioned, cell loss in the medial thalamus is a frequent finding in cases of amnesia. In fact, severe amnesia was described in a patient who, as judged from computer tomography of the brain, had a small lesion confined to the anterior and medial parts of the thalamus on the left side.[6]

It is also possible that the *amygdala* takes part in the learning of certain kinds of associations (as described above). Furthermore, parts of the *prefrontal cortex* are necessary for the ability to retain an internal "picture" of an object that is no longer seen (see Chapter 17). The *cerebellar role in motor learning* has also been mentioned.

In conclusion, different kinds of learning, and later recall, appear to be related to at least partly different regions of the brain.

The hippocampus appears to be crucial only for certain specific aspects of learning and memory.

Permanent Memory Traces Probably Lie in Many Parts of the Cerebral Cortex

As mentioned, the amnesia after lesions of the hippocampus and surrounding structures is predominantly or solely anterograde. This shows that information about events taking place some time before the lesion must be stored in other parts of the brain.

Other clinical observations of patients with damage in various parts of the brain indicate that there is no specific "memory center," but well-consolidated information is stored in a distributed fashion. When a memory is established—presumably in the form of long-term synaptic changes—the hippocampal formation no longer seems to be necessary for storage and recall. The time required to reach this stage is not known, but, again on the basis of observations of patients with damage to medial parts of the temporal lobe, it may perhaps take as long as a year.

The Basal Nucleus (Meynert) and Alzheimer's Disease

The amnesia occurring after localized damage to the temporal lobe is characterized by the absence of significant intellectual impairment. Most commonly, however, amnesia occurs as one of the symptoms of *dementia* (that is, a general mental and intellectual reduction). Dementia may have various causes, but typically there is a pronounced neuronal loss in large parts of the cerebral cortex. Recently, especially the dementia of the *Alzheimer type* (Alzheimer's disease) has attracted much interest. The disease was described just after the turn of the century as a distinct form that, in contrast to ordinary dementia, typically starts before the sixth decade of life (presenile dementia). Alzheimer's disease is characterized by the occurrence of fibrillary tangles (senile plaques) and neuronal loss in the cortex. Clinically, the disease manifests itself with a gradual deterioration of mental and intellectual

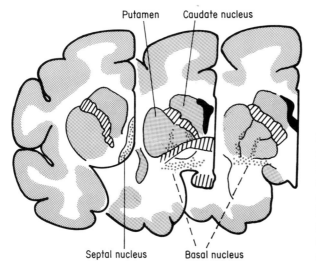

Putamen   Caudate nucleus

Septal nucleus   Basal nucleus

Fig. 16.8. *The basal nucleus (of Meynert).* Frontal section through the left hemisphere (monkey). The cholinergic neurons of the basal nucleus are indicated with red dots. The basal nucleus is continuous anteriorly with the septal nuclei and other cholinergic cell groups of the forebrain. Redrawn from Richardson and DeLong (1988).

faculties, with amnesia for recent events as an early sign.

Some years ago, it was discovered that patients with Alzheimer's disease regularly have marked cell loss in a diffuse cell group at the base of the hemisphere, the *basal nucleus* (of Meynert) (Fig. 16.8). The neurons of the basal nucleus contain choline acetyltransferase (Fig. 16.9) and most likely release *acetylcholine* from their terminals in the cerebral cortex. The basal nucleus fuses anteriorly without demarcation with other cholinergic cell groups, among them the septal nuclei (Fig. 16.8). In patients with Alzheimer's disease, the amount of acetylcholine is reduced both in the basal nucleus and in the cerebral cortex. The efferents from the basal nucleus distribute rather diffusely to large parts of the cortex. Such an arrangement would suggest that the basal nucleus exerts a *modulatory* effect on the excitability of cortical neurons. Most likely, acetylcholine has a slow depolarizing effect on neocortical neurons (like the effect in the hippocampus). Experimental studies show that many neurons of the basal nucleus are continuously active but that they typically increase their activity in conjunction with the animal being rewarded for a particular behavioral response. There is, for example, a stronger increase of neuronal firing when a monkey performs an arm movement that is rewarded than when exactly the same movement is performed without a reward. Other findings, too, suggest that the basal nucleus activity is related to *motivation*. There is, furthermore, some evidence that acetylcholine and the basal nucleus have some relation to the level of consciousness and attention.

The above considerations might suggest a simple explanation of the dementia in Alzheimer's disease: The lack of acetylcholine reduces the excitability of cortical neurons, making it much

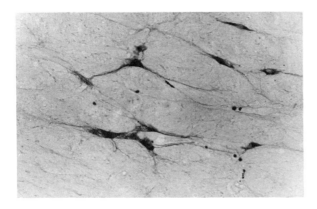

Fig. 16.9. *Cholinergic neurons of the basal nucleus.* Photomicrograph of a section treated to demonstrate immunocytochemically the enzyme choline acetyltransferase. The enzyme is necessary for the synthesis of acetylcholine. Magnification, ×300. Courtesy of Dr. J.-E. Aas.

harder for specific inputs to fire the cells. Furthermore, one might guess that a lack of acetylcholine in the hippocampal formation would be important for the reduction of recent memory. This is so far no more than speculation, however. In fact, further research has shown that conditions in Alzheimer's disease are more complicated than described above. There are, for example, lesions of other parts of the brain in addition to the basal nucleus, and the amounts of many neurotransmitters in addition to acetylcholine are reduced. The cortical cell loss, which is most pronounced in the association areas, the entorhinal area, and the hippocampus (especially CA1 pyramidal cells), by itself can explain the dementia at the later stages of the disease. The lack of effect (so far) of drugs increasing the level of acetylcholine in the brain does not strengthen the acetylcholine theory.

Behavior and the "Limbic System"

The phylogenetically old parts of the brain that we have discussed in this chapter influence complex functions closely related to various aspects of behavior. Even though some structures appear to be especially important for certain functions, there is no sound basis for localizing complex brain functions to smaller, well-defined cell groups or parts of the brain and to use terms such as "centers" for memory, sexual behavior, aggression, and so forth. In general, the more complex a function is, the more distributed the neural network subserving it. Our present knowledge tells us that all complex behavioral reactions engage the amygdala, the septal nuclei, the hippocampal region, the reticular formation, the hypothalamus, and large parts of the cerebral cortex. As witnessed by their numerous interconnections, all of these regions cooperate to exert an integrated influence on the peripheral somatic and autonomic effectors. What the American psychologist Grossman said about the septal nuclei probably holds for the rest of the limbic structures too: "Just about every behavior and/or psychological function which has been investigated to date has been shown to be affected in some way by septal lesions. . . ."

Further studies of the limbic structures are of great importance to improve our understanding of the interplay between conscious, cognitive processes and the emotional and more or less subconscious processes that together determine our behavior. Such knowledge is presumably also of importance for a better understanding of psychiatric diseases, in which emotional disturbances as a rule constitute an important aspect.

NOTES

1. Some authors use the term "limbic system" even more extensively and include the hypothalamus and parts of the basal ganglia (primarily the ventral striatum; see Chapter 10).

2. Only parts of the cingulate gyrus belong to the allocortex; most of it probably belongs to the oldest parts of the neocortex.

3. The region containing the septal nuclei is called the precommissural part of the septum. The postcommissural part is the septum pellucidum, which contains no neurons.

4. Fibers destined for the mammillary nucleus comprise the majority of the fornix fibers. Until the mid-1970s it was held that these fibers come from the hippocampus itself—that is, they were the axons of the pyramidal cells. With the introduction of methods utilizing axonal transport of radioactively labeled amino acids, it was shown, however, that the fibers originate in the subiculum. The old view was based on experiments with anterograde degeneration techniques, which require that the neurons be damaged. To produce lesions of the hippocampus without at the same time affecting the subiculum is virtually impossible.

5. Memory as a concept is not easy to define precisely. Usually, it is used only of stored information that can be consciously recalled (and described). Thus, "motor memory" would not be included with such a restrictive definition. Nevertheless, the same basic cellular mechanisms appear to underlie all kinds of long-term changes in the performances of the nervous system.

6. In this particular case the verbal memory was more severely affected than the visual. The patient could with some difficulty remember objects he had seen some time ago, whereas words heard at the same time were completely forgotten.

17

Cerebral Cortex

The human cerebral cortex consists of between 10 and 20 billion neurons and constitutes more than half of all gray matter of the central nervous system. This gives a rough impression of its functional importance. In lower vertebrates there are only very modest primordia of the cerebral cortex (allocortex), and it is first in mammals, particularly anthropoid apes and humans, that the cerebral cortex comes to dominate the rest of the nervous system quantitatively. This enormous increase in the volume of the cortex has necessitated a marked folding of the surface of the hemisphere. The outer layer of the human cerebral cortex is around 0.2 m², but only one-third of this is exposed on the surface. The *neocortex* constitutes most of the cerebral cortex in higher mammals, and this chapter will deal only with the neocortex.

STRUCTURE OF THE CEREBRAL CORTEX

The Neocortex Consists of Six Layers

All parts of the neocortex share a common basic structure, with the neurons arranged in six *layers* or *laminae* oriented parallel to the surface of the cortex (Figs. 17.1, 17.2, and 17.4). Another general feature is the arrangement of the neurons in rows or *columns* oriented perpendicular to the cortical surface (Fig. 17.2). Both kinds of cellular aggregation are related to functional specializations among the neurons, as we will discuss below. Figure 17.1 shows the main features of the layering. It can be seen that the laminar pattern arises because cells of similar shape and size are collected in more or less distinct layers. The density of perikarya also differs among the layers. About two-thirds of the neurons are cortical *pyramidal cells* (the name refers to the triangular shape of their perikarya). A typical pyramidal cell has a long axon arising from the base of the pyramid and a long *apical dendrite* that extends toward the cortical surface—it thus extends through several layers superficial to the layer in which the perikaryon is located (Figs. 1.1 and 17.5). The fairly large pyramidal cells are found in layers 3 and 5, but many of the smaller cells in the other layers are also pyramidal. The pyramidal cells are also characterized by their large number of *dendritic spines* (Figs. 1.1 and 17.5). The rest of the cortical neurons constitute a heterogenous group whose neurons have in common that their perikarya are not pyramidal; such neurons are therefore lumped together as *nonpyramidal cells.*

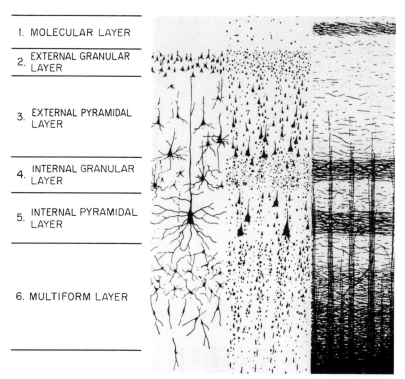

I. MOLECULAR LAYER

2. EXTERNAL GRANULAR LAYER

3. EXTERNAL PYRAMIDAL LAYER

4. INTERNAL GRANULAR LAYER

5. INTERNAL PYRAMIDAL LAYER

6. MULTIFORM LAYER

Fig. 17.1. *The basic six-layered structure of the neocortex.* The three columns show sections perpendicular to the cortical surface subjected to different staining methods. The left column shows the appearance in Golgi-impregnated sections, in which the perikarya and some of the dendrites can be seen. The middle column shows a thionine-stained section, in which only the perikarya are visible. The right column shows the appearance after myelin staining—that is, the main pattern of the myelinated axons is evident, with perpendicular bundles of fibers entering the cortex, and horizontal bundles of fibers interconnecting nearby parts of the cortex. After Brodmann and Vogt.

Their shape and size vary considerably, but all of them are most likely *interneurons.*[1]

The most superficial cortical layer, *layer 1,* the *molecular layer,* is fiber-rich with few neurons (Figs. 17.1 and 17.2). Apart from axons, it contains the apical dendrites of pyramidal cells in the deeper layers. *Layer 2,* the *external granular layer,* contains densely packed, small perikarya.[2] *Layer 4,* the *internal granular layer,* is similarly built. In primary sensory cortical areas, layer 4 is especially well developed, and shows even a further laminar subdivision in the striate area (layer 4A, B, and C; Fig. 17.4). *Layer 3,* the *external pyramidal layer,* can be recognized by its content of medium-sized pyramidal cells, whereas *layer 5,* the *internal pyramidal layer,* also contains many large pyramidal cells. *Layer 6,* the *multiform layer,* contains many cells with spindle-shaped perikarya.

Considering only certain salient features, we can say that *layers 2 and 4* are mainly *receiving*—being most developed in the primary sensory areas—whereas *layers 3 and 5* are mainly *efferent* and send their axons out of the part of the cortex in which they are located. The pyramidal cells of layer 5 send their axons primarily to subcortical nuclei, and this layer is particularly well developed in MI (Figs. 9.3 and 17.2). The layer 3 pyramidal cells send their axons primarily to other areas of the cortex (association and commissural fibers). Layer 6 is also largely efferent and sends many axons to the thalamus.

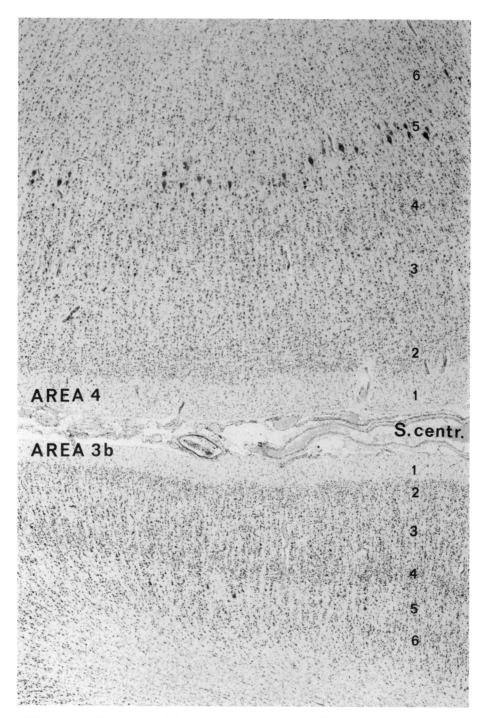

Fig. 17.2. *Cytoarchitectonics of the cerebral cortex.* Photomicrograph of a thionine-stained section through the central region of the human brain. The section is perpendicular to the direction of the central sulcus. The six-layered structure is evident in area 4 (MI) and in area 3b (SI). Note, however, the difference in development and appearance of the various layers in the two areas, especially with regard to layers 4 and 5.

The cortex of the MI in the precentral gyrus is much thicker than that of the SI. This is not because there are more neurons but because of more extensive dendritic trees, more axonal branches and boutons, and perhaps more glial cells. Note also the tendency for the cells to be arranged in vertically oriented rows or columns. See also Figure 9.3 with a corresponding section from the monkey. Magnification, ×170.

The Cerebral Cortex Can Be Divided into Cytoarchitectonic Areas

Even though all parts of the neocortex consist of six cell layers, the thickness and structure of the various layers vary from one area to another. This is most easily observed in sections stained to visualize the perikarya alone (Figs. 1.2, 1.3, 17.2, and 17.4). Such *cytoarchitectonic* differences form the basis of the subdivision of the entire cortex into cytoarchitectonic *areas* (Fig. 17.3), as done around the turn of the century by Brodmann and others (Fig. 17.3). This was briefly described in Chapter 2, and several of the cytoarchitectonic areas were mentioned in previous chapters.

The main importance of the division of the cortex into cytoarchitectonic areas is that these areas have proved in many instances to differ functionally, even though they were initially defined solely on the basis of the size, shape, and arrangement of the neuronal cell bodies. In many cases a cytoarchitectonically defined area is unique also with regard to its afferent and efferent connections and the physiological properties of its cells.

Even though the borders between different cytoarchitectonic areas are sometimes easy to identify, as exemplified in Figure 17.4, more often the differences are rather subtle. Thus, it should not come as a surprise that authors often disagree with regard to the parcellation of the cortex into areas, as a comparison of their published maps will show. Today we try to define a cortical area not only on the basis of cytoarchitectonics but also by additional criteria, such as fiber connections, cellular markers, recordings of single-cell activity, and the behavioral effects of stimulation or ablation of the area in question. We will return to connections and functions of different cortical areas later in this chapter.

With regard to the size of cortical areas, there are surprisingly large individual variations. The volume of the striate area (the most easily identified one) varies by a factor of three among adult humans. Because the volume of the hemispheres does not show similar variations, this implies that in a brain with a large striate area, other areas are relatively smaller. Whether such anatomic differences also have functional significance is unknown, but conceivably they may contribute to the large differences between humans in mental and other capacities.

Projection Neurons and Main Types of Interneurons

The pyramidal cells send their axon toward the white matter to reach other parts of the cortex or subcortical cell groups. Thus, they are the *projection neurons* of the cortex (Fig. 17.5), which most likely constitute more than half of all cortical neurons. The projection neurons send *recurrent collaterals* before the axon leaves the cortex and can thus influence the level of activity among the cortical neurons in their vicinity. The recurrent collaterals may, for example, excite inhibitory interneurons and thereby limit the activity of the parent cell and other pyramidal cells.

All cells belonging to the other main type of cortical neurons, the *nonpyramidal cells*, have locally branching axons that do not reach the white matter—that is, they are the cortical *interneurons* (Fig. 17.6). Such interneurons may be classified into three main types on the basis of the course and branching pattern of their axons. One type has an axon that forms numerous terminal branches close to the perikaryon. It mediates influence mainly to neighboring neurons within the lamina in which the cell body is located. A second type has an axon coursing perpendicularly or *vertically* toward either the cortical surface or the white matter, giving off collaterals on its way. This enables the interneuron to influence neurons in several layers. Finally, the third main type of interneuron sends its axon in a *horizontal* direction (parallel to the cortical surface).

Even though this division into three kinds of cortical interneurons is an oversimplification, it shows the main features of the *intracortical* connections, which permits inter-

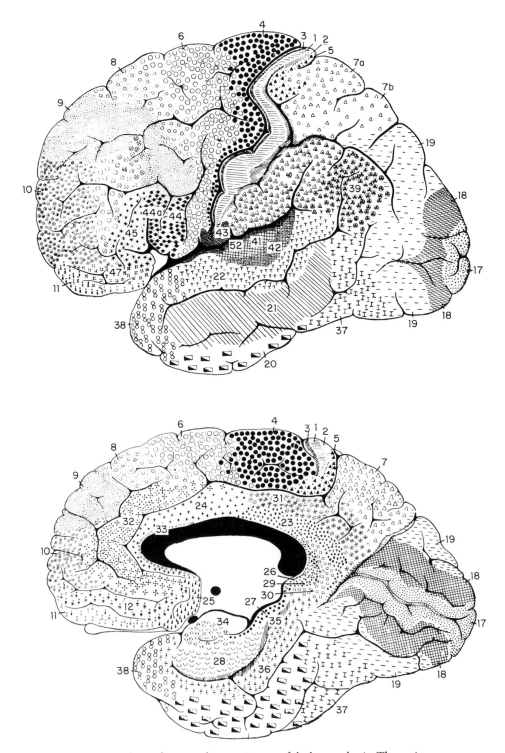

Fig. 17.3. *Brodmann's cytoarchitectonic map of the human brain.* The various areas are labeled with different symbols and numbers.

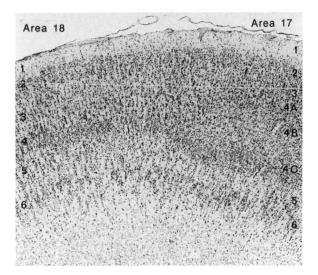

Fig. 17.4. *The transition between area 17 (the striate area) and area 18.* Thionine-stained section from the human visual cortex. Note how the various layers change in cell size, cell density, and thickness at the transition between the two cytoarchitectonic areas. Most areal borders are less clear-cut than this.

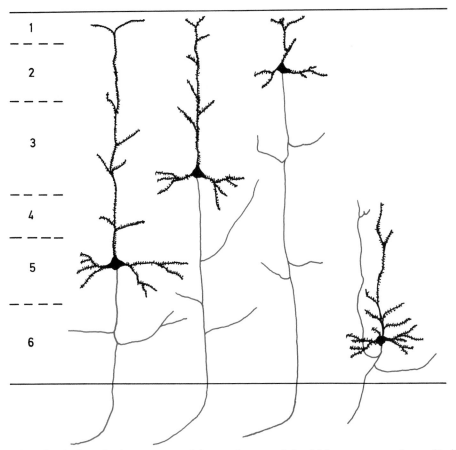

Fig. 17.5. *Cortical projection neurons.* Schematic drawing. The axons, shown in red, give off several recurrent collaterals on their way to the white matter. The dendrites have numerous spines. The larges neurons, with the largest peri- karya and the thickest axons, are located in layer 5. Schematic drawing based on studies by Jones (1988) of the central region of the monkey with the Golgi method.

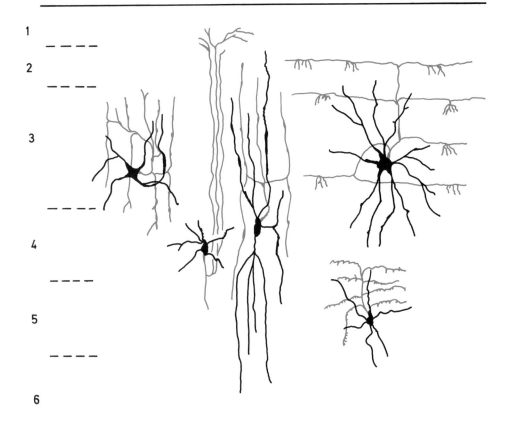

1
2
3
4
5
6

Fig. 17.6. *Main kinds of cortical interneurons.* Note three patterns of axonal distribution (in red): in the immediate vicinity of the perikaryon, horizontally in the layer of the perikaryon, and vertically spanning several layers. Based on Jones (1988).

actions among neighboring neurons, among neurons within different layers, and among neurons located at some distance within the same layer. Vertically oriented axons (from either interneurons or pyramidal cell recurrent collaterals) ensures the communication among neurons within a narrow cortical cylinder or *column*. The horizontal axonal branches mediate communication among neurons in different columns. Most often, such horizontal influences appear to be inhibitory. In sensory cortical areas, the horizontal intracortical connections mediate *lateral inhibition,* which increases the spatial resolution of the sensory information (lateral inhibition is present at several levels of the sensory pathways). The length of horizontal axons is limited to 1–2 mm, however.

Thus, cortical columns that are farther apart than this must communicate by means of projection neurons with an axon coursing in the white matter—that is, association fibers.

Excitation and Inhibition in the Cortex: Neurotransmitters

Most or perhaps all projection neurons contain an *excitatory amino acid neurotransmitter* (glutamate or aspartate). Accordingly, physiological studies show that they have fast, excitatory synaptic actions. A subgroup of cortical interneurons is most likely also excitatory, as judged from, among other things, the kind of synapse they form (asymmetrical synaptic thickening, in contrast to the symmetrical thickening found at most inhibitory cortical synapses). This kind of interneuron has numerous dendritic spines, in this respect resembling the (excitatory) pyramidal cells. Apart from such so-called *spiny stallate cells,* the rest of the interneurons (the "aspiny" ones) are probably inhibitory, with GABA as the predominant neurotransmitter. Some of the GABAergic interneurons also contain one or several neuropeptides (such as VIP, CCK, and others).

There is some evidence that epilepsy may be related to selective loss of GABAergic cortical interneurons (even though this is just one of several possible mechanisms).

Intracortical Connections and Impulse Traffic

Afferent fibers ending in a small volume of the cortex make excitatory synapses with a large number of projection neurons and interneurons. Thus, *one* afferent fiber from the thalamus has been estimated to contact about 5000 cortical neurons. The synaptic contacts are established in certain layers only, but the excitation is propagated to other layers by the pyramidal cell recurrent collaterals and excitatory interneurons (spiny stellate cells). At the same time, numerous inhibitory interneurons are activated. The inhibitory interneurons serve to focus the efferent cortical signals and to terminate the activity of the projection neurons. In addition, the inhibitory interneurons inhibit other inhibitory interneurons, with resulting disinhibition.

The enormous number of neurons and their complex interconnections within even a small volume of cortical tissue explain why we still do not understand the basic rules underlying intracortical information processing. Promising advances have been made, however, especially in the *visual cortex,* with the use of methods enabling the recording of single-cell activity in relation to specific stimuli and subsequent intracellular injection of HRP. Thus, the dendritic and axonal patterns of individual, functionally characterized neurons can be determined. Successful attempts have also been made to abolish the activity of neurons in specific layers and then study how the properties of neurons in other layers are changed. As expected from the known terminal pattern of axons from the lateral geniculate body, neurons are first activated in layer 4 after visual stimuli (in addition, neurons in other lay-

ers with dendrites extending into layer 4 can be influenced). From layer 4, the excitation is propagated to layers 2 and 3, and from there to layers 5 and 6. Some cells in layer 6 send axons upward to layer 4. Presumably, at every step in such a pathway through the cortex some processing of the sensory information takes place, such as integration by one cell of the signals from other functionally different cells. In accordance with this assumption, the functional properties of cells in different layers vary, as shown with microelectrode recordings after natural stimulation of receptors. A projection neuron in layer 5 has quite different properties than a cell in layer 4; for example, the receptive fields of the layer 5 cells are larger (as a sign of convergence of signals from several neurons in layer 4). Other properties of layer 5 cells also suggest that signals from functionally different layer 4 cells converge on layer 5 cells (via processing in layers 2 and 3).

Many cortical neurons react primarily when information about two events reaches them simultaneously, like cells in the visual cortex that respond poorly to signals from one eye only but vigorously to simultaneous signals from both eyes (binocular cells). Like a good detective who has a special eye for *coincidences* (events occurring simultaneously) and disregards numerous trivial bits of information, the cortical neurons respond preferentially to certain coincidences of stimuli that have a survival value. This characteristic property of cortical cells is probably built into the inborn wiring pattern ("hardware") of the brain, but it also needs proper use to be further developed and maintained (see "The Parietal Lobe and the Development of the Ability to Integrate Somatosensory and Visual Information," later in this chapter).

Each Cortical Neuron Integrates Information from Many Other Neurons

The activity (that is, the frequency and pattern of action potentials) of each cortical neuron depends, as we have discussed, on the activity of the numerous other neurons with which it is synaptically connected. This is true of fibers reaching the cortex from other regions (subcortical nuclei and other parts of the cortex) and intracortical connections from cells in the immediate vicinity (within a radius of 1–2 mm in the horizontal direction). One cortical neuron, such as a pyramidal cell of the MI, integrates information from perhaps 600 nearby cortical cells and has been estimated to receive about 60,000 synapses (monkey). Synapses from different sources often end on different parts of the neuron. Thus, as a rule cortical inhibitory synapses are axosomatic, whereas the excitatory synapses are axodendritic (primarily on the dendritic spines of pyramidal cells).

Many cortical cells receive excitatory inputs with a fast synaptic action from the thalamus and from other parts of the cortex (association and commissural fibers). In addition, they are subjected to slow, modulatory synaptic influences from rather diffusely organized fiber systems, which release acetylcholine and monoamines. Last, but not least, the activity of the cortical neurons is influenced by the numerous intracortical fiber connections, of which some are inhibitory and some are excitatory. Inhibitory actions may be fast (mediated by GABA) or slow (mediated by the neuropeptides present together with GABA in many interneurons).

Cortical Microstructure: The Columnar Concept

We have mentioned previously that the cortical cells appear to be organized into small units, formed by cylinders or *columns* of tissue extending perpendicular to the surface of the cortex. A tendency for cortical neurons to be arranged in perpendicular rows is evident from thionine-stained sections (Figs. 17.2 and 17.4). That neurons within such a column share functional properties that differ from those within adjacent columns was first observed by Mountcastle in the monkey SI. He found that when a microelectrode was inserted perpendicular to the cortical surface, the cells encountered as the electrode traversed the thickness of the cortex had very similar receptive fields. They were furthermore similar with regard to their adequate stimulus, as if they were activated by the same kind of receptor. When, in contrast, the microelectrode was inserted obliquely, the receptive fields of the neurons moved with the advancement of the electrode. On the basis of such experiments, it was proposed that SI neurons with similar receptive fields and modalities are grouped together in columns with a diameter of some hundred micrometers. A similar columnar arrangement has been observed in the MI, but with relation to muscles rather than to receptors (neurons within one column act on one or a few synergistic muscles). Interestingly, a pyramidal cell with all its dendrites and recurrent collaterals is contained within a cortical tissue cylinder with a diameter of about

350 μm (of course, hundreds of other neurons are present within the same cylinder).

The relation between the tendency for cortical neurons to be arranged in columns and the physiologically defined functional columns, however, is not clear. Furthermore, the distribution in the cortex of neurons with different properties is less schematic than the columnar concept might imply. In the visual cortex, in which the segregation of functionally different neurons has been most thoroughly investigated, cells sharing functional properties are arranged in bands rather than in cylinders. Another more serious problem with the columnar concept is that neurons in different layers—for example, of the striate area—are not functionally identical (for example, cells that are color-specific and cells that are movement-specific are located in different layers). Thus, the "columns" may not always extend through the depth of the cortex but may be limited to one or a few layers. To apply the columnar concept to such examples of segregation of functionally different cortical neurons is rather confusing.

Afferents from Different Sources End in Different Cortical Layers

The cortical layers differ with regard to the origin of their extrinsic afferents. Schematically, pathways conveying precise sensory information end primarily in layer 4. This concerns thalamocortical fibers from the somatosensory relay nucleus, VPL, and from the relay nuclei of the visual and auditory pathways, the lateral and medial geniculate bodies. Association fibers (that is, from other cortical areas) end preferentially in layers 2–4. Subcortical afferents with modulatory effects end in several layers, notably layer 1. Such fibers arise in the intralaminar thalamic nuclei, in several brain stem nuclei (the raphe nuclei, nucleus locus coeruleus, and dopaminergic cell groups in the mesencephalon), and in the basal nucleus.

CONNECTIONS OF THE CEREBRAL CORTEX

The connections of the cerebral cortex with subcortical structures have been described in several of the previous chapters. We have dealt with the terminal regions of the major sensory pathways and the areas giving origin to the descending pathways involved in motor control. Here we will describe *general aspects of connections between the thalamus and the cerebral cortex* and of the *corticocortical connections* (association and commissural connections). Such knowledge is a necessary basis for the following treatment of the cortical association areas and their functional roles.

A Brief Survey of Cortical Connections

We can classify the *afferent* connections of the cerebral cortex as follows:

1. Precisely, topographically organized connections from the "specific" thalamic nuclei; each thalamic nucleus supplies one particular part of the cortex;
2. Diffusely organized connections from the intralaminar thalamic nuclei and from several other subcortical nuclei (the raphe nuclei, the nucleus locus coeruleus, dopaminergic cell groups in the mesencephalon, and the basal nucleus); such connections do not respect the cytoarchitectonic borders in contrast to the connections from the specific thalamic nuclei;
3. Association fibers—that is, precisely organized connections linking cortical areas within the same hemisphere;
4. Commissural fibers—that is, precisely organized connections between areas in the two hemispheres.

The *efferent* connections of the cerebral cortex can also be divided into subcortical and corticocortical ones (association and commissural connections). The *subcortical* fibers are destined for the thalamus, the striatum, various brain stem nuclei (among them the pontine nuclei projecting to the cerebellum), and the spinal cord. The corticocortical connections are for the most part reciprocal—that is, an area receives fibers from the same areas to which it sends fibers.

Thalamocortical Connections

The thalamus has been mentioned in several contexts (see Chapters 2 and 4 for descriptions of its gross anatomy and main subdivisions). *The thalamus supplies all parts of the neocortex with afferents.* Each part of the cortex receives fibers primarily from one of the specific thalamic nuclei. The main features of this topographic arrangement of the thalamocortical projection are shown in Figure 17.7 (as we believe it is organized in humans). Figures 4.19 and 11.14 show the projection from the ventral thalamic nucleus in more detail, based on experimental studies in monkeys with retrograde degeneration techniques and retrograde and anterograde axonal transport methods.

Conditions are more complex than shown in the diagrams, however. In the first place, the topographic arrangement is much more fine-grained. Thus, the projection from one thalamic nucleus is precisely arranged, with subdivisions of the nucleus supplying minor parts only of the large fields shown in Figure 17.7. As described in Chapters 4 and 5, the thalamocortical connections from the VPL and the lateral geniculate body are somatotopically and retinotopically organized, respectively, with a precision that enables the cortex to extract information about minute spatial details. Furthermore, each thalamic nucleus sends fibers to more than one cortical area. We can take the MD as an example. In the scheme, it is depicted as sending fibers to the prefrontal cortex (without any topographic arrangement). In reality, the MD sends fibers to other parts of the cortex, too, such as parts of the cingulate gyrus. The MD furthermore consists of several subdivisions, each supplying a different part of the prefrontal cortex. The main point emerging from such knowledge is that the MD is not a functional unit. A small lesion, for example, must be expected to produce quite different effects depending on its exact location within the MD.

Some of the specific thalamic nuclei are relay stations in the *pathways for impulses from sensory receptors* (vision, hearing, cu-

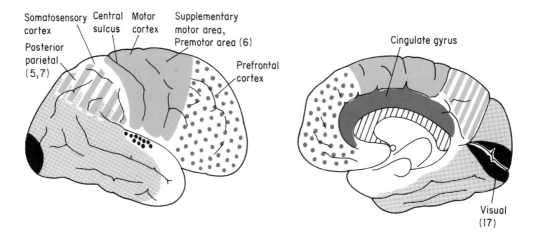

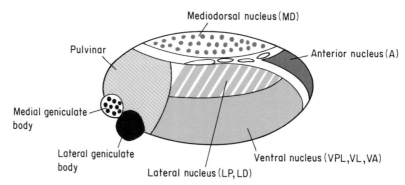

Fig. 17.7. *The thalamocortical projection.* Highly simplified scheme showing the main features of its topographic organization.

taneous sensation, proprioception) to specific cortical areas. The *VPL* receives afferents from the somatosensory pathways and projects to the SI, areas 3, 1, and 2 (Figs. 4.13 and 4.14); the *lateral geniculate body* receives afferents from the retina and projects to the striate area (Fig. 5.11); the *medial geniculate body* is the last subcortical station in the auditory pathways and sends efferents to AI (Figs. 6.9 and 6.10). Other specific thalamic nuclei, the *VL* and *VA*, are relay stations in the pathways from the cerebellum and the basal ganglia to the motor and premotor cortical areas (Fig. 11.14). Other thalamic nuclei relay signals from limbic structures: The *anterior thalamic nucleus* receives afferents from the mammillary nucleus (which receives its main input from the subiculum of the hippocampal formation) and projects to the cingulate gyrus, and the *MD*

can relay signals from the amygdaloid nucleus to the frontal lobes (Chapter 16). The posterior parietal cortex (areas 5 and 7) receives fibers from the posterior part of the thalamus, the *lateral posterior nucleus* (LP), and parts of the *pulvinar* (Figs. 2.15, 2.23, and 17.7). Other parts of the pulvinar projects to the temporal lobe. The LP and the pulvinar receive afferents from nuclei related to vision and eye movements, such as the *superior colliculus* and the *pretectal nuclei,* and may relay such information to the posterior parietal cortex.

The Corticothalamic Connections

All of the thalamic nuclei receive massive connections from the cerebral cortex. In general, the nuclei receive afferents from the cortical areas to which they send their efferents—that is, the thalamocortical and the corticothalamic connections are *reciprocal.* The corticothalamic projections are also precisely, topographically organized. As mentioned, corticothalamic neurons have their perikarya mainly in layer 6, whereas projections to other subcortical nuclei arise mainly in layer 5. This indicates that the information received by the thalamus is not merely a copy of information sent from the cortex to other regions.

In view of the massive corticothalamic connections, the function of the thalamus is probably not limited to mediating information from subcortical cell groups to the cortex. In addition, the thalamus receives and presumably processes vast amounts of information from the cortex and is therefore intimately involved in processes taking place in the cortex itself. That the corticothalamic fibers really influence the information processing in the thalamus is witnessed by observations of the lateral geniculate body; the properties of the relay cells (thalamocortical) of the nucleus are in part determined by signals from the striate area.

The Thalamus Contains Numerous Interneurons: The Reticular Thalamic Nucleus

Inhibitory interneurons (GABA) probably constitute one-fourth or more of all neurons in some of the thalamic nuclei. In the thalamic sensory relay nuclei, the inhibitory interneurons may contribute to the enhancement of stimulus contrasts (by lateral inhibition) and to selection of certain kinds of stimuli by suppressing other kinds (for example, in relation to transmission of signals from nociceptors). Opioid peptides are present in several of the thalamic nuclei, including the sensory nuclei.

The *reticular thalamic nucleus* is unique among the thalamic nuclei because virtually all neurons are GABAergic. The nucleus, which forms a thin shell at the lateral aspect of the thalamus (Fig. 17.8), sends its efferent fibers in the medial direction to end in the other thalamic nuclei (and not to the cortex, differing also in this respect from the other thalamic nuclei). Both the corticothalamic and thalamocortical fibers pass through the reticular nucleus on their way to and from the thalamus and give off numerous collaterals that end in the nucleus. Furthermore, the reticular nucleus receives afferents from the mesencephalic reticular formation and has reciprocal

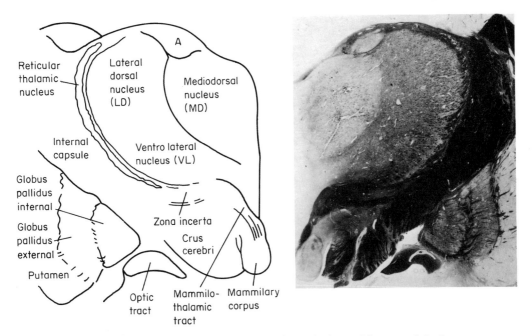

Fig. 17.8. *The thalamus.* Frontal section through the middle part of the human thalamus. Myelin stain. (See also Figs. 2.25 and 2.28.)

connections with the PAG (the latter nucleus is related to, among other things, the control of transmission of signals from nociceptors).

The function of the reticular thalamic nucleus is not clear, but its connections indicate that it can influence the activity of thalamocortical neurons and thus indirectly the activity of the cerebral cortex. Thalamocortical relay cells appear to be inhibited by the reticular nucleus shortly after being activated by sensory impulses.

The Intralaminar Thalamic Nuclei

Modern tracer studies have shown that the cortical projections from each of the intralaminar nuclei end in certain parts of the cortex only; for example, the CL nucleus sends fibers predominantly to the parietal cortex. Nevertheless, the projections are considerably more widespread and diffuse than those from the specific thalamic nuclei and do not respect areal borders (the intralaminar nuclei were formerly termed the unspecific thalamic nuclei). Physiological studies indicate that the intralaminar nuclei exert general effects on the excitability of cortical neurons. Thus, electrical stimulation produces a so-called *recruiting response* in extensive parts of the cortex, which resembles the EEG changes associated with arousal (desynchronization; see Chapter 12).

The tasks of the intralaminar nuclei are not only related to the cerebral cortex, since they have even stronger connections with the *striatum*. Such connections are precisely organized (another fact against the use of the term unspecific thalamic nuclei). We do not know the role of these thalamostriatal connections for the functioning of the basal ganglia.

Extrathalamic, Modulatory Connections to the Cerebral Cortex

Apart from the massive afferent connections to the cerebral cortex from the thalamus, several other subcortical cell groups provide sparser cortical inputs. This concerns the *raphe nuclei* (serotonin), the *nucleus locus coeruleus* (norepinephrine), *dopaminergic cell groups in the mesencephalon* (apart from the substantia nigra), and the *basal nucleus*. As mentioned, all of these groups project to large parts of the cortex with no distinct topographic pattern. Nevertheless, recent studies in monkeys show that each nucleus (and thus fibers with a particular transmitter) projects with a higher density to some than to other parts of the cortex. For example, dopaminergic fibers end with highest density in the prefrontal and temporal neocortex, whereas noradrenergic fibers innervate especially the central region (MI, SI). Furthermore, fibers from the various nuclei end in somewhat different cortical layers. A striking feature of the fibers is that, after having entered the cortex, they run horizontally for a considerable distance (in contrast to the vertical organization of the afferents from the specific thalamic nuclei).

It was formerly assumed that cortical afferents containing biogenic amines terminated in the cortex without forming typical synaptic contacts. More recent electron microscopic studies indicate, however, that many fibers do form synapses with cortical neurons.

Fibers from the above-mentioned nuclei appear to exert a modulatory control over the excitability level of cortical neurons, with relation to wakefulness and phases of sleep. In addition, they probably control more specifically selected neuronal groups in connection with our attention being directed to relevant, novel stimuli (see also Chapter 12 for more information about the ascending activating system, the raphe nuclei, and the nucleus locus coeruleus, and Chapter 16 for more about the basal nucleus).

Association Connections of the Cerebral Cortex

Vast numbers of association fibers ensure the cooperation of various parts of the cortex. The shortest association fibers connect minor parts within one area (so-called U fibers), whereas somewhat longer fibers link together neighboring areas. There are, for example, ample connections between the SI and area 5 posteriorly (Fig. 17.9) and the MI anteriorly. MI furthermore receives association fibers from the PMA and SMA (pre-

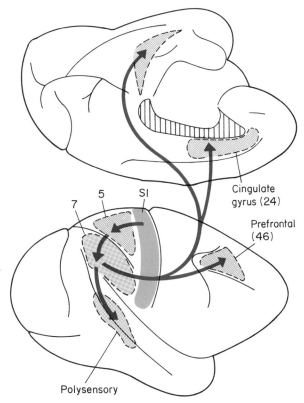

Fig. 17.9. *Association connections of the SI* (monkey). Only some fiber connections are shown, to illustrate the flow of information progressing from SI to the posterior parietal cortical areas, and from there to polysensory areas in the temporal lobe, to the prefrontal cortex, and to limbic cortical regions. Based on Jones and Powell (1970).

motor areas). The longest association fibers interconnect functionally related areas in different lobes. There are, for example, connections from the extrastriatal visual areas and the posterior parietal cortex to the premotor and prefrontal areas (Figs. 17.9 and 17.13).

When we follow the *association connections "outward" from the primary sensory areas (SI, VI, and AI), they progress toward areas that integrate sensory information of different modalities*—somatosensory and visual information converge in one area, visual and auditory in another, and so forth. The areas outside the primary sensory areas (like the areas of the posterior parietal cortex and the extrastriate areas) send their efferent projections not only to their immediate neighbors but also to distant areas in the frontal lobe (premotor and prefrontal areas) and to "limbic" cortical areas (the cingulate gyrus and the parahippocampal gyrus) (Figs. 17.9, 17.10, and 17.12).

The discussion so far may give the impression that the flow of information between various cortical areas goes only in one direction, but this is not the case. As a general rule *the association connections are reciprocal,* enabling areas to exert mutual influences. Certain differences exist, however, between the connections going in opposite directions between two areas. For example, fibers going outward from the striate area to the extrastriate areas end primarily in layer 4, whereas the projections in the opposite direction end in layers 1, 5, and 6. Possibly, the connections that are efferent from the sensory areas are involved in increasing integration and higher-level processing of sensory information, whereas the "backward" connections are of a feedback nature (the term feedback in this connection lacks precise meaning, however).

As a rule, each cortical area establishes association connections with several other

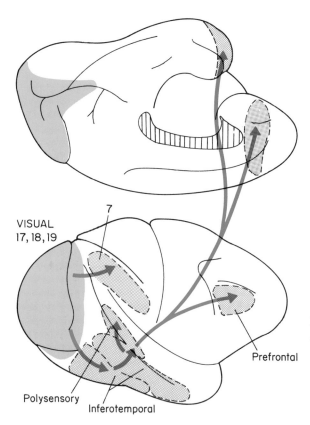

VISUAL
17, 18, 19

7

Prefrontal

Polysensory

Inferotemporal

Fig. 17.10. *Association connections of the visual cortex.* Compare with Figure 17.9 and note similarities with regard to the progression of information outward from the striate area. Only some connections are shown. Based on Jones and Powell (1970).

areas (Fig. 17.10); that is, there is a considerable *divergence* of information. At the same time, there is also considerable *convergence,* since each area receives afferents from several other areas.

Commissural Connections of the Cerebral Cortex

Most commissural fibers are found in the *corpus callosum* (Figs. 2.27 and 2.28). A small fraction (in humans, 1–2%) course in the *anterior commissure.* The latter fibers are believed to belong primarily to the olfactory pathways.[3] As a general rule, commissural fibers interconnect corresponding areas in the two hemispheres. The density of such fibers varies considerably among regions, however. Some regions are almost or totally devoid of commissural fibers (Fig. 17.11). This concerns primarily the striate area and parts of the MI and SI representing distal parts of the extremities (the regions

representing the hands and feet). Thus, regions of the cortex dealing with parts of the body that usually work in a symmetrical fashion (such as the two halves of the back) are amply interconnected, whereas parts that usually work independently (such as the hands) have few commissural fibers. A corresponding organization is present in the somatosensory and the motor pathways; connections related to distal body parts are entirely crossed, whereas connections related to proximal parts are to a greater extent bilateral. It seems possible that commissural connections between, for example, the hand areas, would disturb the independent control of the hands. It should be emphasized, however, that via commissural connections of other cortical areas, information about movement commands and sensory signals pertaining to the distal body parts reach both hemispheres.

We will return to the corpus callosum and the commissural connections later in this

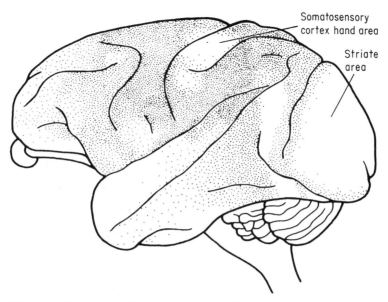

Somatosensory
cortex hand area

Striate
area

Fig. 17.11. *The total distribution of commissural connections* (monkey). Note the absence of commissural fibers to the striate area and the SI hand region. The MI hand region likewise lacks commissural connections but is not seen in the figure because it is largely buried in the central sulcus. From Myers (1965).

chapter when dealing with the sharing of tasks by the two hemispheres.

FUNCTIONS OF THE CEREBRAL CORTEX

Association Areas

For some of the cortical areas, functional aspects have been discussed in previous chapters. This concerns areas related to movement control such as the MI, PMA, and SMA. We have also dealt with the primary sensory areas, SI, VI, and AI, and discussed further processing of sensory information in neighboring areas. Parts of the cortex of importance for control of autonomic functions have been discussed in Chapter 16.

Here we will address primarily functions that can be ascribed to the so-called *association areas* of the cerebral cortex. This term is not precisely defined but is traditionally used of parts of the cortex that neither receive direct sensory information via the major sensory pathways nor send direct fibers to motoneuronal groups. All of the cerebral lobes contain association areas for which such a definition is used.

The connections of the association areas indicate that they are able to integrate information from sensory and "limbic" parts of the cortex and thereafter issue commands to motor cortical areas and (indirectly) to the hypothalamus.

Comparison of the cerebral hemispheres of humans and monkeys (Figs. 17.3, 17.9, 17.10, and 17.13) shows that the association areas occupy a much larger fraction of the total in humans than in monkeys. Comparison of monkeys with other mammals, such as cats and dogs, shows again that the main difference between them with regard to the cerebral cortex is the relative size of the association areas. These parts of the cortex are of importance for what we may loosely call *higher mental functions,* as we will discuss below. One should realize, however, that the individual association areas cannot be regarded as "centers" for specific mental faculties. First, several areas—often located in quite different parts of the hemisphere—participate in one task or function, and, fur-

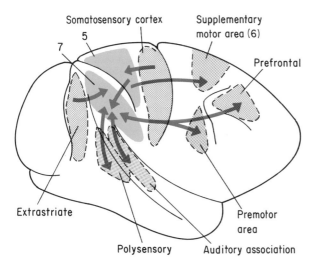

Fig. 17.12. *The association connections of the posterior parietal cortex* (monkey). Connections with the limbic cortical areas are not shown (see Fig. 17.9). Note the convergence of visual and somatosensory information in area 7.

thermore, one area participates more than one function. This is witnessed by the high degree of divergence and convergence of the connections of the association areas. Second, the operations of the association areas cannot be understood if considered in isolation; the intimate connections between the association areas and subcortical cell groups, like the thalamus and the limbic structures, are essential for normal functioning.

Measurements of regional cerebral blood flow and metabolism during the performance of various cognitive tasks indicate that *large parts of the cortex participate in all higher mental functions.* When a person is asked to imagine that she is walking from one place to another in a city she knows, the activity increases in the extrastriate visual areas, in the posterior parietal cortex, in parts of the temporal lobe, and in several prefrontal areas. Solving a mathematical problem activates many of the same cortical areas but with certain differences, and a verbal task activates multiple areas that partly coincide with and partly differ from those activated in the spatial and the mathematical tasks.

Parietal Association Areas

Usually areas 5 and 7—located in the upper and lower parietal lobules, respectively—are considered to constitute the parietal associ-

ation cortex (Figs. 4.19, 17.3, and 17.12).[4] The term *posterior parietal cortex* is also used of this region. Both areas 5 and 7 can be further subdivided into parts differing in connections and functional properties. These areas are intercalated between the visual cortical areas in the occipital lobe and the somatosensory cortex in the anterior parietal cortex. Functionally, as one might expect from this location, areas 5 and 7 process and integrate somatosensory and visual information. From these areas, signals are conveyed to premotor and motor areas (Fig. 17.12), explaining why lesions of the posterior parietal cortex can produce disturbances of voluntary movements. The posterior parietal cortical areas also have ample connections (both ways) with the cingulate gyrus (Fig. 16.3) and the prefrontal cortex. These connections are assumed to mediate the influence of emotions, attention, and motivation on behavior produced by somatosensory and visual stimuli.

Experiments with recording of *single-cell activity* in *area 5* of the monkey indicate that this area is essential for the *proper use of somatosensory information, for goal-directed voluntary movements, and for the manipulation of objects,* as expressed by the Finnish neurophysiologist Hyvärinen. This fits well with the symptoms occurring in humans after damage to the posterior parietal cortex, as will be discussed below.

Single-cell recordings indicate that *area 7* has an important role in the integration of visual and somatosensory stimuli, which is essential for the coordination of the eye and the hand—that is, for visual guidance of movements. Area 7 is also involved in the control of eye movements, as discussed in Chapter 13.

Humans with lesions of the posterior parietal cortex have difficulties with the *transformation of sensory stimuli into adequate motor actions.* The understanding of the meaning of sensory stimuli is seriously impaired (but usually not the mere recognition of a stimulus). This is called *agnosia* (depending on the sensory quality concerned, we use terms such as visual agnosia, tactile agnosia, and so forth). The patient is also unable to use well-known tools and objects. This symptom is called *apraxia.* They furthermore have problems with visually guided movements (such as stretching out the arm to obtain an object). Similar symptoms may occur also after lesions of other parts of the hemisphere, for example apraxia caused by a frontal lobe lesion.

Properties of Single Cells in the Posterior Parietal Cortex

Studies of monkeys with permanently implanted electrodes have demonstrated a wide repertoire of properties among neurons in areas 5 and 7. Common to many is that a task-related increase in firing frequency occurs only when a stimulus is *relevant* and the attention of the animal is directed toward the stimulus. Thus, it is virtually impossible to activate many neurons when the animal is drowsy and inattentive. Some cells respond to stimulation of proprioceptors, but their response is much more vigorous when a movement (stimulating the proprioceptors) is self-initiated by the monkey than when the joint is passively manipulated by the examiner. In area 5, many neurons change their firing frequency in relation to manipulatory hand movements. Other neurons increase their firing in relation to reaching movements, but only when the hand is moved toward an object the monkey wants to obtain (such as an orange). The increase of firing in such neurons starts at the time the animal discovers the object—that is, *before* the arm movement starts—and is therefore not a result of pro-

prioceptive stimulation. Mountcastle, who first described such neurons, suggested that they may function as command neurons for the target-directed exploration of our immediate surrounding extrapersonal space. Such neurons appear to respond to the coincidence of two events: a sensory stimulus (for example, the sight of an orange) and a signal that depends on motivation (whether the monkey is hungry and wants the orange).

Lesions of the Posterior Parietal Cortex in Humans

The most marked symptom produced by bilateral parietal lesions is the inability to grasp and to manipulate objects. Thus, the patient may be unable to *move the hand toward an object* that is clearly seen, even though there are no pareses and no visual defects. Movements that do not require visual guidance, such as buttoning, bringing an object to the mouth, and so forth, are performed normally. When the patient is asked to pour water from a bottle into a glass, he pours the water outside the glass over and over again, even though he can see clearly both the bottle and the glass. Such patients also have severe difficulties with the appraisal of distances and the size of objects. Furthermore, to fix the gaze becomes difficult, especially to direct the gaze toward a point in the periphery of the visual field. The identification of objects is difficult, because of the *inability to attend to more than one detail at a time* (such as seeing a cigarette but not the person who smokes it). This may be a fundamental defect after parietal lobe lesions, perhaps also explaining the difficulties mentioned above with pouring water into a glass (the patient is unable to locate in space the bottle and the glass at the same time).

Patients with parietal lobe lesions typically have difficulties with *drawing* an object or a scene; again the inability to perceive more than one feature at a time is the probable basic defect. The parts of an object are drawn separately, without the proper spatial relations, or the drawing gives an extremely simplified representation. This symptom occurs most often after damage to the right parietal cortex, in cases of unilateral lesions. The *use of tools* is also difficult or impossible: For example, the patient no longer knows how to use a hammer (apraxia).

Unilateral lesions of the right parietal lobe typically produce *negligence of the opposite body half and visual space.* Such a patient behaves as if the left part of his body does not exist. He dresses only the right side, shaves only the right half of the face, and so forth. He may, for example, deny that the left leg belongs to him and claim that it belongs to the person in the adjacent bed. When drawing a face, for example, the right side is drawn normally, whereas the left side is vague or not included in the drawing.

Even though the symptoms mentioned above are most often seen after damage of the posterior parietal cortex, most of them have been described after lesions in other parts of the brain too, especially of the prefrontal cortex, the thalamus, and the basal ganglia (all of these have connections with the parietal cortex).

A peculiar constellation of symptoms, the *Gerstmann syndrome,* can occur after lesions of the parietal lobe at the transition to the temporal lobe (usually of the left hemisphere). The symptoms are as follows: *finger agnosia* (the patient cannot recognize and distinguish the various fingers on her own or other people's hands), *agraphia* (inability to write), sometimes *alexia* (inability to read), *right–left confusion,* and, finally, *dyscalculia* (reduced ability to perform simple calculations, especially to distinguish categories of numbers such as tens, hundreds, and so forth). The most distinctive feature of the syndrome is the finger agnosia, which can occur in isolation. That finger agnosia can be the only symptom of a parietal lobe lesion indicates that a disproportionally large part of the human parietal cortex is devoted to the hand. Thus, the hand has a unique role as an exploratory sense organ and as a tool, and, furthermore, it has a special place in our inner, mental, body image. The British neurologist Critchley expressed it as follows: "The hand is largely an organ of the parietal lobe."

The Parietal Lobe and the Development of the Ability to Integrate Somatosensory and Visual Information

The ability to integrate somatosensory and visual information and to use visual information to guide voluntary movements is not inborn but learned in infancy and early childhood. Persons who were born blind but get back the visual sense as young adults do not manage to coordinate the visual information with the other senses and therefore cannot utilize the "new" sense. They usually continue to use tactile sensation to "see" objects, and the visual information can in fact be more confusing than helpful.

Studies by Hyvärinen and co-workers show that the properties of single cells in the parietal cortex change during the phase in which an infant monkey learns to coordinate visual and somatosensory information. Monkeys were prevented from seeing from birth (by suturing the eyelids) until they were between 6 months and 1 year old. At that time few cells in area 7 responded to visual stimuli, in contrast to the normal situation at that age. An abnormally large fraction of the cells were activated by passive somatosensory stimuli and by active movements. Most striking was the almost total absence of cells that could be activated by both somatosensory and visual stimuli. Even 2 years after reestablishment of normal vision, the single-cell properties of area 7 remained virtually unaltered, with very few cells responding to visual stimuli. Properties of cells of the extrastriate cortex (area 19) were also altered in the visually deprived monkeys; some cells were, for example, activated by somatosensory stimuli (which never occurred in normal monkeys), and there were fewer than normal visually driven cells.

Behaviorally, the monkeys were blind after opening of the eyes, and no improvement occurred during the next month. They bumped into obstacles, fell off tables, and were unable to retrieve food by sight alone. They were not frightened by threatening faces, in contrast to normal monkeys at the same age. One monkey that was observed for 3 years improved to some extent, but it never regained the full use of the visual sense.

The above data indicate that the functional properties of neurons in the association areas, and thus the capacity of the areas to contribute to certain tasks, are determined to a large extent in early childhood. Furthermore, there is only a limited possibility of regaining the proper function of these regions at a later stage.

The experiments also show that when one kind of sensory information is lacking during an early stage of development, other sensory modalities take over parts of the cortex not normally used for processing that kind of sensory information.

Frontal Association Areas

In this context we use the term *association cortex* only about the prefrontal cortex—that is, the parts of the frontal lobe in front of areas 6 (PMA, SMA) and 8 (the frontal eye

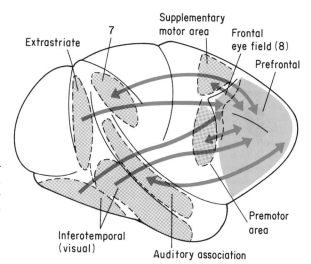

Fig. 17.13. *The association connections of the prefrontal cortex* (monkey). Note the convergence of all kinds of processed sensory information and the connections with PMA and SMA. Connections with limbic cortical areas are not shown (see Figs. 16.3 and 16.4).

field) (Fig. 17.3). The prefrontal cortex consists of several different cytoarchitectonic areas, each with a specific set of connections. Together, the areas receive strong connections from areas in the occipital, parietal, and temporal lobes and, in addition, from the cingulate gyrus (Fig. 17.13). Thalamic afferents come from the MD (Fig. 17.7), which in turn receives afferents from the amygdala (among other places). Together, the prefrontal cortex appears to *receive information about all sensory modalities* and also about *the motivational and emotional state* of the individual. The prefrontal cortex sends fibers back to most of the areas from which it receives afferents, among them the *SMA* and the *PMA*. In addition, many prefrontal efferents reach the caudate nucleus of the *striatum* (Fig. 10.5). Finally, some efferents reach the *hypothalamus*.

The symptoms that occur in humans and monkeys with *lesions of the prefrontal cortex* are at least partially different from those occurring after lesions of other parts of the hemispheres. For example, there are usually changes of mood and personality. Commonly, large lesions produce apathy, indifference, and emotional leveling-off. The patient appears to be uncritical compared with before the damage. He may, for example, behave in a complacent and boastful manner, which he would never have done before. The

ability to alter the behavior on the basis of experience from previous actions appears to be reduced. Clear-cut symptoms occur usually only after bilateral damage to the prefrontal cortex.

More About Symptoms After Lesions of the Prefrontal Cortex

A striking defect after bilateral lesions of the dorsolateral prefrontal cortex is the lack of the so-called *delayed response*. A monkey sees that food is put into one of two bowls. Then the sight of the bowls is blocked for up to 10 minutes before the monkey is allowed to choose one of the two. In contrast to normal monkeys, the lesioned ones do not remember which bowl contained the food (even though they do not show reduced performance in other more complicated memory tests). The dorsolateral parts of the prefrontal cortex thus appear to be necessary for the *ability to form and retain an inner conception of the existence of an object in time and space* when the object is no longer seen. Interestingly, humans manage a similar test first at the age of about 1 year. Before that age, everything that is not seen or felt is presumably nonexistent for the infant.

A characteristic symptom in humans with prefrontal lesions is the *inability to alter the response when the stimulus changes*—they continue to make the same response even though it is no longer adequate. This phenomenon is called *perseveration*. The so-called Wisconsin card sort test is often used to reveal such a defect. The person is asked to sort cards in accordance with certain general rules, such as color, number, shape, and so forth. The correct rule to be applied is indicated by the response given by the examiner to the first attempts at sorting the cards. The rules can be changed without warning. Normal persons understand fairly quickly that the rule has been changed and alter their responses accordingly, whereas patients with prefrontal lesions continue sorting in accordance with the first rule, in spite of repeated warnings that they are making mistakes.

Emotional and personality changes after frontal lobe lesions are difficult to evaluate, and the premorbid personality of the patients appears to play a decisive role. Nevertheless, a general tendency is for the patients to become less emotional and to show reduced emotional reactions to events. They also have difficulties in extracting the salient features from a complex situation, making their responses unpredictable and often inadequate. A test designed for such symptoms utilizes drawings of complex situations, in part with a dramatic content, such as a man who has fallen through the ice on a lake and is in danger of drowning. Patients with frontal lesions usually attend only to details, saying, for example, "Since there is a sign saying 'Careful!' on the beach, there may be a high-voltage cable nearby." This kind of reduction results in inability to foresee the consequences of one's own actions, and poor insight into other people's circumstances. This leads to poor social adaptation, with isolation as the final result.

The reduced capacity to retain inner conceptions is most likely the reason why such patients have increased distractibility, with reduced ability to perform tasks that require continuous activity and attention. Motor hyperactivity, which can be a symptom, may perhaps result from the increased distractibility. Thus, in monkeys with prefrontal lesions, the hyperactivity disappears when they are placed in an environment with few stimuli.

In humans with frontal lobe tumors (for example, a glioma or a metastasis from a malignant tumor elsewhere), a depressive disorder has been observed. This may rather be a condition of deemotionalization and social isolation.

The Frontal Lobes and Psychiatric Disease

Ever since the first accurate description of psychiatric diseases such as schizophrenia, it has been postulated that the disease is caused by alteration of the frontal lobes. This assumption was partly based on similarities between the symptoms in schizophrenia and in cases of frontal lobe damage. Whether the symptoms of schizophrenia are caused by organic brain changes, however, is still not clarified. Other parts of the brain than the frontal lobes have been implicated, too, such as certain limbic structures.

The fact that the drugs commonly used for the treatment of psychotic disorders are antidopaminergic gave rise to the hypothesis that schizophrenia is caused by disturbances of dopamine actions pre- or postsynaptically (alterations of other biogenic amines may play a role, too). The problem with examining the brains of schizophrenic patients after their death is that they almost always have been treated with antidopaminergic drugs for a long time. Thus, observed changes of, for example, dopamine receptor density and dopamine content can therefore be a result of the treatment and not of the disease. The same reservations hold for the interpretation of postmortal structural changes.

Various morphological changes have been observed in the brains of schizophrenic patients, including cell loss in the frontal lobes and in limbic structures, but often such findings are not confirmed by later studies. Measurements of regional blood flow lend some support to the theory that the frontal lobes may be involved in some manner. Thus, many schizophrenics have been reported to have abnormally low blood flow in the prefrontal cortex, and various tasks that give increased flow in normal people failed to do so in these patients. Even these results are controversial, however.

The Temporal Association Cortex

A unitary functional role is even less evident for the temporal association areas than for those in the parietal and frontal lobes. Apart from the auditory cortex (areas 41 and 42) (Fig. 6.10) and the phylogenetically old parts at the medial aspect (Fig. 16.1), the temporal lobe consists largely of areas 20, 21, and 22, which here are considered the association areas (Fig. 17.3).

The cortex of the *superior temporal gyrus* is characterized by its *connections with the auditory cortex,* whereas the inferior parts of the temporal lobe—the *inferotemporal cortex*—are dominated by *processed visual information* from the extrastriate visual areas.

In addition, there are strong connections with *limbic structures* such as the hippocampal formation (via the entorhinal area) and the amygdala (Figs. 16.4 and 16.7). Finally, long association fibers interconnect the temporal association areas with the *prefrontal cortex* (Fig. 17.13).

Bilateral damage of the temporal lobes produces pronounced *amnesia*, which can be ascribed largely to the destruction of the hippocampal region (there are also symptoms caused by the concomitant destruction of the amygdala located in the tip of the temporal lobe). These aspects were discussed in Chapter 16. In addition, the patients become very *distractible*—they have difficulties in maintaining their attention on a certain stimulus or task. Finally, psychic blindness or *visual agnosia* is a typical symptom of temporal lobe lesions affecting the inferotemporal parts. The patient is unable to recognize objects and persons she sees, even though her vision is normal. As for other association areas, it is the interpretation of sensory information that is deficient, not the sensory experience as such.

Experimental Studies of the Temporal Association Cortex

Electrical stimulation of the temporal association cortex in awake humans can recall memories of past events or produce dreamlike sequences of imagined events. Such data come largely from pioneer studies made by the Canadian neurosurgeon Penfield, in which he stimulated the temporal lobe and other parts of the cortex in awake patients (in whom the cortex was exposed under local anesthesia for therapeutic reasons). In monkeys, some single neurons of the temporal cortex respond only when the monkey sees, for example, a face or a hand. Some neurons respond preferentially to one particular face, whereas other neurons respond to any face. A neuron that responds briskly when the monkey is shown a drawing of a face may stop firing when important features are removed, such as the mouth or the eyes.

The inferotemporal cortex is especially of importance for the interpretation of complex visual stimuli, as judged from experiments in monkeys. Thus bilateral removal of these regions makes the monkeys unable to recognize and distinguish complex visual patterns. These and other observations lead to the conclusion that the inferotemporal cortex is of special importance for the *categorization of complex visual stimuli.*

Stimulation of the *insula,* which is hidden at the bottom lateral fissure (Fig. 2.30), produces mostly chewing movements, changed respiratory pattern, abdominal sensations, altered peristaltic movements of the gut, and other vegetative phenomena.

Language Functions and "Speech Areas" of the Cerebral Cortex

Clinical observations in the past century led to the identification of two so-called speech areas in the left hemisphere (Fig. 17.14). That speech depends almost entirely on only one hemisphere—in most people, the left— is the most marked and best-known example of *laterlization* (of function) or *hemispheric dominance.* We will return to the topic of lateralization below.

What are termed speech areas should,

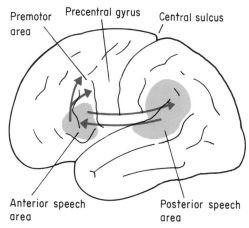

Fig. 17.14. *Speech areas of the human brain.* Lesions of the anterior speech area (of Broca) produce predominantly motor aphasia, whereas lesions of the posterior speech area produce mainly sensory aphasia. The posterior speech area as shown here comprises parts of the inferior parietal lobulus that were not included in the area described by Wernicke. Note the long association fibers interconnecting the two areas. These connections explain why a lesion in between the two speech areas can produce aphasia (so-called conductance aphasia).

more correctly, be termed "areas of aphasia," since we know that their destruction produces various disturbances of language functions (aphasia), but we know little of how these areas contribute to the normal production of language and speech.

Very schematically, there are two main types of aphasia.[5] The simplest type is the so-called *motor aphasia*. This occurs most often after destruction of an area in front of the precentral (MI) face area, called *Broca's area* or the anterior speech area. The patient more or less completely loses the ability to speak, and typically produces only single words in a sort of telegram style. The few words used may also be applied wrongly. Other names used of this type are *nonfluent aphasia* (because the speech becomes stuttering) and *expressive aphasia*. The understanding of language is usually preserved, whereas the production of speech is deficient. Nevertheless, there are no signs of pareses of the muscles involved in speech production. Often, motor aphasia is combined with *agraphia*—the inability to express language in writing.

In patients with *sensory or receptive aphasia,* the lesion usually affects more posterior parts of the hemisphere at the junction between the parietal, temporal, and occipital lobes (Fig. 17.14). This region is called *Wernicke's* or the *posterior speech area*. Typically, the comprehension of language is most severely affected. The various elementary sounds are not properly put together to form meaningful words and sentences. Words that are heard cannot be repeated. In contrast to motor aphasia, spontaneous speech is fluent, but sounds are often put together into meaningless words, and proper words lack relation to each other ("word–salad"). Usually, sensory aphasia is combined with *alexia*—the inability to read.

In reality, pure forms of aphasia as described above are very seldom encountered; in most patients there is a mixture of motor and sensory symptoms, with one or the other dominating. Often there are other symptoms as well, since lesions of the hemispheres are very seldom confined to the speech areas. There are, furthermore, similarities between word blindness (alexia, dyslexia) and visual agnosia, which may be caused by lesions of the parietal lobe and the inferotemporal cortex. On the other hand, elementary symptoms of aphasia—such as agraphia or alexia—may sometimes occur in isolation or in combination with other kinds of symptoms (cf. Gerstmann's syndrome, described above).

It should also be emphasized that the relationship between specific aphasic symptoms and the anatomic location of a brain lesion is not absolute. Virtually all forms of aphasia have been described after lesions in unexpected parts of the brain. Thus, we can only say that the probability of speech disturbances is highest when the lesion affects one or both of the areas depicted in Figure 17.14 (or the association fibers interconnecting the anterior and posterior speech areas).

The Function of the Commissural Connections: The Corpus Callosum

The fact that the two hemispheres are connected by afferent and efferent fiber tracts with the opposite body half is proof that there is a division of tasks between the hemispheres. This does not mean, of course, that the two hemispheres are independent units—the *commissural connections* ensure that information reaching one hemisphere also reaches the other and that commands issued to lower parts of the brain also are known to both hemispheres. Complex functions are often carried out by cooperation of the two hemispheres, and we have mentioned examples above that lesions of the association areas often have to be bilateral to produce clear-cut functional deficits.

We will mention a few examples of the significance of the commissural connections. When the optic nerve fibers that cross in the chiasma are cut (Figs. 5.11 and 5.17), impulses from one eye reach only the hemisphere of the same side. After such an operation, monkeys are trained in a visual discrimination task (to distinguish a triangle and a circle to obtain a fruit reward) with a patch occluding vision in the left eye. The learning must depend on processes taking place in the right hemisphere, which receives visual information from the right eye. When the monkey has learned the task with the right eye, the occlusion is reversed. Nevertheless, even when using the left eye, the monkey solves the task as well as when using the right eye. Thus, the left hemisphere must also have learned the task. This must be dependent on an effective transmission of visual information from one hemisphere to the other, as can be demonstrated by cutting also the corpus callosum (and the anterior commissure) before the discrimination training starts. Then the animal learns the task only with the right hemisphere when the left eye is occluded. The transmission of visual information from one hemisphere to the other in this experiment must depend on commissural connections between the extrastriate and probably the inferotemporal areas, since the striate area lacks commissural fibers (Fig. 17.11).

Corresponding experiments have shown that tactile and kinesthetic sensations are also transferred through the corpus callosum. A monkey with transection of the corpus callosum (and the anterior commissure) is trained to open a box with the right hand only (without being allowed to see the box). After some training, the opening is performed swiftly. If, however, the monkey then is prevented from using the right hand, the task has to be learned over again with the left hand—no learning had taken place in the right hemisphere (which controls the left hand). A monkey with an intact corpus callosum uses both hands with identical dexterity to solve this task, even though only one hand was used during the training period.

There is a certain topographic arrangement of the commissural fibers within the corpus callosum. As one might expect, the posterior parts are necessary for the transfer of visual information, whereas the anterior and middle parts are necessary for transfer of somatosensory signals.

The ample commissural connections make it possible for the two hemispheres to specialize and to share tasks between them. Both are not required to be equally good at all tasks. Nevertheless, they keep each other constantly informed (just as one would expect of hospital specialists sharing the responsibility for one patient). The brain, even though in a sense consisting of two anatomic parts, functions as a unit for the whole body and our extrapersonal space. The degree of hemispheric specialization or lateralization of functions can be studied only after eliminating the callosal transfer of information.

Cerebral Lateralization and Dominance

A wealth of information on this topic has been provided by the study of patients in whom the corpus callosum has been transected (this is done in severe cases of epilepsy, to prevent spread of the abnormal discharges from one hemisphere to the other). The American Sperry was awarded the Nobel Prize in 1981 for his pioneering studies of so-called *split brain* patients. Even though lateralization is probably most marked in humans, there is much evidence that it occurs also in animals (for example, the ability to sing depends on cell groups in the left side of the brain in birds). Certain anatomic differences between the two hemispheres appear to exist in most humans. Thus, in about 70% the upper face of the temporal lobe (the temporal plane) in the vicinity of the auditory cortex is more extensive on the left than on the right side. The difference appears to be present before birth,[6] and recent studies indicate that the lateralization of language functions is determined prenatally. It is well known that early brain damage (in infancy, before language has been acquired) has less severe effects on language functions than lesions occurring later. Since, obviously, in such early cases of brain damage the right hemisphere can take over the language functions, it was concluded that language function is not initially lateralized. However, a more likely interpretation is that even though there is an inborn tendency for lateralization of speech, at an early stage the right hemisphere has not been fully occupied by other tasks and therefore can substitute for the left hemisphere. At later stages, both hemispheres are fully used and specialized for specific tasks and therefore unable to take over new complex functions.

Patients who have been subjected to so-called commissurotomy (transection of the corpus callosum) manage well in everyday life, mainly because visual information reaches both hemispheres (because we move the gaze constantly) and there are some bilateral sensory and motor pathways. They get into trouble, however, if, for example, somatosensory information is not supplemented with visual information. The above example of the commissurotomized monkey and tactile learning is relevant for split-brain patients, too. In some situations conflicts may arise between commands issued from the two hemispheres; the left hemisphere may, for example, command the right hand to start dressing, whereas the left hand is ordered to undress.

When one hemisphere is most important for a certain function, we say that it is *dominant* for that function, whereas the other hemisphere is recessive. The most clear-cut example of such cerebral dominance—or, in other words, lateralization of function—is *speech,* as mentioned above.[7] Thus, for most people, even for most left-handed persons, the left hemisphere is responsible for language functions. Various investigations have confirmed the lateralization of language. Studies of split-brain patients are especially instructive in this respect. They confirm, among other things, that the right hemisphere is mute in most people (even though it may express single words when strong emotions are aroused). When a split-brain patient is asked to identify with the right hand an object that is not seen, he can easily tell the name of the object, what it is used for, and so forth. This is because the tactile information comes to the left, speech-dominant hemisphere. When the left hand is used for the same test, however, the patient is unable to name the object, because the in-

formation reaches only the "mute" right hemisphere. The patient nevertheless shows signs of adequate emotional reactions to the object. That the right hemisphere "understands" the nature of the object is further supported by other experiments in which the right hemisphere is presented with a picture of, for example, a key. Even though the patient cannot say anything about the object, he nevertheless picks out with the left hand a key among several objects (which are not seen).

Not *all* aspects of language function are necessarily localized to the dominant hemisphere. The modulation and melody of the sounds of speech, *prosody,* may be localized to the right hemisphere, as witnessed by several clinical reports. Thus, in some patients who have had a stroke without aphasia, prosody has been reported to be changed or reduced. Since prosody is, at least in part, emotional expression, the dominance of the right hemisphere would fit with other observations of right-hemisphere specialization.

With regard to *lateralization of hand functions,* the hemispheric differences are less clear-cut than for language. It is of course not a question of the ability to use the hand, but a matter of preference of one hand for most or all tasks. Even though hand preference is inheritable, there are also strong social factors that contribute to the final outcome of hand preference, for example, in writing. There is most likely a gradual transition with regard to the strength of hand preference, from those with a strong tendency to use the right hand for all tasks if possible (writing, drawing, use of tools, eating, and so forth) to those with an equally strong tendency to use the left hand. The latter group probably constitutes 2% to 3% of the total population. Hand preference starts to become expressed from the second year of life and is usually finally established at the age of 5 to 6.

There is not a strong correlation between the lateralization of speech and hand preference. Thus, for about 95% of the population, the left hemisphere is dominant for speech, whereas the corresponding number for left-handedness is 70%. Thus, only about 30% of left-handed people have right-hemisphere speech dominance.

Whereas many studies show that the left hemisphere usually is superior with regard to analytical and logical thinking as expressed verbally and in numbers, the right hemisphere is superior with regard to spatial abilities, the comprehension of complicated patterns, and drawing. Observations of split-brain patients furthermore indicate that the right hemisphere is dominant with regard to the expression of emotions.[8]

Studies of split-brain patients raise interesting questions, such as whether the two hemispheres have independent consciousness and what the relation is between consciousness and language and between intelligence and language. No simple answers are available to such questions addressing phenomena in the transition zone between neuroscience, philosophy, and religion. To argue that man consists of two personalities, one in each of the hemispheres, is of course a gross oversimplification. The normal cooperation and interaction between the hemispheres is so intimate that our mental life and behavior are caused by their collective activities.

Further Examples of Lateralization

A certain degree of "ear dominance" exists in most people, which correlates well with the speech lateralization—that is, the right ear is dominant for most people. This phenomenon can be studied by use of so-called *dichotic listening*. Two words are presented at the same time, one to each ear. Afterwards, most people say that they heard the word presented to the right ear.

It has proved difficult to localize the ability to appreciate and express *music* to one of the two hemispheres. *Amusia* most often occurs together with aphasia, but it has also been reported to occur in isolation. It has been customary to say that the right hemisphere is dominant with regard to, for example, the perception of a melody and that with high-level musical training (professional musicians), the left hemisphere becomes increasingly important. Studies of musicians after brain strokes have not confirmed such assumptions, however.

Visual field dominance has been described in studies in which different visual stimuli are presented to the two hemispheres simultaneously. With regard to written words and letters, there is a tendency to prefer those presented in the right visual field (that is, those transferred to the left hemisphere). For the recognition of faces, the reverse situation appears to exist for most people, as can be demonstrated by the presentation of so-called chimeric portraits composed of two left halves and two right halves, respectively. The person is asked which of the chimeric portraits most resembles the original (authentic) portrait. Most persons claim that the chimeric portrait consisting of two right facial halves most resembles the original. This is taken to suggest that the right hemisphere dominates in the analysis of faces and other complex visual patterns. Another indication of this is that when the shape of letters is made sufficiently ornate, the right hemisphere appears to become necessary for their interpretation.

Lateralization and Sex Differences

Some studies have been taken to show that men, on the average, have better visuospatial abilities than women. This has furthermore been interpreted as related to another alleged sex difference—namely that men have stronger lateralization of visuospatial functions, whereas women to a higher extent use both hemispheres for such tasks (it is not obvious, however, that a strong lateralization gives a higher visuospatial ability—the reverse might just as well be the case). It was then studied whether there might be sex differences in the cross-sectional area of the corpus callosum, which would correlate with differences in lateralization; that is, a corpus callosum with relatively few fibers was expected to correlate with a high degree of lateralization. Indeed, some studies reported that the corpus callosum is relatively larger in cross section in women than in men.

Neither of the above points has been confirmed by further and more comprehensive studies, however. Thus, there are about as many reports of no sex differences with regard to visuospatial abilities as there are reports of differences, and even the reported differences constitute merely a few percent of the individual variations among members of the same sex. Furthermore, the sex differences in the size of the corpus callosum are at best very small, whereas the individual variations again are surprisingly large. One report claimed in fact that the corpus callosum is about 10% larger in left-handers (and persons using both hands equally) than in right-handers. This does not support a correlation between superior visuospatial abilities, strong lateralization, and a small corpus callosum. Thus, left-handedness is most common among boys, and it is usually considered that left-handers have better visuospatial (and mathematical) abilities than right-handers.

In conclusion, the available data do not support firm conclusions as to possible relations among sex, hand dominance, and visuospatial abilities.

NOTES

1. Some of the nonpyramidal cells are multipolar and are called *stellate cells*. Others are called *basket cells* because their axonal branches form a wickerwork around the perikarya of pyramidal cells. There are in addition several other varieties, given names that as a rule reflect the shape of the neuron.

2. Formerly, the term *granule cells* was used of the small cortical neurons, explaining the names of layers 2 and 4, which contain mainly small perikarya. Many of the so-called granule cells are in fact small pyramidal cells, and the term granule cell should therefore not be used of cortical neurons.

3. In the monkey the anterior commissure contains about 5% of all commissural fibers, many of which link corresponding parts of the temporal lobes.

4. There is some disagreement in the literature with regard to the parcellation of the posterior parietal cortex in humans. Brodmann (Fig. 17.3) placed areas 5 and 7 in the superior parietal lobule, whereas the inferior lobule contained areas 39 and 40. Vogt (and others), however, described area 5 as located in the superior parietal lobule and area 7 in the inferior—that is, corresponding to the situation in monkeys.

5. There is an enormous literature dealing with the disturbances of speech and language, and there are numerous classifications of aphasias. Also, there is no lack of hypotheses, whereas understanding of the basic mechanisms underlying language and speech is still limited. This should come as no surprise, however, considering the complexity of the function in question.

6. It should be noted, however, that in more than 90% of persons the language function depends on the left hemisphere. Thus, the relationship between speech lateralization and anatomic asymmetry is not absolute.

7. It was formerly often assumed that one hemisphere, usually the left, was dominant for all functions and that the right hemisphere was recessive in all respects. It was also assumed that dominance for speech and for hand functions was closely linked.

8. Some studies indicate that patients with strokes affecting the left hemisphere tend to have more depressive reactions than patients with corresponding right-sided lesions (the "emotional" right hemisphere understands the agony of the left?). Right hemisphere lesions, especially when they affect the frontal lobe, appear to have a stronger tendency to produce a somewhat inadequate elevation of mood.

LITERATURE

TEXTBOOKS AND REFERENCE WORKS

Adelman, G. *Encyclopedia of neuroscience.* Birkhauser, 1987.

Brodal, A. *Neurological anatomy in relation to clinical medicine.* Oxford University Press, 1981.

Carpenter, M. B., and Sutin, J. *Human neuroanatomy,* 8th ed. Williams and Wilkins 1983.

Heimer, L. *The human brain and spinal cord. Functional neuroanatomy and dissection guide.* Springer-Verlag, 1983.

Kandel, E., et. al. *Principles of neural science,* 3d ed. Elsevier, 1991.

Kuffler, S. W., et al. *From neuron to brain. A cellular approach to the function of the nervous system,* 2nd ed. Sinauer Associates, 1984.

Martin, J. H. *Neuroanatomy. Text and atlas.* Elsevier, 1989.

Matthews, G. *Cellular physiology of nerve and muscle.* Blackwell, 1985.

McGeer, P. L., and Eccles, J. C. *Molecular neurobiology of the mammalian brain,* 2nd ed. Plenum Press, 1987.

Ottoson, D. *Physiology of the nervous system.* Macmillan Press, 1983.

Paxinos, G. *The human nervous system.* Academic Press, 1990.

Rauber/Kopsch. *Anatomie des Menschen. Band III. Nervensystem. Sinnesorgane.* Georg Thieme Verlag, 1987.

Schmidt, R. F. *Fundamentals of neurophysiology,* 3rd ed. Springer-Verlag, 1985.

Schmidt, R. F. *Fundamentals of sensory physiology,* 3rd ed. Springer-Verlag, 1986.

Shepherd, G. M. *Neurobiology,* 2nd ed. Oxford University Press, 1988.

Smith, C. U. M. *Elements of molecular neurobiology.* John Wiley & Sons, 1989.

ATLASES

DeArmond, S. J. et al. *Structure of the human brain. A photographic atlas,* 3rd ed. Oxford University Press, 1989.

Gouaze, A., and Salomon, G. *Brain anatomy and magnetic resonance imaging.* Springer-Verlag, 1988.

Haines, D. E. *Correlative neuroanatomy. The anatomical basis for some common neurological deficits.* Urban & Schwarzenberg, 1985.

Haines, D. E. *Neuroanatomy. An atlas of structures, sections, and systems,* 2nd ed. Urban & Schwarzenberg, 1987.

Miller, R. A., and Burack, E. *Atlas of the central nervous system in man,* 3rd ed. Williams & Wilkins, 1983.

Nieuwenhuys, R. *Chemoarchitecture of the brain.* Springer-Verlag, 1985.

Nieuwenhuys, R., Voogd, J., and van Huijzen, C. *The human central nervous system. A synopsis and atlas,* 3rd ed. Springer-Verlag, 1988.

Olszewski, J. *Cytoarchitecture of the human brain stem.* Karger, 1954.

Roberts, M. P. *Atlas of the human brain in section.* Lea & Febiger, 1987.

CHAPTER 1

Structure and Function of Nervous Tissue

Atwood, H. L., and Lnenicka, G. A. Structure and function in synapses: Emerging correlations. Trends Neurosci. 9:248–250, 1986.

Cajal, R. Y. *Histologie du systeme nerveux,* Vol. I–II, Instituto Ramon Y Cajal, 1952.

Calcium and neuronal excitability (Special issue). Trends Neurosci. 11(10), 1988.

Calcium effector mechanisms (Special issue). Trends Neurosci. 12(11), 1989.

Clarke, K. A. *Neurophysiology. Applications in the behavioral and biomedical sciences.* Ellis Horwood, 1990.

Eccles, J. C. *The physiology of synapses.* Springer-Verlag, 1964.

Edelman, G. M., et al. *Synaptic function.* John Wiley & Sons, 1987.

Emson, P. C. *Chemical neuroanatomy.* Raven Press, 1983.

Guy, H. R., and Conti, F. Pursuing the structure and function of voltage-gated channels. Trends Neurosci. 13:201–206, 1990.

Hille, B. Ionic channels of excitable membranes. Blackwell, 1984.

Jacobs, M. Microfilaments and cell movement. Trends Neurosci. 5:369–374, 1982.

Jones, E. G. The nervous tissue. In: *Cell and tissue biology,* Weiss, L., ed. Urban & Schwarzenberg, 1988, pp 279–350.

Kandel, E. Cellular biology of neurons. In: *Handbook of physiology,* Section 1: *The nervous system.* American Physiological Society, 1977.

Kimelberg, H. K., and Norenberg, M.D. Astrocytes. Sci. Am. 260:44–55, 1989.

Kuffler, S. W., et al. *From neuron to brain. A cellular approach to the function of the nervous system,* 2nd ed. Sinauer Associates, 1984.

Levitan, I. B. Modulation of ion channels in neurons and other cells. Annu. Rev. Neurosci. 11:119–136, 1988.

Matus, A. Microtubule-associated proteins: Their potential role in determining neuronal morphology. Annu. Rev. Neurosci. 11:29–44, 1988.

Meyer, F. B. Calcium, neuronal hyperexcitability and ischemic injury. Brain Res. Rev. 14:227–243, 1989.

Peters, A., et al. *The fine structure of the nervous system.* Oxford University Press, 1991.

Riederer, P., et al. *An introduction to neurotrans-mission in health and disease,* Oxford University Press, 1990.

Schwartz, J. H., and Greenberg, S. M. Molecular mechanisms for memory: Second-messenger induced modifications of protein kinases in nerve cells. Annu. Rev. Neurosci. 10:459–476, 1987.

Searle, J. R. Is the brain's mind a computer program? Sci. Am. 262:20–25, 1990.

Shepherd, G. M. *The synaptic organization of the brain.* 3rd ed. Oxford University Press, 1990.

Smith, C. U. M. *Elements of molecular neurobiology.* John Wiley & Sons, 1989.

Tolbert, L. P., and Oland, L. A. A role for glia in the development of organized neuropilar structures. Trends Neurosci. 12:70–75, 1989.

Vallee, R. B., and Bloom, G. S. Mechanisms of fast and slow axonal transport. Annu. Rev. Neurosci. 14:59–92, 1991.

Vallee, R. B., et al. The role of dynein in retrograde axonal transport. Trends Neurosci. 12:66–70, 1989.

Vizi, E. S. *Non-synaptic interactions between neurons. Modulation of neurochemical transmission, pharmacological and clinical aspects.* John Wiley & Sons, 1984.

Walz, W. Role of glial cells in the regulatiom of the brain ion microenvironment. Prog. Neurobiol. 33:309–333, 1989.

Zucker, R. S. Short-term synaptic plasticity. Annu. Rev. Neurosci. 12:13–31, 1989.

Neurotransmitters

Bobker, D. H., and Williams, J. T. Ion conductances affected by 5-HT receptor subtypes in mammalian neurons. Trends Neurosci. 13:169–173, 1990.

Choi, D. W., and Rothman, S. M. The role of glutamate neurotoxicity in hypoxic–ischemic neuronal death. Annu. Rev. Neurosci. 13:171–182, 1990.

Dunant, Y. On the mechanism of acetylcholine release. Prog. Neurobiol. 26:55–92, 1986.

Excitatory amino acids in the brain—focus on NMDA receptors (Special issue). Trends Neurosci. 10(7), 1987.

Garthwaite, J. Glutamate, nitric oxide and cell-cell signalling in the nervous system. Trends Neurosci. 14:60–67, 1991.

Julius, D. Molecular biology of serotonin receptors. Annu. Rev. Neurosci. 14:335–360, 1991.

Lodge, D. *Excitatory amino acids in health and disease.* John Wiley & Sons, 1988.

Mansour, A., et al. Anatomy of CNS opioid receptors. Trends Neurosci. 11:308–314, 1988.

Mason, T. Noradrenaline in the brain: progress in theories of behavioural function. Prog. Neurobiol. 16:263–303, 1981.

Matsumoto, R. R. GABA receptors: Are cellular differences reflected in function? Brain Res. Rev. 14:203–225, 1989.

Maycox, P. R., et al. Amino acid neurotransmission: Spotlight on synaptic vesicles. Trends Neurosci. 13:83–87, 1990.

Schofield, P. R., et al. The role of receptor subtype diversity in the CNS. Trends Neurosci. 13:8–11, 1990.

Telegdy, G. *Neuropeptides and brain function.* Karger, 1987.

van Ree, J. M., and Matthysse, S. Psychiatric disorders: Neurotransmitters and neuropeptides. Prog. Brain Res. 65:1–228, 1986.

Development, Plasticity, and Restitution

Bignami, A., et al. *Central nervous system plasticity and repair.* Raven Press, 1985.

Conel, J. L. *The postnatal development of the human cerebral cortex,* Vols. 1–6. Harvard University Press, 1939–1959.

Constantine-Paton, M., et al. Patterned activity, synaptic convergence, and the NMDA receptor in developing visual pathways. Annu. Rev. Neurosci. 13:129–154, 1990.

Cragg, B. G. The development of synapses in the cat visual cortex. Invest. Ophthal. 11:377–389, 1972.

Davies, A. M., and Lumsden, A. Ontogeny of the somatosensory system: Origins and early development of primary sensory neurons. Annu. Rev. Neurosci. 13:61–73, 1990.

Frank, E. The influence of neuronal activity on patterns of synaptic connections. Trends Neurosci. 10:188–190, 1987.

Giaquinto, S. *Aging and the nervous system.* John Wiley & Sons, 1988.

Goldberger, M. E., and Murray, M. Recovery of movement and axonal sprouting may obey some of the same laws. In: *Neuronal plasticity.* Cotman, C. W., Ed. Raven Press, 1978, pp. 73–96.

Hamilton, W. J., et al. *Human embryology. Prenatal development of form and function,* 4th ed. Williams & Wilkins, 1972.

Harris, W. A., and Holt, C. E. Early events in the embryogenesis of the vertebrate visual system: Cellular determination and pathfinding. Annu. Rev. Neurosci. 13:155–69, 1990.

Hatten, M. E. Riding the glial monorail: A common mechanism for glial-guided neuronal migration in different regions of the developing mammalian brain. Trends Neurosci. 13:179–184, 1990.

Herschman, H. R. Polypeptide growth factors and the CNS. Trends Neurosci. 9:53–57, 1986.

Jacobson, M. *Developmental neurobiology,* 2nd ed. Plenum Press, 1978.

Jan, Y. N. and Jan, L. Y. Genes required for specifying cell fates in *Drosophila* embryonic sensory nervous system. Trends Neurosci. 13:483–498, 1990.

Jessel, T. M., et al. Carbohydrate and carbohydrate-binding proteins in the nervous system. Annu. Rev. Neurosci. 13:227–255, 1990.

Kalil, R. E. Synapse formation in the developing brain. Sci. Am. 261:38–45, 1989.

Korsching, S. The role of nerve growth factor in the CNS. Trensd Neurosci. 9:570–573, 1986.

Learning and memory (Special issue). Trends Neurosci. 11(4), 1988.

Liestøl, K., et al. Selective synaptic connections: Significance of recognition and competition in mature sympathetic ganglia. Trends Neurosci. 9:21–24, 1986.

Nicholls, J. G. *Repair and regeneration of the central nervous system.* Springer-Verlag, 1982.

Oppenheim, R. W. Cell death during development of the nervous system. Annu. Rev. Neurosci. 14:453–502, 1991.

Purves, D., and Lichtman, J. W. *Principles of neural development.* Sinauer, 1985.

Sanes, J. R. Extracellular matrix molecules that influence neural development. Annu. Rev. Neurosci. 12:491–516, 1989.

Schwartz, J. H., and Greenberg, S. M. Molecular mechanisms for memory: Second-messenger induced modifications of protein kinases in nerve cells. Annu. Rev. Neurosci. 10:459–476, 1987.

Wall, J. T. Variable organization in cortical maps of the skin as an indication of the lifelong adaptive capacities of the circuits in the mammalian brain. Trends Neurosci. 11:549–558, 1988.

Williams, R. W., and Herrup, K. The control of neuron number. Annu. Rev. Neurosci. 11:423–453, 1988.

Zucker, R. S. Short-term synaptic plasticity. Annu. Rev. Neurosci. 12:13–31, 1989.

CHAPTER 2

Abbott, N. J. The neuronal microenvironment. Trends Neurosci. 9:3–6, 1986.

Bargman, W. A., et al. Meninges, choroid plexuses, ependyma, and their relations. In: *Histology and histopathology of the nervous system*. Haymaker. W., and Adams, R. D., Eds. Thomas, 1982.

Brown, A. G. *Organization in the spinal cord. The anatomy and physiology of identified neurones*. Springer-Verlag, 1981.

Dudley, A. W. Cerebrospinal blood vessels: Normal and diseased. In: *Histology and histopathology of the nervous system*. Haymaker, W., and Adams, R. D., Eds. Thomas, 1982.

Heimer, L. *The human brain and spinal cord. Functional neuroanatomy and dissection guide*. Springer-Verlag, 1983.

Landon, D. N. *The peripheral nerve*. Chapman and Hall, 1976.

Olesen, J., and Edvinsson, L. Migraine: A research field matured for the basic sciences. Trends Neurosci. 14:3–5, 1991.

Rechthand, E., and Rapoport, S. I. Regulation of the microenvironment of peripheral nerve: Role of the blood–nerve barrier. Prog. Neurobiol. 28:303–343, 1987.

Rexed, B. The cytoarchitectonic organization of the spinal cord in the cat. J. Comp. Neurol. 96:415–495, 1952.

Scheibel, M. E., and Scheibel, A. Terminal axonal patterns in cat spinal cord. I. The lateral corticospinal tract. Brain Res., 2:333–350, 1966.

Risau, W., and Wolburg, H. Development of the blood–brain barrier. Trends Neurosci. 13:174–184, 1990.

Walz, W. Role of glial cells in the regulation of the brain ion microenvironment. Prog. Neurobiol. 33:309–333, 1989.

Wood, J. H. *Neurobiology of cerebrospinal fluid* (2 vols.). Plenum Press, 1983.

CHAPTER 3

Bolz, J., et al. Pharmacological analysis of cortical circuitry. Trends Neurosci. 12:292–296, 1989.

Damasio, H., and Damasio, A. R. *Anatomical correlates of neuropsychological disorders. A neuroimaging approach*. Oxford University Press, 1989.

Heimer, L., and Zaborsky, L. *Neuroanatomical tract-tracing methods. 2. Recent progress*. Plenum Press, 1989.

Kuhar, M. J., et al. Neurotransmitter receptor mapping by autoradiography and other methods. Annu. Rev. Neurosci. 9:27–59, 1986.

Martin, J. B. Molecular genetic studies in the neuropsychiatric disorders. Trensd Neurosci. 12:130–137, 1989.

Mesulam, M. M. Tracing neural connections with horseradish peroxidase. John Wiley & Sons, 1982.

Mora, B. M., et al. In vivo functional localization of the human cortex using positron emission tomography and magnetic resonance imaging. Trends Neurosci. 12:282–284, 1989.

Mountcastle, V. B. The neural mechanisms of cognitive functions can now be studied directly. Trends Neurosci. 9:505–508, 1986.

Olesen, J. Migraine and cerebral blood flow. Trends Neurosci. 8:318–321, 1985.

Ottersen, O. P. Quantitative electron microscopic immunocytochemistry of neuroactive amino acids. Anat. Embryol. 180:1–15, 1989.

Shallice, T. *From neuropsychology to mental structure*. Cambridge University Press, 1988.

Sharif, N. A., and Lewis, M. E. *Brain imaging. Techniques and applications*. John Wiley & Sons, 1989.

Stahl, S. M., et al. Imaging neurotransmitters and their receptors in living human brain by positron emission tomography. Trends Neurosci. 9:241–245, 1986.

Swash, M., and Kennard, C. Scientific basis of clinical neurology. Churchill Livingstone, 1985.

Valentino, K. L., et al. Applications of monoclonal antibodies to neuroscience research. Annu. Rev. Neurosci. 8:199–223, 1985.

Young, S. W. In situ hybridization histochemistry and the study of the nervous system. Trends Neurosci. 9:549–551, 1986.

CHAPTER 4

Receptors and Pathways

Brown, A. G. *Organization in the spinal cord. The anatomy and physiology of identified neurones*. Springer-Verlag, 1981.

Gordon, G. *Active touch. The mechanism of recognition of objects by manipulation. A multi-disciplinary approach*. Pergamon Press, 1978.

Hasan, Z., and Stuart, D. G. Animal solutions to problems of movement control: The role of proprioceptors. Annu. Rev. Neurosci. 11:199–223, 1988.

Keegan, J. J., and Garrett, F. D. The segmental distribution of cutaneous nerves in the limbs of man. Anat. Rec. 102:409–437, 1948.

Lynn, B., and Hunt, S. P. Afferent C-fibres: Physiological and biochemical correlations. Trends Neurosci. 7:186–188, 1984.

Mapp, P. I., et al. Substance P-, calcitonin gene-related pepetide and c-flanking peptide of neuro-pepetide Y are present in normal synovium. Neuroscience 37:143–153, 1990.

Matthews, P. B. C. Evolving views on the internal operation and functional role of the muscle spindle. J. Physiol. 320:1–30, 1981.

Maxwell, D. J., and Rethelyi, M. Ultrastructure and synaptic connections of cutaneous afferent fibres in the spinal cord. Trends Neurosci. 10:117–123, 1987.

McMahon, S. B., and Koltzenburg, M. New classes of nociceptors: Beyond Sherrington. Trends Neurosci. 13:199–201, 1990.

Nathan, P. W., et al. Sensory effects in man of lesions of the posterior columns and of some other afferent pathways. Brain 109:1003–1041, 1986.

Proske, U., et al. Joint receptors and kinaesthesia. Exp. Brain Res. 72:219–224, 1988.

Roland, P. E., and Mortensen, E. Somatosensory detection of microgeometry, macrogeometry and kinesthesia in man. Brain Res. Rev. 12:1–42, 1987.

Rudomin, P. Presynaptic inhibition of muscle spindle and tendon organ afferents in the mammalian spinal cord. Trends Neurosci. 13:499–505, 1990.

Sinclair, D. Mechanisms of cutaneous sensation. 2nd ed. Oxford University Press, 1981.

Vallbo, Å. B., and Johansson, R. S. The tactile sensory innervation of the glabrous skin of the human hand. In: Active touch, pp. 29–54. Pergamon Press, 1978.

Vallbo, Å. B., et al. Somatosensory, proprioceptive and autonomic activity in human peripheral nerves. Physiol. Rev. 59:919–957, 1979.

Thalamus and Cortex

Albe-Fessard, D., et al. Diencephalic mechanisms of pain sensation. Brain Res. Rev. 9:217–296, 1985.

Gordon, G. Active Touch. The mechanism of recognition of objects by manipulation. A multi-disciplinary approach. Pergamon Press, 1978.

Hyvärinen, J. The parietal cortex of monkey and man. Springer-Verlag, 1982.

Jeannerod, M. The neural and behavioural organization of goal-directed movements. Oxford University Press, 1988.

Jones, E. G. The thalamus. Plenum Press, 1985.

Linsker, R. Perceptual neural organization: Some approaches based on network models and information theory. Annu. Rev. Neurosci. 13:257–281, 1990.

Macchi, G., et al. Somatosensory integration in the thalamus. Elsevier, 1990.

Phillips, C. G. Movements of the hand. Liverpool University Press, 1986.

Roland, P. E. Somatosensory detection of macrogeometry, macrogeometry and kinesthesia after localized lesions of the cerebral hemispheres in man. Brain Res. Rev. 12:43–94, 1987.

Sinclair, D. Mechanisms of cutaneous sensation, 2nd ed. Oxford University Press, 1981.

Van Buren, J. M. Sensory responses from stimulation of the inferior Rolandic and Sylvian regions in man. J. Neurosurg. 59:119–130, 1983.

Woolsey, C. N. Cortical localization as defined by evoked potential and electrical stimulation studies. In: Cerebral localization and organization, pp. 17–32. Schaltenbrand, G., and Woolsey, C. N., Eds. University of Wisconsin Press, 1964.

Pain

Akil, H., and Lewis, J. W. Neurotransmitters and pain control. Karger, 1987.

Akil, H., et al. Endogenous opioids: Biology and function. Annu. Rev. Neurosci. 7:223–255, 1984.

Besson, J.-M., et al. Thalamus and pain. Excerpta Medica, 1987.

Fields, H. L. Neural mechanisms of opiate analgesia. In: Advances in pain research and therapy, Vol. 9. Fields, H. L., et al., Eds. Raven Press, 1985, pp. 479–486.

Fields, H. L., et al. Neurotransmitters in nociceptive modulatory circuits. Annu. Rev. Neurosci. 14:219–246, 1991.

Fitzgerald, M. Monoamines and descending control of nociception. Trends Neurosci. 9:51–52, 1986.

Fitzgerald, M. Pain and analgesia in neonates. Trends Neurosci. 10:344–346, 1987.

Fitzgerald, M. c-Fos and the changing face of pain. Trends Neurosci. 13:439–440, 1990.

Gybels, J. M., and Sweet, W. H. Neurosurgical treatment of persistent pain. Physiological and pathological mechanisms of human pain. Karger, 1989.

Mansour, A., et al. Anatomy of CNS opioid receptors. Trends Neurosci. 11:308–314, 1988.

Melzack, R. Phantom limbs and the concept of neuromatrix. Trends Neurosci. 13:88–92, 1990.

Melzack, R. The tragedy of needless pain. Sci. Am. 262:19–25, 1990.

Wall, P. D., and McMahon, S. B. The relationship of perceived pain to afferent nerve impulses. Trends Neurosci. 9:254–255, 1986.

Wall, P. D., and Melzack, R. *Textbook of pain*, 2nd ed. Churchill Livingstone, 1988.

CHAPTER 5

Darian-Smith, I. Sensory processes. In: *Handbook of physiology*, Section 1: *The nervous system*. American Physiological Society, 1984.

Daw, N. W., et al. Rod pathways in mammalian retina. Trends Neurosci. 13:110–115, 1990.

Dowling, J. *The retina: An approachable part of the brain*. Harvard University Press, 1987.

Holmes, G. Disturbancies of vision by cerebral lesions.In: *Selected papers of Gordon Holmes,* Phillips, C. G., Ed. Chap. 6. Oxford University Press, 1979, pp. 337–367.

Hubel, D., and Wiesel, T. Receptive fields, binocular interaction and functional architecture in the cat's visual cortex. J. Physiol. 160:106–154, 1962.

Information processing in the retina (Special issue). Trends Neurosci. 9(5), 1986.

Kaas, J. H. Why does the brain have so many visual areas? J. Cogn. Neurosci. 1:121–135, 1989.

Kennard, C., and Clifford Rose, F. *Physiological aspects of clinical neuro-ophthalmology*. Chapman and Hall Medical, 1988.

Kuffler, S. W., et al. *From neuron to brain. A cellular approach to the function of the nervous system,* 2nd ed. Sinauer Associates, 1984.

Livingston, M. S., and Hubel, D. H. Psychophysical evidence for separate channels for the perception of form, color, movement, and depth. J. Neurosci. 7:3416–3468, 1987.

Martin, K. A. C. From enzymes to visual perception: A bridge too far? Trends Neurosci. 11:280–387, 1988.

Mishkin, M., et al. Object vision and spatial vision: Two cortical pathways. Trends Neurosci. 6:414–417, 1983.

Mora, B. M., et al. In vivo functional localization of the human visual cortex using positron emission tomography and magnetic resonance imaging. Trends Neurosci. 12:282–284, 1989.

Peterhans, E., and von der Heydt, R. Subjective contours—bridging the gap between psychophysics and physiology. Trends Neurosci. 14:112–119, 1991.

Shapley, R., and Perry, V. H. Cat and monkey retinal ganglion cells and their visual functional roles. Trends Neurosci. 9:229–235, 1986.

van Essen, D. C. Functional organization of primate visual cortex. In: *Cerebral cortex,* Vol. 3. Peters, A., Jones, E. G., Eds. Plenum Press, 1985.

CHAPTER 6

Bisiach, E., et al. Disorders of perceived auditory lateralization after lesions of the right hemisphere. Brain 107:37–52, 1984.

Corwin, J. T., and Warchol, M. E. Auditory hair cells: Structure, function, development and regeneration. Annu. Rev. Neurosci. 14:301–333, 1991.

Creutzfeldt, O., et al. *Hearing mechanisms and speech*. Springer-Verlag, 1979.

Darian-Smith, I. Sensory processes. In: *Handbook of physiology*. Section 1: *The nervous system*. American Physiological Society, 1984.

Edelman, G. M., et al. *Auditory function. Neurobiological bases of hearing*. John Wiley & Sons, 1988.

Loeb, G. E. Cochlear prosthesics. Annu. Rev. Neurosci. 13:357–371, 1990.

Penfield, W., and Perot, P. The brain's record of auditory and visual experience. Brain 86:596–696, 1963.

Pickles, J. O. *An introduction to the physiology of hearing,* 2nd ed. Academic Press, 1988.

CHAPTER 7

Carr, W. E. S., et al. The role of perireceptor events in chemosensory processes. Trends Neurosci. 13:212–215, 1990.

Dionne, V. E. How do you smell? Principle in question. Trends Neurosci. 11:188–199, 1988.

Finger, T. E., and Silver, W. L. *Neurobiology of taste and smell*. John Wiley & Sons, 1987.

Haberly, L. B., and Bower, J. M. Olfactory cortex: Model circuit for study of associative memory. Trends Neurosci. 12:258–264, 1989.

Kauer, J. S. Contributions of topography and parallel processing to odor coding in the vertebrate olfactory pathway. Trends Neurosci. 14:79–85, 1991.

Margolis, F. L., and Getchel, T. V. *Molecular neurobiology of the olfactory system: Molecular, membranous, and cytological studies*. Plenum Press, 1988.

Snyder, S. H., et al. Molecular mechanisms of olfaction. Trends Neurosci. 12:35–38, 1989.

CHAPTER 8

Basmajian, J. V. *Muscles alive. Their functions revealed by electromyography,* 5th Ed. Williams & Wilkins, 1985.

Cody, F. J. W., et al. Observations on the genesis of

the stretch reflex in Parkinsons' disease. Brain 109:229–249, 1986.

Cody, F. J. W., et al. Stretch and vibration reflexes of wrist flexor muscles in spasticity. Brain 110:433–450, 1987.

Corcos, D. M., et al. Movement deficits caused by hyperexcitable stretch reflexes in spastic humans. Brain 109:1043–1058, 1986.

Fawcett, J. W., and Keynes, R. J. Peripheral nerve regeneration. Annu. Rev. Neurosci. 13:43–60, 1990.

Granit, R. *The basis of motor control. Integrating the activity of muscles, alpha and gamma motoneurons and their leading control system.* Academic Press, 1970.

Hammond, P. H. The influence of prior instruction to the subject on an apparently involuntary neuromuscular response. J. Physiol. (Lond.) 132: 17–18P, 1956.

Henneman, E., et al. Rank order of motoneurons within a pool: Law of combination. J. Neurophysiol. 37:1338–1349, 1974.

Jenny, A. B., and Inukai, J. Principles of motor organization of the monkey cervical spinal cord. J. Neurosci. 3:567–575, 1983.

Liddell, E. G. T. *The discovery of reflexes.* Oxford University Press, 1960.

Matthews, P. B. C. Muscle spindles and their motor control. Physiol. Rev. 44:219–288, 1964.

Matthews, P. B. C. The human stretch reflex and the motor cortex. Trends Neurosci. 14:87–91, 1991.

Marsden, C. D., et al. Stretch reflex and servo action in a variety of human muscles. J. Physiol. (Lond.) 259:531–560, 1976.

Peachey, L. D. Skeletal muscle. *Handbook of physiology,* Section 10. American Physiological Society, 1983.

Sherrington, C. S. *The integrative action of the brain.* Cambridge University Press, 1947.

Swash, M., et al. Focal loss of anterior horn cells in the cervical cord in motor neuron disease. Brain 109:939–952, 1986.

Van der Meché, F. G. A., and Van Gijn, J. Hypotonia: An erronous clinical concept? Brain 109:1169–1178, 1986.

Evarts, E., and Wise, S. P. *The motor system in neurobiology* (A collection of articles from Trends in Neurosciences). Eslevier, 1985.

Foerster, O. Motorische Felder and Bahnen. Hdb. d. Neurol. 6:1–448, 1936.

Goodwin, A. W., and Darian-Smith, I. *Hand function and the neocortex.* Springer Verlag, 1985.

Granit, R. *The basis of motor control. Integrating the activity of muscles, alpha and gamma motoneurons and their leading control systems.* Academic Press, 1970.

Jeannerod, M. *The neural and behavioural organization of goal-directed movements.* Oxford University Press, 1988.

Kennedy, P. R. Corticospinal, rubrospinal and rubro-olivary projections: A unifying hypothesis. Trends Neurosci. 13:474–478, 1990.

Monrad-Krohn, G. H. *The clinical examination of the nervous system,* 10th ed. H. K. Lewis & Co., 1954.

Phillips, C. G. *Movements of the hand.* Liverpool University Press, 1986.

Phillips, C. G., and Porter, R. *Corticospinal neurones. Their role in movement.* Academic Press, 1977.

Prochazka, A. Sensorimotor gain control: A basic strategy of motor systems? Prog. Neurobiol. 33:281–307, 1989.

Quinn, N., and Jenner, P. *Disorders of movement. Clinical, pharmacological and physiological aspects.* Academic Press, 1989.

Ralston, D. D., and Ralston, H. J. III. The terminations of corticospinal tract axons in the macaque monkey. J. Comp. Neurol. 242:325–337, 1985.

Rothwell, J. C. *Control of human voluntary movement.* Croom Helm, 1987.

Sherrington, C. S. *The integrative action of the brain.* Cambridge University Press, 1947.

Sjölund, B., and Björklund, A. *Brain stem control of spinal mechanisms.* Elsevier, 1982.

Woolsey, C. N. Organization of somatic sensory and motor areas of the cerebral cortex. In: *Biological and biochemical bases of behavior.* Harlow, H. F., and Woolsey, C. N., Eds. University of Wisconsin Press, 1958.

CHAPTER 9

Armstrong, D. M. The supraspinal control of mammalian locomotion. J. Physiol. 405:1–37, 1988.

Asanuma, H. *The motor cortex.* Raven Press, 1989.

Brooks, V. B. *The neural basis of motor control.* Oxford University Press, 1986.

CHAPTER 10

Albin, R. L., et al. The functional anatomy of basal ganglia disorders. Trends Neurosci. 12:366–375, 1989.

Alexander, G. E., et al. Parallel organization of functionally segregated circuits linking basal ganglia and cortex. Annu. Rev. Neurosci. 9:357–381, 1986.

Basal ganglia research (Special Issue). Trends Neurosci. 13(7), 1990.

Brandt, J., and Butters, N. The neuropsychology of Huntington's disease. Trends Neurosci. 9:118–120, 1986.

Brooks, V. B. *The neural basis of motor control*. Oxford University Press, 1986.

Brown, R. G., and Marsden, C. D. Cognitive function in Parkinson's disease: From description to theory. Trends Neurosci. 13:21–29, 1990.

Carpenter, M. B., and Jayaraman, A. *The basal ganglia. II. Structure and function—current concepts.* Plenum Press, 1987.

Chevalier, G., and Deniau, J. M. Disinhibition as a basic process in the expression of striatal functions. Trends Neurosci. 13:277–280, 1990.

Dray, A. The physiology and pharamcology of mammalian basal ganglia. Prog. Neurobiol. 14:221–235, 1980.

Evarts, E., and Wise, S. P. *The motor system in neurobiology* (A collection of articles from Trends in Neurosciences). Elsevier, 1985.

Gerfen, C. R. The neostriatal mosaic: Compartmentalization of corticostriatal input and striatonigral output systems. Nature 311:461–464, 1984.

Groves, P. M. A theory of the functional organization of the neostriatum and the neostriatal control of voluntray movement. Brain Res. Rev. 5:109:132, 1983.

Poirier, L. J., et al. *The extrapyramidal system and its disorders*. Raven Press, 1979.

Riederer, P., et al. *An introduction to neurotransmission in health and disease*. Oxford University Press, 1990.

Schieber, M. H. How might the motor cortex individuate movements? Trends Neurosci. 13:440–444, 1990.

Wexler, N. S. Molecular approaches to hereditary diseases of the nervous system: Huntington's disease as a paradigm. Annu. Rev. Neurosci. 14:503–529, 1991.

Yurek, D. M., and Sladek, J. R. Dopamine cell replacement: Parkinson's disease. Annu. Rev. Neurosci. 13:415–440, 1990.

CHAPTER 11

Brooks, V. B. *The neural basis of motor control*. Oxford University Press, 1986.

Dow, R. S., and Moruzzi, G. *The physiology and pathology of the cerebellum*. University of Minnesota Press, 1958.

Eccles, J. C., Ito, M., and Szentágothai, J. *The cerebellum as a neuronal machine*. Springer-Verlag, 1967.

Holmes, G. The cerebellum. In: *Selected papers of Gordon Holmes*, Chap. 5. Phillips, C. G., Ed. Oxford University Press, 1979, pp. 186–247.

Ito, M. *The cerebellum and neural control*. Raven Press, 1984.

Ito, M. Long-term depression. Annu. Rev. Neurosci. 12:85–102, 1989.

King, J. S. *New concepts in cerebellar neurobiology*. Alan R. Liss, 1987.

Leiner, H. C., et al. Does the cerebellum contribute to mental skills? Behav. Neurosci. 100:443–454, 1986.

Llinás, R., and Sasaki, K. The functional organization of the olivo-cerebellar system as examined by multiple Purkinje cell recordings. Eur. J. Neurosci. 1:587–602, 1989.

Optican, L. M., and Robinson, D. A. Cerebellar-dependent adaptive control of primate saccadic system. J. Neurophysiol. 44:1058–1076, 1980.

Ross, C. A., et al. Messenger molecules in the cerebellum. Trends Neurosci. 13:216–222, 1990.

CHAPTER 12

Brodal, A. *The reticular formation of the brain stem. Anatomical aspects and functional correlations.* Oliver and Boyd, 1957.

Fields, H. L. Neural mechanisms of opiate analgesia. In: *Advances in pain research and therapy*, Vol. 9. Fields, H. L., et al., Eds. Raven Press, 1985, pp. 479–486.

Foote, S. L., and Morrison, J. H. Extrathalamic modulation of cortical function. Annu. Rev. Neurosci. 10:67–95, 1987.

Horne, J. *Why we sleep: The functions of sleep in humans and other mammals*. Oxford University Press, 1988.

Lagercrantz, H. Neuromodulators and respiratory control during development. Trends Neurosci. 10:368–372, 1987.

McGinty, D., and Szymusiak, R. Keeping cool: A hypothesis about the mechanisms and fucntions of slow-wave sleep. Trends Neurosci. 13:480–487, 1990.

Miller, K. W. Are lipids or proteins the target of general anaesthetic action? Trends Neurosci. 9:49–51, 1986.

Moruzzi, G., and Magoun, H. W. Brain stem reticular formation and activation of the EEG. Electroenceph. Clin. Neurophysiol. 1:455–473, 1949.

Saper, C. B. Function of the locus coeruleus. Trends Neurosci. 10:343–344, 1987.

Scheibel, M. E., and Scheibel, A. B. structural substrates for integrative patterns in the brain stem reticular core. In: *Reticular formation of the brain*, pp 31–55. Little Brown, 1958.

Siegel, J. M., and Rogawski, M. A. A function of REM sleep: Regulation of noradrenergic receptor sensitivity. Brain Res. Rev. 13:213–233, 1988.

Sjölund, B., and Björklund, A. Brain stem control of spinal mechanisms. Elsevier, 1982.

Steriade, M., and McCarley, R. W. *Brainstem control of wakefulness and sleep.* Plenum Press, 1990.

van Dongen, P. A. M. The human locus coeruleus in neurology and psychiatry. Prog. Neurobiol. 17:97–139, 1981.

Winson, J. The meaning of dreams. Sci. Am. 263:42–48, 1990.

CHAPTER 13

Bender, M. B. Brain control of conjugate horizontal and vertical eye movements. A survey of the structural and functional correlates. Brain 103:23–69, 1980.

Brodal, A. *The cranial nerves. Anatomy and anatomico-clinical correlations,* 2nd ed. Munksgaard, 1967.

Büttner-Ennever, J. A. (ed.) *Neuroanatomy of the oculomotor system.* Elsevier, 1988.

Carpenter, R. H. S. *Movements of the eyes,* 2nd ed. Pion Limited, 1988.

Dean, P., Redgrave, P., and Westby, G. V. M. Event or emergency? Two systems in the mammalian superior colliculus. Trends Neurosci. 12:137–147, 1989.

Finger, T. E., and Silver, W. L. *Neurobiology of taste and smell.* John Wiley & Sons, 1987.

Kennard, C., and Clifford Rose, F. *Physiological aspects of clinical neuro-ophthalmology.* Chapman and Hall Medical, 1988.

Kinnamon, S. C. Taste transduction: A diversity of mechanisms. Trends Neurosci. 11:491–496, 1988.

Latto, R. The role of the inferior parietal cortex and the frontal eye-fields in visuospatial discriminations in the macaque monkey. Behav. Brain Res. 22:41–52, 1986.

Lindeman, H. H. Anatomy of the Otolith organs. Adv. Oto-Rhino-Laryng. 20:405–433, 1973.

Lisberger, S. G., et al. Visual motion processing and sensory-motor integration of smooth pursuit eye movements. Annu. Rev. Neurosci. 10:97–129, 1987.

Monrad-Krohn, G. H. *The clinical examination of the nervous system,* 10th ed. H. K. Lewis & Co., 1954.

Mumenthaler, M. *Neurologie,* 6th ed. Thieme Verlag, 1979.

Optican, L. M., and Robinson, D. A. Cerebellar-dependent adaptive control of primate saccadic system. J. Neurophysiol. 44:1058–1076, 1980.

Roper, S. D. The cell biology of vertebrate taste receptors. Annu. Rev. Neurosci. 12:329–354, 1989.

Samii, M., and Janetta, P. J. *The cranial nerves. Anatomy, pathology, pathophysiology, diagnosis, treatment.* Springer-Verlag, 1981.

Sparks, D. L., and Mays, L. Signal transformations required for the generation of saccadic eye movements. Annu. Rev. Neurosci. 13:309–336, 1990.

Travers, J. B., et al. Gustatory neural processing in the hindbrain. Annu. Rev. Neurosci. 10;595–632, 1987.

Wilson, V. J., and Melvill Jones, G. *Mammalian vesitbular physiology.* Plenum Press, 1979.

CHAPTER 14

Andersson, K.-E., and Sjögren, C. Aspects of the physiology and pharmacology of the bladder and urethra. Prog. Neurobiol. 19:71–89, 1982.

Appel, N. M., and Elde, R. P. The intermediolateral cell column of the thoracic spinal cord is comprised of target-specific subnuclei: Evidence from retrograde transport studies and immunohistochemistry. J. Neurosci. 8:1767–1775, 1988.

Burnstock, G. The changing face of autonomic neurotransmission. Acta Physiol. Scand. 126:67–91, 1986.

Cervero, F., and Morrison, J. F. B. Visceral sensation. *Progress in brain research,* Vol. 67. Elsevier, 1986.

Cervero, F., and Sharkey, K. A. More than just gut feelings about visceral sensation. Trends Neurosci. 8:188–190, 1985.

Creazzo, T., et al. Neural regulation of the heart. A model for modulation of voltage-sensitive channels and regulation of cellular metabolism by neurotransmitters. Trends Neursci. 6:430–433, 1983.

Gabella, G. *Structure of the autonomic nervous system.* Chapman and Hall, 1976.

Gybels, J. M., and Sweet, W. H. *Neurosurgical treatment of persistent pain. Physiological and pathological mechanisms of human pain.* Karger, 1989.

Haymaker, W., and Woodhall, B. *Peripheral nerve*

injuries. Principles of diagnosis. W. B. Saunders, 1945.

Laskey, W., and Polosa, C. Characteristics of the sympathetic preganglionic neuron and its synaptic input. Prog. Neurobiol. 31:47–84, 1988.

Loewy, A. D., and Spyer, K. M. *Central regulation of autonomic functions.* Oxford University Press, 1990.

Pick, J. *The autonomic nervous system. Morphological, comparative, clinical and surgical aspects.* Lippincott, 1970.

Simmons, M. A. The complexity and diversity of synaptic transmission in the prevertebral sympathetic ganglia. Prog. Neurobiol. 24:43–93, 1985.

Wallin, B. G., and Fagius, J. The sympathetic nervous system in man—aspects derived from microelectrode recordings. Trends Neurosci. 9:63–67, 1986.

CHAPTER 15

Arnold, A. P., and Gorski, R. A. Gonadal steroid induction of structural sex differences in the central nervous system. Annu. Rev. Neurosci. 7:413–442, 1984.

Bloom, F. E. Intrinsic regulatory systems of the brain. In: *Handbook of physiology.* Section 1: *The nervous system.* American Physiological Society, 1986.

Breedlove, M. Regional sex differences in steroid accumulation in the nervous system. Trends Neurosci. 6:403–406, 1983.

Cassone, V. M. Effects of melatonin on vertebrate circadian systems. Trends Neurosci. 13:457–464, 1990.

Ciriello, J., et al. *Organization of the autonomic nervous system: Central and peripheral mechanisms.* Alan R. Liss, 1987.

Clark, Le Gros W. E., et al. *The hypothalamus. Morphological, functional, clinical, and surgical aspects.* Oliver and Boyd, 1936.

Cross, B. A., and Leng, G. The neurohypophysis: Structure, function and control. *Progress in brain research,* vol. 60. Elsevier, 1983.

DeVoogd, T. J. Androgens can affect the morphology of mammalian CNS neurons in adulthood. Trends Neurosci. 10:341–342, 1987.

Ganten, D., and Pfaff, D. Central cardiovascular control. Basic and clinical aspects. Current Topics in Neuroendocrinology, Vol. 3. Springer-Verlag, 1985.

Ganten, D., and Pfaff, D. Actions of progesterone in the brain. Current Topics in Neuroendocrinology, Vol. 4. Springer-Verlag, 1985.

Ganten, D., and Pfaff, D. Morphology of hypothalamus and its connections. Current Topics in Neuroendocrinology, Vol. 7. Springer-Verlag, 1986.

Kuhar, M. J. Neuroanatomical substrates of anxiety: A brief survey. Trends Neurosci. 9:307–310, 1986.

Lagercrantz, H. Neuromodulators and respiratory control during development. Trends Neurosci. 10:368–372, 1987.

McGinty, D., and Szymusiak, R. Keeping cool: A hypothesis about the mechanisms and functions of slow-wave sleep. Trends Neurosci. 13:480–487, 1990.

Reisine, T., et al. New insights into the molecular mechanisms of stress. Trends Neurosci. 9:574–579, 1986.

Riederer, P., et al. *An introduction to neurotransmission in health and disease.* Oxford University Press, 1990.

Rusak, B., and Bina, K. G. Neurotransmitters in the mammalian circadian system. Annu. Rev. Neurosci. 13:387–401, 1990.

Smith, O., and DeVito, J. L. Central neural integration for the control of autonomic responses associated with emotions. Annu. Rev. Neurosci. 7:43–65, 1984.

Yoshimura, F., and Gorbman, A. Pars distalis of the pituitary gland. Structure, function and regulation. International Congress Series 673. Elsevier, 1986.

CHAPTER 16

Alkon, D. L., et al. Learning and memory. Brain Res. Rev. 16:193–220, 1991.

Amaral, D. G., and Witter, M. P. The three-dimensional organization of the hippocampal formation: A review of anatomical data. Neuroscience 31:571–591, 1989.

Andersen, P., et al. Lamellar organization of hippocampal excitatory pathways. Exp. Brain Res. 13:222–238, 1971.

Brown, T. H., et al. Hebbian synapses: Biophysical mechansims and algorithms. Annu. Rev. Neurosci. 13:475–511, 1990.

Buzsaki, G. Two-stage model of memory trace formation: A role for "noisy" brain states. Neuroscience 31:551–570, 1989.

Chan-Palay, V., and Köhler, C. *The hippocampus. New vistas.* Alan R. Liss, 1989.

Changeux, J.-P. *The neural and molecular bases of learning.* John Wiley & Sons, 1987.

Doane, B. K., and Livingston, K. E. *The limbic sys-*

tem. Functional organization and clinical disorders. Raven Press, 1985.

Dudai, Y. *The neurobiology of memory. Concepts, findings, trends.* Oxford University Press, 1989.

Excitatory amino acids in the brain—focus on NMDA receptors (Specital issue). Trends Neurosci. 10(7), 1987.

Fisher, R. S. Animal models of the epilepsies. Brain Res. Rev. 14:245–278, 1989.

Grossman, S. P. Behavioral functions of the septum: A re-analysis. In: *The septal nuclei,* pp. 361–422. Plenum Press, 1976.

Henderson, A. S., and Henderson, J. H. *Etiology of dementia of Alzheimer type.* John Wiley & Sons, 1988.

Isaacson, R. L. *The limbic system,* 2nd ed. Plenum Press, 1982.

Kuhar, M. J. Neuroanatomical substrates of anxiety: A brief survey. Trends Neurosci. 9:307–310, 1986.

Laitinen, L. V., and Livingston, K. E. *Surgical approaches to psychiatry.* University Park Press, 1973.

Learning and memory (Special issue). Trends Neurosci. 11(4), 1988.

Linden, D. L., and Routtenberg, A. The role of protein kinase C in long-term potentiation: A testable model. Brain Res. Rev. 14:279–296, 1989.

Madison, D. V., et al. Mechanisms underlying long-term potentiation of synaptic transmission. Annu. Rev. Neurosci. 14:379–397, 1991.

McEntee, W. J., and Mair, R. G. The Korsakoff syndrome: A neurochemical perspective. Trends Neurosci. 13:340–344, 1990.

O'Keefe, J., and Nadel, L. *The hippocampus as a cognitive map.* Clarendon Press, 1978.

Richardson, R. T., and DeLong, M. R. A reappraisal of the functions of the nucleus basalis of Meynert. Trends Neurosci. 11:264–267, 1988.

Schwartz, J. H., and Greenberg, S. M. Molecular mechanisms for memory: Second-messenger induced modifications of protein kinases in nerve cells. Annu. Rev. Neurosci. 10:459–476, 1987.

Scoville, W. B., and Milner, B. Loss of recent memory after bilateral hippocampal lesions. J. Neurol. Neurosurg. Psychiat. 20:11–21, 1957.

Shallice, T. *From neuropsychology to mental structure.* Cambridge University Press, 1988.

Squire, L. R. *Memory and brain.* Oxford University Press, 1987.

Stewart, M., and Fox, S. E. Do septal neurons pace the hippocampal theta rhythm? Trends Neurosci. 13:163–169, 1990.

Zola-Morgan, S., et al. Human amnesia and the medial temporal region: Enduring memory impairment following a bilateral lesion limited to field CA1 of the hippocampus. J. Neurosci. 6:2950–2967, 1986.

Zucker, R. S. Short-term synaptic plasticity. Annu. Rev. Neurosci. 12:13–31, 1989.

CHAPTER 17

Structure, Function, and Development

Bentivoglio, M., and Sperafico, R. *Cellular thalamic mechanisms.* Excepta Medica, 1988.

Barlow, H. The mechanical mind. Annu. Rev. Neurosci. 13:15–24, 1990.

Bolz, J., et al. Pharmacological analysis of cortical circuitry. Trends Neurosci. 12:292–296, 1989.

Bressler, S. L. The gamma wave: A cortical information carrier? Trends Neurosci. 13:161–162, 1990.

Brodmann, K. *Vergleichende Lokalisationslehre der Grosshirnrinde.* J. A. Barth, 1909.

Conel, J. L. *The postnatal development of the human cerebral cortex,* Vols. 1–6. Harvard University Press, 1939–1959.

Connor, B. W., and Gutnik, M. J. Intrinsic firing patterns of diverse neocortical neurons. Trends Neurosci. 13:99–104, 1990.

Creutzfeldt, O. D. *Cortex Cerebri. Leistung, strukturelle und funktionelle organisation der Hirnrinde.* Springer-Verlag, 1983.

Foote, S. L., and Morrison, J. H. Extrathalamic modulation of cortical function. Annu. Rev. Neurosci. 10:67–95, 1987.

Jones, E. G. *The thalamus.* Plenum Press, 1985.

Jones, E. G., and Peters, A. *Functional properties of cortical cells. Cerebral cortex,* Vol. 2. Plenum Press, 1984.

Jones, E. G., and Powell, T. P. S. An anatomical study of converging sensory pathways within the cerebral cortex of the monkey. Brain 93:793–820, 1970.

Macchi, G., Rustioni, A., and Spreafico, R. *Somatosensory integration of the thalamus.* Elsevier, 1990.

Myers, R. E. Phylogenetic studies of commissural connexious. In: *Functions of the corpus callosum.* Ciba Foundation Study Group, No. 20, pp. 138–142, Churchill, 1965.

Olesen, J., and Edvinsson, L. Migraine: A research field matured for the basic sciences. Trends Neurosci. 14:3–5, 1991.

Parnavelas, J. G., and Papadopolous, G. C. The monoaminergic innervation of the cerebral cortex is not diffuse and nonspecific. Trends Neurosci. 12:315–319, 1989.

Penfield, W., and Rasmussen, T. *The cerebral cortex of man.* Macmillan, 1950.

Perrett, D. I. Visual neurones responsive to faces. Trends Neurosci. 10:358–364, 1987.

Peters, A. Morphological correlates of epilepsy: Cells in the cerebral cortex. In: *Antiepileptic drugs: Mechanisms of action.* Glaser, G. H., et al., Eds. Raven Press, 1980, pp. 21–48.

Peters, A., and Jones, E. G. *Cellular components of the cerbral cortex. Cerebral cortex,* Vol. 1. Plenum Press, 1984.

Peters, A., and Jones, E. G. *Development and maturation of cerebral cortex.* Cerebral cortex, Vol. 7. Plenum Press, 1988.

Rakic, P., and Singer, W. *Neurobiology of neocortex.* John Wiley & Sons, 1988.

Searle, J. R. Is the brain's mind a computer program? Sci. Am. 262:20–25, 1990.

Swindale, N. V. Is the cerebral cortex modular? Trends Neurosci. 13:487–492, 1990.

Wall, J. T. Variable organization in cortical maps of the skin as an indication of the lifelong adaptive capacities of the circuits in the mammalian brain. Trends Neurosci. 11:549–558, 1988.

Association Areas

The frontal lobes—uncharted provinces of the brain (Special issue). Trends Neurosci. 7(11), 1984.

Creutzfeldt, O. D. *Cortex Cerebri. Leistung, strukturelle und funktionelle organisation der Hirnrinde.* Springer-Verlag, 1983.

Critchley, M. *The parietal lobes.* Edward Arnold, 1953.

Damasio, A. R., et al. Face agnosia and the neural substrates of memory. Annu. Rev. Neurosci. 13:89–109, 1990.

Damasio, A. R. Category-related recognition defects as a clue to the neural substrates of knowledge. Trends Neurosci. 13:95–98, 1990.

Fuster, J. *The prefrontal cortex. Anatomy, physiology, and neuropsychology of the frontal lobe,* 2nd ed. Raven Press, 1989.

Goldman-Rakic, P. S. Topography of cognition: Parallel and distributed networks in primate association cortex. Annu. Rev. Neurosci. 11:137–156, 1988.

Hyvärinen, J. *The parietal cortex of monkey and man.* Springer-Verlag, 1982.

Jeannerod, M. *The neural and behavioural organization of goal-directed movements.* Oxford University Press, 1988.

Linsker, R. Perceptual neural organization: Some approaches based on network models and information theory. Annu. Rev. Neurosci. 13:257–281, 1990.

Pandya, D. N., and Selzer, B. Association areas of the cerebral cortex. Trends Neurosci. 5:386–390, 1982.

Posner, M. I., and Petersen, S. E. The attention system of the human brain. Annu. Rev. Neurosci. 13:25–42, 1990.

Language and Lateralization

Bleier, R., et al. Can the corpus callosum predict gender, handedness, or cognitive differences? Trends Neurosci. 9:391–394, 1986.

Brust, J. C. M. Music and language. Musical alexia and agraphia. Brain 103:367–392, 1980.

Bryden, M. P. *Laterality. Functional assymmetry in the intact brain.* Academic Press, 1982.

Caramazza, A. Some aspects of language processing revealed through the analysis of acquired aphasia: The lexical system. Annu. Rev. Neurosci. 11:395–421, 1988.

Damasio, A. R. Category-related recognition defects as a clue to the neural substrates of knowledge. Trends Neurosci. 13:95–98, 1990.

Geschwind, N., and Galaburda, A. M. *Cerebral lateralization. Biological mechanisms, associations and pathology.* MIT press, 1986.

Glass, A. *Individual differences in hemispheric specialization.* Plenum Press, 1987.

Lecours, A. R., et al. *Aphasiology.* Bailliere Tindall, 1983.

Ottoson, D. *Duality and unity of the brain. Unified functioning and specialization of the hemispheres.* Plenum Press, 1987.

Penfield, W., and Roberts, L. *Speech and brain mechanisms.* Princeton University Press, 1959.

Poizner, H., et al. Biological foundations of language: Clues from sign language. Annu. Rev. Neurosci. 13:283–307, 1990.

Ross, E. D. Right hemisphere's role in language, affective behavior and emotion. Trends Neurosci. 7:342–346, 1984.

Sperry, R. W. Lateral specialization in the surgically separated hemispheres. In The Neurosciences. Third study program, pp. 5–19. MIT Press, 1974.

Springer, S. P., and Deutsch, G. *Left brain, right brain.* Freeman, 1989.

Weiskrantz, L. *Thought without language.* Oxford University Press, 1988.

Woods, B. T. Is the left hemisphere specialized for

language at birth? Trends Neurosci. 6:115–117, 1983.

The Cerebral Cortex and Mental Disease

Andreasen, N. C. *Can schizophrenia be localized in the brain?* American Psychiatric Press, 1986.

Helmchen, H., and Henn, F. A. Biological perspectives of schizophrenia. Dahlem workshop report 40. Wiley, 1987.

McEntee, W. J., and Mair, R. G. The Korsakoff syndrome: A neurochemical perspective. Trends Neurosci. 13:340–344, 1990.

Miller, R. Schizophrenia as a progressive disorder: Relation to EEG, CT, neuropathological and other evidence. Prog. Neurobiol. 33:17–44, 1989.

Reynolds, E. H., and Trimble, M. R. *The bridge between neurology and psychiatry.* Churchill Livingston, 1989.

Roberts, G. W. Schizophrenia: The cellular biology of a functional psychosis. Trends Neurosci. 13:207–211, 1990.

van Ree, J. M., and Matthysse, S. Psychiatric disorders: Neurotransmitters and neuropepetides. Prog. Brain Res. 65:1–228, 1986.

Weinberger, D. Schizophrenia and the frontal lobes. Trends Neurosci. 11:367–370, 1988.

INDEX

Page numbers in *italics* refer to illustrations.

A cell (retina), 166
A fibers (sensory), 130
AI (primary auditory area), 190
AII (second auditory area), 190
Abdominal organs, innervation of
    parasympathetic, 309–11
    symapthetic, 352, 359
Abducens (abducent) nerve. *See* Nerve
Abducens nucleus. *See* Nucleus
Accessory nerve. *See* Nerve
Accommodation
    of the lens, 158
    reflex. *See* Reflex
Acetylcholine. *See* Neurotransmitters
Acetylcholine esterase (AchE), 39, 203
Acoustic
    agnosia, 191
    neuroma, 190
Actin filaments, 9
Action potential(s), 24–25
    conduction of, 27–29
    definition, 21
Activating system (of the brain stem), 294, 296
Activation of the EEG, 297
Activity, and development of the nervous system,
    48–50
Acuity (visual), 163
Acupuncture, 150
Adaptation
    dark (photoreceptors), 160

receptors, of, 110
    stretch reflexes, of, 214
    vestibulo-ocular reflex of, 322
Adequate stimulus, 110
Adrenal medulla, 353, 362
Adrenergic receptors. *See* Receptors (molecules)
Agnosia, 415
    acoustic, 191
    finger, 416
    visual, 175, 419
Aggression (rage)
    amygdala and, 386
    cingulate gyrus and, 385
    hypothalamus and, 379
    septal nuclei and, 388
Agraphia, 416, 420
Akinesia, 258
Alar plate, 305
Alcohol (ethanol)
    ADH secretion, and, 380 *n* 2
    cerebellar disease, and, 279
Alexia (dyslexia), 416, 420
Allocortex, 381
Alpha(α)
    axons (fibers). *See* Motoneurons
    motoneurons. *See* Motoneurons
    waves (of the EEG), 297
Alpha(α)-gamma(γ) coactivation, 124, 216
Alzheimer's disease, 395
Amacrine cell, 163, *158*

Amino acid(s)
  as transmitters, 37
  axonal transport of, 101
Amnesia, 393–95
Amplification (of sound waves), 182
Ampulla (of semicircular duct), 313
Ampullar crista, 313
Amygdala (amygdaloid nucleus), 386–88
  and behavior, 387
  connections, 386
  and learning and memory, 388
  and olfaction, 194
  and psychosurgery, 388
Analgesia, 132, 149, 150
Anesthesia, general, 301
Animal experiments and neuroscience, 98
Anions, 23–24
Ansa
  cervicalis, 309
  lenticularis, 261 *n* 4
Anterior
  chamber (of the eye), 157
  commissure, 76
Anterograde
  amnesia, 393
  axonal transport, 9, 101
  degeneration, 101
Anticholinergic drugs. *See* Drugs
Antidromic impulses, 366
Anxiety (fear), 388
Aphasia, 420
Apical dendrite, 398
Apraxia, 242, 415
Aqueduct (cerebral), 72, 90
Arachnoid, 83
  granulations, 90
  villi, 90
Arbor vitae, 82
Arc, reflex, 210
Archicerebellum, 263
Area(s)
  cerebral cortex, of. *See* Cerebral cortex
  entorhinal, 389, 392
Arousal, 296
Arterioles, innervation of, 357
Artery
  anterior cerebral, 92
  anterior spinal, 94
  basilar, 93
  internal carotid, 92
  middle cerebral, 92
  ophthalmic, 92
  posterior cerebral, 93
    communicating artery, 94

  inferior cerebellar, 93
  spinal, 94
  vertebral, 93
Aspartate, 37
Association
  areas of cerebral cortex, 413–19
  connections (fibers) of cerebral cortex, 75, 410
Astrocytes (astroglia), 18
  and blood-brain barrier, 92
Asynergia, 280
Ataxia
  cerebellum, and, 279
  lesions of the dorsal columns, after, 142
  speech, 280
Athetosis, 259
ATP (adenosine triphosphate), 8
  as neurotransmitter, 35, 361
ATPase (in muscle), 205
Atrophy, of muscle, 209
Atropine, 362
Attention
  amygdala and, 387
  deficit after posterior parietal lesions, 415
  focusing of, 299
Auditory
  cortex (AI), 78, 190
  pathways, 185–89
    descending control of transmission, 189
    lesions, 190
  reflexes. *See* Reflex(es)
Aura (epileptic), 171
Auricle, 182
Auricular ramus (of the vagus nerve), 312
Auriculotemporal nerve. *See* Nerve
Autogenic inhibition. *See* Inhibition
Autonomic nervous system
  cerebral cortex, influence from, 384–86
  ganglia. *See* Ganglion
  general features, 345–48
  neurons. *See* Neuron(s)
  neurotransmitters in, 345, 347, 361
  noncholinergic and nonadrenergic transmission
    in, 361
  parasympathetic system. *See* Parasympathetic
  and Parkinson's disease, 258
  plexuses in. *See* Plexus(es)
  sympathetic system. *See* Sympathetic
Axoaxonic synapses, 6, 32
Axodendritic synapses, 6
Axon(s), 5
  alpha(α). *See* Motoneurons
  beta(β), 125
  collaterals. *See* Collaterals
  gamma(γ). *See* Gamma(γ) fibers

impulse conduction in, 27
initial segment of, 30
myelinated,
    impulse conduction in, 28
    structure of, *10*, 12
myelination of, 14, 19
unmyelinated,
    impulse conduction in, 27
    structure of, *10*, 12, 14
transport in, 9, 101
Axonal reflex. *See* Reflex
Axonal transport. *See* Axon(s)
Axosomatic synapses, 6

B cell (retina), 166
Babinski, sign of, 244
Barbiturates, 37
Baroreceptors. *See* Receptors
Basal ganglia, 79
    afferent connections, 248
    cell types, 249
    diseases, 257
    disinhibition in, 252
    efferent connections, 251
    functions, 257
    interneurons, 250
    matrix, 251
    mosaic arrangement, 249
    parallel circuits, 255
    striosomes, 250
    subdivisions, 79, 246
    transmitters, 252
    transplantation and, 260
Basal nucleus (Meynert). *See* Nucleus
Basal plate, 305
Basilar membrane, 180
    frequency discrimination and, 184
Basket cells
    cerebellum in, 273
    hippocampus in, 389
Basolateral nuclear group (of amygdala), 386
Behavior
    amygdala and, 387
    cingulate gyrus and, 385
    feeding, 374
    hormones and, 378
    hypothalamus and, 368, 373, 379
    limbic system and, 397
    septal nuclei and, 388
    sexual, 378, 388
Belt projection (of auditory pathways), 188
Bergman cells, 53 *n* 2
Beta(β)
    axons, 125

blockers, 363
    endorphin, 149
    waves (of the EEG), 297
Betz cells, 224, *400*
Bilateral connections, 44
Binocular cells, 169
Biofeedback (EMG), 221 *n* 4, 241
Biogenic amines (monoamines). *See*
    Neurotransmitters
Bipolar cells (retina), 159, 161
Bladder, innervation of, 356
    transmission from nociceptors, 367 *n* 5
Blind spot (of the eye), 165
Blink reflex. *See* Reflex(es), corneal
Blobs (in striate area), 173
Blood-brain barrier, 91
    hormones and, 370, 380 *n* 2
    regions without, 370
Blood-cerebrospinal fluid barrier, 88
Blood flow
    axonal reflex and, 145
    regional. *See* Regional
Blood pressure
    baroreceptors and, 313
    vasomotor reflexes, and, 360
Body
    ciliary, 157
    lateral geniculate (nucleus). *See* Thalamus
    mammillary. *See* Hypothalamus
    medial geniculate (nucleus). *See* Thalamus,
    temperature control of, 374
        vasomotor reflexes, and, 360
    trapezoid, *187*, 188
Bone conduction (of sound), 182
Bony spiral lamina, 182
Botulinum toxin, 203
Bouton(s), 6, 8
    en passage 6, 9
    postsynaptic, 10
    presynaptic, 10
Brachium
    conjunctivum, 81
    inferior collicular, 186
    pontis, 81
Bradykinesia, 258
Brain-derived neurotrophic factor (BDNF), 48
Brain stem, 65–75
    definition, 283
Bridging veins, 96
Broca's area, 420
Brodmann's areas. *See* Cerebral cortex
Bulb, olfactory. *See* Olfactory
Bundle, medial forebrain. *See* Medial
Burst neurons (in PPRF), 339

CA1-3 (of hippocampus), 391, 394, 398
Calcium ion(s)
    action potentials and, 26
    channels and EEG, 298
    ischemic cell damage and, 51
    NMDA receptors and, 37
    presynaptic inhibition and, 32
    release of transmitter and, 29
    signal molecules as, 26
Caloric test (of the vestibular labyrinth), 323
cAMP (cyclic adenosine monophosphate), 26
CAMs (cell adhesion molecules), 47
Canal, hypoglossal, 307
Capacity (of axonal membrane), 27
Capsular hemiplegia, 243
Carotid sinus, 312
Cations, 23
Cauda equina, 57, 59
Caudate nucleus, 80, 246; *see also* Striatum
    afferent connections, 249
Causalgia, 366
CD4 antigen, 53 *n* 2
Celiac ganglion. *See* Ganglion
Center(s)
    horizontal eye movements for, 339
    hypothalamic, 373
    locomotor movements for, 237
    vertical eye movements for, 340
Central
    canal, 56
    cervical nucleus, 267
    paresis(es). *See* Paresis
    sulcus. *See* Sulcus
Centromedian nucleus. *See* Thalamus
Cerebellar
    cortex, 263, 270
        interneurons, 273
        layers, 270
    hemispheres. *See* Hemispheres
    hypotonia, 280
    lobes. *See* Lobe(s)
    nuclei (deep, intra-). *See* Nucleus
    peduncles. *See* Peduncles
    tentorium, 85
Cerebellomedullary cistern, 84
Cerebellopontine angle, 313
Cerebellum
    archi-, 263
    afferents
        catecholaminergic, 281 *n* 3
        cerebral cortex, 267
        spinal cord, 265
        vestibular, 264
    decerebrate rigidity, and, 235

    efferents, 274
        red nucleus, 231, 276
    functions, 278
    intermediate zone, 264, 269
    learning, and, 280
    lesions of, 278
    main structure, 80–82, 263
    neo-, 264
    paleo-, 264
    somatotopic organization, 263, 277
    stimulation of, therapeutic, 282 *n* 6
    subdivisions, 263
    symptoms in disease, 279–80
Cerebral
    aqueduct. *See* Aqueduct
    palsy and cerebellar stimulation, 282 *n* 6
    peduncle. *See* Peduncles
    ventricles. *See* Ventricular system
Cerebral cortex
    afferents
        thalamocortical, 407
        extrathalamic (modulatory), 410
    association areas, 413
        frontal, 416; *see also* Cerebral cortex, prefrontal
        parietal, 414; *see also* Parietal
        polysensory, 392, 410–11
        temporal, 418
    association connections, 407, 410
    columnar organization, 404, 406
    commissural connections, 407, 412
    function of, 420
    connections, brief survey, 407
    cytoarchitectonic areas, 79
        3,1 & 2 (SI), 140, 144, 150, *400*
        4 (MI), 223, *225*, 239, *400*
        5 & 7 (posterior parietal), 153, 414
        6 (PMA & SMA), 241, 242
        8 (frontal eye field), 232, 256, 340
        17 (striate), 167, *403*
        18 & 19 (extrastriate), 172, *403*
        28 (olfactory), 194
        41 (auditory), 190
    definition, 75
    efferents
        corticothalamic, 408; *see also* Tract(s), cortico-
    hypothalamus, afferents from, 372
    interneurons, 79, 401
    intracortical connections, 401–5
    language functions, 419
    lateralization and dominance. *See* Lateralization
    layers (laminae), 78, 398

termination of fibers from different sources, 406
neurotransmitters, 404
numbers of cell types, relative, 398
pain and, 152
prefrontal, 416
  basal ganglia and, 256
  lesions of, 417
  hypothalamus and, 371
  psychiatric disease and, 418
projection neurons, 401
sex differences, 423
structure, main features, 78–79
Cerebrocerebellum, 264
Cerebrospinal fluid, 56, 83, 87
  circulation and drainage, 90
  function, 89
  production, 88
Cerebrospinal nervous system, xiv
Cerebrum, 75
Cervical nerves, 58
cGMP (cyclic guanosine monophosphate), 161
CGRP (calcitonin gene-related peptide). *See* Neurotransmitters
Channels. *See* Ion channels
Chemoaffinity, 47
Chemoreceptors, definition, 111
Chiasm, optic. *See* Optic
Chimeric portraits, 423
Chloride ions (Cl⁻)
  equilibrium potential for, 23
  inhibition and, 31
  membrane potential and, 23
Choline acetyltransferase (ChAT), 35, 104
Cholinergic neurons and receptors, 35; *see also* Neurotransmitters, acetylcholine
Chorda tympani, 325, 329, *355*
Chordotomy, 144, 154 *n* 7
Chorea (Huntington), 258, 260
Choroid
  of the eye, 155, *159*
  plexus. *See* Plexus
Chromaffin cells, 353
Cilia, 313
Ciliary
  body (corpus ciliare), 157
  muscle. *See* Muscle
Cingulotomy, 385
Circadian rhythms, 374
Circle of Willis, 94
Circuit of Papez, 384
Circulation
  autonomic nervous system and, 357, 360
  control from reticular formation, 296

Cisterna magna (cerebellomedullary cistern), 84
Clark's column (column of Clark), 266
Claustrum, *247*, 260 *n* 1
Climbing fibers, 271, 273
Clonus, 244
Coccygeal nerves, 58
Cochlea, 179–85
Cochlear
  duct, 180
  nerve. *See* Nerve
  nuclei. *See* Nucleus
Coexistence of neurotransmitters. *See* Colocalization
Cognitive; *see also* Mental
  map (in hippocampus), 393
  tasks
    basal ganglia and, 252
    cerebral cortex and, 414
Collagen fibers, in nerves, 15
Collateral(s)
  axonal, 6, 15
  recurrent, 215, 401
  Schaffer, 391
  sprouting, 51, 209
Colliculus
  inferior, 72, 186
    brachium of, 186
    auditory reflexes, and, 190
  superior, 72, 167, 233
    efferents to pulvinar, 176
Colocalization (coexistence) of neurotransmitters, 35, 38
  autonomic nervous system in, 361–62
  basal ganglia in, 250
  cerebral cortex, 405
Color-specific cells (in striate area), 173
Color vision, 161, 173
Column
  of Clark, 266
  intermediolateral cell, 60, 349
Columnar organization
  of cerebral cortex, 173, 406
  of motoneurons, 201
Commissural connections (fibers)
  anterior commissure, 76, 194, 412
  of cerebral cortex, 75
  corpus callosum, 75, 412, 420
  definition, 45
  of hippocampus, 390
Communicating rami. *See* Ramus
Comparative studies, 99
Competition (during development of neuronal connections), 48, 177
Concentration gradient, of ions, 22–23

Conditioned responses (reflexes), 221 *n* 5
  cerebellum and, 281
  vagus nerve and, 311
Conductance, 53 *n* 5
Conduction
  axons, in, 27
  bone, of sound waves, 182
  deafness, 182
  velocity (in axons), 29
    relation to receptors, 130–31
Cones (retina) 160
Confluence (of sinuses), 95
Conjugate eye movements. *See* Movement(s)
Conscious sensation
  of pain, 145
    central control of, 147
  receptors, and, 112, 118, 131
  somatosensory area, stimulation of, 140
  vestibular signals, and, 320
Consciousness, 296–97, 301 *n* 5
Conus (medullary), 56
Convergence of connections, 41
  in retina, 161, 164
  spinothalamic cells on, 145
  visceral and somatic structures, from, 145
Coordination, 262, 279
Core projection (of auditory pathways), 188
Cornea, 156
Corneal reflex. *See* Reflex
Corpus
  callosum, 75, 412, 420
  cerebelli, 264
  striatum, 247
Corresponding points (in retina), 156, *169*
  strabismus and, 176
Cortex
  cerebellar. *See* Cerebellar cortex
  cerebral. *See* Cerebral cortex
Corti. *See* Organ of Corti
Corticobulbar tract. *See* Tract
Corticomedial nuclear group (of amygdala), 386
Corticoreticular tract. *See* Tract
Corticoreticulospinal pathway, 231
Corticorubrospinal tract (pathway), 231
Corticospinal tract. *See* Pyramidal tract
Coverings of the brain (meninges), 82
Cranial
  nerve ganglia. *See* Ganglion
  nerve nuclei, 303–5; *see also* Nucleus
  nerves, 66, 302–41; *see also* Nerve(s)
    kinds of fibers in, 302
Crista, ampullar, 313
Critical periods of development, 50
Crus cerebri, 72

CT (computed tomography), 108
Cuneate fascicle, 138
Cuneate nucleus. *See* Nucleus
Cuneate tubercle, 71
Cupula, 315
Curare, 203
Cutaneous
  hyperesthesia. *See* Hyperesthesia
  sensation, 113–119; *see also* Receptors
Cytoarchitectonic(s)
  areas in cerebral cortex, 79, 401; *see also*
    Cerebral cortex
  definition, 79
  laminae in spinal cord, 63
Cytochrome oxidase, 173
Cytoskeleton, 9

Dark adaptation, 160
dB (decibel), 191 *n* 1
Deafness
  conduction, 182
  lesions of central pathways, and, 190
  noise exposure, and, 184
Decerebrate rigidity, 234
Decerebration, 234
Decibel (dB), 191 *n* 1
Decomposition of movements, 280
Deep sensation, 119
Degeneration
  anterograde, 101
  retrograde, 100
  transneuronal, 101, 169
Deiters' nucleus. *See* Nucleus
Déjà vu, 194, 388
Delayed response, 417
Dementia
  Alzheimer's disease and, 395
  Huntington's disease and, 260
Demyelinating diseases, 14
Dendrite(s), 5
Dendrodendritic synapse, 34
Dentate
  gyrus. *See* Gyrus
  nucleus. *See* Nucleus
Denticulate ligaments, 85
Deoxyglucose (method), 107, 173
Depolarization, 24–25
Depression
  frontal lobe lesions and, 418
  stroke and, 424 *n* 8
Dermatomes, 132
Desynchronization (of EEG), 296
Development of the nervous system
  cranial nerve nuclei, 305

external morphology, 55, *88*
general, 45–50
ventricular system, *88*
Diabetes insipidus, 376
Diencephalon, 65, 72
Differentiation, 46
Diplopia, 334
Direction selectivity, 173
Discrimination
roughness, 141
two-point, 119, 142
Discriminative sensation, 119
dorsal column-medial lemniscus system and, 142
olfaction and, 193
Disinhibition, 43
in basal ganglia, 252
in spinal cord, 215
in retina, 161
Divergence of connections, 41
Dominance
cerebral. *See* Lateralization
ocular, 173
Dopamine, 36; *see also* Neurotransmitters
Dorsal
column-medial lemniscus system. *See* Somatosensory
column nuclei. *See* Nucleus
columns, 138, 141
postsynaptic neurons in, 141
horn, 59, 130, 143
root(s), 57, 129–31
dorsal columns and, 138, 141
spinothalamic cells and, 143
spinocerebellar tract, 266
Dorsolateral fasciculus, 143
Double-labeling experiments, 103
Dreamy state, 194
Drugs (acting on the nervous system), 40
amphetamine, 300
anticholinergic, 259, 362
narcolepsy, and, 300
autonomic nervous system, 362
basal ganglia, 259
motor system, 37, 203, 259
tricyclic antidepressants, 300
Duct(s)
cochlear, 180
semicircular, 313, 315
Dura mater, 84
Dural sac, 84
Dynamic sensitivity
joint receptors of, 126

muscle spindles of, 122
vestibular receptors, 315, 316
Dynorphin, 149
Dyscalculia, 416
Dysdiadochokinesia, 280
Dyskinesia, 258
Dyslexia, 416, 420
Dysmetria, 280
Dyspnea, 365

Ear, 180
Eardrum, 182
Ectoderm, 55
Edema of brain, 51, 85, 90
EEG. *See* Electroencephalography
Effector, definition, xiii
Efferent innervation of sense organs
muscle spindles, 121, 123
organ of Corti, 183, 186, 189
vestibular apparatus, *318*, 341 *n* 4
Electrical stimulation, 107
Electroencephalography (EEG), 296–97
Electron microscopy (of nervous tissue), 103
Elimination of axon collaterals, 48
EMG (electromyography), 208
Emotional reactions, 379, 388
Emotions
basic kinds, 380
facial expression and, 325
frontal lobe lesions, disturbance of, 418
hypothalamus and, 379
sympathetic innervation of the skin and, 360
Encephalitis, 91
Endolymph, 179, 315
composition, 191 *n* 2
Endoneurium, 15
Endoplasmic reticulum, rough, 9–11
Endorphins. *See* Neuropeptides
End plate
motor, 202
potential, 202
Enkephalins, 149
Enlargements (of spinal cord), 67
Enteric nervous system, 356
Enteroceptors. *See* Receptors (sense organs)
Entorhinal area. *See* Area
Ependyma, *19*, 53 *n* 2, 55
innervation from raphe nuclei, 288
Epidural plexus (venous), 94
Epigenetic factors, 46
Epilepsy
amygdala and, 388
aura, 171
cerebellar stimulation and, 282 *n* 6

Epilepsy (*continued*)
  Jacksonian fits, 140, 245 *n* 4
  motor cortex and, 245 *n* 4
  somatosensory cortex and, 140
  uncinate fits, 194
Epineurium, 15
EPSP, 31
Equilibrium
  cerebellum and, 279
  potential for ions, 23
  sense of, 313
Error
  signal (cerebellum), 273
  sources of, in research, 99
Eustachian tube, 182
Excitability, definition, 21
Excitatory
  postsynaptic potential (EPSP), 31
  synapses, 31
  transmitters, 31, 37
Exocytosis, 38
External
  auditory meatus, 182
  cuneate nucleus. *See* Nucleus
  ear, 182
  eye muscles. *See* Muscle(s), extraocular
  granular layer, 399
  pyramidal layer, 399
  segments (of photoreceptors), 160
Exteroceptors. *See* Receptors (sense organs)
Extrafusal muscle fibers, 119
Extraocular muscles. *See* Muscle(s)
Extrapyramidal system, 222
Eye
  far point of, 158
  movements. *See* Movement(s)
  muscles. *See* Muscle(s)
  near point of, 158
  structure of the eye ball, 155, 156

Facial nerve. *See* Nerve
Facial nucleus. *See* Nucleus
Facilitation, 31, 32
Facilitatory region of the reticular formation, 294
Falx cerebri, 85
Far point (of the eye), 158
Fascicle(s)
  anterolateral, 143
  cuneate, 138
  dorsolateral, 143
  gracile, 138
  peripheral nerves, in, 15
Fasciculus
  lenticularis, 261 *n* 4

medial longitudinal, 70, 320, 338
  lesion of, 339
  thalamicus, 261 *n* 4
Fast twitch (FT) muscle fibers, 205
Fastigial nucleus. *See* Nucleus
Feedback connections, 44
  hypothalamus and, 370
Fiber(s)
  muscle, 204
  nerve. *See* Axon
  types (muscle), 204, *206*
Fibrillary tangles, 395
Fictive locomotion, 237
Filaments, 9
Final common path, 41, 199
Fissure (fissura)
  calcarine, 77, 78
  definition, 76
  hippocampal, 78
  lateral cerebral (Sylvian), 76
  longitudinal cerebral, 75
  parieto-occipital, 78
  primary, 264
  rhinal, *194*
  ventral median, 57
Flaccid paresis, 209
Flavors, and taste receptors, 327
Flocculonodular lobe. *See* Lobe
Flocculonodular syndrome. *See* Syndrome
Flocculus, *65*, 81, 281
Fluorescent substances
  demonstration of calcium influx, 26
  tracing of neuronal connections, for, 103
Folium (folia), 81, 263
Foramen
  interventricular (of Monro), 75, 90
  jugular, 309
  of Luschka, 90
  of Magendie, 90
  stylomastoid, 323
Fornix, 75, 371, *390*
  origin of fibers, 397 *n* 4
  termination of fibers, 373
Fourth ventricle, 86
Fovea (centralis), 163, *156*
Foveola, 164
Frequency coding, 25
Fractured somatotopy, 278
Frontal eye field (area 8), 232, 340
Funiculi (columns), *58*, 60, *349*
Fusimotor fibers. *See* Gamma(γ) fibers
Fusion (of visual images), *169*, 176

GAD (glutamic acid decarboxylase), 104

Gait ataxia, 279
Galanin. *See* Neuropeptides
Gamma(γ) fibers, 121
   dynamic and static, 124
   functional properties of, 123–24, 217
   motoneurons. *See* Motoneurons
Ganglion (ganglia)
   autonomic, 345, 351
   celiac, 353
   cell layer (retina), 160
   cells
      cranial nerve, 303
      retinal, 158
      spinal, 61, 129, 130
   cervical (sympathetic), 350
   definition, 17
   geniculate, 325
   jugular, 309, 312
   nodose, 309, 311
   otic, 313
   paravertebral (sympathetic), 349, 352
   petrous, 312
   prevertebral (sympathetic), 351, 353
   pterygopalatine, 325, *355*
   semilunar (trigeminal), 328
   spinal, 58
   spiral, 186
   stellate, 350
   submandibular, 325, *355*
   superior, 312
   vestibular, 313
Gap junction, 34
General somatic afferent nerve fibers,
      304
Geniculate
   bodies (medial and lateral). *See* Thalamus
   ganglion. *See* Ganglion
Genital organs, innervation of
   parasympathetic, 356, 360
   sympathetic, 353, 359
   transmission from nociceptors in, 367 *n* 5
Giant cells of Betz. *See* Betz cells
Gigantocellular reticular formation, *286*
Gland(s)
   lacrimal, 323, 325
   nasal, 325
   parotid, 312
   salivary, 312, 323, 325
   sweat, 359
Glial cells (glia), 5, 18–20
Globus pallidus, 80, 247, 251
Glossopharyngeal nerve. *See* Nerve
Glutamate, 37; *see also* Neurotransmitters
Glycogen depletion technique, 221 *n* 3

Golgi, 100
   cell (cerebellar cortex), 273
   complex, 9
   method, 7, *16*, *64*, 100
   tendon organ, 125
   type 1 and 2 neurons, 15
Gracile fascicle. *See* Fascicle
Gracile nucleus. *See* Nucleus
Gracile tubercle, 71
Gradient(s)
   concentration, 22
   voltage, 22
Granular layer(s)
   cerebellum, 270
   cerebral cortex, 399
Granule cells
   cerebellar cortex, in, 271
   dentate gyrus, in, 389
Grasp reflex. *See* Reflex(es)
Gray matter, 18
   spinal cord, of, 59
Groups of afferent (sensory) fibers
   Ia, 121
   Ib, 125
   II, 121
   A & C, 130
Growth cone (of axon), 9
Guidance of axons during growth, 47
Gyrus (gyri), 76–78
   cingulate, 77
      cerebellum, and, 269
      connections, 385–86
      effects of stimulation, 385
      hypothalamus, and, 371, 372–73, 386
   dentate, 389
   lingual, 175
   parahippocampal, 78, 389
   postcentral, 78, 150, *225*
   precentral, 78, 223, 239

Hair cells
   cochlear, 183, 184
   vestibular, 313
Heart
   cardiac muscle cells, properties of, 358
   innervation of, 311, 358, 360
Hemianopsia
   bitemporal, 177
   homonymous, 178
Hemiballismus, 258
Hemiplegia (hemiparesis), 243
Hemispheres
   cerebral, 75
   cerebellar, 81, 264

Hemispheric dominance. *See* Lateralization
Hemorrhage, intracranial, 90
　subarachnoid, 91
　subdural (hematoma), 96
Herniation
　temporal lobe, 85, 90, 244
　　oculomotor nerve, and, 335
　tonsillar, 90
Herpes zoster, 133
Higher mental functions. *See* Mental
High-threshold units (HT), 144
Hippocampal formation, 389–92
　functions of, 392
　hypothalamus, and, 371
Hippocampal region, 389
Hippocampus, 78, 389
　amnesia, and, 394
　cognitive map theory, 393
　long-term potentiation (LTP), and, 394
　memory, and, 393
　neurotransmitters, in, 391
Histamine, 36, 367; *see also* Neurotransmitters
HIV-1, 53 *n* 3
Homeostasis, 373
Horizontal cell, 163, *158*
Hormone(s)
　adrenocorticotrophic (ACTH), 376, 380 *n* 1
　angiotensin, 370
　antidiuretic (ADH), 376, 380 *n* 2
　acting on the hypothalamus, 370, 378
　beta(β)-lipotropin, 380 *n* 1
　corticotrophin-releasing (CRH), 377
　epinephrine, 362
　gonadotrophic (FSH, LH), 376
　growth (GH), 375
　inhibiting (factors), 377
　prolactin, 376
　pro-opiomelanocortin (pro-ACTH/endorphin),
　　380 *n* 1
　receptors for, 370
　　sex hormones, in amygdala, 288
　releasing (factors), 377
　sex, 370
　somatostatin, 377
　thyroid, 370
　thyroid stimulating (TSH), 375
　thyrotrophin-releasing (TRH), 377
Horner's syndrome, 360
Horseradish peroxidase (HRP), 101
Huntington's disease (chorea), 258, 260
Hydrocephalus, 91
Hyperactive children, psychosurgery and, 388
Hyperalgesia, 115
Hypercalcemia, 26

Hyperesthesia, 145, 366
Hyperkinetic disorders (of basal ganglia), 261 *n* 5
Hyperpolarization, 24–25
　photoreceptors, of, 161
Hyperreflexia, 243
Hypertonus (of muscle), 220
Hypesthesia, 134
Hypnotics, 37
Hypocalcemia, 26
Hypoglossal
　canal, 307
　nerve. *See* Nerve
　nucleus. *See* Nucleus
Hypokinetic disorders (of basal ganglia), 261 *n* 5
Hypophyseal portal system, 377
Hypophysis. *See* Pituitary
Hypothalamus, 75, 368–80
　afferents, 370
　and biological rhythms, 374
　and body temperature, 374
　and digestion and feeding, 374
　efferents, 372
　and endocrine system, 375–77
　functions, 373–75
　hormonal actions on, 370, 378
　and immune system, 378
　mammillary body (nucleus), 75, 369, 373
　　cerebellum, connections with, 269
　　function, 373
　　and memory, 395
　and mental functions, 378
　neurotransmitters in, 370
　olfactory connections, 194, 370
　psychosomatic interrelations, 378
　and psychosurgery, 388
　and sleep, 299, 374
　subdivisions, nuclei, 369
Hypotonus (hypotonia) of muscle, 220
　and cerebellar disease, 280

Immune system, nervous system and, 378
Immunocytochemistry, 104
Implanted electrodes, 107
Impulse conduction (in axons), 27–28
In situ hybridization, 104
Inactivation of Na$^+$ channels, 25
Incus, 182
Induction, 46
Inferior
　colliculus. *See* Colliculus
　olive (olivary nucleus), 70, 266, 270, 271
　　learning and, 273, 280
Inferotemporal cortex, 418
Infundibulum (stalk of pituitary), 75, 377

Inhibition
  autogenic, 217, 221 *n* 6, 229
  lateral, 163, 405
  postsynaptic, 31
  presynaptic, 32
  reciprocal, 213
    spasticity and, 243
  recurrent, 43, 215
    spasticity and, 244
Inhibitory
  interneurons, 43
    in cerebellar cortex, 273
    in cerebral cortex, 405
    in lateral geniculate body, 171
    in retina, 163
    spasticity and, 244
    in spinal cord, 213, 215
    in thalamus, 409
  postsynaptic potential (IPSP), 31, 33
  reticular formation, regions of, 294
  synapses, 31
  transmitters, 31, 37
Initial segment (of axon), 30
Injury
  glial cells and, 20
  pain and, 145, 156
Inner
  hair cells (cochlea), 183
  nuclear layer (retina), 160
  plexiform layer (retina), 160
  synaptic layer (retina), 160
Insomnia, 301
Insula, 76, 419
Insulation (of axons), 12
Intentional tremor, 280
Intermediary filaments, 9
Intermediate zone (cerebellum), 264, 269
Intermediolateral cell column, 60, 349
Internal
  granular layer, 399
  medullary lamina, 74, 137
  pyramidal layer, 399
Internal capsule, 72
  lesion of, 167, 226, 243
  localization of
    auditory pathway, 186
    optic radiation, 167
    pyramidal tract, 225
Interneurons. *See* Neuron(s)
Interposed nuclei. *See* Nucleus
Intracerebellar nuclei. *See* Cerebellar nuclei
Intrafusal muscle fibers, 119
Intralaminar thalamic nuclei 137, 410
  arousal and, 410

basal ganglia and 248
pain transmission and 144
reticular formation and, 290, 299
Ion(s), 21
Ion channels, 21
  calcium, 29, 26, 37
  chloride, 37
  potassium, 36, 37
  sodium, 24, 37
    photoreceptors in, 161
  taste buds and, 327
  transmitter(ligand)-gated, 22
  voltage-gated, 22, 25, 29
Ipsilateral connections, 45
IPSP (inhibitory postsynaptic potential), 31
Iris, 157
Ischemic cell damage, 51
Isoprenaline (isoproterenol), 363

Joint receptors. *See* Receptors
Joint sensation (sense). *See* Kinesthesia
Jugular ganglion. *See* Ganglion
Junctional folds, 202

Kainate receptors, 37
Kinesthesia, 127
  dorsal column-medial lemniscus system and,
    142, 153 *n* 5
Kinocilium, 317
Korsakoff's psychosis, 395

Labyrinth, 179, 313
Labyrinthine reflexes. *See* Reflex(es)
Lacrimal gland. *See* Gland
Lamellae,
  in hippocampus, 391
  myelin, 13
Lamina(e)
  bony spiral, 182
  cerebral cortex of. *See* Cerebral cortex
  cribrosa, 193
  of spinal cord. *See* Spinal cord
Langerhans cells, 53 *n* 3
Lateral
  cervical nucleus, 146
  corticospinal tract, 226; *see also* Pyramidal tract
  geniculate body (nucleus). *See* Thalamus
  hypothalamic area, 369
  horn (of spinal gray matter), 60
  inhibition. *See* Inhibition
  reticular nucleus. *See* Nucleus
  ventricles, 86
  vestibulospinal tract. *See* Tract
Lateralization (hemispheric dominance), 421–24

Lateralization (*continued*)
anatomic asymmetry, 421
auditory, 423
emotions, 422
handedness, 422
language, 419
sex differences in, 423
visual, 423
Law of specific nerve energies (Müller), 110
Layer(s)
cerebellar cortex, 270
cerebral cortex. *See* Cerebral cortex
Learning
hippocampus and, 392
long-term potentiation (LTP) and, 394
motor, 273, 280
synaptic change and, 26, 31, 50
Lemniscus
lateral, 186
medial, 70, 138–42
Length sensitivity, of muscle spindle, 124
Lens, 157
changes with age, 158
Lentiform nucleus, 80
Lesion experiments, 106
L-dopa, 259
Light reflex. *See* Reflex
Limbic structures
basal ganglia and, 257
Limbic system, 381, 383
Limiting membrane, 19
Lingual nerve. *See* Nerve
Lipid bilayer of cell mebrane, *21*
Lissauer, tract of, 143, 154 *n* 6
Lobe(s)
anterior (of cerebellum), 264
lesion, 279
of cerebral hemisphere, 76; *see also* Cerebral
cortex
flocculonodular, 263, 264
lesions, 279
posterior (of cerebellum), 264
Localization
retinotopic, 169
somatotopic, 135
tonotopic, 184
Locomotion, 236
Locus coeruleus. *See* Nucleus
Long-term potentiation (LTP), 394
Longitudinal zones (cerebellum), 277
Long-loop stretch reflex, 215
Long-term memory, 393–94
Lower motor
neurons, 199, 222
syndrome, 243

Lumbar
nerves, 58
puncture, 84
Lungs, innervation of, 358, 361, 365
Luschka, foramen of, 90
Lymphocytes (and hypothalamus), 378

M cell (retina), 165
Macrophage-like cells, 53 *n* 3
Macula
lutea (retina), 163
saccular, 315, 317
utricular, 315, 316, 317–18
Magendie, foramen of, 90
Magnocellular
layers (of the lateral geniculate), 167
red nucleus, part of, 231
Main (principal) trigeminal nucleus. *See* Nucleus
Malleus, 182
Mammillary body (nucleus). *See* Hypothalamus
Mandibular nerve. *See* Nerve
MAPs (microtubule-associated proteins), 9
Maxillary nerve. *See* Nerve
Meatus
external auditory, 182
internal auditory (acoustic), 186, 313, 323
Mechanoreceptors
definition, 111
Medial
forebrain bundle, 369, 391
lemniscus. *See* Lemniscus
longitudinal fasciculus. *See* Fasciculus
vestibulospinal tract, 233, 319, *320*
Median eminence, 377
Medium spiny neuron, 250, *256*
Medulla oblongata, 65, 69–71
Medullary
conus, 56
tractotomy, trigeminal, 329
Meissner corpuscles, 116
Membrana limitans, 19
Membrane
basilar. *See* Basilar
capacity, 27
limiting, 19
permeability, 22
potential, 22–24
resistance, 27
structure, *21*
synovial, 127
tectorial, 183
tympanic, 182
vestibular, 182
Membranous labyrinth, 313

Memory
  and amygdala , 388
  and hippocampus, 393–94
  kinds of, 392
  and mammillary nucleus, 395
  and basal nucleus (Meynert), 395
Meningeal ramus, 64
Meninges, 82–85
Meningitis, 91
Mental functions (higher)
  and basal ganglia, 252, 256
  and cerebral cortex, 413
  and reticular formation, 300
Merkel's disk, 116
Mesencephalic
  locomotor region, 237, 252
  trigeminal nucleus. See Nucleus
Mesencephalon, 65, 69, 72
Mesolimbic dopaminergic system, 261 n 3
Metaraminol, 363
Microelectrodes, 107
Microfilaments, 9
Microglial cells (microglia), 18
Microneurography
  autonomic efferent fibers, 360
  cutaneous afferents, 118
  muscle spindle afferents, 124
Microtubules, 9
Microzones (cerebellum), 278
Middle
  ear, 182
  temporal visual area (MT), 176
Migration (of neurons during development), 46
Milk ejection reflex. See Reflex
Mimetic muscles. See Muscle(s)
Miniature EPSP, 38
Miosis, 360
Mirror movements, 216
Mitochondria, 8
Mitral cells, 193
Modality (of sensory experience), 110
Modality-specific neurons, 141
Modiolus, 183
Modular (columnar) organization; see also
      Columnar
  striate area, 173
  SI, 406
Molecular layer
  cerebellar cortex, 270
  cerebral cortex, 399
Monoamines (biogenic amines). See
      Neurotransmitters
Monocular cells, 169
Monocytes, 20
Monro, foramen of, 90

Mood; see also Emotions
  hypothalamus and, 378
  L-dopa and, 259
Morphine, 149
Mossy fibers
  in cerebellum, 271, 273
  in dentate gyrus, 391
Motivation
  basal ganglia and, 257
  basal nucleus (Meynert) and, 396
  monoaminergic pathways to the cord and, 233
Motoneurons, 60
  alpha(α), 199
    phasic and tonic, 202
  columns of, 201
  gamma(γ), 124, 199, 217
  somatotopic organization of, 201–2
Motor
  end plate, 202
  learning. See Learning
  neurons. See Motoneurons
  program, 238
    basal ganglia, and, 257
  trigeminal nucleus. See Nucleus
  unit(s), 206–8
    fiber types and, 207
Motor areas (cortex)
  premotor (PMA), 238, 242
  primary (MI), 78, 223, 239
  supplementary (SMA), 239, 241
    grasp reflex, and, 236
Movement(s)
  automatic, 197
  ballistic, 196
  classification of, 196
  disorders
    and basal ganglia, 257
    and central motor pathways, 242
    and cerebellar lesions, 278
    dorsal columns, lesions of, 142
    and peripheral motor neurons, 208, 220
  eye, 331–34, 336
    brain stem centers for, 338
    cerebellum, and, 279, 337
    conjugate, 177, 334, 339
    control of, 336–40
    cortical centers for, 340
    horizontal, 331, 338
    nystagmus. See Nystagmus
    optokinetic, 337, 340
    saccadic, 321
    smooth pursuit, 321
    vergence, 337
    vertical, 331, 340
    voluntary, 337, 340

Movement(s) (*continued*)
 fractionated, 230
 head and eyes, 232
 locomotor, 236
 mirror, 216
 orienting, 231
 ramp, 196
 translatory, 315
 visually guided, 242, 269
 voluntary, 196, 237–42
  and posterior parietal cortex, 242
MRI (magnetic resonance imaging), 108
MT (area), 176
Müller cells, 53 *n* 2, 160
Multiform layer, 399
Multiunit (smooth muscle), 347
Multiple sclerosis, 14
Muscarinic receptors, 36
Muscle(s)
 buccinator, 324
 ciliary, 157
 contraction, 204
  cutaneous receptors and, 218
  reflex adjustment, 217
 extraocular, 331–35
  muscle spindles in, 333
 fascia, 206
 fiber types, 204–6
 force, control of, 207
 inferior
  oblique, 333
  rectus, 332
 intrinsic
  of the eye, 335
  of the hand, 228
 lateral rectus, 332
 levator
  palpebrae superioris, 335, *332*
  veli palatini, 312
 masticatory, 328, 330
 medial rectus, 332
 mimetic (facial), 324
 orbicularis oculi, 324
 pupillary dilatator, 157
 sphincter
  external (of bladder), *356*
  pupillae, 157, 335
 spindles. *See* Receptors (sense organs)
 stapedius, 190
 stiffness, 219
 superior
  oblique, 33
  rectus, 332
 tension, 219

 tensor tympani, 157
 tone, 218
  changes in disease, 220
  anterior lobe, and, 279
  reticular formation and, 294
Myasthenia gravis, 203
Mydriasis, 362
Myelin, 12
 sheath, 12
 staining, *68*, 100
Myelinated axons. *See* Axons
Myelination, 19
Myoglobin, 205
Myosin ATPase, 205

Naloxone, 150
Narcolepsy, 300
Natural killer cells (and hypothalamus), 378
Near point (of the eye), 158
Neck reflexes, 234, 235
Negligence (of body parts), 415
Neocerebellum, 264
Neocortex, 381
Neostriatum. *See* Striatum
Nerve(s) (nervus)
 abducens (abducent), 71, 331, 334
 accessory, 70, 309
 cochlear, 185
  efferent fibers in, 186
 cranial. *See* Cranial
 definition, 17
 facial, 71, 323–26
  pareses of, 324
 glossopharyngeal, 70, 312
 greater petrosal, 325
 hypoglossal, 70, 307–9
 impulse, 5
 intermediate, 323, 325, 327
 lingual, 325
 mandibular, 328
 maxillary, 328
 oculomotor, 72, 331, 334
  lesion of, 335
 olfactory, 67, 193
 ophthalmic, 328
 optic, 72, 166
  lesions of, 177
  number of axons, 15
 pelvic, 357
 recurrent laryngeal, 311
 spinal (peripheral) 57
 splanchnic (greater and lesser), 353
 structure, 15
 trigeminal, 70, 328–31

trochlear, 72, 331, 334
vagus, 70, 309–12
  lesion of, 312
vestibulocochlear, 71
vestibular, 313–23
  efferent fibers in, 341 *n* 4
Nerve growth factor (NGF), 48
Neural groove, 55
Neural tube, 55
Neuroactive substances. *See* Neurotransmitters
Neurofibrils, 9
Neurofilaments, 9
Neuromuscular
  junction, 202
  transmission, 203
Neuron(s)
  bipolar, 16
  definition, 5
  interneurons, 15, 43
    basal ganglia, 250, *256*
    cerebellar cortex, 273
    cerebral cortex, 401, 404–5
    spinal cord, 62, 135, 143, 148, 215
    retina, 159, 163
  medium spiny (striatum), 250, *256*
  multipolar, 16
  organelles of, 8–9, *10*
  postganglionic, 345
    axonal terminations, 345
    parasympathetic, 356–57, 360
    sympathetic, 352–54
  preganglionic, 345
    parasympathetic, 354
    sympathetic, 349
  projection, 15
    basal ganglia, 250
  pseudounipolar, 16
  types of, 15–16
Neuropeptides
  beta(β) endorphin, 149
  CCK (cholecystokinin), 132, 361
  CGRP (calcitonin gene-related peptide), 132
    motoneurons, in, 200, 221 *n* 1
  dynorphin, 149
  enkephalin, 149,
    basal ganglia, in, 250
  galanin, 132, 221 *n* 2
  general, 37, 39
  hyperesthesia and, 145
  opioid, 148
  somatostatin, 250, 361
  SP (substance P), 132, 145
    airways, in, 365

autonomic nervous system, in, 361
  basal ganglia, in, 250
VIP (vasoactive intestinal peptide), 38, 132, 145
  autonomic nervous system, in, 361
Neurosecretory cells, 376
Neurotransmitter(s), 34–40
  acetylcholine 35, 39
    Alzheimer's disease and, 396
    in autonomic nervous system, 361
    in basal ganglia, 250, *256*
    drugs and, 362
    in lateral geniculate body, 171
    and neuromuscular transmission, 202–3
    receptors, 36, 202
    and sleep, 300
  amino acids, 37
  aspartate, 37
    in cerebellum, 271
  ATP, 359
    in dorsal root fibers, 132
    in autonomic nervous system, 361
  classification, 34
  colocalization (coexistence). *See* Colocalization
  definition, 6
  dopamine, 36, 39
    in basal ganglia, 248, 253, 259
    receptors, 250, 253
  epinephrine (adrenaline), 36
    autonomic nervous system and, 362
  excitatory, 31, 37
  GABA (gamma-aminobutyric acid), 37
    in auditory nuclei, 189
    in basal ganglia, 250, 252
    in cerebellum, 271, 273
    in cerebral cortex, 405
    in lateral geniculate body, 171
  glutamate, 37
    in basal ganglia, 252, 254
    in dorsal root fibers, 132
    in retina, 161
    in cerebellum, 271
    in pyramidal tract, 231
  glycine, 37, 189
  histamine, 36, 40
  inhibitory, 31, 37
  modulatory, 34
  monoamines (biogenic amines), 36
  neuropeptides. *See* Neuropeptides
  nitric oxide (NO), 361
  norepinephrine (noradrenaline), 36, 39
    autonomic nervous system in, 361, 363
    pain and, 154 *n* 8

Neurotransmitter(s) (*continued*)
    sleep and, 300
    in spinal cord afferents, 233
    in sensory fibers (spinal ganglion cells), 131
    serotonin (5HT), 36, 39
      in basal ganglia, 249
    degradation and removal of, 39
      pain transmission and, 148
      release of, 38
      sleep and, 300
    synthesis of, 38
Nicotinic receptors, 36
Night
    blindness, 161
    vision, 160
Nissl
    bodies, 9
    staining, 7, 100
NMDA (N-methyl-D-Aspartate) receptor. *See*
      Receptors (molecules)
Nociceptors. *See* Receptors (sense organs)
Node of Ranvier, 13, 28
Nodose ganglion. *See* Ganglion
Noncholinergic and nonadrenergic transmission
      (in autonomic nervous system), 361
Nonpyramidal cells, 398
Norepinephrine (noradrenaline), 36; *see also*
      Neurotransmitters
Nuclear bag fibers, 119, 153 *n* 1
Nuclear chain fibers, 120
Nuclear layers (of retina), 160
Nucleus (nuclei)
    accessory, 309
    abducens, 71, 334, 339
    ambiguus, 311
    amygdaloid (amygdala). *See* Amygdala
    arcuate (infundibular), 369, 377
    basal (Meynert), 39, 395
    central
      amygdaloid, 386
      cervical, 267
      lateral (CL). *See* Thalamus
    centromedian (CM). *See* Thalamus
    cerebellar, 81, 274–77
    cochlear (dorsal and ventral), 185–86, 188
    corticomedial, 194
    cuneate, 70, 71, 138
    definition, 17
    of Deiters, 282 *n* 4, 318
    dentate, 274, 276
    descending (inferior) vestibular, 318
    dorsal column, 70, 138–39
    dorsomedial (hypothalamic), 369
    external cuneate, 267

    Edinger-Westphal, 334
    facial, 323
    fastigial, 274, 277
    gracile, 70, 71, 138
    hypoglossal, 307
      lesion of, 308
    inferior
      olivary (inferior olive), 70, 266, 270, 271
      salivatory, 313
      vestibular, 318
    infundibular (arcuate), 369
    interposed (anterior and posterior), 274, 276
    interstitial, of Cajal, 340
    intralaminar. *See* Thalamus
    lateral
      cervical, 146
      geniculate (body). *See* Thalamus
      reticular, 267, 281 *n* 1, 290
      vestibular (Deiters), 318
    laterodorsal tegmental, 300
    locus coeruleus, 39, 285, 289
      facilitation of spinal motoneurons, 233
      and hypothalamus, 371
      and sleep, 300
    mammillary. *See* Hypothalamus
    medial vestibular, 318
    motor trigeminal, 330
    oculomotor, 72, 334
    parabrachial, 300
    paramedian reticular, 290
    paraventricular, 369, 376
    pedunculopontine (PPN), 252, 300
    perihypoglossal, 338
    posterior (hypothalamic), 369
    precerebellar, 281 *n* 1, 290
    prepositus, 338
    pretectal, 167
      light reflex and, 335
      inferior olive, and, 270
    raphe, 39, 285, 287–88
      and cerebral cortex, 288, 407, 410
      facilitation of spinal motoneurons, 233
      and hypothalamus, 371
      and pain transmission, 148
      and sleep, 300
    red, 72, 230–31
    reticular tegmental, 281 *n* 1, 290
      thalamic. *See* Thalamus, nuclei
    riMLF (rostral interstitial nucleus of the medial
      longitudinal fasciculus), 340
    sensory trigeminal, 70–71, 329–31
      main (principal), 329
      mesencephalic, 329, 330
      spinal, 329

septal, 388, 397
  olfaction and, 194
of solitary tract, 304, 311
  and hypothalamus, 371
submedius. *See* Thalamus
subthalamic, 253
superior
  salivatory, 325
  vestibular, 318, 320
suprachiasmatic, 374
supraoptic, 369, 376
thalamic. *See* Thalamus
trochlear, 334
tuberomammillary, 40
vagus, dorsal motor, 309
ventral anterior (VA). *See* Thalamus
  lateral (VL). *See* Thalamus
ventromedial (hypothalamic), 369
Nystagmus
  cerebellum, and, 279
  definition, 282 *n* 5, 321
  optokinetic, 337
  spontaneous, 323
  vestibular, 321, 322

Object identification (visual), 175
Ocular dominance columns, 48, 173
Oculomotor
  nerve. *See* Nerve
  nucleus. *See* Nucleus
Odorant, 192
Off-center retinal ganglion cells, 162
Ohm's law, 53 *n* 5
Olfactory
  bulb, 67, 193
  cortex, 78, 194
  epithelium, 192
  nerve. *See* Cranial, nerves
  receptors, 192
  reflexes. *See* Reflex(es)
  tract. *See* Tract
Oligodendrocytes, 13, 18–19
Olive (olivary nucleus)
  inferior. *See* Inferior olive
  superior, 186, 189
Olivocochlear bundle, 189
On-center retinal ganglion cells, 162
Ophthalmic nerve. *See* Nerve
Opioid peptides, 149
Opsin, 160
Optic
  chiasm, 75, 166
  nerve. *See* Nerve
  papilla, *156, 165*

radiation, 167
tract. *See* Tract
Organ of Corti, 182, 183–85
Orientation selectivity, 173
Osmoreceptors. *See* Receptors (sense organs)
Ossicles (of the ear), 182
Otic ganglion. *See* Ganglion
Otoliths, 315
Outer
  hair cells, 183
  nuclear layer (retina), 160
  plexiform layer (retina), 160
  synaptic layer (retina), 160
Oval window, 182

P cell (retina), 165
Pacemaker properties, 43
  cerebellar nuclear cells, 276
Pacinian corpuscles. *See* Receptors
Pain
  acupuncture and, 150
  central control of, 147–49
  deafferentation, 146
  definition, 146
  frontal lobes and, 146
  intralaminar thalamic nuclei and, 146
  raphe magnus nucleus (NRM) and, 148
  opioid peptides (endorphins) and, 148
  periaqueductal gray (PAG) and, 148–49
  pathways. *See* Somatosensory pathways
  referred, 145, 366
  receptors. *See* Receptors, nociceptors
  and serotonin, 148
  and stress, 149, 150
  thalamic, 146
  transcutaneous nerve stimulation (TNS) and, 150
  visceral, 365, 367 *n* 5
Paleocerebellum, 264
Paleostriatum. *See* Globus pallidus
Pallidum. *See* Globus pallidus
Papez, circuit of, 384
Papilla (optic), *156, 165*
Paradoxical sleep, 299
Parallel
  fibers, 270
  pathways, 44
Paralysis agitans, 258
Paramedian reticular nucleus. *See* Nucleus
Parasympathetic
  ganglia, location of, 310, 347, 354
  system, general aspects, 345–48
    cranial nerves and, 303–5, 354
    hypothalamic influence on, 372, 374

Parasympathetic (*continued*)
  sacral part, 356
  vagus nerve and, 309–11
Parasympathicomimetic drugs, 362
Paravertebral ganglia. *See* Ganglion
Paresis (paralysis)
  cancer and, 203
  central, 242
    contractile properties and, 243
    spasticity and, 243
  peripheral, 208
Parietal association areas (posterior parietal), 414
  integration of somatosensory and visual
      information, 416
  lesions, 415
  properties of single cells, 415
Parkinsonism, 258
Parkinson's disease, 220, 258
  and transplantation, 260
Parotid gland, innervation of, 312
Pars compacta and reticulata (of s. nigra), 254
Parvocellular
  layers (of the lateral geniculate), 167
  red nucleus, part of, 231
Patch clamp, 108
Peduncle(s)
  cerebellar, 72, 80, 263
  cerebral, 72, 96 *n* 3
Pedunculopontine nucleus (PPN). *See* Nucleus
Pelvic nerves. *See* Nerve(s)
Peptidase, 39
Perception. *See* Conscious sensation
Perforant path, 391
Periaqueductal gray (PAG), 72, 148–50
Perihypoglossal nuclei. *See* Nucleus
Perikaryon, 5
Perilymph, 179, *315*
  composition, 191 *n* 2
Perineurium, 15
Peripheral nerve(s), 15, 17
Permeability, 22, 53 *n* 5
Perseveration, 242, 417
PET (positron emission tomography), 108
Petrosal nerve (greater). *See* Nerve, greater
      petrosal
Phagocytes (in the brain), 19, 53 *n* 3
Phasic
  alpha(α) motoneurons, 202
  stretch reflex, 213
Phentolamine, 363
Photopigment, 160
Photoreceptors, 160
  definition, 111
  properties, 160
  neurotransmitters, 161

Pia mater, 82
Pigment epithelium (of the retina), 158
Pillar cell, 183
Piloerection, 359
Piriform cortex, 194
Pituicytes, 53 *n* 2
Pituitary (hypophysis), 75
  anterior lobe (adenohypophysis), 375, 376–77
  hormones, 375–76
  hypophyseal portal system, 377
  posterior lobe (neurohypophysis), 375, 377
  releasing hormones (factors) and, 377
Place-specific neurons, 141
Plantar reflex. *See* Reflex(es)
Plasticity, 46
Plaques, in multiple sclerosis, 14
Plexiform layers (of retina), 160
Plexus(es)
  autonomic, 345, 357
  brachial, *200*
  cardiac, 357
  celiac, 357
  choroid, 87
  hypogastric, 357
  mesenteric (superior and inferior), 357
  myenteric, 356
  pelvic, 357
  prevertebral, 354
  renal, 357
  of spinal nerves, 64, 199, *200*
  submucous, 356
Polarization, of vestibular receptors, 317
Poliomyelitis, 201
Poliovirus, 201
Polymodal nociceptors, 115
Polyneural innervation, 48
Pontocerebellum, 264
Posterior chamber (of the eye), 157
Posterior complex. *See* Thalamus
Posterior parietal cortex. *See* Parietal association
      areas
Postganglionic neurons. *See* Neurons
Postrotational past pointing, 322
Postsynaptic
  dorsal column neurons (units), 141
  excitation, 31
  inhibition, 31
  membrane, 6
  potentials, 31
Postural reflexes. *See* Reflex(es)
Posture, 196, 231
  Parkinson's disease, in, 258
Potassium channels
  acetylcholine and, 36
Potassium ions (K$^+$)

equilibrium potential for, 23
  inhibition and, 31
  membrane potential and, 23
  refractory period and, 26
Potential(s)
  equilibrium, 23
  membrane, 22
  readiness, 238
  resting, 22
PPRF (paramedian pontine reticular formation), 339
Precerebellar nuclei. See Nucleus
Prefrontal cortex. See Cerebral cortex
Preganglionic neurons. See Neuron(s)
Premenstrual syndrome, 378
Premotor area (PMA), 238, 242
Premotor centers (cell groups) in the reticular formation, 296
  for eye movements, 338–40
Prepositus nucleus. See Nucleus
Presbyopia, 158
Presynaptic
  facilitation, 32
  inhibition, 32
  membrane, 6, 8
  neuron, 6
  receptors. See Receptors
Pretectal nuclei. See Nucleus
Prevertebral ganglia. See Ganglion
Primary
  afferent fibers. See Sensory fibers
  fissure, 264
  motor area (cortex). See Motor areas
  sensory ending (of the muscle spindle), 121
    neuron, definition of, 125
  somatosensory area (SI). See Somatosensory
  vestibular afferents, 264, 318
Principal (main) trigeminal nucleus. See Nucleus
Projection neuron, 15
Proliferation (of neurons during development), 46
Proprioceptors. See Receptors (sense organs)
Prosody, 422
Psychiatric disease, 395, 418
Psychic processes. See Mental functions
Psychosis. See Psychiatric disease
Psychosurgery, 385, 388
Propriospinal neurons, 62, 96 n 2
Pterygopalatine ganglion. See Ganglion
Pulvinar. See Thalamus
Punctate cutaneous sensation, 119
Pupil (of the eye) 155, 157
Pupillary
  dilatator muscle. See Muscle(s)
  reflex (light reflex). See Reflex, light
  sphincter muscle. See Muscle(s)

Purkinje cell layer, 270
Purkinje cells, 270
Putamen, 80, 246; see also Striatum
  afferent connections, 249
Putative transmitters, 35
Pyramid, 70
Pyramidal cells, 6
  cerebral cortex, in, 398
  hippocampus, in, 389
Pyramidal decussation, 70
Pyramidal layers (cerebral cortex), 399
Pyramidal tract, 70, 222–30
  conduction velocities, 227
  control of head muscles, 226
  crossed and uncrossed fibers, 245 n 1
  function, 229
  lesions
    and emotion, expression of, 324
    humans, 243
    monkeys, in, 230
  myelination, 245 n 5
  origin of, 223
  somatotopic localization, 225, 227
  spasticity and, 230, 243–44
  spinal reflexes and, 229
  syndrome, 244
  termination of fibers, 227

Quiscalate receptors. See Receptors
Quantal release of neurotransmitters, 38

Radiation, optic. See Optic
Radioactively labeled amino acids, 101
Ramus, communicating (sympathetic)
  gray, 352
  white, 350
Ramus, meningeal, 64
Ramus of spinal nerves, 64
Ranvier, node of, 12, 28
Raphe nuclei. See Nucleus
Rapid eye movements (REM), 299
Readiness potential, 238
Receptive fields
  cutaneous receptors, of, 117
  retinal ganglion cells, of, 162, 163–64, 166
  visual cortical neurons, of, 162, 172
Receptors (molecules)
  acetylcholine (AchR), 36, 202, 361
  adrenergic (α and β), 361
    fat and liver cells, in, 362
  dopamine (D_1 and D_2), 37, 253, 259
  endorphins, 149
  GABA, 37
  for hormones, 362, 370
  kainate, 37

Receptors (molecules) (*continued*)
  localization of, 105
  muscarinic, 36
    and narcolepsy, 300
  for neurotransmitters, 35–37
  nicotinic, 36
  NMDA, 37, 394
  opiate, 149
  presynaptic, 362
  serotonin, 36
  quiscalate, 37
Receptors (sense organs)
  auditory, 179, 183–85
  adaptation, 110
  adequate stimulus, 110
  baro-, 311, 313, 360
  chemo-, 111
  definition, 109
  efferent innervation of
    muscle spindles, 121, 123
    organ of Corti, 183, 186, 189
  encapsulated, 115
  enteroceptors, 111
  exteroceptors, 111
  free, 115, 117
  joint, 125
    central transmission of signals, 153 *n* 5
  juxtapulmonary (J-receptor), 365
  mechanoreceptors, 111
    high-threshold, 115
    low-threshold, 116, 179
    in skin, 116
  Meissner corpuscle, 116
  Merkel's disk, 116
  muscle spindle, 119–25
    extraocular muscles, in, 333
    functional properties, 121
    reticular formation and, 294
    structure, 119
  nociceptors, 112, 115
    definition, 145
    and pain perception, 145
  osmo-, 376
  Pacinian corpuscles, 117
    in visceral organs, 367 *n* 4
  photoreceptors, 111, 158–60
  postural reflexes, for, 234, 236
  proprioceptors, 111, 119–27
    cortical projection of, 224
  Ruffini corpuscles, 116
  smell (olfactory), 192
  tendon organ (Golgi), 125
  thermoreceptors, 111, 115
  vestibular, 313–15, 317
  in visceral organs, 364

Reciprocal inhibition, 213
Recovery after brain damage. *See* Restitution
Recruiting response, 410
Recruitment (of motor units), 207
  size principle of, 208, 221 *n* 4
Recurrent
  collaterals. *See* Collaterals
  inhibition. *See* Inhibition
  laryngeal nerve. *See* Nerve
Red
  muscle (fibers), 204
  nucleus. *See* Nucleus
Referred pain, 145, 366
Reflex(es)
  accommodation, 335
  arc, 210
  auditory, 189
  autonomic, 364
    coordination of, 368
  axon(al), 145, 366
  brain stem, 210, 305
  conditioned. *See* Conditioned responses
  corneal (blink), 325
  cough, 365
  dystrophy, 367
  emptying, of bladder and rectum, 364
  fixation, 340
  flexion, 211
  general aspects, 209–11
  grasp, 236
  Hering-Breuer, 365
  labyrinthine, 234, 335
  light, 335
  masseter, 330
  milk ejection, 377, 378
  monosynaptic, 210
  olfactory, 194
  patellar, 210
  plantar, 243, 245 *n* 5
  polysynaptic, 210
  postural, 234–36
    neck and labyrinthine, 234, 235
    in Parkinson's disease, 258
  sneeze, 330
  spinal, 210
    pyramidal tract and, 229
  stapedius, 325
  stretch, 212
    function of, 216
    long latency (loop), 213, 215
    monosynaptic, 213
    tonic, 219
  sucking, 330
  tone, 219
  vasomotor, 360, 365

vestibular, 321
vestibulo-ocular, 321–22, 337
    and cerebellum, 280, 322
visceral, 311, 360, 364–65
vomiting, 364
Refraction (of light), 155
Refractory period, 26
Regeneration of peripheral axons, 209
Regional blood flow (cerebral cortex), 108, 241, 414
    and schizophrenia, 418
REM sleep, 299
Renshaw cells, 215
    spasticity and, 244
Repolarization, 25
rER, 9–11
Resistance
    against disease, hypothalamus and, 378
    internal (axonal), 27
    membrane, 27
Resolution, spatial, 161
Resonance theory of Helmholtz, 185
Respiration
    control from reticular formation, 296
Response properties
    of dorsal column neurons, 141
    of spinothalamic neurons, 144
Resting
    potential, 22
    tremor, 258
Restitution, after brain damage, 50–52
Retardation (of movements), 243
Reticular
    formation, 67, 285–301
        afferents, 293
        and circulation, 296
        and consciousness, 296–97
        and EEG, 296–97
        efferents, 290
        facilitatory and inhibitory regions, 294
        functions, 294–301
        and mammillary nucleus, 373
        and muscle tone, 294
        and respiration, 296
        and sensory information, 293, 299
        and sleep, 299
        subdivisions, 285, 286
    tegmental nucleus. See Nucleus
Reticulospinal tracts. See Tract
Reticulothalamocortical pathway, 299
Retina, 156, 158–66
    cell types, 158
    interneurons, 158, 163
    layers, 158
    receptive fields, 162

Retinal
    ganglion cells. See Ganglion cells
    interneurons. See Neurons
Retinene, 160
Retinotopic localization, 169
Retrograde
    amnesia, 393
    axonal transport, 9, 101
    degeneration, 100
Rexed's laminae, 62
    termination of dorsal root fibers in, 129, 130, 143
    motoneurons and, 200
Rhinencephalon, 192, 383
Rhodopsin, 160
Rhomboid fossa, 71
Rhythm generator, central, 237
Right-left confusion, 416
Rigidity, 220
    decerebrate, 234
    gamma(γ), 235
    in Parkinson's disease, 258
riMLF. See Nucleus
Rootlets, 57
Roots of spinal nerves, 57
Roughness discrimination, 141
Round window, 182
Rubrospinal tract. See Tract
Ruffini corpuscles, 116

Saccule (sacculus), 313, 316, 341 n 5
Sacral nerves, 58
Satellite cells, 19
Saliva, secretion of, 325
Scala vestibuli & tympani, 182
    media. See Cochlear duct
Schaffer collaterals, 391
Schizophrenia, 418
Schwann cells, 13, 115
Sciatica, 133
Sclera, 156
Scotoma, 178
Secondary
    sensory ending (of the muscle spindle), 121
    sensory neuron, definition of, 135
    somatosensory area (SII). See Somatosensory
    vestibular afferents, 265
Secretion of tears and saliva, 325
Segments. See Spinal cord
Segmental
    arrangement, in dorsal columns, 138
    innervation, 132
Selective
    permeability, 22
    cell death, 47

Selectivity
  color, 173
  direction, 173
  orientation, 173
Semicircular ducts, 313, 315
Semilunar (trigeminal) ganglion. *See* Ganglion
Senile plaques, 395
Sensitization
  in autonomic nervous system, 362
  of nociceptors, 115
Sensory
  fibers, 61
    transmitters in, 131
  trigeminal nucleus, 329
  unit, 117
Septal nuclei. *See* Nucleus
Serotonin (5HT), 36; *see also* Neurotransmitters
Set-point theory (hypothalamic function), 374
Sex hormones. *See* Hormones
Sham rage, 379
Shingles, 133
Short-term memory, 393
Sign of Babinski, 244
Single unit (smooth muscle), 347
Sinus (venous)
  cavernous, 94
  node (heart), 358
  sigmoid, 94
  straight, 95
  superior sagittal, 94
  transverse, 94
Size principle of recruitment (Henneman), 208
Skin, structure of, 113
Sleep, 299
  L-dopa and, 259
Slow twitch (ST) muscle fibers, 205
Smile, social and spontaneous, 325
Snake poisons, 203
Sodium ions (Na$^+$), 21
  action potential and, 24–25
  equilibrium potential for, 24
  impulse conduction and, 27
Sodium-potassium pump, 23
Solitary tract nucleus. *See* Nucleus
Soma, 5
Somatic afferent and efferent
  cranial nerve nuclei, 303
  nerve fibers, 302
Somatosensory area (cortex)
  primary (SI), 78, 140, 150
    lesions of, 153
    pain perception and, 153
    termination of fibers in the cord, 227
  secondary (SII), 140, 150

Somatosensory pathways
  descending control of transmission, 147–49
  dorsal column-medial lemniscus system, 136, 138
    function of, 140–42
    lesion experiments, 141
    motor symptoms after lesions of, 142
    trigeminal nucleus, fibers from, 330
  from face and head, 307, 330
  general features, 135–138
  spinocervicothalamic tract, 146
  spinoreticulothalamic tract, 146
  spinothalamic tract, 136, 143
    classification of units, 144
    dorsal root fibers and, 143
    function of, 144–45
    location of cell bodies in the cord, *139*, 143
    thalamic termination of, 144
    trigeminal nucleus, fibers from, 330
Somatotopic organization (localization), 135
  cerebellum, 265, 278
  dorsal columns, in, 138
  epilepsy and, 140, 245 *n* 4
  motoneurons, 201–2
  motor cortex, 225
  pyramidal tract, 225, *227*
Sound
  localization, 189
  waves, frequency of, 179
Spasticity, 220, 243
  mechanisms responsible, 244
Spatial
  memory, 373
  resolution, 161
  summation, 30
Special somatic afferent nerve fibers, 304
Specific thalamic nuclei, 138
Specificity of neural connections, 46
Speech areas, 420
Spinal cord, 54, 56–65
  enlargements, 57
  dorsal horn
    different parts of SI, fibers from, 227
    different receptors, fibers from, 130, 143
  ganglion. *See* Ganglion
  ganglion cells. *See* Ganglion
  interneurons. *See* Neurons
  monoaminergic afferents, 233
  neuronal types, 60–62, 148, 200–2, 215
  reflexes. *See* Reflex(es)
  Rexed's laminae, 62
    dorsal root fibers, termination in, *129*, 130, 143
    motoneurons and, 200–2

spinothalamic tract cells and, *139*, 143
segments, 59, 64, 132
tract of the trigeminal nerve, 329
trigeminal nucleus. *See* Nucleus
Spine(s), 5
Spinocerebellum, 264
afferents, 265
efferents, 277
Spinocerebellar tracts, 265, 266
Spinocervicothalamic tract. *See* Somatosensory
pathways
Spinoreticular tract (neurons)
pain and, 146
Spinoreticulothalamic tract. *See* Somatosensory
pathways
Spinothalamic tract. *See* Somatosensory pathways
Spiny stellate cell (cerebral cortex), 405
Spiral ganglion. *See* Ganglion
Splanchnic nerves. *See* Nerve(s)
Split-brain patients, 421, 423
Spontaneous nystagmus, 279
Sprouting (of axonal collaterals) 51, 209
Squint, 177, 334
Stabilization of nervous function, 44
Stapedius muscle. *See* Muscle
Stapes, 182
Startle response, 189
Static
labyrinth, 316
sensitivity
of joint receptors, 126
of muscle spindles, 122
vestibular receptors, 316
Stellate
cell, 273, 424 *n* 1
ganglion. *See* Ganglion
Stereochemical theory of smell, 193
Stereocilia, 183, 317
Stiffness (of muscle), 219
Stimulation-induced analgesia, 149, 150
Strabismus (squint), 177, 334
Stress-induced analgesia, 149, 150
Stria terminalis, 387
Striate area (area 17). *See* Visual cortical areas
Striatum, 247
afferent connections, 248–49
ventral, 248, 257, 261 *n* 2
amygdala, fibers from, 386
Strychnine, 37
Subarachnoid space, 83–84
Subdural
hematoma, 96
space, 84
Subfornical organ, 370, 380 *n* 2

Subiculum, 289, 397 *n* 4
Submandibular
ganglion. *See* Ganglion
gland. *See* Gland
Substance P. *See* Neuropeptides
Substantia
gelatinosa, *63*, 143
nigra, 72, 247, 254
and disease, 258
Subthalamic
nucleus. *See* Nucleus
region, locomotion and, 237
Sulcus
anterior lateral, 57
central, 76, 78,
hypothalamic, 75
limitans, 305
posterior lateral, 57
posterior median, 57
Summation,
muscle contraction, 204
postsynaptic potentials, 30
Superior
colliculus. *See* Colliculus
olivary complex, 186, 189
salivatory nucleus. *See* Nucleus
Supplementary motor area (SMA). *See* Motor
areas
Supramotor areas, 239
Sweat glands. *See* Glands
Sylvian fissure, 76
Sympathectomy, 366
Sympathetic
ganglia, 349–50
postganglionic fibers, 352
system, peripheral parts, 349–54
hypothalamic influence of, 372, 374
tone (tonus), 360
trunk, 349
Sympathicomimetic drugs, 363
Synapse(s)
axoaxonic, 6, 32
axodendritic, 6
axosomatic, 6
definition, 6
dendrodendritic, 34
electrotonic, 34
excitatory, 31
formation, use-dependent, 50
inhibitory, 31
modulatory, 34
Synaptic
cleft, 6
layers (of retina), 160

Synaptic (*continued*)
  potentials, 29
  transmission, 29
  vesicles, 6, *8*, 29
Synchronization (of EEG), 296
Syndrome
  anterior lobe, 279
  flocculonodular, 279
  Gerstmann, 418
  Horner's, 360
  lower motor, 243
  neocerebellar, 279
  premenstrual, 378
pyramidal tract, 244
Synovial membrane, innervation of, 127

Taste
  buds, 312, 313, 326
  elementary qualities, 327
  pathways, 327
Tears, secretion of, 325
Tectorial membrane, 183
Tectospinal tract. *See* Tract
Tegmental area, ventral, 261 *n* 3
Tegmentum, 96 *n* 3
Tela choroidea, 87
Teleceptive impulses, 111
Temporal
  plane, 421
  summation, 30
Tendon organ, 125
Tension (of muscle), 219
Tensor tympani muscle. *See* Muscle
Tentorium, cerebellar, 85
Terminal bouton, 6
Tertiary sensory neuron, definition of, 135
Tetanic contraction, 204
Tetanus
  fused and unfused (muscle contraction), 204
  toxin, 37
Thalamocortical neurons, functional states of, 298
Thalamus, 73, 137, 407–9
  corticothalamic connections, 408
  EEG, and, 298
  internal medullary lamina, 137
  interneurons, 409
  lateral geniculate body, 75, 167, 170
  medial geniculate body, 75, 186, 188
  nucleus (nuclei)
    anterior (A), 74, 373, 408
    central lateral (CL), 144
    centromedian (CM), 249, 251
    intralaminar. *See* Intralaminar
    lateral, 74
    lateral posterior (LP), 408

    medial, 74
    mediodorsal (MD), 372, 387, 407
    reticular thalamic, 409
    specific, 138
    submedius, 144
    ventral anterior (VA), 251, 408
    ventral lateral (VL), 251, 408
    ventral posterolateral (VPL), 140, 408
    ventral posteromedial (VPM), 328, 330
  pulvinar, 75, 408
    visual pathways and, 176
  thalamocortical connections, 407
Thermoreceptors
  definition, 111
Thermosensitive units, 144
Third ventricle, 86
Thoracolumbar system, 349
Tinnitus, 190
TNS (transcutaneous nerve stimulation) 150
Tonic alpha(α) motoneurons, 202
Tonotopic localization, 184
Tracing of neuronal connections, 101
Tractotomy, medullary trigeminal, 329
Tract(s)
  corticobulbar, 223, 307
  corticopontine, 268
  corticoreticular, 231, *291*, 293
  corticoreticulospinal, 231, *291*
  corticorubrospinal, 231
  corticospinal. *See* Pyramidal tract
  definition, 17, 62
  hippocamposeptal, 388
  lateral vestibulospinal, 233, 319, *320*
  Lissauer, of, 143, 154 *n* 6
  mammillotegmental, 373
  mammillothalamic, 75, 373
  medial vestibulospinal, 319
  olfactory, 78, 193
  optic, 75, 167
    lesions, 178
    pontocerebellar, 267
  pyramidal. *See* Pyramidal tract
  reticulospinal, 231, 232, 290
  rubrospinal, 230
  septohippocampal, 388, 391
  spinal, of the trigeminal nerve, 329
  spinocerebellar, 265, 266
  spinocervicothalamic, 146
  spinoreticular, 147, 293
  spinoreticulothalamic, 146
  spinothalamic. *See* Somatosensory pathways
  supraopticohypophysial, 375
  tectospinal, 232
  tuberoinfundibular, 375, 377
  ventral corticospinal, 226, 245 *n* 1

vestibulospinal (lateral and medial), 233, 319, *320*

Transcutaneous nerve stimulation (TNS), 150

Transmitter substance. *See* Neurotransmitter

Transmitter systems, 39

Transneuronal degeneration, 101

Transplantation (of dopaminergic neurons), 260

Trapezoid body, *187*, 188

Tremor
  intentional, 280
  resting, 258

Trigeminal
  nerve. *See* Nerve
  neuralgia, 329
  nucleus (nuclei). *See* Nucleus
  tractotomy, medullary, 329

Tuber cinereum, 75

Tubercles (tuberculum)
  gracile and cuneate, 71

Twitch, 204

Two-point discrimination, 119

Tympanic cavity, 182

Tympanic membrane, 182

Type 1 and 2 muscle fibers, 205

Tyrosine hydroxylase, 104

Uncinate fits, 194

Uncus, 78, 194

Unmyelinated axons. *See* Axons

Upper motor
  neurons, 222
  syndrome, 243

Uptake mechanisms, for neurotransmitters, 39

Utricle (utriculus), 313, 316, 341 *n* 5

Utricular macula. *See* Macula

Vagus nerve. *See* Nerve

Varicosities (of postganglionic fibers), 346

Vasoconstriction, 357

Vasodilation (vasodilatation), 258

Vasopressin, 376

Vein(s)
  great cerebral, 94
  innervation of, 358
  internal jugular, 95
  portal, hypophyseal, 377

Ventral
  corticospinal tract, 226; *see also* Tract
  horn, 59, 60, 200
  posterolateral nucleus (VPL). *See* Thalamus
  posteromedial nucleus (VPM). *See* Thalamus
  roots, 57–58
    sensory fibers in, 129
  spinocerebellar tract, 266
  striatum, 248, 257

tegmental area, 261 *n* 3

Ventricular system, *56*, 67, 86–87
  development, 55, *88*

Vermis, 81, *83*, 264
  afferents, 265
  efferents, 277

Vertigo, 334

Vestibular
  apparatus, 313
  membrane, 182
  nerve. *See* Nerve
  nuclei, 318–20; *see also* Nucleus
  receptors. *See* Receptors (sense organs)
  reflexes. *See* Reflex(es)

Vestibulocerebellum, 264

Vestibulocochlear nerve. *See* Nerve

Vestibulo-ocular reflex. *See* Reflex(es)

Vestibulospinal tracts. *See* Tract(s)

Vibration
  muscle spindles and, 128, 216
  receptors for, 117

Visceral
  afferent and efferent
    cranial nerve nuclei, 303
    nerve fibers, 302
  organs, innervation
    parasympathetic, 356–57
    sensory, 363–65
    sympathetic, 352, 357–59
    vagus nerve, by, 310
  pain, 365
  reflexes. *See* Reflex(es)
  sensation, central pathways for, 364

Viscoelastic properties of muscle, 220

Visual
  acuity, 163
  axis (of the eye), *156*, 163
  cortical areas
    striate area (area 17), 78, 167, 171–76
    extrastriate areas, 172, 174–76
    lesions of, 175, 176, 178
    middle temporal (MT), 176
  field, 157
    defects of, 177

Visually guided movements. *See* Movements

Vitamin A, 160

Vitreous body, 157

Voltage clamp, 108

Vomiting, 311

W cell (retina), 166

Wheat germ agglutinin (WGA), 101

Wernicke's area, 420

White
  matter, 18

White (*continued*)
    spinal cord, of, 59
   muscles (fibers), 204
Wide dynamic range units (WDR), 144
Windows of the labyrinth, 182
Wisconsin Card Sort Test, 417

X cell (retina), 166

Y cell (retina), 166

Zones in the cerebellar cortex, 277